MODERN Essentials™
HANDBOOK

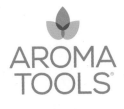

AROMA TOOLS®

aromatools.com

Published and Distributed by:

AromaTools®
144 W. 1900 North
Spanish Fork, UT 84660

Phone: 1-866-728-0070 • 801-798-7921

Internet: www.AromaTools.com

E-mail: Webmaster@AromaTools.com

ISBN Number:

978-1-937702-89-2

Disclaimer:

This book has been designed to provide information to help educate the reader in regard to the subject matter covered. It is sold with the understanding that the publisher and the authors are not liable for the misconception and misuse of the information provided. It is not provided in order to diagnose, prescribe, or treat any disease, illness, or injured condition of the body. The authors and publisher shall have neither liability nor responsibility to any person or entity with respect to any loss, damage, or injury caused, or alleged to be caused, directly or indirectly by the information contained in this book. The information presented herein is in no way intended as a substitute for medical counseling. Anyone suffering from any disease, illness, or injury should consult a qualified health care professional.

Printed and Bound in the U.S.A.

Table of Contents

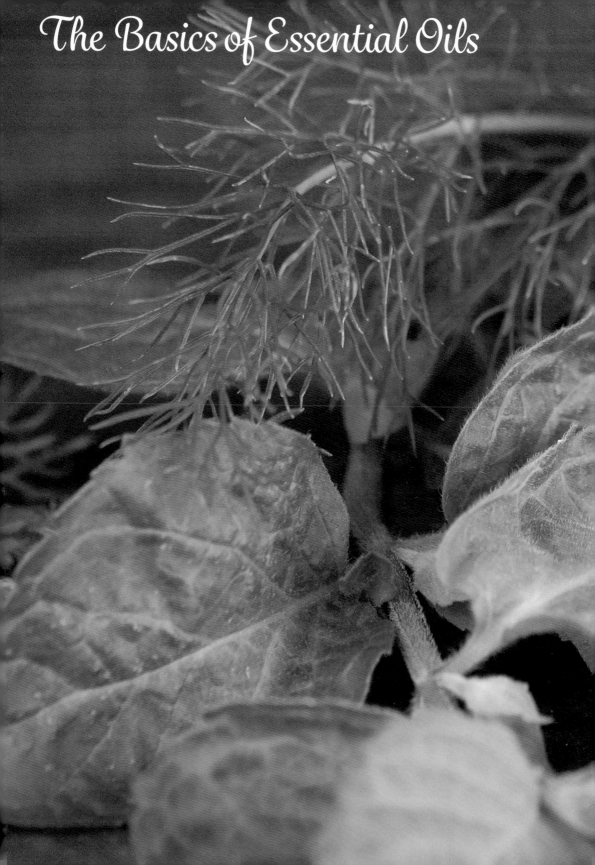

The Basics of Essential Oils

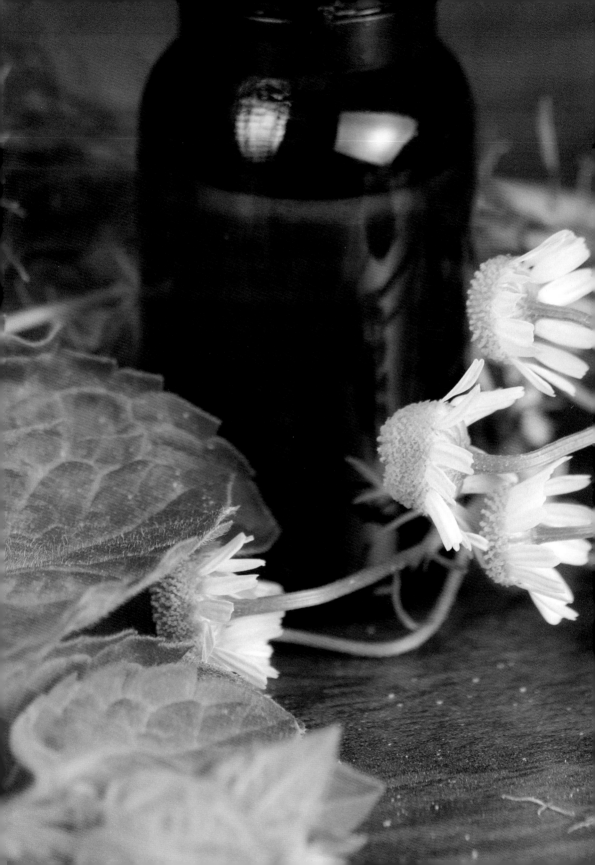

Essential Oils: A Natural Choice

In today's world of artificially high healthcare costs and artificial drugs, millions of people are returning to nature to find relief from everyday health concerns. While plants have been used for millennia to fight disease and to help ease pain and discomfort, individuals are just now beginning to rediscover some of the amazing health benefits of pure, natural essential oils.

Why Plants Make Essential Oils

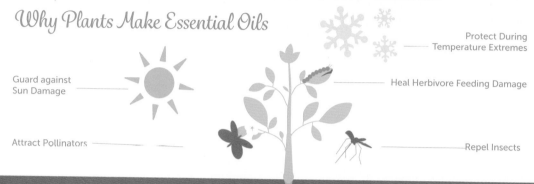

Guard against Sun Damage

Attract Pollinators

Protect During Temperature Extremes

Heal Herbivore Feeding Damage

Repel Insects

Assist during Periods of Low Nutrients

Resist Microbial Attack

What Are Essential Oils?

- Natural substances created by plants
- Aromatic molecules that give plants their distinct aroma
- Small, light molecules that are steam-distilled (or pressed) from plants
- Oil-soluble substances that mix with oils and not water

- Highly concentrated blends of natural substances that have been used for thousands of years and are currently being studied for their profound health benefits, including their antiseptic properties and their ability to help lessen pain, ease feelings of depression, enhance memory, and decrease inflammation, among many other amazing benefits

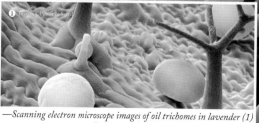

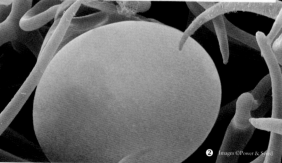

—Scanning electron microscope images of oil trichomes in lavender (1) and rosemary (2) plants.

Many essential oil–producing plants store these oils in special storage structures called trichomes. Others secrete the oils onto the surface of the plant or into special cells or cavities within the plant.

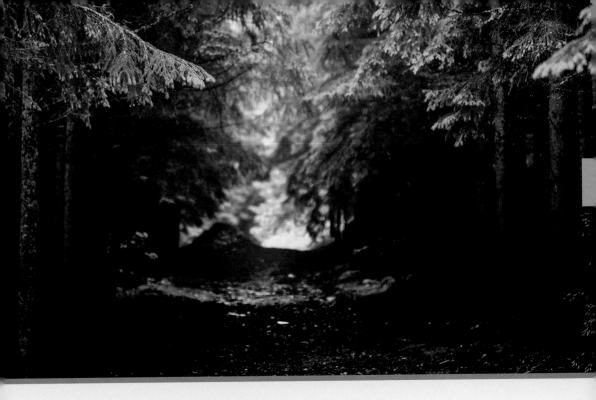

Essential Oils: Direct from Nature

If you've ever been enchanted by the aroma of a pine forest, or been tempted by the sweet smell of a rose, or been uplifted by the crisp scent of a fresh-cut lemon, you have already experienced the amazing benefits of aromatic essential oils directly from nature.

By gently steam-distilling or pressing the plant material, skilled artisans can capture these unique essences to be used in our homes.

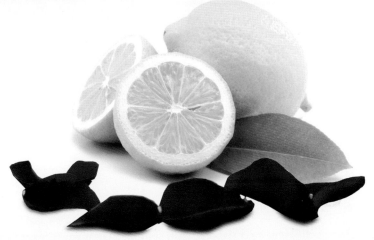

What Benefits Do Essential Oils Have?

Natural Body Support

How Do Essential Oils Support a Healthy Body?

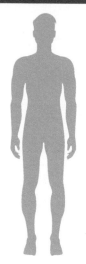

MIND
Promote Relaxation | Calm Tension and Nerves | Increase Positive
Feelings and Help Decrease Stress

IMMUNE
Support Healthy Immune Function | Protect Against Environmental
and Seasonal Threats

CARDIOVASCULAR
Maintain Healthy Circulation | Support Healthy Respiratory Function

DIET
Promote Healthy Digestion | Help Reduce Occasional Stomach Upset
Promote Healthy Metabolism

PHYSICAL ACTIVITY
Support Muscle and Joint Function | Support Energy and Stamina

BODY SYSTEMS
Improve Appearance of the Skin | Soothe Occasional Skin Irritations
Provide Antioxidants | Purify the Body's Systems| Repel Insects

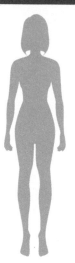

Joy

Why We Use Oils...
Here are some of the many
reasons why millions of people
have chosen to make essential
oils part of their everyday lives.

I LOVE THE HOW CALM
AND RELAXED I FEEL.

Kids

MY PETS
STAY
HEALTHY
FROM PURE
ESSENTIAL
OILS.

THEY HELP
SUPPORT ME
EMOTIONALLY.

ESSENTIAL
OILS HAVE
POWERFUL
MENTAL
HEALTH
BENEFITS.

I ENJOY BETTER
SLEEP WHEN I USE
ESSENTIALS OILS.

HAVING A
NATURAL WAY TO
SUPPORT MY KIDS
IS SO FULFILLING.

Mood

I TRUST
OILS
FOR MY
FAMILY'S
HEALTH.

ESSENTIAL OILS ARE
PURE & NATURAL.

How Can Essential Oils Have So Many benefits?

Since there are so many different essential oils, each comprised of many different natural constituents
with various properties, essential oils can affect the body and mind in diverse ways.

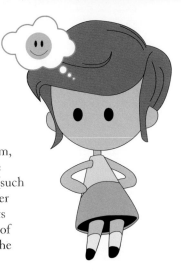

Emotions come in response to what we see, smell, hear, feel, taste, think, or have experienced and can affect our future thoughts and behavior. While much is still being discovered about the complex psychological and physiological processes involved in emotions, researchers have discovered that emotions involve many different systems in the body, including the brain, the sensory system, the endocrine/hormonal system, the autonomic nervous system, the immune system, and the release or inhibition of neurotransmitters (such as dopamine) in the brain. Recent research has also begun to uncover compelling evidence that various essential oils and their components have the ability to affect each one of these systems, making the use of essential oils an intriguing tool for helping to balance emotions in the human body.

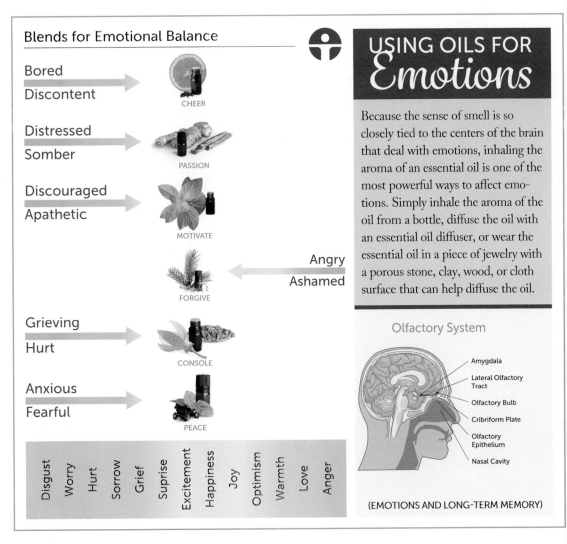

Blends for Emotional Balance

Bored / Discontent → CHEER

Distressed / Somber → PASSION

Discouraged / Apathetic → MOTIVATE

Angry / Ashamed → FORGIVE

Grieving / Hurt → CONSOLE

Anxious / Fearful → PEACE

Disgust · Worry · Hurt · Sorrow · Grief · Suprise · Excitement · Happiness · Joy · Optimism · Warmth · Love · Anger

USING OILS FOR Emotions

Because the sense of smell is so closely tied to the centers of the brain that deal with emotions, inhaling the aroma of an essential oil is one of the most powerful ways to affect emotions. Simply inhale the aroma of the oil from a bottle, diffuse the oil with an essential oil diffuser, or wear the essential oil in a piece of jewelry with a porous stone, clay, wood, or cloth surface that can help diffuse the oil.

Olfactory System

Amygdala
Lateral Olfactory Tract
Olfactory Bulb
Cribriform Plate
Olfactory Epithelium
Nasal Cavity

(EMOTIONS AND LONG-TERM MEMORY)

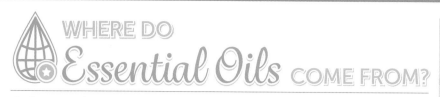

WHERE DO Essential Oils COME FROM?

Only an estimated 10% of the world's plants produce essential oils. These plants can usually be recognized by the aroma that they produce. The plants used to make essential oils originate from all over the world and are cultivated from many locations in North and South America, Europe, Africa, Asia, and Australia.

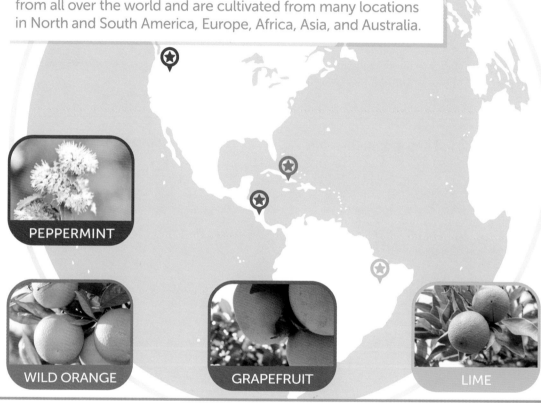

PEPPERMINT

WILD ORANGE

GRAPEFRUIT

LIME

How Are Essential Oils Extracted from Plants?

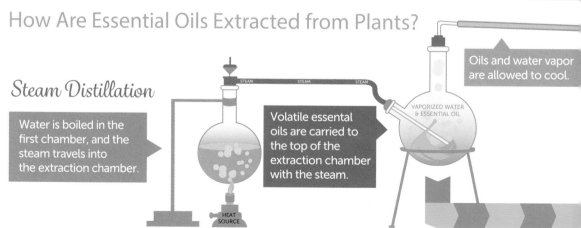

Steam Distillation

Water is boiled in the first chamber, and the steam travels into the extraction chamber.

Volatile essential oils are carried to the top of the extraction chamber with the steam.

Oils and water vapor are allowed to cool.

STEAM   STEAM   STEAM

VAPORIZED WATER & ESSENTIAL OIL

HEAT SOURCE

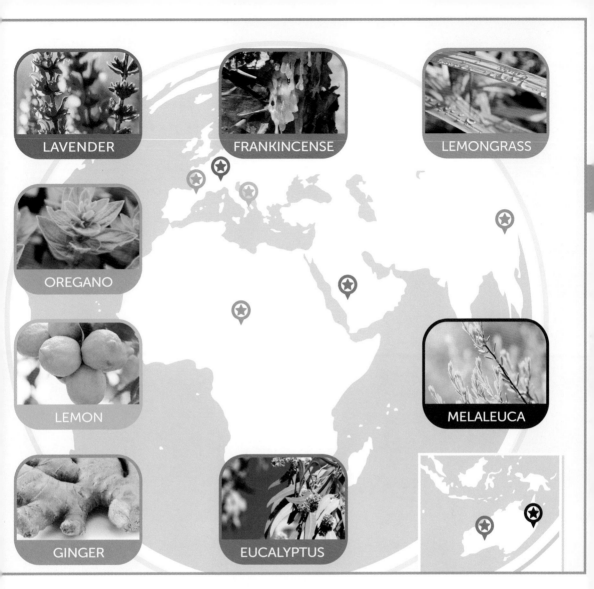

LAVENDER

FRANKINCENSE

LEMONGRASS

OREGANO

LEMON

MELALEUCA

GINGER

EUCALYPTUS

Hydrophobic oils rise to the top of the water, where they can be easily separated.

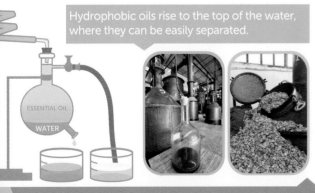

ESSENTIAL OIL

WATER

Plant material is placed inside the extraction chamber.

Cold Expression

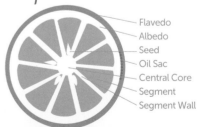

Flavedo
Albedo
Seed
Oil Sac
Central Core
Segment
Segment Wall

Cold expression, or cold pressing, is the method used commonly to produce oils from citrus fruits. Mechanical pressure is applied to the plant material, most often the peel or rind, and the oil is "pressed" out.

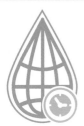

TIMELINE OF AROMATIC PLANTS &
Essential Oils

Aromatic plants have long played an important role in human civilizations. They have been a part of religion, marriage ceremonies, dating and courtship, cosmetics, funerary services, medicine, and many other aspects of human life. Although the use of essential oils has evolved over the years, the basic principles remain the same. From the beginning of time, oils extracted from aromatic plants have been recognized as the most effective medicine known to mankind.

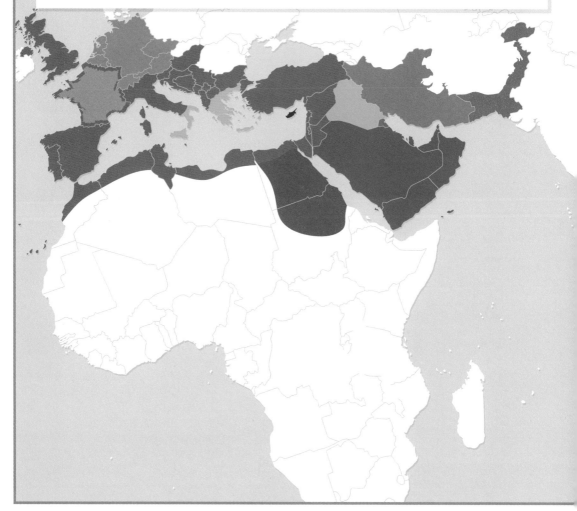

4000–3000 BC: The Sumerians leave the first known perfume recipes on clay cuneiform tablets.

3000 BC: Terra-cotta stills and containers are used to create and store perfumes in the Indus Valley Civilization.

2500 BC: Chinese emperor Shen Nung (Shennong) identifies medicinal uses for over 300 plants.

1850 BC: Ancient perfume makers on the island of Cyprus use hydrodistillation to create perfume from plant extracts.

1550 BC: The Ebers Papyrus is written, detailing how ancient Egyptians used frankincense and other aromatics for many purposes, including religious rituals and curing ailments.

1000–400 BC: Frankincense is the largest trade commodity in ancient Arabia, and a trade route called the Frankincense Trail stretches 2,400 miles from Omar to Petra.

800–150 BC: Greek physicians use aromatic plants medicinally, believing they are divine inventions of the gods.

430 BC: Hippocrates fumigates the city of Athens using aromatic essences to fight the plague.

70 BC: Dioscorides publishes *De Materia Medica*, a text on herbal medicine and the medicinal uses of many different plants.

27 BC–395: Ancient Romans use aromatic oils to scent their baths, homes, and bodies.

1000: Persian philosopher and physician Avicenna is credited with the invention of the steam distillation process.

1500: German physician Hieronymus Brunschwig publishes *Liber de Arte Distillandi*, one of the first printed books on essential oil distillation.

1937: French chemist René-Maurice Gattefossé publishes *Aromathérapie*, which emphasizes the therapeutic value of essential oils, especially lavender.

Topical Application

Topical application refers to placing essential oils on some area of the body, including the skin, hair, nails, or teeth. There are many benefits from topical application. Therapeutic effects can occur both at the site of application and throughout the bloodstream to affect different organs inside the body.

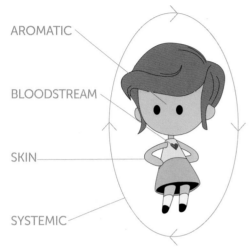

AROMATIC

BLOODSTREAM

SKIN

SYSTEMIC

Many oils can be applied "neat"—or without dilution—but some contain concentrated constituents that may irritate if they are applied directly on sensitive skin. Diluting oils with a pure vegetable oil, referred to as a carrier oil, can make even the most concentrated oils safe and comfortable for topical application. Diluting an oil can also spread the effects of a drop or two of an essential oil over a much larger area.

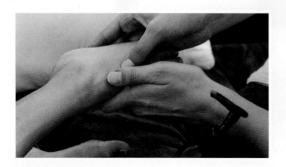

Methods

Direct Application: the simplest method of topical application; refers to applying oils directly to the area of concern. Usually, 1–3 drops of essential oil is more than enough for direct application. A few drops of oil can be added to a carrier oil, and oils can also be mixed or applied on top of one another.

Massage: the stimulation of muscle, skin, and connective tissues. Adding massage to essential oils can enhance their invigorating, relaxing, stimulating, or soothing effects and promote healing and balance. Anyone who is not a certified massage therapist should use only light to medium strokes and avoid the spine or other sensitive areas of the body. To create a massage oil, add 10 drops of essential oil or blend to 1 Tbs. (15 ml) of carrier oil.

Balancing Touch Massage Technique: is a simple, effective way that both beginners and experts alike can apply essential oils with meaningful results. See page 26 for more information.

Baths: can help topically apply oils. Adding essential oils to bathwater helps drive the oils into the skin. Though oils can be added directly to the water, they will rise to the top and might irritate sensitive areas of the body. It is better to blend 2 Tbs. (25 ml) carrier oil with 15 drops essential oil in a small container. Adding 1 tsp. (5 ml) of this blend to a warm bath can be a great way to topically apply essential oils.

Compresses: can help relieve pain and soothe muscles. To create a compress, fill a basin with 2 quarts (2 L) of hot or cold water and the desired essential oils. Place a towel in the basin, and allow it to soak up the oils. Wring out the water and place the damp, oil-saturated towel on the affected area. For a hot compress, cover with a dry towel and hot water bottle. For a cold compress, cover with a piece of plastic wrap.

Reflexology/Reflex Therapy: is a method of applying oils to contact points or nerve endings in the feet or hands. For more details, refer to the reflex hand and foot charts on page 34.

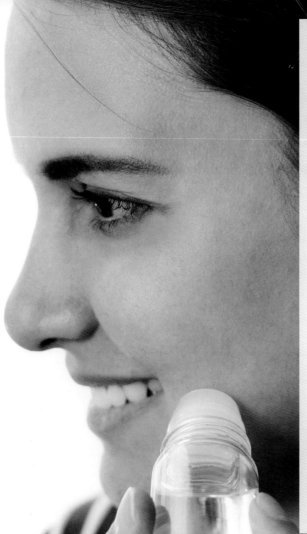

Bath Blends

Soothe Your Troubles

4 drops Roman chamomile   4 drops lavender

4 drops cedarwood   3 drops lemongrass

Up and at 'Em

8 drops pepperment   4 drops grapefruit

3 drops rosemary

Massage Oil

Relaxing

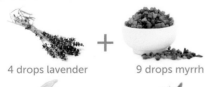

4 drops lavender   9 drops myrrh

5 drops ylang ylang   4 drops Roman chamomile

Invigorating

2 drops lemon   2 drops grapefruit

2 drops white fir   3 drops peppermint

Aromatherapy can have many benefits on the body and mind because our sense of smell is closely tied to the part of the brain controlling emotions and long-term memory. Inhaling the aroma or diffused mist of an essential oil can powerfully affect these areas of the body as well as the respiratory system.

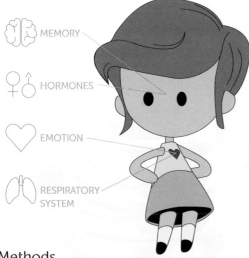

MEMORY

HORMONES

EMOTION

RESPIRATORY SYSTEM

Methods

Direct Inhalation: a simple way to inhale an essential oil. Oils can be inhaled straight from the bottle or applied to the hands and cupped over the mouth and nose to quickly affect moods and emotions.

Diffusion: the easiest way to spread essential oils throughout an entire room. A diffuser can do this with any favorite essential oil or blend of oils.

Perfumes or Colognes: can be made using essential oils and worn daily to provide emotional support and an incredible scent. Simply apply 1–2 drops of an essential oil or blend to the wrists or neck.

Fans or Vents: can spread the aroma of an essential oil in a small space by placing a few drops of essential oil on a cotton ball and attaching it to a standing fan, ceiling fan, or air vent. This can work especially well in a car's air vent.

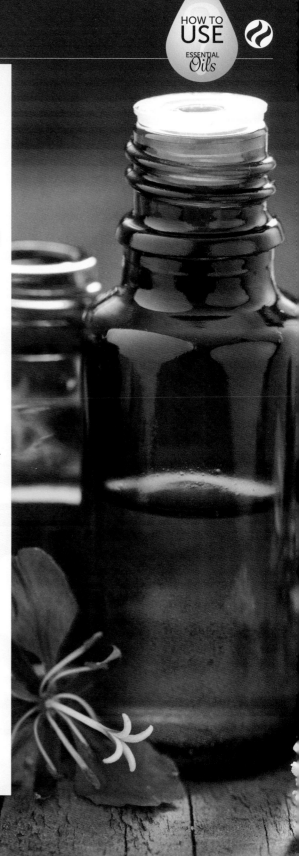

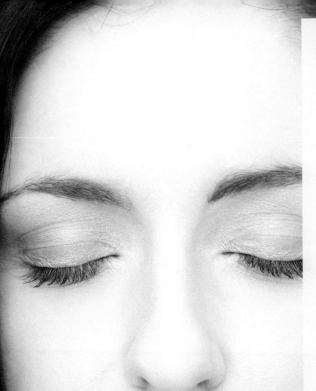

Perfume Blends

Romance

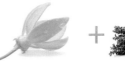

5 drops ylang ylang

4 drops clary sage

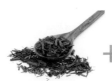

4 drops sandalwood

2 drops lemongrass

Oriental Nights

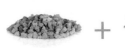

7 drops frankincense

5 drops white fir

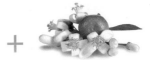

3 drops orange

Diffuser Blends

Stress Less

2 drops lemon

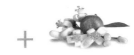

2 drops orange

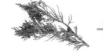

2 drops cedarwood

2 drops clove

Energizing

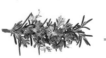

1 drop rosemary

3 drops orange

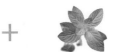

3 drops peppermint

Internal application refers to consuming oils. Taking certain essential oils internally affects the digestive system, and many oils are able to pass into the bloodstream this way and travel quickly to many areas of the body.

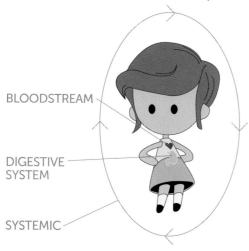

BLOODSTREAM

DIGESTIVE SYSTEM

SYSTEMIC

Only the highest quality oils are meant for internal use. Some essential oils may be diluted or processed using harmful chemicals. Fragrance oils or any other oil that is not labeled as safe for internal use should never be used internally.

Methods

Sublingual: placing a drop or two of essential oil underneath the tongue. This is one of the most effective ways to take essential oils internally. Some stronger oils may need to be diluted before being taken sublingually.

Capsules: take 1–10 drops of essential oil inside an empty capsule. This allows the ingestion of some oils that have a potent or unpleasant taste. Because essential oils are so potent, most should be diluted with a carrier oil like olive oil when used in capsules.

Beverages: an easy way to take essential oils internally. Simply place 1 drop of essential oil in 1–4 cups (250–1000 ml) of a favorite beverage (water, milk, and almond milk all work great).

Cooking: using essential oils to substitute for many different herbs and flavorings. Only very small amounts are needed for cooking—oftentimes just a toothpick dipped into the oil and stirred into the food. See the "Essential Living" chapter for more information on cooking with essential oils.

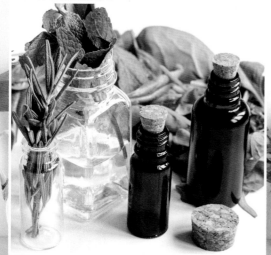

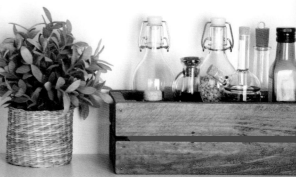

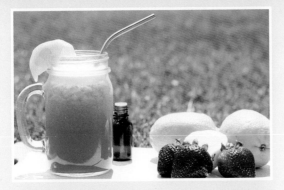

Recipes

Strawberry Lemon Essential Oil–Flavored Water

Add a few slices of fresh strawberries and 1 drop lemon essential oil to your water.

1 drop lemon

Hot Chocolate with Essential Oil

Add 1–2 drops peppermint essential oil into hot chocolate.

1–2 drops peppermint

Chocolate Peppermint Pretzels

Stir 5 drops peppermint essential oil into 2 bags of melted milk chocolate chips. Dip pretzels in chocolate mixture, and let cool. Enjoy!

5 drops peppermint

More recipes and guidelines for cooking and internal use can be found in the "Essential Living" chapter of this book.

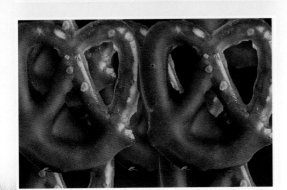

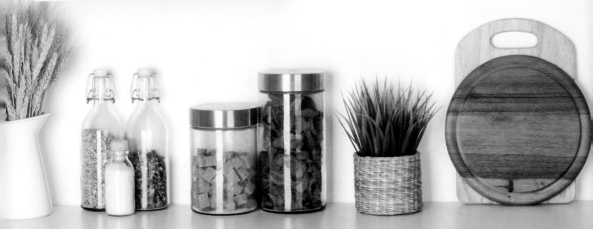

Essential Oil Quality

There are many different options to consider when purchasing essential oils; however, not all manufacturers produce oils with the same high standards. If essential oils are diluted with chemical additives or even packaged improperly, the therapeutic benefits of the oils can be greatly reduced—and can sometimes even be countered by harmful effects.

For this reason, it is important to use only essential oils that are pure, therapeutic grade. To meet this level of quality, the producer must maintain the highest standards, from the plants they use to their production methods and packaging.

Source

Plants from which essential oils are derived should be grown in appropriate climates to develop the right balance of constituents. Pesticides and other chemicals that could affect the chemical composition of the oils should never be used.

Essential oils should also be sourced from the correct species of plant. For instance, essential oils from *Lavandula angustifolia* and *Lavandula latifolia* are often both called lavender oil, but these essential oils actually have different chemical constituents and therapeutic properties. Be certain that the label lists the correct species of plant for the desired essential oil.

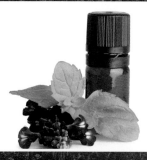

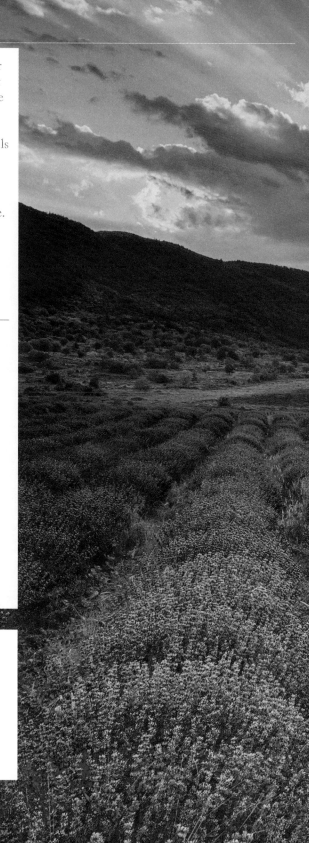

Production

Pure essential oils should be steam-distilled (or pressed from the rind), not chemically extracted. Anything labeled as an extract or fragrance oil is not the same as therapeutic-grade essential oil. Proper distillation techniques are a crucial part of creating high-quality essential oils. It is also important that plants are distilled during the right time of year, at the right age, and after the right amount of time from harvest to ensure that they contain the right balance of chemical constituents. Distillers who understand this will distill the plant material under optimal circumstances for the best therapeutic properties.

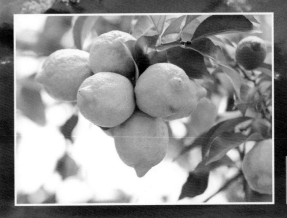

Testing

One of the most important qualities of therapeutic-grade oils is purity from synthetic fragrances or other additions or dilutions that are used to cut costs. Essential oil producers committed to creating the highest-quality oils will not add other materials to them. Rigorous testing should be done to ensure essential oils have the correct balance of constituents and that they are truly pure. Types of testing can include the following:

Sensory Evaluation: There is a difference between the scent of pure essential oils and synthetic fragrances, and experts have trained their senses to detect inconsistencies in aroma as well as color and texture. Physical tests, such as measuring the specific gravity, refractive index, or optical rotation of the oil can also be used to help determine the chemical makeup and purity of essential oils.

Chemical Analysis: This type of testing is used to assess qualities that cannot be determined by the senses or physical tests alone. Two methods (Gas Chromatography Mass Spectrometry and Fourier Transform Infrared Spectroscopy) are used for modern chemical analysis. These processes allow scientists to measure the chemical composition of an essential oil and determine the concentration of each of its constituents.

Pricing

One last quality to look for is a fluctuation in prices between different essential oils. Some essential oils require much more plant matter and are much more difficult to produce than others, and these naturally have a higher cost. If two essential oils like frankincense and lemon are priced similarly, it is a sign that the manufacturer uses methods to cut production costs and the oil is not therapeutic grade.

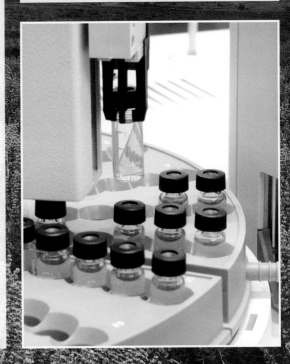

Safe and Effective Use of Essential Oils

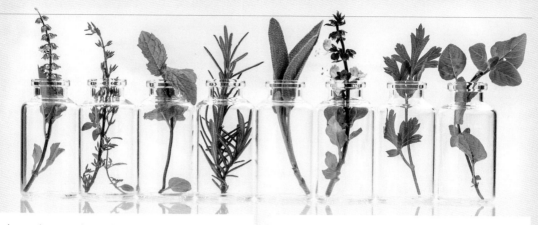

As with any other substance that affects the body, it is important to use essential oils properly to ensure safe use and to maximize their benefits. The "Essential Oils" chapter in this handbook provides information on proper essential oil use, including circumstances in which certain oils or methods are not advised. Essential oils are natural, wonderful, and safe, but common sense is still important. The following points are some basic essential oil usage tips to keep in mind.

Using the Right Amount

More is not always better when it comes to essential oils. For example, drinking one or two glasses of cool water at a time on a hot day can provide relief and needed nourishment for the body. However, drinking 30 or 40 glasses all at once would not be wise, and could even make the body sick. The same concept applies to essential oils. Because essential oils are so concentrated, 1–3 drops (or even less) at a time is almost always sufficient.

Using small amounts of essential oils consistently over time with proper oil dilution will conserve essential oils, increase their benefits, and ensure safe and proper use.

Understanding What Each Essential Oil is Meant to Do

Each essential oil is unique. Each can affect the body differently and have very different benefits. At the same time, not all essential oils can be used in the same way. Refer to the "Essential Oils" chapter for specific application instructions for each oil.

Sensitive Areas

There are some areas of the body where essential oils should not be applied. These include the eyes and any other sensitive tissues, such as the inside of the nose, ear canal, or mucous membranes. Applying oils in these areas can cause severe discomfort or damage these tissues. Flush with a carrier oil if essential oils are causing discomfort in these areas.

Essential Oils and Water Don't Mix

If an essential oil causes discomfort when applied to sensitive skin, or if they get into the eyes or on a sensitive area of the body, never use water to dilute an essential oil or to attempt to wash it away. Because essential oils and water do not mix, applying water can drive the oil deeper into the tissue, increasing discomfort. Instead, use a carrier oil, like fractionated coconut oil, olive oil, or another vegetable oil, to dilute the oil and relieve discomfort.

Dilution of Essential Oils

Certain oils should be diluted before using on the skin as they may irritate or cause discomfort on sensitive skin or other sensitive tissues. See the "Essential Oils" chapter for specific dilution recommendations for each essential oil.

Photosensitivity

Some essential oils—including certain citrus oils—contain substances that can cause the skin to be more sensitive to UV radiation. Avoid direct sunlight and UV lights after applying these oils on the skin for up to 72 hours. See the "Essential Oils" chapter for information on specific essential oils.

Internal Use of Essential Oils

Only certain essential oils are recommended for internal use or ingestion. Only pure, therapeutic-grade essential oils should ever be ingested, as less expensive alternatives may contain harmful chemical additives or may not ensure safe internal use. If an essential oil does not have a supplement label on the bottle, it is probably not meant for internal use. See the "Essential Oils" chapter for specific information on internal use for each essential oil.

Pregnancy & Nursing

Essential oils can be a great benefit during pregnancy, labor, delivery, and motherhood. However, some oils should be heavily diluted or may even need to be avoided by pregnant and nursing women. Check the "Essential Oils" and "Essential Oil Blends" chapters in this handbook for specific information on safe and proper use of specific essential oils or blends.

Kids

Essential oils are great for natural kids' recipes, home remedies, and more. However, it is important that children always use essential oils under the supervision of a trusted adult. Children often require heavier oil dilutions, and some oils should not be used for children under the age of 6. Oils should be stored where children cannot reach them to avoid accidental ingestion or contact with the eyes.

Special care should be taken on newborn infants as their skin is thin and not fully developed. This can allow more of an essential oil to be absorbed, increasing its effects. Heavy dilution is often recommended, and certain oils should be avoided. See the "Children and Infants" section of the "My Usage Guide" chapter, and also the "Essential Oils" chapter of this book for more information on using oils with children.

Animals

Animals can also benefit from the power of essential oils. However, each animal has a different physiology, and the effects of essential oils differ between different animals. For smaller animals, such as small dogs and cats, heavy dilution may be necessary, and certain oils should be avoided. Refer to the "Animals" section in the "My Usage Guide" chapter of this handbook for information on how to use essential oils with your favorite animals.

Medical Conditions/Drug Interactions

Some essential oils constituents may enhance or block the effects of certain types of pharmaceutical drugs. It is recommended that you consult with a health care professional before using an essential oil if suffering from a medical condition or using a medication.

Essential oils are amazing substances and can be used in a myriad of ways on their own. However, having a few tools can maximize the use of essential oils and bring their full range of benefits, allowing for easy application and the ability to create many natural products for cleaning, personal care, healthy living, and more.

Carrier Oils

Carrier oils are vegetable oils (like fractionated coconut oil) that are used to dilute essential oils and to spread a drop or two of essential oil over a larger area when applying topically. Carrier oils are especially beneficial when applying essential oils on those with sensitive skin, children, and pregnant women. Carrier oils are great to use when making essential oil roll-ons, massage oils, and other natural body care essentials like lotions and lip balms. Examples of carrier oils include fractionated coconut oil, jojoba oil, sesame seed oil, sweet almond oil, and other vegetable oils.

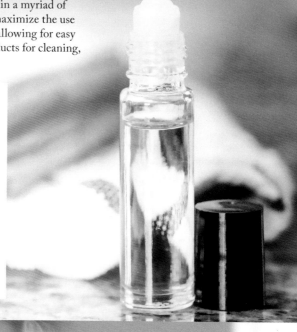

Aromatherapy Diffuser

An aromatherapy diffuser disperses essential oils into the air for inhalation and aromatherapy and is the easiest way to spread an oil throughout the room or other space. The simplest diffusers place essential oils on a porous surface where they are allowed to evaporate. This method can be used to create a personal diffuser from a porous material fashioned into pendants, bracelets, or other jewelry. Often, heat or air movement is used to accelerate the evaporation of the oil into the air. More sophisticated mechanical diffusers break the oil into tiny droplets that are then dispersed into the air. These mechanical diffusers include ultrasonic and nebulizing diffusers.

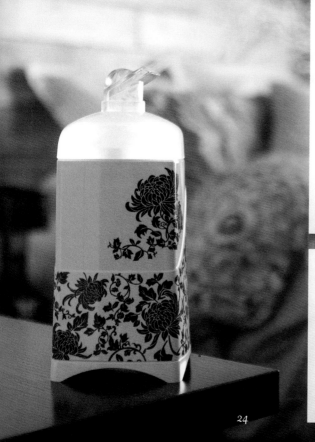

Carrying Cases

There are many cases available meant specifically for storing and transporting oils. Larger cases can store oil collections at home, while smaller ones can be used to bring favorite oils along while traveling.

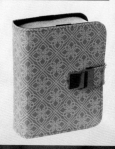

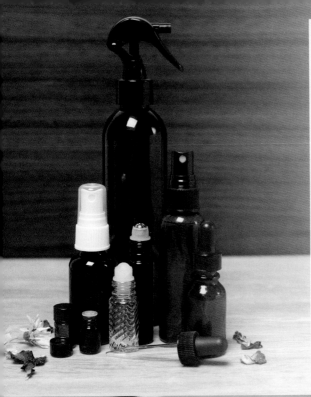

Oil Bottles

With so many diverse ways to use essential oils, specialized bottles can be an easy way to fulfill each purpose.

DROPPER BOTTLES are especially useful for measuring a specific number of drops, such as when applying oils, making oil blends, or following a recipe.

ROLL-ON BOTTLES make it easy to topically apply essential oils. Oils can be diluted and blended directly in the bottle so they're ready for application.

SPRAY BOTTLES are great for making many natural household essentials like disinfecting sprays, glass cleaners, cooking sprays, linen sprays, air fresheners, and natural perfumes. Glass spray bottles will allow you to use your essential oils to create many of these household necessities.

SAMPLE BOTTLES come in handy for small amounts of essential oil to carry or to give to a friend. These bottles are conveniently sized for portability and come in handy for traveling, everyday use, emergency kits, and office use.

Glass/Stainless Steel Water Bottle

Some essential oils can be used to create flavored drinks by adding 1–2 drops into water, almond milk, or another beverage. Glass and stainless steel water bottles are a good choice for making essential oil–flavored beverages.

Capsules

Another easy way to take essential oils internally is with empty capsules. These capsules can be filled with a small amount of an essential oil or blend and a carrier oil meant for internal use (like olive oil). Taking essential oil capsules is a good way to avoid the taste of certain oils while still benefiting from internal application. Some capsules also inhibit digestion until the oils reaches the intestines. Only essential oils meant for internal consumption should be taken this way.

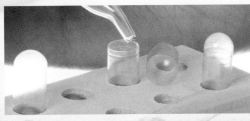

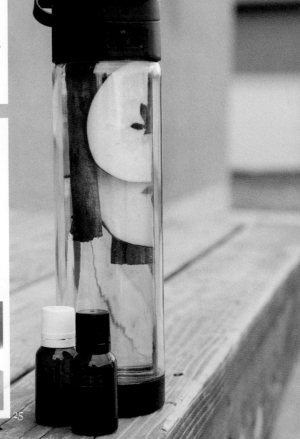

Aroma Touch™ Massage Technique

This technique is a simple, yet effective, way that both beginners and experts alike can apply essential oils with meaningful results.

This effective technique utilizes eight individual essential oils and oil blends that have demonstrated profound effects on four conditions that constantly challenge the ability of the body's systems to function optimally: stress, increased toxin levels, inflammation, and autonomic nervous system imbalance.

This system is comprised of simple application methods that enable these powerful essential oils to reach the optimal areas within the body where they are able to help combat stress, enhance immune function, decrease inflammation, and balance the autonomic nervous system within the recipient.

Stress:

Stress refers to the many systemic changes that take place within the body as it responds to challenging situations. Stress comes not only from difficult, new, and pressured circumstances but also from the body being challenged to cope with things such as abnormal physical exertion, a lack of proper nutrients in the diet, disease-causing microorganisms, and toxic chemicals that make their way into the body. While the systems within a healthy body can typically deal with most short-term challenges, having constant or chronic stress on these systems can overly fatigue them, limiting their abilities to respond to future challenges.

Toxic Insult:

The body is constantly working to cope with a vast array of toxins that continually bombard it. These toxins can come from many different sources, including chemical-laden foods, pollution in the air and water, and pathogenic microorganisms that invade the body. As the environment of the world becomes increasingly saturated with toxins and a rising number of resistant pathogens, the cells, tissues, and systems of the body are forced to work harder to process and eliminate these threats in order to maintain health.

Inflammation:

Inflammation is an immune system response that allows the body to contain and fight infection or to repair damaged tissue. This response dilates the blood vessels and increases vascular permeability to allow more blood to flow to an area with injured or infected tissue. It is characterized by redness, swelling, warmth, and pain. While a certain amount of inflammation can be beneficial in fighting disease and healing injuries, chronic inflammation can actually further injure surrounding tissues or cause debilitating levels of pain.

Autonomic Imbalance:

The autonomic nervous system is comprised of nerves that are connected to the muscles, organs, tissues, and systems that don't require conscious effort to control. The autonomic system is divided into two main parts that each have separate, balancing functions: the sympathetic nervous system and the parasympathetic nervous system. The sympathetic nervous system functions to accelerate heart rate, increase blood pressure, slow digestion, and constrict blood vessels. It activates the "fight or flight" response in order to deal with threatening or stressful situations. The parasympathetic nervous system functions to slow heart rate, store energy, stimulate digestive activity, and relax specific muscles.

Maintaining a proper balance within the autonomic nervous system is important for optimal body function and maintenance.

Oils Used in the Balancing Touch Technique:

For additional information on the oils and blends used in this technique, see the Single Essential Oils and Essential Oil Blends sections of this book.

Stress-Reducing Oils:

Balance: is an oil blend formulated from oils that are known to bring a feeling of calmness, peace, and relaxation. It can aid in harmonizing the various physiological systems of the body and promote tranquility and a sense of balance.

Lavender: has been used for generations for its calming and sedative properties.

Immune Enhancement Oils:

Melaleuca: has potent antifungal, antibacterial, and anti-inflammatory properties.

On Guard: is a blend of oils that have been studied for their strong abilities to kill harmful bacteria, mold, and viruses.

Inflammatory Response–Reducing Oils:

AromaTouch: is a blend of oils that were selected specifically for their ability to relax, calm, and relieve the tension of muscles, soothe irritated tissue, and increase circulation.

Deep Blue: is a blend containing oils that are well known and researched for their abilities to soothe inflammation, alleviate pain, and reduce soreness.

Autonomic Balancing Oils:

Orange: has antidepressant properties and is often used to relieve feelings of anxiety and stress. Its aroma is uplifting to both the body and mind.

Peppermint: has invigorating and uplifting properties.

Applying the Oils: Step One—Stress Reduction

Balance:

Apply Oil: Apply Balance from the base (top) of the sacrum to the base of the skull, distributing the oil evenly along the spine. Use the pads of your fingers to lightly distribute the oils over the length of the spine.

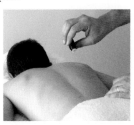

Palm Circles and Connection: With the palms down and fingers overlapping, make three clockwise circles over the heart area; hold the hands briefly in that area, and then slide one hand to the base of the sacrum and the other hand to the base of the skull.

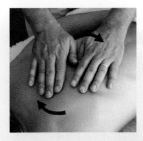

Hold as long as necessary to form a connection, balance, and feeling of trust.

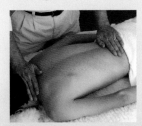

Lavender

Apply Oil: Apply lavender oil from the base of the sacrum to the base of the skull, distributing the oil evenly along the spine. Use the pads of your fingers to lightly distribute the oils over the length of the spine.

Alternating Palm Slide: Standing at the recipient's side, place both hands next to the spine on the opposite side of the back at the base of the sacrum, with the palms down and the fingers pointing away from you. Slide one hand away from the spine toward the side using a mild pressure; then repeat using alternating hands. Continue with this sliding motion as you slowly work your hands from the base of the sacrum to the base of the skull.

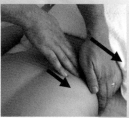

Repeat this step two more times on one side of the back; then move around the person to the opposite side, and repeat three times on that side.

5–Zone Activation: Standing at the head, place both hands together with the fingertips on either side of the spine at the base of the sacrum.

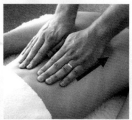

Using a medium downward pressure, pull the hands toward the head through zone 1; then continue through the neck and up to the top of the head.

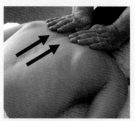

Return the hands to the base of the sacrum, and pull the hands in a similar manner through zone 2 to the shoulders.

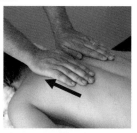

When the hands arrive at the shoulders, push the hands out to the points of the shoulders.

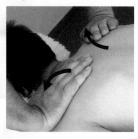

Rotate the hands around the points so that the fingers are on the underside of the shoulders.

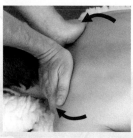

Pull the hands back to the neck, and continue up to the top of the head.

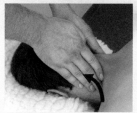

Repeat the steps for zone 2 through zones 3, 4, and 5, ending each pull at the top of the head.

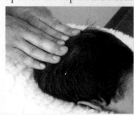

Auricular Stress Reduction: Grip each earlobe between the thumb and forefinger; using gentle pressure, work your fingers in small circles along the ear to the top.

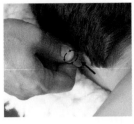

Slide your thumbs with gentle pressure along the backs of the ears returning to the lobes. Repeat this ear massage 3 times.

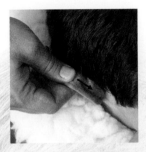

Step Two—Immune Enhancement

Melaleuca

Apply Oil: Apply melaleuca oil from the base of the sacrum to the base of the skull, distributing the oil evenly along the spine. Use the pads of your fingers to lightly distribute the oils over the length of the spine.

Alternating Palm Slide: Perform as outlined under Lavender above.

5–Zone Activation: Perform as outlined under Lavender above.

On Guard

Apply Oil: Apply On Guard from the base of the sacrum to the base of the skull, distributing the oil evenly along the spine. Use the pads of your fingers to lightly distribute the oils over the length of the spine.

Alternating Palm Slide: Perform as outlined under Lavender above.

5–Zone Activation: Perform as outlined under Lavender above.

Thumb Walk Tissue Pull: Place the hands with palms down on either side of the spine at the base of the sacrum, with the thumbs in the small depression between the spine and the muscle tissue. Using a medium pressure, move the pads of the thumbs in small semi-circles, pulling the tissue up, away, and then down from the spine.

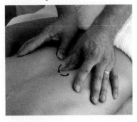

Gradually move each thumb up the spine in alternating fashion until you reach the base of the skull. Repeat this step two more times.

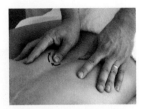

Step Three—Inflammation Reduction

AromaTouch:

Apply Oil: Apply AromaTouch from the base of the sacrum to the base of the skull, distributing the oil evenly along the spine. Use the pads of your fingers to lightly distribute the oils over the length of the spine.

Alternating Palm Slide: Perform as outlined under Lavender above.

5–Zone Activation: Perform as outlined under Lavender above.

Deep Blue:

Apply Oil: Apply Deep Blue from the base of the sacrum to the base of the skull, distributing the oil evenly along the spine. Use the pads of your fingers to lightly distribute the oils over the length of the spine.

Alternating Palm Slide: Perform as outlined under Lavender above.

5–Zone Activation: Perform as outlined under Lavender above.

Thumb Walk Tissue Pull: Perform as outlined under On Guard above.

Step Four—Autonomic Balance

Orange and Peppermint

Apply Oils to Feet: Place drops of orange oil on the palm of your hand, and apply this oil evenly over the entire bottom of the foot.

Apply peppermint oil in the same manner.

Hold the foot with both hands. Beginning in region 1 at the point of the heel and using a medium pressure, massage the foot using first the pad of one thumb and then the pad of the other thumb. Continue this process, alternating thumbs, back and forth through region 1 to thoroughly relax all of the tissue in that region. Repeat through regions 2 and 3.

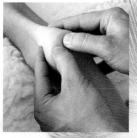

Beginning in zone 1 at the point of the heel, walk the pads of the thumbs through zone 1 using a medium pressure. Continue this process using alternating thumbs and working in a straight line through zone 1 to the tip of the big toe to thoroughly stimulate all of the tissue in that zone.

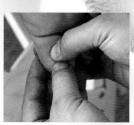

Repeat through zones 2–5.

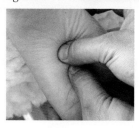

Using a medium pressure with the pad of your thumb, pull the tissue in zone 1—beginning at the point of the heel and ending at the toe. Repeat two additional times through zone 1, using alternate thumbs each time. Repeat this tissue pull process in zones 2–5 on the same foot.

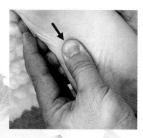

Repeat this entire process, beginning with the application of orange oil, on the opposite foot.

Apply Oils to Back: Apply first orange and then peppermint oils from the base of the sacrum to the base of the skull, distributing the oils evenly along the spine. Use the pads of your fingers to lightly distribute the oils over the length of the spine.

Alternating Palm Slide: Perform as outlined under Lavender above.

Lymphatic Stimulation:

Gentle Body Motion: Standing at the feet, grasp the feet so that the palms of your hands are against the soles of the recipient's feet and your arms are in a straight line with the recipient's legs. Use a repeated, gentle pressure on the feet that allows the recipient's body to translate (move) back and forth naturally on the table. Repeat this process for two or three 15–30 second intervals.

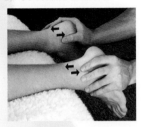

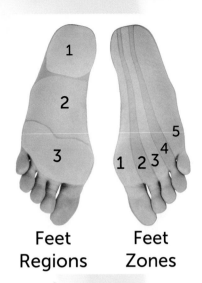

Feet Regions

Feet Zones

Zones of the Back and Head

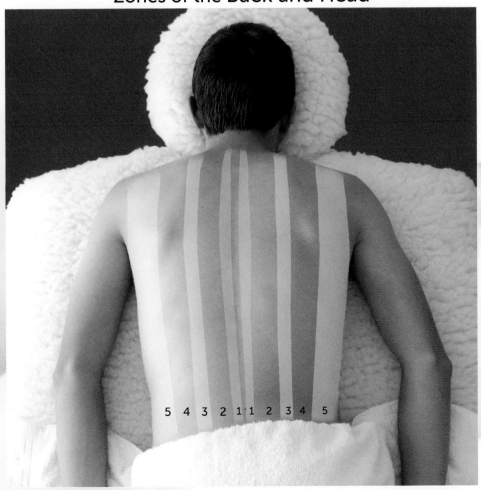

Autonomic Nervous System

Sympathetic Nervous System

Parasympathetic Nervous System

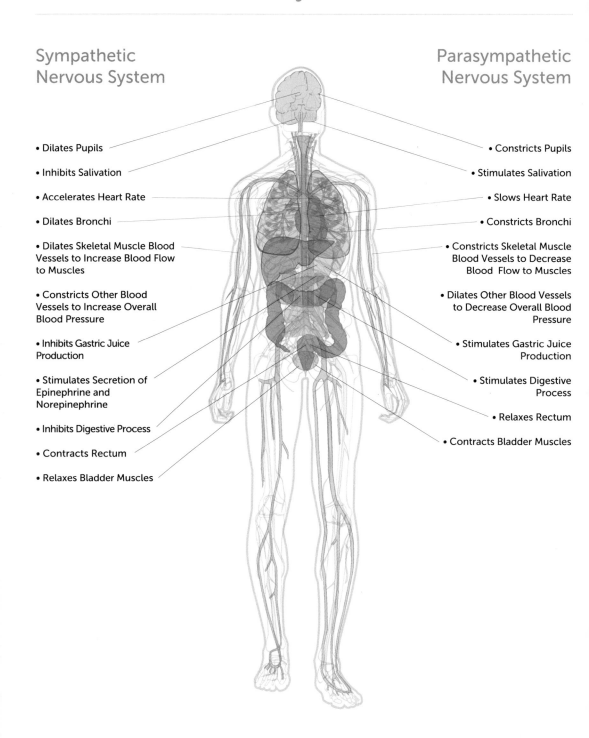

Sympathetic Nervous System
- Dilates Pupils
- Inhibits Salivation
- Accelerates Heart Rate
- Dilates Bronchi
- Dilates Skeletal Muscle Blood Vessels to Increase Blood Flow to Muscles
- Constricts Other Blood Vessels to Increase Overall Blood Pressure
- Inhibits Gastric Juice Production
- Stimulates Secretion of Epinephrine and Norepinephrine
- Inhibits Digestive Process
- Contracts Rectum
- Relaxes Bladder Muscles

Parasympathetic Nervous System
- Constricts Pupils
- Stimulates Salivation
- Slows Heart Rate
- Constricts Bronchi
- Constricts Skeletal Muscle Blood Vessels to Decrease Blood Flow to Muscles
- Dilates Other Blood Vessels to Decrease Overall Blood Pressure
- Stimulates Gastric Juice Production
- Stimulates Digestive Process
- Relaxes Rectum
- Contracts Bladder Muscles

Auricular Internal Body Points

Auricular therapy refers to applying a small amount of oils to various points on the ear related to internal body parts. After applying the oil, the point is stimulated with the fingers or a glass probe.

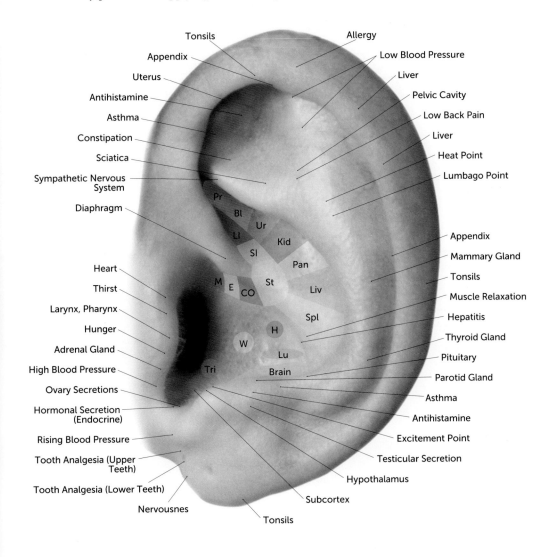

Labels (top, going around):
- Tonsils
- Appendix
- Uterus
- Antihistamine
- Asthma
- Constipation
- Sciatica
- Sympathetic Nervous System
- Diaphragm
- Heart
- Thirst
- Larynx, Pharynx
- Hunger
- Adrenal Gland
- High Blood Pressure
- Ovary Secretions
- Hormonal Secretion (Endocrine)
- Rising Blood Pressure
- Tooth Analgesia (Upper Teeth)
- Tooth Analgesia (Lower Teeth)
- Nervousnes
- Tonsils
- Subcortex
- Hypothalamus
- Testicular Secretion
- Excitement Point
- Antihistamine
- Asthma
- Parotid Gland
- Pituitary
- Thyroid Gland
- Hepatitis
- Muscle Relaxation
- Tonsils
- Mammary Gland
- Appendix
- Lumbago Point
- Heat Point
- Liver
- Low Back Pain
- Pelvic Cavity
- Liver
- Low Blood Pressure
- Allergy

Abbreviations on ear: Pr, Bl, Ur, LI, Kid, SI, Pan, M, St, E, CO, Liv, Spl, H, W, Lu, Tri, Brain

Bl: Bladder	Liv: Liver	Spl: Spleen
CO: Cardiac Orifice	Lu: Lungs	St: Stomach
E: Esophagus	M: Mouth	Tri: Triple Warmer
H: Heart	Pan: Pancreas	Ur: Ureter
Kid: Kidney	Pr: Prostate	W: Windpipe/Trachea
LI: Large Intestine	SI: Small Intestine	

Reflex Therapy Hand and Feet Charts

Reflex points on this hand chart correspond to those on the feet. Occasionally the feet can be too sensitive for typical reflex therapy. Working with the hands will not only affect the specific body points but may also help to provide some pain relief to the corresponding points on the feet.

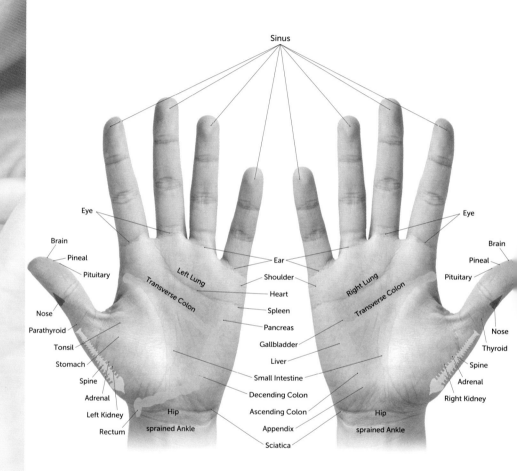

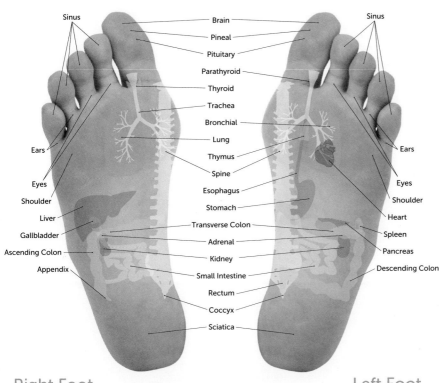

Sinus — Brain — Sinus

Pineal

Pituitary

Parathyroid

Thyroid

Trachea

Bronchial

Ears — Lung — Ears

Thymus

Eyes — Spine — Eyes

Shoulder — Esophagus — Shoulder

Liver — Stomach — Heart

Gallbladder — Transverse Colon — Spleen

Ascending Colon — Adrenal — Pancreas

Appendix — Kidney — Descending Colon

Small Intestine

Rectum

Coccyx

Sciatica

Right Foot   Left Foot

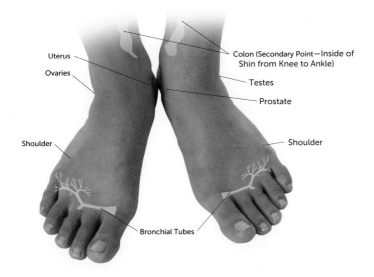

Uterus — Colon (Secondary Point—Inside of Shin from Knee to Ankle)

Ovaries — Testes

Prostate

Shoulder — Shoulder

Bronchial Tubes

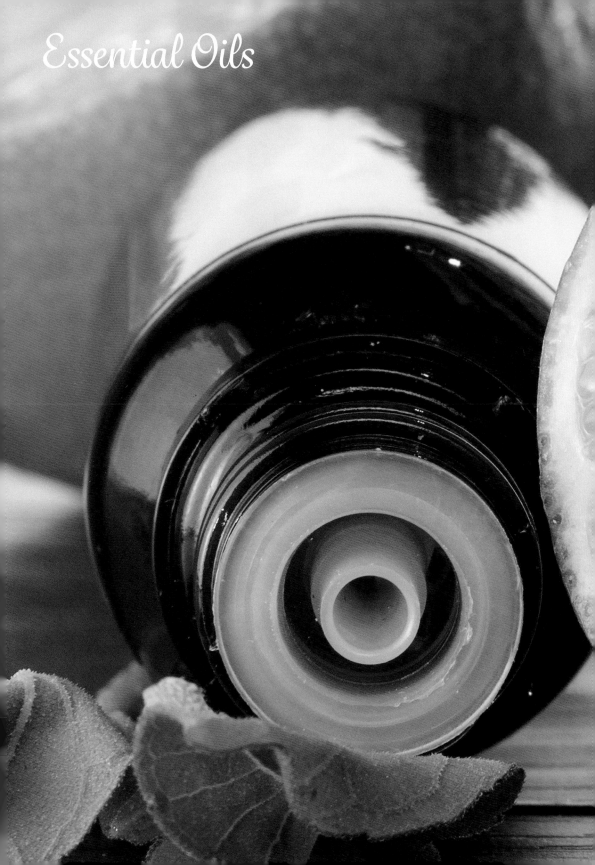

Essential Oils

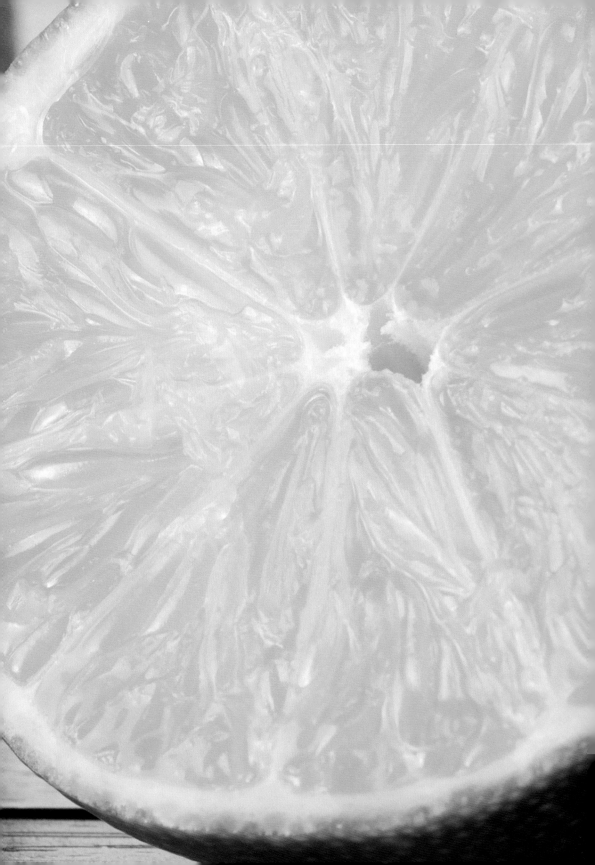

Single Essential Oils

Look for this symbol throughout this section for additional information on several essential oils that are an essential part of any oils tool kit.

Symbols and Colors Used in This Section

Topical	Neat (can be used without dilution)
Aromatic	Dilute for children and those with sensitive skin
Internal	Dilute
Cleaning/Disinfecting	Body System(s) Affected
Avoid sunlight for up to 12 hours after use	See Additional Research
Avoid sunlight for up to 72 hours after use	

See My Usage Guide section for more details. ●=Neat, ●=Dilute for Children/Sensitive Skin, ●=Dilute

Arborvitae *Thuja plicata*

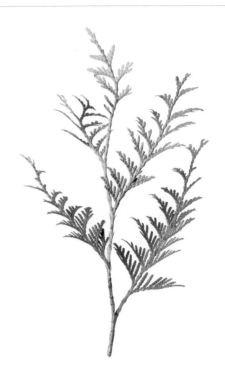

Properties: Antibacterial, antifungal, antiseptic, anticancer⬤, antitumor, astringent, expectorant, insect repellent, and stimulant (nerves, immune system, uterus, and heart muscles).

Historical Uses: The arborvitae, or western red cedar, has been referred to as the "Tree of Life." It has been used by ancient civilizations to enhance their potential for spiritual communication during rituals and other ceremonies. It has also been used for coughs, fevers, intestinal parasites, cystitis, and venereal diseases.

Other Possible Uses: This oil may help with hair loss, inflammation⬤[4], skin (nourishing), rheumatism, sun protection⬤[5], warts, and psoriasis. It has powerful effects on the subconscious and unconscious mind.

⊕ **Body System(s) Affected:** Emotional Balance, Respiratory System, Skin.

Aromatic Influence: It is calming and may help enhance spiritual awareness or meditation.

Oral Use As Dietary Supplement: None.

Safety Data: Use with caution during pregnancy. For topical and aromatic use only. Use sparingly and dilute.

Blend Classification: Enhancer and Equalizer.

Blends With: Birch, cedarwood, cassia, eucalyptus.

Odor: Type: Top to Middle Notes (10–20% of the blend); Scent: Intense, medicinal, woody, earthy; Intensity: 5.

---

‡See Application section beginning on page 14 for more details.   ⬒=Topical, ⬒=Aromatic, ⬤=Internal

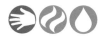

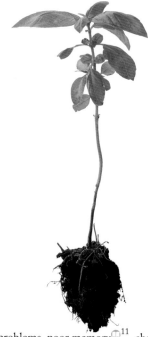

Quick Facts

Botanical Family: Lamiaceae or Labiatae (mint)

Extraction Method: Steam distillation of leaves, stems, and flowers

Common Primary Uses*: ⬤Amenorrhea, ⬤Autism, ⬤Bee/Hornet Stings, ⬤Bites/Stings, ⬤⬤Bronchitis⬤[6], ⬤Bursitis, ⬤Carpal Tunnel Syndrome, ⬤⬤Chronic Fatigue, ⬤⬤Cramps (Abdominal), ⬤Cuts, ⬤Earache, ⬤Frozen Shoulder, ⬤Greasy/Oily Hair, ⬤Healing, ⬤Hiatal Hernia, ⬤Incisional Hernia, ⬤Induce Sweating, ⬤⬤Infertility, ⬤Lactation (Increase Milk Production), ⬤⬤Mental Fatigue, ⬤⬤Migraines, ⬤Mouth Ulcers, ⬤Muscle Spasms, ⬤Muscular Dystrophy, ⬤⬤Olfactory Loss (Sense of Smell), ⬤⬤Ovarian Cyst, ⬤Schmidt's Syndrome, ⬤Snake Bites, ⬤Spider Bites, ⬤Transition (Labor), ⬤⬤Viral Hepatitis, ⬤Wounds

Common Application Methods‡:

⬤: Can be applied neat (with no dilution) when used topically. Dilute with carrier oil for sensitive skin and for children over 6. Apply to temples, tip of nose, reflex points, and/or directly on area of concern.

⬤: Diffuse, or inhale the aroma directly.

⬤: Take in capsules, or use as a flavoring in cooking.

Properties: Antibacterial⬤[7], antifungal⬤[8], anti-infectious, anti-inflammatory, antioxidant⬤[9], antispasmodic (powerful), antiviral, decongestant (veins, arteries of the lungs, prostate), diuretic, disinfectant (urinary/pulmonary), stimulant (nerves, adrenal cortex), and uplifting. Basil is also anticatarrhal, antidepressant, energizing, and restorative.

Historical Uses: Basil was used anciently for respiratory problems, digestive and kidney ailments, epilepsy, poisonous insect or snake bites, fevers, epidemics, and malaria.

Other Possible Uses: This oil may be used for alertness, anxiety, chills, chronic colds, concentration, nervous depression, digestion, fainting, headaches, hiccups, insect bites (soothing), insect repellent⬤[10], insomnia (from nervous tension), intestinal problems, poor memory⬤[11], chronic mucus, prostate problems, rhinitis (inflammation of nasal mucous membranes), vomiting, wasp stings, and whooping cough.

⬤ **Body System(s) Affected:** Cardiovascular and Skeletal Systems and Muscles.

Aromatic Influence: Helps one maintain an open mind and increases clarity of thought.

Oral Use As Dietary Supplement: Basil oil is generally recognized as safe (GRAS) for human consumption by the FDA (21CFR182.20). Dilute 1 drop oil in 1 tsp. (5 ml) honey or in ½ cup (125 ml) of beverage (e.g., soy/rice milk). Not for children under 6 years old; use with caution and in greater dilution for children 6 years old and over.

Safety Data: Avoid during pregnancy. Not for use by people with epilepsy. It may also irritate sensitive skin (test a small area first).

Blend Classification: Enhancer and Equalizer.

Blends With: Bergamot, cypress, white fir, geranium, helichrysum, lavender, lemongrass, marjoram, peppermint, and wintergreen.

Odor: Type: Top to Middle Notes (20–80% of the blend); Scent: Herbaceous, spicy, anise-like, camphorous, lively; Intensity: 4.

*See My Usage Guide section for more details.   ⬤=Neat, ⬤=Dilute for Children/Sensitive Skin, ⬤=Dilute

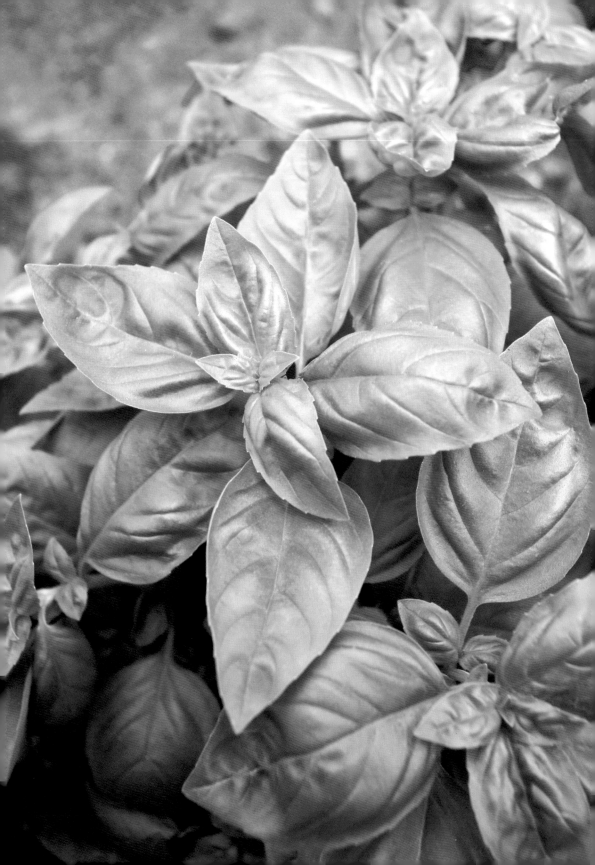

Bergamot *Citrus bergamia*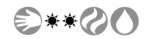

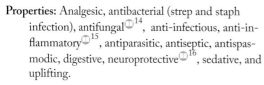
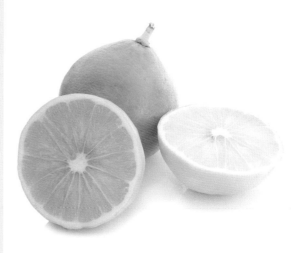

Properties: Analgesic, antibacterial (strep and staph infection), antifungal[14], anti-infectious, anti-inflammatory[15], antiparasitic, antiseptic, antispasmodic, digestive, neuroprotective[16], sedative, and uplifting.

Historical Uses: Bergamot was used by the Italians to cool and relieve fevers, protect against malaria, and expel intestinal worms.

Other Possible Uses: This oil may help acne, anxiety, appetite regulation, boils, bronchitis, carbuncles, cold sores, oily complexion, coughs, cystitis, digestion, eczema, emotions, endocrine system, fever, gallstones, gonorrhea, infectious disease, insect bites, soothe lungs, psoriasis, respiratory infection[—], scabies, sore throat, nervous tension, thrush, acute tonsillitis, ulcers, urinary tract infection, spot varicose veins, and wounds.

Body System(s) Affected: Digestive System, Emotional Balance, Skin.

Aromatic Influence: It may help to relieve anxiety[17], depression, stress, and tension. It is uplifting and refreshing.

Oral Use As Dietary Supplement: Bergamot oil is generally recognized as safe (GRAS) for human consumption by the FDA (21CFR182.20). Dilute 1 drop oil in 1 tsp. (5 ml) honey or in ½ cup (125 ml) of beverage (e.g., soy/rice milk). Not for children under 6 years old; use with caution and in greater dilution for children 6 years old and over.

Safety Data: Repeated use may result in extreme contact sensitization. Avoid direct sunlight or ultraviolet light for up to 72 hours after use.

Blend Classification: Equalizer, Modifier, and Enhancer.

Blends With: Cypress, eucalyptus, geranium, lavender, lemon, and ylang ylang.

Odor: Type: Top Note (5–20% of the blend); Scent: Sweet, lively, citrusy, fruity; Intensity: 2.

Birch *Betula lenta*

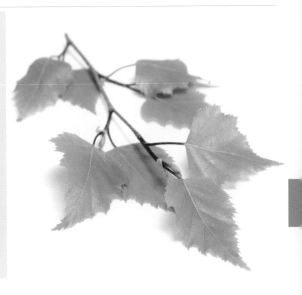

Properties: Analgesic, anti-inflammatory, antirheumatic, antiseptic ⬤[18], antispasmodic, disinfectant, diuretic, stimulant (bone, liver), and warming.

Historical Uses: Birch oil has a strong, penetrating aroma that most people recognize as wintergreen. Although birch (*Betula lenta*) is completely unrelated to wintergreen (*Gaultheria procumbens*), the two oils are almost identical in chemical constituents. The American Indians and early European settlers enjoyed a tea that was flavored with birch bark or wintergreen. According to Julia Lawless, "this has been translated into a preference for 'root beer' flavourings [sic]." A synthetic methyl salicylate is now widely used as a flavoring agent, especially in root beer, chewing gum, toothpaste, etc.

Other Possible Uses: This oil may be beneficial for acne, bladder infection, cystitis, dropsy, eczema, edema, reducing fever, gallstones, gout, infection, reducing discomfort in joints, kidney stones, draining and cleansing the lymphatic system, obesity, osteoporosis, skin diseases, ulcers, and urinary tract disorders. It is known for its ability to alleviate bone pain. It has a cortisone-like action due to the high content of methyl salicylate.

⬤ **Body System(s) Affected:** Skeletal System and Muscles.

Aromatic Influence: It influences, elevates, opens, and increases awareness in the sensory system (senses or sensations).

Oral Use as a Dietary Supplement: None.

Safety Data: Avoid during pregnancy. Not for use by people with epilepsy. Some people are very allergic to methyl salicylate. Test a small area of skin first.

Blend Classification: Personifier and Enhancer.

Blends With: Basil, bergamot, cypress, geranium, lavender, lemongrass, marjoram, and peppermint.

‡See Application section beginning on page 14 for more details. ⬤=Topical, ⬤=Aromatic, ⬤=Internal

Black Pepper *Piper nigrum*

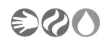

Properties: Analgesic, anticatarrhal, anti-inflammatory, antiseptic, antispasmodic, antitoxic, aphrodisiac, expectorant, laxative, rubefacient, and stimulant (nervous, circulatory, digestive)[20].

Historical Uses: Pepper has been used for thousands of years for malaria, cholera, and several digestive problems.

Other Possible Uses: This oil may increase cellular oxygenation, support digestive glands, stimulate the endocrine system, increase energy, and help rheumatoid arthritis. It may also help with loss of appetite, catarrh, chills, cholera, colds, colic, constipation, coughs, diarrhea, dysentery, dyspepsia, dysuria, flatulence (combine with fennel), flu, heartburn, influenza, nausea, neuralgia, poor circulation, poor muscle tone, quinsy, sprains, toothache, vertigo, viruses, and vomiting.

Body System(s) Affected: Digestive and Nervous Systems.

Aromatic Influence: Pepper is comforting and stimulating.

Oral Use As Dietary Supplement: Black pepper oil is generally regarded as safe (GRAS) for human consumption by the FDA. Dilute 1 drop oil in 1 tsp. (5 ml) honey or in ½ cup (125 ml) of beverage (e.g., soy/rice milk). Not for children under 6 years old; use with caution and in greater dilution for children 6 years old and over.

Safety Data: Can cause extreme skin irritation.

Blend Classification: Enhancer.

Blends With: Fennel, frankincense, lavender, marjoram, rosemary, sandalwood, and other spice oils.

Odor: Type: Middle Note (50–80% of the blend); Scent: Spicy, peppery, musky, warm, with herbaceous undertones; Intensity: 3.

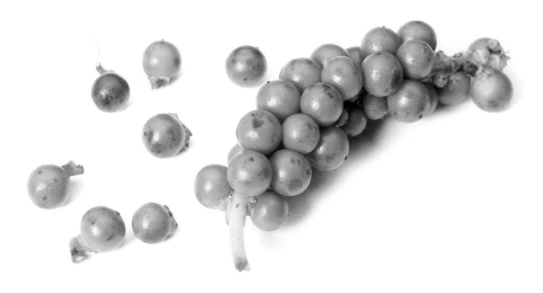

Blue Tansy *Tanacetum annuum*

Quick Facts

Botanical Family: Compositae (daisy)

Extraction Method: Steam distillation from leaves and flowers

Common Primary Uses*: 🕉️💧Anxiety, 🕉️💧Calming, 💧Wounds

Common Application Methods‡:

💧: Apply to reflex points and/or directly on area of concern.

🕉️: Diffuse, or inhale the aroma directly.

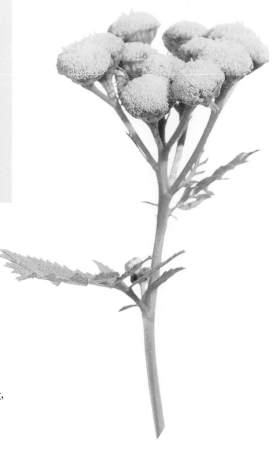

Properties: Analgesic, antibacterial, antifungal📖[21], anti-inflammatory, antihistamine, hypotensive, hormone-like, nervine.

Historical Uses: Anciently, tansy was used to help heal wounds, as a diuretic, and for dealing with kidney issues.

Other Possible Uses: Blue tansy may help raise blood pressure, relieve itching, reduce pain, and sedate the nerves.

🧠 **Body System(s) Affected:** Nervous System.

Aromatic Influence: Blue tansy is uplifting, refreshing, and calming to a troubled mind. It may also help instill confidence and enthusiasm.

Oral Use As Dietary Supplement: None.

Safety Data: Consult a physician before using if taking medications.

Blend Classification: Personifier and Modifier.

Blends With: Most oils; perfumers in France have found that wild tansy has a greater fixative capability than any other oil.

Odor: Type: Middle Note (50–80% of the blend); Scent: Camphoraceous, sweet, herbaceous; Intensity: 4.

‡*See Application section beginning on page 14 for more details.* 💧=Topical, 🕉️=Aromatic, ⭕=Internal

Cardamom *Elettaria cardamomum*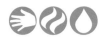

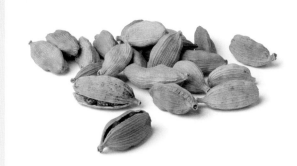

Quick Facts

Botanical Family: Zingiberaceae (ginger)

Extraction Method: Steam distillation from seeds

Common Primary Uses*: ❷Coughs,
O❸Digestive Support, ❸Headaches, ❷❷In-
flammation[22], ❸Muscle Aches, ❷ONausea,
❸❷Respiratory Ailments[23]

Common Application Methods‡:

❸: Apply to reflex points and/or directly on area of
concern. Dilute with base oil, and massage over
the stomach, solar plexus, and thighs. This oil is
excellent as a bath oil.

❷: Diffuse, or inhale the aroma directly.

O: Place 1 drop under the tongue, or take oil in capsules. Use as a flavoring in cooking or in beverages.

Properties: Antibacterial[24], anti-infectious, anti-inflammatory[25], antiseptic, antispasmodic, aphrodisiac, decongestant, diuretic, expectorant, stomachic,
and tonic.

Historical Uses: Anciently, cardamom was used for
epilepsy, spasms, paralysis, rheumatism, cardiac
disorders, all intestinal illnesses, pulmonary disease, fever, and digestive and urinary complaints.
It is said to be able to neutralize the lingering odor
of garlic.

Other Possible Uses: Cardamom may help with appetite (loss of), bronchitis, colic, debility, dyspepsia,
flatulence, halitosis, mental fatigue, pyrosis (or
heartburn), sciatica, ulcers[26], and vomiting. It
may also help with menstrual periods, menopause,
and nervous indigestion.

❸ **Body System(s) Affected:** Digestive and Respiratory Systems.

Aromatic Influence: Cardamom is uplifting, refreshing, and invigorating. It may be beneficial for
clearing confusion.

Oral Use As Dietary Supplement: Generally regarded as
safe (GRAS) for human consumption by the FDA.
Dilute 1 drop oil in 1 tsp. (5 ml) honey or in ½ cup
(125 ml) of beverage (e.g., soy/rice milk). Not for
children under 6 years old; use with caution and in
greater dilution for children 6 years old and over.

Blend Classification: Personifier and Modifier.

Blends With: Bergamot, cedarwood, cinnamon, clove,
orange, rose, and ylang ylang.

Odor: Type: Middle Note (50–80% of the blend);
Scent: Sweet, spicy, balsamic, with floral undertones; Intensity: 4.

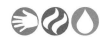

Quick Facts

Botanical Family: Lauraceae (laurel)

Extraction Method: Steam distillation from bark

Common Primary Uses*: ◑Antiseptic⊕, ◐Cooking

Common Application Methods‡:

◑: Dilute heavily with a carrier oil or blend with milder essential oils before applying on the skin. Apply to forehead, muscles, reflex points, and/or directly on area of concern.

◐: Diffuse with caution: it will irritate the nasal membranes if it is inhaled directly from the diffuser.

◐: Use as a flavoring in cooking (similar to cinnamon but has a stronger, more intense flavor).

Properties: Antibacterial⊕[27], antifungal⊕[28], anti-inflammatory⊕[29], and antiviral.

Historical Uses: Has been used extensively as a domestic spice. Medicinally, it has been used for colds, colic, flatulent dyspepsia, diarrhea, nausea, rheumatism, and kidney and reproductive complaints.

Other Possible Uses: This oil can be extremely sensitizing to the dermal tissues. Can provide some powerful support to blends when used in very small quantities.

Oral Use As Dietary Supplement: Cassia oil is generally recognized as safe (GRAS) for human consumption by the FDA (21CFR182.20). Dilute 1 drop oil in 2 tsp. (10 ml) honey or in 1 cup (250 ml) of beverage (e.g., soy/rice milk). May need to increase dilution even more due to this oil's potential for irritating mucous membranes. Not for children under 6 years old; use with caution and in greater dilution for children 6 years old and over.

Safety Data: Repeated use can result in extreme contact sensitization. Avoid during pregnancy. Can cause extreme skin irritation. Diffuse with caution; it will irritate the nasal membranes if it is inhaled directly from the diffuser.

Blend Classification: Personifier and Enhancer.

Blends With: All citrus oils, cypress, frankincense, geranium, juniper berry, lavender, rosemary, and all spice oils.

Odor: Type: Middle Note (50–80% of the blend); Scent: Spicy, warm, sweet; Intensity: 5.

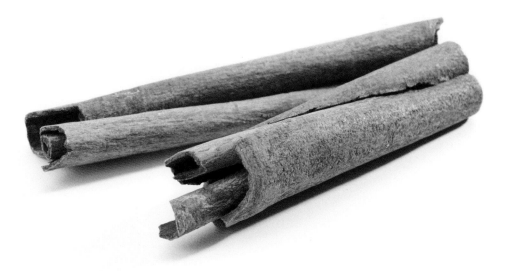

Cedarwood *Juniperus virginiana*

Quick Facts

Botanical Family: Cupressaceae (conifer: cypress)

Extraction Method: Steam distillation from wood

Common Primary Uses*: 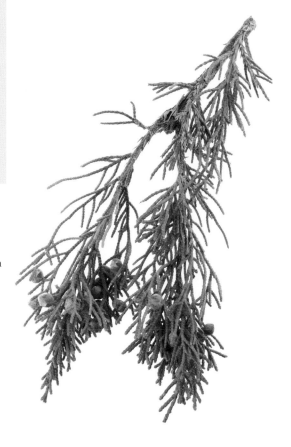Calming, Tension, Tuberculosis, Urinary Infection, Yoga

Common Application Methods‡:

: Dilute with a carrier oil for children and for those with sensitive skin. Apply to reflex points and/or directly on area of concern.

: Diffuse, or inhale the aroma directly.

Properties: Antifungal, anti-infectious, antiseptic (urinary and pulmonary), astringent, diuretic, insect repellent, and sedative.

Historical Uses: This variety of cedarwood (also known as red or Virginian cedarwood) has been used for its strong antiseptic, diuretic, calming, and insect-repelling[30] properties.

Other Possible Uses: This oil may help acne, anxiety, arthritis, congestion, coughs, cystitis, dandruff, inflammation[31], psoriasis, purification, sinusitis, skin diseases, stroke[32], and water retention. It may also help to reduce oily secretions.

Body System(s) Affected: Nervous and Respiratory Systems.

Oral Use As Dietary Supplement: None.

Safety Data: Use with caution during pregnancy.

Blend Classification: Enhancer and Equalizer.

Blends With: Bergamot, clary sage, cypress, eucalyptus, floral oils, juniper, resinous oils, rosemary.

Odor: Type: Base Note (5–20% of the blend); Scent: Warm, soft, woody; Intensity: 3.

Cilantro *Coriandrum sativum L.*

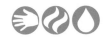

Quick Facts

Botanical Family: Umbelliferae (parsley)

Extraction Method: Steam distillation from leaves (same plant as coriander oil, which is distilled from the seeds)

Common Primary Uses*: ✿Anxiety, ○Cooking

Common Application Methods‡:

✿: Can be applied neat (with no dilution) when used topically. Apply to reflex points and directly on area of concern.

✿: Diffuse, or inhale the aroma directly.

○: Use as a flavoring in cooking.

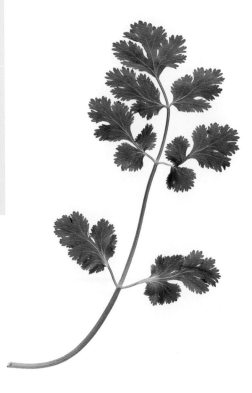

Properties: Antibacterial, antifungal⊡[33].

Historical Uses: Cilantro leaves have been used since the times of ancient Greece as an herb for flavoring. Its aroma has also been used for anxiety and insomnia.

Other Possible Uses: Mainly used as a flavoring in cooking. May also help with liver conditions⊡[34], and with protecting the skin⊡[35].

Oral Use As Dietary Supplement: Cilantro oil is generally recognized as safe (GRAS) for human consumption by the FDA (21CFR182.20). Dilute 1 drop oil in 1 tsp. (5 ml) honey or in ½ cup (125 ml) of beverage (e.g., soy/rice milk). Not for children under 6 years old; use with caution and in greater dilution for children 6 years old and over.

Safety Data: May cause irritation on sensitive or damaged skin.

Blend Classification: Personifier and Modifier.

Blends With: Lime, lemon.

Odor: Scent: Herbaceous, citrusy, fresh.

‡*See Application section beginning on page 14 for more details.*   ✿=Topical, ✿=Aromatic, ○=Internal

49

Cinnamon *Cinnamomum zeylanicum*

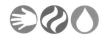

Quick Facts

Botanical Family: Lauraceae (laurel)

Extraction Method: Steam distillation from bark

Common Primary Uses*: Airborne Bacteria, Bacterial Infections, Bites/Stings, Breathing, Diabetes[36], Diverticulitis, Fungal Infections, General Tonic, Immune System (Stimulates), Infection, Libido (Low), Mold, Pancreas Support, Physical Fatigue, Pneumonia, Typhoid, Vaginal Infection, Vaginitis, Viral Infections, Warming (Body)

Common Application Methods‡:

: Dilute 1:3 (1 drop essential oil to at least 3 drops carrier oil) before using topically. Apply directly on area of concern or on reflex points.

: Diffuse with caution; it may irritate the nasal membranes if it is inhaled directly from a diffuser.

: Use as a flavoring in cooking.

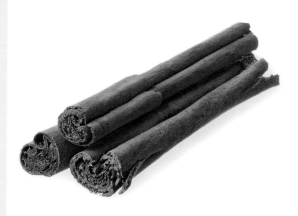

Properties: Antibacterial[37], antidepressant, antifungal[38], anti-infectious (intestinal, urinary), anti-inflammatory, antimicrobial, antioxidant, antiparasitic, antiseptic, antispasmodic (light), antiviral, astringent, immune stimulant, purifier, sexual stimulant, and warming. It also enhances the action and activity of other oils.

Historical Uses: This most ancient of spices was included in just about every prescription issued in ancient China. It was regarded as a tranquilizer, tonic, and stomachic and as being good for depression and a weak heart.

Other Possible Uses: This oil may be beneficial for circulation, colds, coughs, digestion, exhaustion, flu, infections, rheumatism[39], and warts. This oil fights viral and infectious diseases, and testing has yet to find a virus, bacteria, or fungus that can survive in its presence.

 Body System(s) Affected: Immune System.

Oral Use As Dietary Supplement: Cinnamon oil is generally recognized as safe (GRAS) for human consumption by the FDA (21CFR182.20). Dilute 1 drop oil in 2 tsp. (10 ml) honey or in 1 cup (250 ml) of beverage (e.g., soy/rice milk). May need to increase dilution even more due to this oil's potential for irritating mucous membranes. Not for children under 6 years old; use with caution and in greater dilution for children 6 years old and over.

Safety Data: Repeated use can result in extreme contact sensitization. Avoid during pregnancy.

Blend Classification: Personifier and Enhancer.

Blends With: All citrus oils, cypress, frankincense, geranium, juniper berry, lavender, rosemary, and all spice oils.

Odor: Type: Middle Note (50–80% of the blend); Scent: Spicy, warm, sweet; Intensity: 5.

---

*See My Usage Guide section for more details. ●=Neat, ●=Dilute for Children/Sensitive Skin, ●=Dilute

Clary Sage *Salvia sclarea*

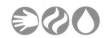

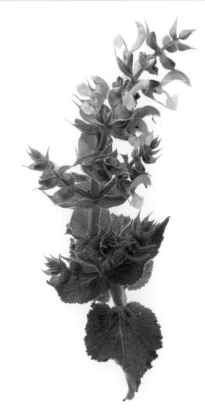

Botanical Family: Labiatae (mint)

Extraction Method: Steam distillation from flowering plant

Common Primary Uses*: ⊜⊘Aneurysm, ⊜Breast Enlargement, ⊜Cholesterol, ⊜Convulsions, ⊜Cramps (Abdominal), ⊜Dysmenorrhea①[40], ⊘⊜Emotional Stress, ⊜Endometriosis, ⊜Epilepsy, ⊜Estrogen Balance, ⊘⊜Frigidity, ⊜Hair (Fragile), ⊜⊘Hormonal Balance, ⊜Hot Flashes, ⊜OImpotence, ⊜⊘Infection, ⊜⊘Infertility, ⊘⊜Insomnia (Older Children), ⊜Lactation (Start Milk Production), ⊘Mood Swings, ⊜Muscle Fatigue, ⊜Parkinson's Disease, ⊜⊘PMS①, ⊘⊜Postpartum Depression, ⊜Premenopause, ⊜Seizure

Common Application Methods‡:

⊜: Can be applied neat (with no dilution) when used topically. Apply to reflex points and/or directly on area of concern.

⊘: Diffuse, or inhale the aroma directly.

O: Take in capsules, or use as a flavoring in cooking.

Properties: Anticonvulsant, antifungal, antiseptic ①[41], antispasmodic, astringent, nerve tonic, sedative, soothing ①[42], tonic, and warming.

Historical Uses: Nicknamed "clear eyes," it was famous during the Middle Ages for its ability to clear eye problems. During that same time, it was widely used for female complaints, kidney/digestive/skin disorders, inflammation, sore throats, and wounds.

Other Possible Uses: This oil may be used for amenorrhea, cell regulation, circulatory problems, depression, insect bites, kidney disorders, dry skin, throat infection, ulcers, and whooping cough.

⊕ **Body System(s) Affected:** Hormonal System.

Oral Use As Dietary Supplement: Clary sage oil is generally recognized as safe (GRAS) for human consumption by the FDA (21CFR182.20). Dilute 1 drop oil in 1 tsp. (5 ml) honey or in ½ cup (125 ml) of beverage (e.g., soy/rice milk). Not for children under 6 years old; use with caution and in greater dilution for children 6 years old and over.

Safety Data: Use with caution during pregnancy. Not for babies. Avoid during and after consumption of alcohol.

Blend Classification: Personifier.

Blends With: Bergamot, citrus oils, cypress, geranium, and sandalwood.

Odor: Type: Middle to Base Notes (5–60% of the blend); Scent: Herbaceous, spicy, hay-like, sharp, fixative; Intensity: 3.

---

‡*See Application section beginning on page 14 for more details.*
⊜=Topical, ⊘=Aromatic, O=Internal

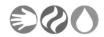

Quick Facts

Botanical Family: Myrtaceae (shrubs and trees)

Extraction Method: Steam distillation from bud and stem

Common Primary Uses*: ◐Addictions (Tobacco), ◐Antioxidant, ◐◐Blood Clots[43], ◐◐Candida, ◐Cataracts, ◐Corns, ◐Disinfectant, ◐Fever, ◐◐Fungal Infections, ◐Herpes Simplex, ◐Hodgkin's Disease, ◐Hormonal Balance, ◐◐Hypothyroidism, ◐◐Liver Cleansing, ◐Lupus, ◐Macular Degeneration, ◐◐Memory, ◐Metabolism Balance, ◐◐Mold, ◐Muscle Aches, ◐Muscle Pain, ◐Osteoporosis, ◐◐Plague, ◐Rheumatoid Arthritis, ◐◐Termites, ◐◐Thyroid Dysfunction, ◐Toothache (Pain), ◐◐Tumor (Lipoma), ◐◐Viral Infections, ◐Warts, ◐Wounds

Common Application Methods‡:

◐: Dilute 1:1 (1 drop essential oil to 1 drop carrier oil) before topical use. Apply to reflex points and/or directly on area of concern. Rub directly on the gums surrounding an infected tooth. Place on tongue with finger to remove desire to smoke, or place on back of tongue to fight against tickling cough.

◐: Diffuse with caution; it may irritate the nasal membranes if it is inhaled directly from a diffuser.

◐: Place 1 drop under the tongue, or take in capsules. Use as a flavoring in cooking.

Properties: Analgesic, antibacterial[44], antifungal[45], anti-infectious, anti-inflammatory[46], antiparasitic, strong antiseptic, antitumor[47], antiviral[48], disinfectant, antioxidant, and immune stimulant.

Historical Uses: Cloves were historically used for skin infections, digestive upsets, intestinal parasites, childbirth, and most notably for toothache. The Chinese also used cloves for diarrhea, hernia, bad breath, and bronchitis.

French Medicinal Uses: Impotence, intestinal parasites, memory deficiency, pain, plague, toothache, wounds (infected).

Other Possible Uses: Clove is valuable as a drawing salve—it helps pull infection from tissues. It may also help amebic dysentery, arthritis[49], bacterial

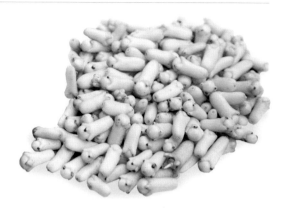

colitis, bones, bronchitis, cholera, cystitis, dental infection, diarrhea, infectious acne, fatigue, flatulence (gas), flu, halitosis (bad breath), tension headaches, hypertension, infection (wounds and more), insect bites and stings, insect control (insecticidal)[50], nausea, neuritis, nettles and poison oak (takes out sting), rheumatism, sinusitis, skin cancer, chronic skin disease, smoking (removes desire), sores (speeds healing of mouth and skin sores), tuberculosis, leg ulcers, viral hepatitis, and vomiting.

✛ **Body System(s) Affected:** Cardiovascular, Digestive, Immune, and Respiratory Systems.

Aromatic Influence: It may influence healing, improve memory (mental stimulant), and create a feeling of protection and courage.

Oral Use As Dietary Supplement: Clove oil is generally recognized as safe (GRAS) for human consumption by the FDA (21CFR182.20). Dilute 1 drop oil in 1 tsp. (5 ml) honey or in ½ cup (125 ml) of beverage (e.g., soy/rice milk). Not for children under 6 years old; use with caution and in greater dilution for children 6 years old and over.

Safety Data: Repeated use can result in extreme contact sensitization. Use with caution during pregnancy. Can irritate sensitive skin.

Blend Classification: Personifier.

Blends With: Basil, bergamot, cinnamon, clary sage, grapefruit, lavender, lemon, orange, peppermint, rose, rosemary, and ylang ylang.

Odor: Type: Middle to Base Notes (20–80% of the blend); Scent: Spicy, warming, slightly bitter, woody, reminiscent of true clove buds but richer; Intensity: 5.

See My Usage Guide section for more details.   ●=Neat, ●=Dilute for Children/Sensitive Skin, ●=Dilute

Copaiba *Copaifera officinalis, C. reticulata, C. coriacea, C. langsdorffii*

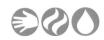

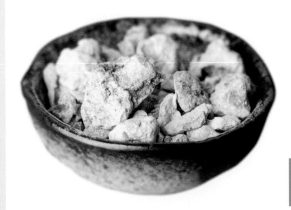

Quick Facts

Botanical Family: Leguminosae (flowering plants)

Extraction Method: Steam distillation from resin

Common Primary Uses*: Acne[51], Antioxidant[52], Anxiety[53], Inflammation[54], Muscle Aches, Pain[55]

Common Application Methods‡:

: Can be applied neat (with no dilution) when used topically. Apply directly on area of concern or to reflex points.

: Diffuse, or inhale the aroma directly.

: Take 1 drop in a beverage or in a capsule.

Properties: Analgesic, powerful anti-inflammatory, antibacterial[56], antiseptic, antioxidant[57] and stimulant (circulatory, pulmonary systems).

Historical Uses: The oleoresin has traditionally been used for inflammation (internal and external), skin disorders[58], respiratory problems including bronchitis and sinusitis, and urinary tract problems including cystitis and bladder/kidney infections. It has also been used for bleeding, gonorrhea, hemorrhages, herpes, incontinence, insect bites, pain, pleurisy, sore throats, stomach ulcers, syphilis, tetanus, tonsillitis, tuberculosis, and tumors[59].

Other Possible Uses: Copaiba may also help with colds, constipation, diarrhea, dyspepsia, edema, flatulence, flu, hemorrhoids, muscular aches and pains, nervous exhaustion, piles, poor circulation, stiffness, and wounds.

Body System(s) Affected: Cardiovascular, Respiratory, Skeletal, and Nervous Systems, Muscles, Emotional Balance, and Skin.

Aromatic Influence: Copaiba helps to elevate the mood and lift depression. It also helps to combat nervous tension, stress problems, and anxiety[60].

Oral Use As Dietary Supplement: Copaiba oil is generally recognized as safe (GRAS) for human consumption by the FDA (21CFR182.20). Dilute 1 drop oil in 1 tsp. (5 ml) honey or in ½ cup (125 ml) of beverage (e.g., soy/rice milk). Not for children under 6 years old; use with caution and in greater dilution for children 6 years old and over.

Safety Data: Repeated use may result in contact sensitization. May irritate sensitive skin in some individuals.

Blends With: Cedarwood, cinnamon, citrus oils, clary sage, jasmine, rose, ylang ylang.

Odor: Type: Base Note (5–20% of the blend); Scent: Soft, sweet, balsamic; Intensity: 3.

---

‡See Application section beginning on page 14 for more details.   =Topical, =Aromatic, =Internal

Coriander *Coriandrum sativum L.*

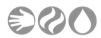

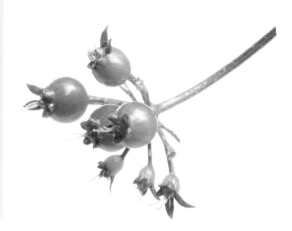

Quick Facts

Botanical Family: Umbelliferae (parsley)

Extraction Method: Steam distillation from seeds

Common Primary Uses*: ☾Cartilage Injury, ☾Degenerative Disease⊕61, ☾Muscle Aches, ☾Muscle Development, ☾Muscle Tone, ☾Whiplash

Common Application Methods‡:

☾: Can be applied neat (with no dilution) when used topically. Apply directly on area of concern or to reflex points.

☾: Diffuse, or inhale the aroma directly.

☾: Use as a flavoring in cooking.

Properties: Analgesic, antibacterial, antifungal, antioxidant, antirheumatic, antispasmodic⊕62, and stimulant (cardiac, circulatory, and nervous systems). It also has anti-inflammatory and sedative properties.

Historical Uses: The Chinese have used coriander for dysentery, piles, measles, nausea, toothache, and painful hernias.

Other Possible Uses: Coriander may help with anorexia, arthritis, colds, colic, diarrhea, digestive spasms, dyspepsia, flatulence, flu, gout, infections (general), measles, migraine, nausea, nervous exhaustion, neuralgia, piles, poor circulation, rheumatism, skin (oily skin, blackheads, and other impurities), and stiffness. It may also help during convalescence and after a difficult childbirth. It may regulate and help control pain⊕63 related to menstruation.

Body System(s) Affected: Digestive and Hormonal Systems.

Aromatic Influence: Coriander is a gentle stimulant for those with low physical energy. It also helps one relax during times of stress, irritability, and nervousness. It may also provide a calming influence to those suffering from shock or fear.

Oral Use As Dietary Supplement: Coriander oil is generally recognized as safe (GRAS) for human consumption by the FDA (21CFR182.20). Dilute 1 drop oil in 1 tsp. (5 ml) honey or in ½ cup (125 ml) of beverage (e.g., soy/rice milk). Not for children under 6 years old; use with caution and in greater dilution for children 6 years old and over.

Safety Data: Use sparingly, as coriander can be stupefying in large doses.

Blend Classification: Personifier and Modifier.

Blends With: Bergamot, cinnamon, clary sage, cypress, ginger, sandalwood, and other spice oils.

Odor: Type: Middle Note (50–80% of the blend); Scent: Woody, spicy, sweet; Intensity: 3.

Cypress *Cupressus sempervirens*

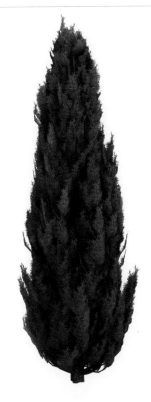

Quick Facts

Botanical Family: Cupressaceae (conifer: cypress)

Extraction Method: Steam distillation from branches

Common Primary Uses*: 🖐️🌀Aneurysm, 🖐️Bone Spurs, 🖐️Bunions, 🖐️Bursitis, 🖐️Carpal Tunnel Syndrome, 🖐️🌀Catarrh, 🖐️🌀Circulation, 🖐️Concussion, 🖐️Dysmenorrhea, 🖐️Edema, 🖐️Endometriosis, 🖐️🌀Environmental Stress, 🖐️🌀Flu (Influenza), 🖐️Greasy/Oily Hair, 🖐️Hemorrhoids, 🖐️Hernia (Hiatal), 🖐️Incontinence, 🖐️Lou Gehrig's Disease, 🖐️🌀Lymphatic Decongestant, 🖐️Menopause, 🖐️Menorrhagia, 🖐️Muscle Fatigue, 🖐️Muscle Tone, 🖐️Pain (Chronic), 🖐️🌀Pleurisy, 🖐️🌀Preeclampsia, 🖐️Prostatitis, 🖐️🌀Raynaud's Disease, 🖐️Retina (Strengthen), 🖐️Rheumatoid Arthritis, 🖐️Skin (Revitalizing), 🖐️🌀Stroke, 🖐️Swollen Eyes, 🖐️🌀Toxemia, 🖐️🌀Tuberculosis, 🖐️Varicose Veins

Common Application Methods‡:

🖐️: Can be applied neat (with no dilution) when used topically. Apply to reflex points and directly on area of concern.

🌀: Diffuse, or inhale the aroma directly.

Properties: Antibacterial[64], anti-infectious, antimicrobial, mucolytic, antiseptic, astringent, deodorant, diuretic, lymphatic and prostate decongestant, refreshing, relaxing, and vasoconstricting.

Historical Uses: It was used anciently for its benefits on the urinary system and in instances where there is excessive loss of fluids, such as perspiration, diarrhea, and menstrual flow. The Chinese valued cypress for its benefits to the liver and to the respiratory system.

Other Possible Uses: This oil may be beneficial for asthma, strengthening blood capillary walls, reducing cellulite, improving the circulatory system, colds, strengthening connective tissue, spasmodic coughs, diarrhea, energy, fever, gallbladder, bleeding gums, hemorrhaging, influenza, laryngitis, liver disorders[65], lung circulation, muscular cramps, nervous tension, nose bleeds, ovarian cysts, increasing perspiration, skin care, scar tissue, whooping cough, and wounds.

🔱 **Body System(s) Affected:** Cardiovascular System, Muscles, and Skeletal System.

Aromatic Influence: It influences and strengthens and helps ease the feeling of loss. It creates a feeling of security and grounding.

Oral Use As Dietary Supplement: None.

Safety Data: Use with caution during pregnancy.

Blend Classification: Equalizer.

Blends With: Bergamot, clary sage, lavender, lemon, orange, and sandalwood.

Odor: Type: Middle Note (50–80% of the blend); Scent: Fresh, herbaceous, slightly woody with evergreen undertones; Intensity: 3.

‡See Application section beginning on page 14 for more details. 🖐️=Topical, 🌀=Aromatic, ⭕=Internal

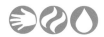
Quick Facts

Botanical Family: Umbelliferae (parsley)

Extraction Method: Steam distillation from whole plant

Common Primary Uses*: ❍❍Cholesterol[66], ❍Flavoring

Common Application Methods‡:

❍: Can be applied neat (with no dilution) when used topically. Apply to reflex points on the feet and/or directly on area of concern. A drop or two on the wrists may help remove addictions to sweets.

❷: Diffuse, or inhale the aroma directly.

❍: Take in a capsule. Use as a flavoring in cooking.

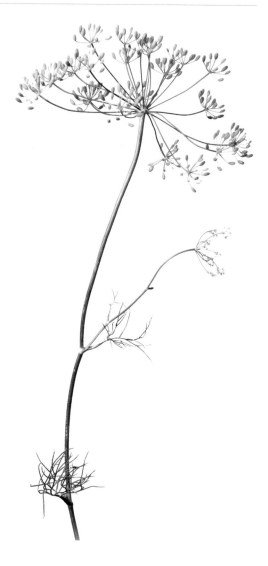

Properties: Antispasmodic, antibacterial, expectorant, and stimulant.

Other Possible Uses: This oil may help with bronchial catarrh, colic, constipation, dyspepsia, flatulence, headaches, indigestion, liver deficiencies, lowering glucose levels, nervousness, normalizing insulin levels, promoting milk flow in nursing mothers, supporting pancreas function, and clearing toxins[67]. It may also act as an insect repellent[68].

⊕ Body System(s) Affected: Digestive & Cardiovascular Systems.

Aromatic Influence: It helps calm the autonomic nervous system and, when diffused with Roman chamomile, may help fidgety children.

Oral Use As Dietary Supplement: Generally regarded as safe (GRAS) for human consumption by the FDA. Dilute 1 drop oil in 1 tsp. (5 ml) honey or in ½ cup (125 ml) of beverage (e.g., soy/rice milk). Not for children under 6 years old; use with caution and in greater dilution for children 6 years old and over.

Safety Data: Use with caution if susceptible to epilepsy.

Blend Classification: Enhancer.

Blends With: Citrus oils.

Odor: Type: Middle Note (50–80% of the blend); Scent: Fresh, sweet, herbaceous, slightly earthy; Intensity: 2

Douglas Fir *Pseudotsuga menziesii*

Quick Facts

Botanical Family: Pinaceae (conifer)

Extraction Method: Steam distillation from twigs and needles

Common Primary Uses*: ⚕⚗Asthma, ⚗⚕Bronchitis⊞[69], ⚗⚕Congestion, ⚗⚕Coughs, ⚕Disinfectant (skin), ⚗⚕Flu (Influenza), ⚗Focus, ⚗⚕Infection

Common Application Methods‡:

⚕: Can be applied neat (with no dilution) when used topically. Dilute 1:1 (1 drop essential oil to at least 1 drop carrier oil) for children and for those with sensitive skin. Apply directly on area of concern or to reflex points.

⚗: Diffuse, or inhale the aroma directly.

Properties: Antiseptic, astringent, diuretic, expectorant, sedative (nerves), and tonic.

Historical Uses: The Douglas fir is highly regarded for its fragrant scent. Douglas fir has also been valued through the ages for its ability to help support the body with respiratory complaints, fever, and muscular and rheumatic pain.

Other Possible Uses: Douglas fir may be beneficial for anxiety, catarrh, colds, respiratory weakness, rheumatism, tension (nervous), and wounds. It

is soothing to sore muscles and can help soothe overworked or tired muscles and joints.

✚ **Body System(s) Affected:** Respiratory and Skeletal Systems and Muscles.

Aromatic Influence: This beautiful aroma can help create a feeling of grounding and anchoring and promotes a sense of focus. It can help balance the emotions and stimulate the mind while allowing the body to relax.

Oral Use As Dietary Supplement: None.

Safety Data: Can irritate sensitive skin.

Blend Classification: Equalizer.

Blends With: Cedarwood, eucalyptus, frankincense, juniper, lavender, lemon, orange, and sandalwood.

Odor: Type: Middle Notes (50–80% of the blend); Scent: Fresh, woody, earthy, sweet; Intensity: 3.

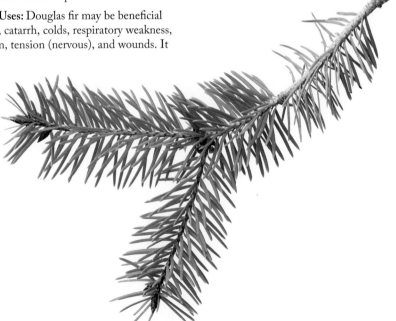

Eucalyptus *Eucalyptus radiata*

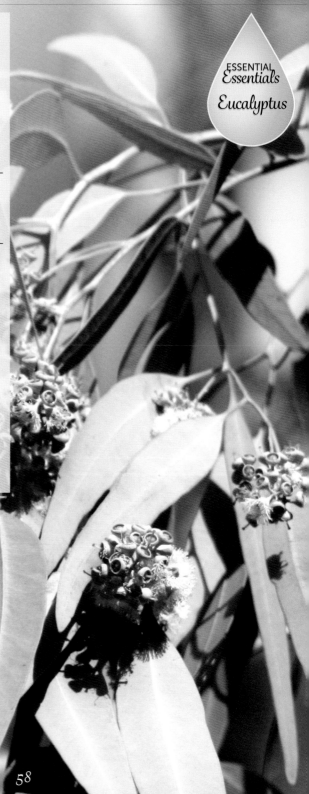

Biography

Australian Aboriginals used eucalyptus leaves to bind wounds, noting its antibacterial and anti-infectious properties. Today, this oil is steam-distilled from the same leaves and is often used to treat inflammation and other concerns.

Eucalyptus is still grown and cultivated in its native home of Australia.

: Scent

- Slightly Camphoric
- Sweet
- Fruity

: Body Systems Affected

Respiratory System   Skin

Top Uses

Respiratory Ailments: To help relieve inflammation within the respiratory system, add 1–2 drops to a bowl of hot water or a humidifier, and inhale vapors.

Muscle Aches/Pains: Add 1–2 drops to a warm bath for muscle relaxation. Add 2–4 drops eucalyptus to 1 Tbs. (15 ml) fractionated coconut oil, and massage on location.

Inflammation: Add 3–4 drops to 1 Tbs. (15 ml) fractionated coconut oil, and massage on inflamed location.

ESSENTIAL
Essentials
Eucalyptus

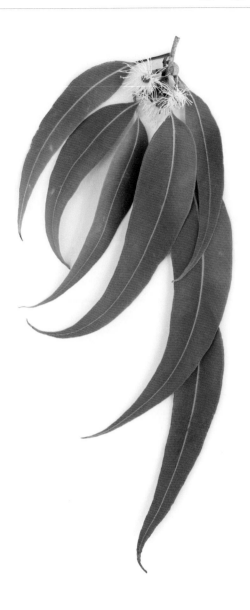

Quick Facts

Botanical Family: Myrtaceae (Myrtle shrubs and trees)

Extraction Method: Steam distillation from leaves

Common Primary Uses*: ⬡Arterial Vasodilator, ⬡⬡Asthma, ⬡Brain Blood Flow, ⬡⬡Bronchitis⊕[70], ⬡⬡Congestion, ⬡⬡Cooling (Body), ⬡⬡Coughs, ⬡⬡Diabetes, ⬡Disinfectant, ⬡Dysentery, ⬡Ear Inflammation, ⬡⬡Emphysema, ⬡⬡Expectorant, ⬡Fever, ⬡⬡Flu (Influenza), ⬡Hypoglycemia, ⬡Inflammation, ⬡Iris Inflammation, ⬡Jet Lag, ⬡Kidney Stones, ⬡Lice⊕[71], ⬡⬡Measles, ⬡Neuralgia, ⬡Neuritis, ⬡Overexercised Muscles, ⬡Pain, ⬡⬡Pneumonia, ⬡Respiratory Viruses, ⬡⬡Rhinitis, ⬡Shingles, ⬡⬡Sinusitis, ⬡Tennis Elbow, ⬡⬡Tuberculosis

Common Application Methods‡:

⬡: Can be applied neat (with no dilution), or dilute 1:1 (1 drop essential oil to at least 1 drop carrier oil) for children and for those with sensitive skin when using topically. Apply to reflex points and/or directly on area of concern.

⬡: Diffuse, or inhale the aroma directly.

Properties: Analgesic⊕[72], antibacterial⊕[73], anticatarrhal, anti-infectious, anti-inflammatory⊕[74], antiviral⊕[75], insecticidal⊕[76], and expectorant.

Other Possible Uses: This oil, when combined with bergamot, has been used effectively on herpes simplex. It may also help with acne, endometriosis, hay fever, high blood pressure⊕[77], nasal mucous membrane inflammation, and vaginitis.

⊕ **Body System(s) Affected:** Respiratory System, Skin.

Oral Use As Dietary Supplement: None.

Safety Data: Use with caution with very small children.

Blend Classification: Enhancer.

Blends With: Geranium, lavender, lemon, sandalwood, juniper berry, lemongrass, melissa, thyme.

Odor: Type: Middle Note (50–80% of the blend); Scent: Slightly camphorous, sweet, fruity; Intensity: 3.

---

‡See Application section beginning on page 14 for more details.   ⬡=Topical, ⬡=Aromatic, ⬡=Internal

Fennel (Sweet) *Foeniculum vulgare*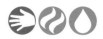

Quick Facts

Botanical Family: Umbelliferae (parsley)

Extraction Method: Steam distillation from the crushed seeds

Common Primary Uses*: ⬥Benign Prostatic Hyperplasia, OⲐⲐBlood Clots, ⬥Bruises, OⲐⲐDigestive System Support, ⲐOGastritis, OIBS[78], ⬥Kidney Stones, ⬥Lactation (Increase Milk Production), ⲐⲐPancreas Support, OⲐParasites, ⬥Skin (Revitalizing), ⬥Tissue (Toxin Cleansing), ⬥Wrinkles

Common Application Methods‡:

⬥: Can be applied neat (with no dilution), or dilute 1:1 (1 drop essential oil to at least 1 drop carrier oil) for children and for those with sensitive skin when using topically. Apply directly on area of concern or to reflex points.

Ⲑ: Diffuse, or inhale the aroma directly.

O: Place 1–2 drops under the tongue, or take in a capsule. Use as a flavoring in cooking.

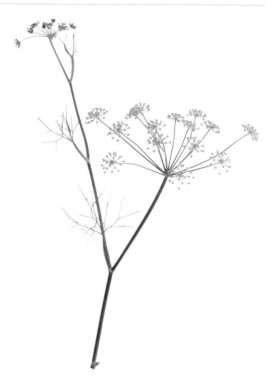

Properties: Antiparasitic, antiseptic, antispasmodic[79], antitoxic, diuretic, and expectorant.

Historical Uses: The ancient Egyptians and Romans awarded garlands of fennel as praise to victorious warriors because fennel was believed to bestow strength, courage, and longevity. It has been used for thousands of years for snakebites, to stave off hunger pains, to tone the female reproductive system, for earaches, eye problems, insect bites, kidney complaints, lung infections, and to expel worms.

Other Possible Uses: Fennel oil may be used for menopause problems[80], colic[81], stimulating the cardiovascular system, constipation, digestion (supports the liver), balancing hormones, nausea, obesity, PMS[82], and stimulating the sympathetic nervous system[83].

Body System(s) Affected: Digestive and Hormonal Systems.

Aromatic Influence: It increases and influences longevity, courage, and purification.

Oral Use As Dietary Supplement: Fennel oil is generally recognized as safe (GRAS) for human consumption by the FDA (21CFR182.20). Dilute 1 drop oil in 1 tsp. (5 ml) honey or in ½ cup (125 ml) of beverage (e.g., soy/rice milk). Not for children under 6 years old; use with caution and in greater dilution for children 6 years old and over.

Safety Data: Repeated use can possibly result in contact sensitization. Use with caution if susceptible to epilepsy. Use with caution during pregnancy.

Blend Classification: Equalizer and Modifier.

Blends With: Basil, geranium, lavender, lemon, rosemary, and sandalwood.

Odor: Type: Top to Middle Notes (20–80% of the blend); Scent: Sweet, somewhat spicy, licorice-like; Intensity: 4.

See My Usage Guide section for more details.   ⬤=Neat, ⬤=Dilute for Children/Sensitive Skin, ⬤=Dilute

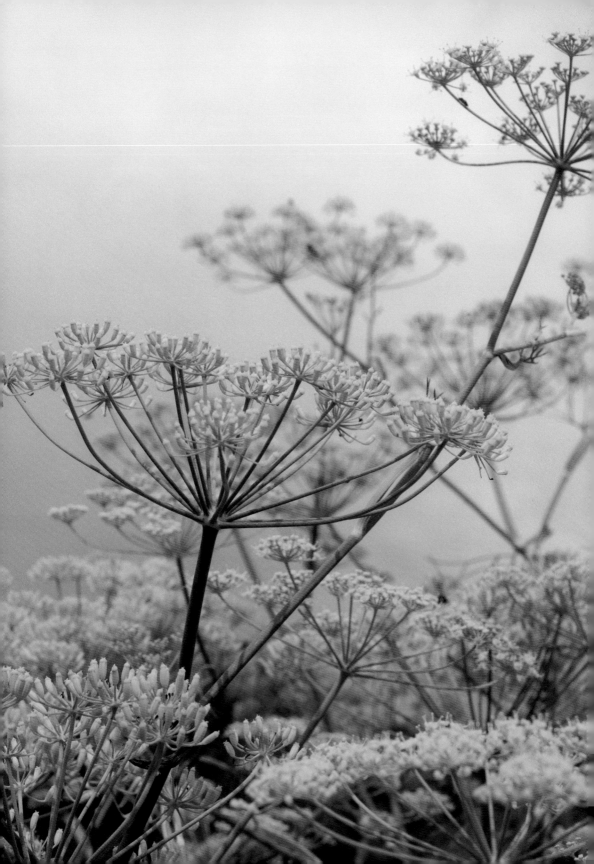

Frankincense _Boswellia frereana, Boswellia carteri, Boswellia sacra_

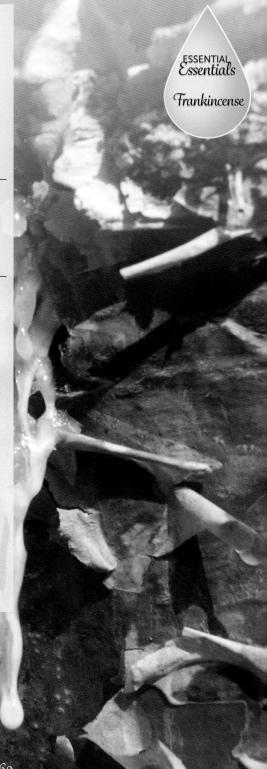

Biography

Created through steam distillation of the resin, frankincense oil has been a traditional remedy for thousands of years. It is used for a myriad of purposes, including cosmetics, perfumes, skincare, and a wide range of medicines.

An ancient treasure in biblical times, frankincense is still grown natively in Africa and the Middle East.

ESSENTIAL
Essentials

Frankincense

Ⓢ : Scent

- Rich
- Deep
- Warm
- Balsamic
- Sweet

ⓣ : Body Systems Affected

- Emotional Balance
- Immune System
- Nervous System
- Skin

Top Uses

Arthritis: Gently massage affected joints with a blend of 3 drops frankincense, 4 drops peppermint, 2 drops marjoram, and 1 Tbs. (15 ml) fractionated coconut oil.

Depression: Apply neat to temple or forehead, add 5–10 drops to 1 Tbs. (15 ml) fractionated coconut oil to use as a massage oil, or add 1–3 drops to a warm bath. Frankincense can also be inhaled directly from the bottle or diffused.

Mental Fatigue: To help relax, apply neat to temples, back of neck, liver area, or feet.

Inflammation: Mix 3 drops frankincense and 2 drops lavender in a bowl of cold water. Dampen a washcloth, and apply to affected area for 15–30 minutes.

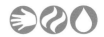

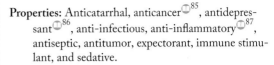

Quick Facts

Botanical Family: Burseraceae (resinous trees and shrubs)

Extraction Method: Steam distillation from gum/resin

Common Primary Uses*: 🌿🌀Alzheimer's Disease, 🌀🌿Aneurysm, 🌀🌿Arthritis[84], 🌀🌿Asthma, 🌿🌀Balance, 🌀🌿Brain (Aging), 🌀🌿Brain Injury, 🌀🌿Breathing, 🌀🌀🌿Cancer, 🌿Coma, 🌀🌿Concussion, 🌀Confusion, 🌀🌿Coughs, 🌀🌿Depression, 🌿Fibroids, 🌿Genital Warts, 🌿🌀Hepatitis, 🌿🌀Immune System Support, 🌿Improve Vision, 🌿🌀Infected Wounds, 🌿🌀Inflammation, 🌿🌀Liver Cirrhosis, 🌿🌀Lou Gehrig's Disease, 🌀🌿Memory, 🌀🌿Mental Fatigue, 🌿Miscarriage (After), 🌿Moles, 🌿MRSA, 🌿🌀Multiple Sclerosis, 🌿🌀Nasal Polyp, 🌀🌿Parkinson's Disease, 🌿🌀Plague, 🌀🌿Postpartum Depression, 🌿Scarring (Prevention), 🌿🌀Tumor (Lipoma), 🌀🌿Ulcers, 🌿Uterus Tissue Regeneration, 🌿Virus of Nerves, 🌿Warts, 🌿Wrinkles

Common Application Methods‡:

🌿: Can be applied neat (with no dilution) when used topically. Apply directly on area of concern or to reflex points.

🌀: Diffuse, or inhale the aroma directly.

🌀: Place 1–2 drops under the tongue, or take in a capsule.

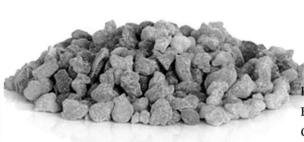

Properties: Anticatarrhal, anticancer[85], antidepressant[86], anti-infectious, anti-inflammatory[87], antiseptic, antitumor, expectorant, immune stimulant, and sedative.

Historical Uses: Frankincense is a holy oil in the Middle East. As an ingredient in the holy incense, it was used anciently during sacrificial ceremonies to help improve communication with the creator.

Other Possible Uses: This oil may help with aging, allergies, bites (insect and snake), bronchitis, carbuncles, catarrh, colds, diarrhea, diphtheria, gonorrhea, headaches, healing, hemorrhaging, herpes, high blood pressure, jaundice, laryngitis, meningitis, nervous conditions, prostate problems, pneumonia, respiratory problems, sciatic pain, sores, spiritual awareness, staph, strep, stress, syphilis, T.B., tension, tonsillitis, typhoid, and wounds. It contains sesquiterpenes, enabling it to go beyond the blood-brain barrier. It may also help oxygenate the pineal and pituitary glands. It increases the activity of leukocytes, defending the body against infection. Frankincense may also help a person have a better attitude, which may help to strengthen the immune system.

Body System(s) Affected: Emotional Balance, Immune and Nervous Systems, Skin.

Aromatic Influence: This oil helps to focus energy, minimize distractions, and improve concentration. It eases hyperactivity, impatience, irritability, and restlessness and can help enhance spiritual awareness and meditation.

Oral Use As Dietary Supplement: Frankincense oil in general is approved by the FDA (21CFR172.510) for use as a Food Additive (FA) and Flavoring Agent (FL). Dilute 1 drop oil in 1 tsp. (5 ml) honey or in ½ cup (125 ml) of beverage (e.g., soy/rice milk). Not for children under 6 years old; use with caution and in greater dilution for children 6 years old and over.

Blend Classification: Enhancer and Equalizer.

Blends With: All oils.

Odor: Type: Base Note (5–20% of the blend); Scent: Rich, deep, warm, balsamic, sweet, with incense-like overtones; Intensity: 3.

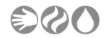

Quick Facts

Botanical Family: Geraniaceae

Extraction Method: Steam distillation from leaves

Common Primary Uses*: Agitation (Calms), Airborne Bacteria, Autism, Bleeding, Breasts (Soothes), Bruises, Calcified Spine, Cancer, Capillaries (Broken), Diabetes, Diarrhea, Dysmenorrhea, Endometriosis, Environmental Stress, Gallbladder Stones, Hair (Dry), Hernia (Incisional), Impetigo, Insomnia (Older Children), Jaundice, Jet Lag, Libido (Low), Menorrhagia, Miscarriage (After), MRSA, Osteoarthritis, Osteoporosis, Pancreas Support, Paralysis, Pelvic Pain Syndrome, Physical Stress, PMS, Post Labor, Rheumatoid Arthritis, Skin (Dry), Skin (Sensitive), Ulcer (Gastric), Varicose Ulcer, Vertigo, Wrinkles

Common Application Methods‡:

: Can be applied neat (with no dilution) when used topically. Apply directly on area of concern or to reflex points.

: Diffuse, or inhale the aroma directly.

: Take in capsules.

Properties: Antibacterial[88], anticonvulsant[89], antidepressant, anti-inflammatory[90], antiseptic, astringent, diuretic, insect repellent[91], refreshing, relaxing, sedative, and tonic.

Historical Uses: Geranium oil has been used for dysentery, hemorrhoids, inflammations, heavy menstrual flow, and possibly even cancer (if the folktale is correct). It has also been said to be a remedy for bone fractures, tumors, and wounds.

Other Possible Uses: This oil may be used for acne, bleeding (increases to eliminate toxins, then stops), burns, circulatory problems (improves blood flow), depression, digestion, eczema, hormonal imbalance, insomnia, kidney stones, dilating biliary ducts for liver detoxification, menstrual problems, neuralgia (severe pain along the nerve), regenerating tissue and nerves, pancreas (balances), ringworm, shingles, skin (may balance the sebum, which is the fatty secretion in the sebaceous glands of the skin that keeps the skin supple. It is good for expectant mothers. It works as a cleanser for oily skin and may even liven up pale skin), sores, sore throats, and wounds.

Body System(s) Affected: Emotional Balance, Skin.

Aromatic Influence: It may help to release negative memories and take a person back to peaceful, joyful moments. It may also help ease nervous tension and stress, balance the emotions, lift the spirit, and foster peace, well-being, and hope.

Oral Use As Dietary Supplement: Geranium oil is generally recognized as safe (GRAS) for human consumption by the FDA (21CFR182.20). Dilute 1 drop oil in 1 tsp. (5 ml) honey or in ½ cup (125 ml) of beverage (e.g., soy/rice milk). Not for children under 6 years old; use with caution and in greater dilution for children 6 years old and over.

Safety Data: Repeated use can possibly result in some contact sensitization.

Blend Classification: Enhancer and Equalizer.

Blends With: All oils.

Odor: Type: Middle Note (50–80% of the blend); Scent: Sweet, green, citrus-rosy, fresh; Intensity: 3.

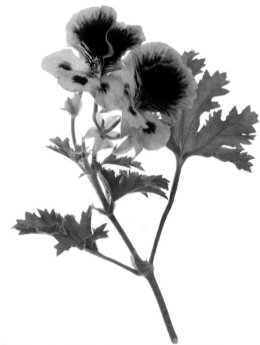

*See My Usage Guide section for more details. ●=Neat, ●=Dilute for Children/Sensitive Skin, ●=Dilute

Ginger *Zingiber officinale*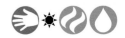

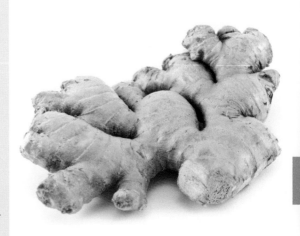

Properties: Antiseptic, laxative, stimulant, tonic, and warming.

Historical Uses: Anciently esteemed as a spice and recognized for its affinity for the digestive system, it has been used in gingerbread (up to 4,000 years ago in Greece), in Egyptian cuisine (to ward off epidemics), in Roman wine (for its aphrodisiac powers), in Indian tea (to soothe upset stomachs), and in Chinese tonics (to strengthen the heart and to relieve head congestion). It was also used in Hawaii to scent clothing, to cook with, and to cure indigestion. The Hawaiians also added it to their shampoos and massage oils.

Other Possible Uses: Ginger may be used for alcoholism, loss of appetite, arthritis⊙, broken bones, catarrh (mucus), chills, colds, colic, congestion, coughs, cramps, digestive disorders, fevers, flu, impotence, indigestion, infectious diseases, memory, motion sickness, muscular aches/pains, rheumatism, sinusitis, sore throats, and sprains. Ginger may also be used in cooking.

⊕ Body System(s) Affected: Digestive and Nervous Systems.

Aromatic Influence: The aroma may help influence physical energy, love, money, and courage.

Oral Use As Dietary Supplement: Ginger oil is generally recognized as safe (GRAS) for human consumption by the FDA (21CFR182.20). Dilute 1 drop oil in 1 tsp. (5 ml) honey or in ½ cup (125 ml) of beverage (e.g., soy/rice milk). Not for children under 6 years old; use with caution and in greater dilution for children 6 years old and over.

Safety Data: Repeated use can possibly result in contact sensitization. Avoid direct sunlight for 3 to 6 hours after use.

Blend Classification: Personifier and Equalizer.

Blends With: All spice oils, all citrus oils, eucalyptus, frankincense, geranium, and rosemary.

Odor: Type: Middle Note (50–80% of the blend); Scent: Sweet, spicy-woody, warm, tenacious, fresh, sharp; Intensity: 4.

Grapefruit *Citrus x paradisi*

Biography

Grapefruit has been enjoyed by many as an energizing, stress-relieving oil. It is also often used to help quell cravings as an appetite suppressant. It is cold-pressed from the rind.

Native to tropical Asia and the West Indies, grapefruit is now cultivated in many areas of the world, including Florida, China, Spain, Mexico, and South Africa.

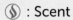 : Scent

- Clean   • Fresh   • Bitter   • Citrusy

⊕ : Body Systems Affected

🫀 Cardiovascular System

Top Uses

Appetite Control: To help quell cravings, diffuse grapefruit in an aromatherapy diffuser.

Energy: Inhale from the bottle for a quick boost of energy.

Stress: Diffuse grapefruit in an aromatherapy diffuser to help relieve stress.

ESSENTIAL
Essentials

Grapefruit

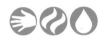

Quick Facts

Botanical Family: Rutaceae (hybrid between *Citrus maxima* and *Citrus sinensis*)

Extraction Method: Cold expressed from rind

Common Primary Uses*: ⬬⬭Addictions (Drugs), ⬭Anorexia, ⬭Appetite Suppressant, ⬭Bulimia, ⬬Cellulite, ⬭⬬Dry Throat, ⬬⬭Edema, ⬬Gallbladder Stones, ⬬⬭Hangovers, ⬬⬭Lymphatic Decongestant, ⬭⬬Mental Stress, ⬬Miscarriage (After), ⬭⬭Obesity⊕[94], ⬭Overeating, ⬬⬭Performance Stress, ⬬⬭PMS, ⬭⬭Slimming/Toning, ⬬⬭Stress, ⬬⬭Withdrawal

Common Application Methods‡:

⬬: Can be applied neat (with no dilution) when used topically. Apply directly on area of concern or to reflex points. Because grapefruit oil has many of the same uses as other citrus oils, it can be used in their place when immediate exposure to the sun is unavoidable. This is because grapefruit oil does not cause as much photosensitivity as the other citrus oils.

⬭: Diffuse, or inhale the aroma directly.

⬭: Take 1–2 drops in a beverage or in capsules. Use as a flavoring in cooking.

Properties: Antidepressant, antiseptic, disinfectant, diuretic, stimulant, and tonic.

Other Possible Uses: Grapefruit oil may help with cancer⊕[95], depression, eating disorders, fatigue, jet lag, liver disorders, migraine headaches, premenstrual tension, stress, and sympathetic nervous system stimulation⊕[96]. It may also have a cleansing effect on the kidneys, the lymphatic system, and the vascular system.

⬭ Body System(s) Affected: Cardiovascular System.

Aromatic Influence: It is balancing and uplifting to the mind and may help to relieve anxiety⊕[97].

Oral Use As Dietary Supplement: Grapefruit oil is generally recognized as safe (GRAS) for human consumption by the FDA (21CFR182.20). Dilute 1 drop oil in 1 tsp. (5 ml) honey or in ½ cup (125 ml) of beverage (e.g., soy/rice milk). Not for children under 6 years old; use with caution and in greater dilution for children 6 years old and over.

Blend Classification: Modifier and Enhancer.

Blends With: Basil, bergamot, cypress, frankincense, geranium, lavender, peppermint, rosemary, and ylang ylang.

Odor: Type: Top Note (5–20% of the blend); Scent: Clean, fresh, bitter, citrusy; Intensity: 2.

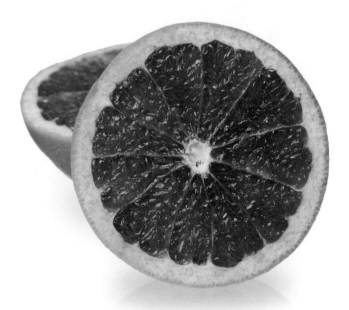

Green Mandarin *Citrus nobilis*

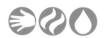

Quick Facts

Botanical Family: Rutaceae (citrus)

Extraction Method: Cold pressed from peel

Common Primary Uses*: ⬤⬤⬤Nausea, ⬤⬤Calming, ⬤GERD⊕⁹⁸, ⬤Skin (Toning)⊕⁹⁹, ⬤⬤⬤Soothing

Common Application Methods‡:

⬤: Can be applied neat (with no dilution) when used topically. Apply directly on area of concern or to reflex points. Avoid UV light for up to 12 hours after using on skin.

⬤: Diffuse, or inhale the aroma directly.

⬤: Take in capsules or in a beverage (add 1 drop to 1 cup (250 ml). Use as a flavoring in cooking.

Properties: Anticoagulant, anti-inflammatory⊕¹⁰⁰, antimicrobial, antispasmodic, antitumor⊕¹⁰¹, antiviral, expectorant, laxative, and sedative.

Historical Uses: Green mandarin essential oil is distilled from the green, unripened fruit of the mandarin tree. Distilling at this time gives the oil a brighter, fresher aroma. Mandarin trees are native to Asia, but they are now cultivated around the world.

Other Possible Uses: This oil may help wth cellulite, circulation, constipation, diarrhea, digestive system disorders, dizziness, fat digestion, fear, flatulence, gallbladder (gallstones), heartburn, insomnia, intestinal spasms, irritability, limbs (tired and aching), liver problems, lymphatic system congestion (helps stimulate drainage), obesity, parasites, sadness, stomach (tonic), stress, stretch marks (smooths when blended with lavender), swelling, and water retention (alleviates edema).

⊕ **Body System(s) Affected:** Emotional Balance, Digestive System, Immune System, Skin.

Aromatic Influence: The bright, fresh aroma of green mandarin is effective for soothing strong emotions such as anger, grief, and shock. It can also be sedating and calming to the nervous system while promoting courage and quiet strength.

Oral Use As Dietary Supplement: Green mandarin oil is generally regarded as safe (GRAS) for human consumption by the FDA. Dilute 1 drop oil in 1 tsp. (5 ml) honey or in ½ cup (125 ml) of beverage (e.g., soy/rice milk). Not for children under 6 years old; use with caution and in greater dilution for children 6 years old and over.

Safety Data: Old or oxidized oil may irritate highly sensitive skin. Consult with a physician before use if taking medications, pregnant, or nursing.

Blend Classification: Personifier and Enhancer.

Blends With: Basil, bergamot, clary sage, frankincense, grapefruit, lavender, lemon, marjoram, orange, Roman chamomile, sandalwood, spearmint.

Odor: Type: Top Note (5–20% of the blend); Scent: Bright, citrusy, fresh, sweet, herbal; Intensity: 3.

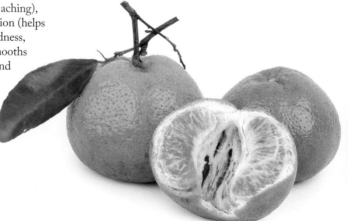

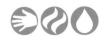

Quick Facts

Botanical Family: Santalaceae (sandalwood)

Extraction Method: Steam distillation from heartwood

Common Primary Uses*: 🤚👃Alzheimer's Disease, 🤚👃Aphrodisiac, 👃Back Pain, 👃Cancer, 👃Cartilage Repair, 👃Confusion, 👃Exhaustion, 🤚👃Fear, 👃Hair (Dry), 🤚👃Hiccups, 🤚👃Laryngitis, 🤚👃Lou Gehrig's Disease, 👃Meditation, 👃Moles, 🤚👃Multiple Sclerosis, 👃Rashes, 👃Skin (Dry), 👃Ultraviolet Radiation, 👃Vitiligo, 👃Yoga

Common Application Methods‡:

🤚: Can be applied neat (with no dilution) when used topically. Apply directly on area of concern or to reflex points.

👃: Diffuse, or inhale the aroma directly.

⚫: Take in capsules.

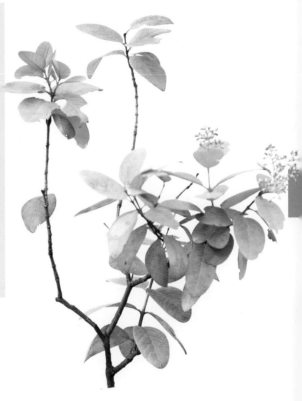

Properties: Antidepressant, antiseptic, antitumor⬚102, aphrodisiac, astringent, calming, sedative, and tonic.

Historical Uses: Hawaiian sandalwood was traditionally used to help clear dandruff, repel insects, and to help heal diseases of the reproductive organs.

Other Possible Uses: Sandalwood may support the cardiovascular system and relieve symptoms associated with lumbago and the sciatic nerves. It may also be beneficial for acne, regenerating bone cartilage, catarrh, circulation (similar in action to frankincense), coughs, cystitis, depression, hiccups, lymphatic system, menstrual problems, nerves (similar in action to frankincense), nervous tension, increasing oxygen around the pineal and pituitary glands, skin infection and regeneration, and tuberculosis.

Body System(s) Affected: Emotional Balance, Muscles, Skeletal and Nervous Systems, Skin.

Aromatic Influence: Calms, harmonizes, and balances the emotions. It may help enhance meditation.

Oral Use As Dietary Supplement: While this specific species of sandalwood has not yet been approved for oral use by the FDA, regular *Santalum album* oil is approved by the FDA (21CFR172.510) for use as a Food Additive (FA) and Flavoring Agent (FL) and possesses a similar chemical profile.

Dilute 1 drop oil in 1 tsp. (5 ml) honey or in ½ cup (125 ml) of beverage (e.g., soy/rice milk). Not for children under 6 years old; use with caution and in greater dilution for children 6 years old and over.

Blend Classification: Modifier and Equalizer.

Blends With: Cypress, frankincense, lemon, myrrh, and ylang ylang.

Odor: Type: Base Note (5–20% of the blend); Scent: Soft, woody, spicy, sweet, earthy, balsamic, tenacious; Intensity: 3.

‡See Application section beginning on page 14 for more details.
🤚=Topical, 👃=Aromatic, ⚫=Internal

Helichrysum *Helichrysum italicum*

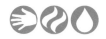

Quick Facts

Botanical Family: Compositae

Extraction Method: Steam distillation from flowers

Common Primary Uses*: ⬡Abscess (Tooth), ⬡⬡AIDS/HIV, ⬡⬡Aneurysm, ⬡⬡Bleeding, ⬡Bone Bruise, ⬡Broken Blood Vessels, ⬡Bruises, ⬡⬡Catarrh, ⬡Cholesterol, ⬡Cleansing, ⬡⬡Colitis, ⬡Cuts, ⬡Dermatitis/Eczema, ⬡Detoxification, ⬡⬡Earache, ⬡Fibroids, ⬡Gallbladder Infection, ⬡Hematoma, ⬡Hemorrhaging, ⬡Herpes Simplex, ⬡Incisional Hernia, ⬡⬡Liver Stimulant, ⬡Lymphatic Drainage, ⬡Nose Bleed, ⬡Pancreas Stimulant, ⬡⬡Phlebitis, ⬡Psoriasis, ⬡Sciatica, ⬡Shock, ⬡Staph Infection, ⬡⬡Stroke, ⬡Sunscreen, ⬡Swollen Eyes, ⬡Taste (Impaired), ⬡Tennis Elbow, ⬡Tinnitus, ⬡Tissue Pain, ⬡Tissue Repair, ⬡Vertigo, ⬡⬡Viral Infections, ⬡Wounds

Common Application Methods‡:

⬡: Can be applied neat (with no dilution) when used topically. Apply directly on area of concern or to reflex points.

⬲: Diffuse, or inhale the aroma directly.

⬤: Take in capsules.

Properties: Antibacterial⬤[103], anticatarrhal, anticoagulant, antioxidant⬤[104], antispasmodic, antiviral⬤[105], expectorant, and mucolytic.

Historical Uses: Helichrysum has been used for asthma, bronchitis, whooping cough, headaches, liver ailments, and skin disorders.

Other Possible Uses: This oil may help with anger management, bleeding, circulatory functions, hearing, detoxifying and stimulating the liver cell function, pain (acute), relieving respiratory conditions, reducing scarring, scar tissue, regenerating tissue, and varicose veins.

Body System(s) Affected: Cardiovascular and Skeletal Systems and Muscles.

Aromatic Influence: It is uplifting to the subconscious and may help calm feelings of anger.

Oral Use As Dietary Supplement: Helichrysum oil is generally recognized as safe (GRAS) for human consumption by the FDA (21CFR182.20). Dilute 1 drop oil in 1 tsp. (5 ml) honey or in ½ cup (125 ml) of beverage (e.g., soy/rice milk). Not for children under 6 years old; use with caution and in greater dilution for children 6 years old and over.

Blend Classification: Personifier.

Blends With: Geranium, clary sage, rose, lavender, spice oils, and citrus oils.

Odor: Type: Middle Note (50–80% of the blend); Scent: Rich, sweet, fruity, with tea and honey undertones; Intensity: 3.

See My Usage Guide section for more details.   ⬤=Neat, ⬤=Dilute for Children/Sensitive Skin, ⬤=Dilute

Hinoki *Chamaecyparis obtusa*

Quick Facts

Botanical Family: Cupressaceae (conifer: cypress)

Extraction Method: Steam distillation from wood

Common Primary Uses*: 🌀🍃Calming, 🍃Cleaning, 🌀🍃Colds, 🍃Cuts/Scrapes, 🍃Rashes

Common Application Methods‡:

🍃: Can be applied neat (with no dilution) when used topically. Apply directly on area of concern or to reflex points. Add 1–2 drops to bathwater before bathing. Use in massage oil.

🌀: Diffuse, or inhale the aroma directly.

Properties: Antibacterial[106], antifungal, anti-infectious, anti-inflammatory[107], antiseptic, antiviral, disinfectant, and insecticidal.

Historical Uses: Hinoki wood has long been used in Japan for building royal palaces and sacred baths because of its beautiful look, wonderful smell, and natural properties for resisting insects, bacteria, and fungi—allowing the wood to last for hundreds of years.

Other Possible Uses: Hinoki may be beneficial for respiratory conditions such as colds, coughs, and bronchitis. It is also often used as an antiseptic to help clean and aid in tissue healing from abrasions, cuts, scrapes, and rashes. It may also be an effective insect repellent. It can be used to clean and polish wood.

Body System(s) Affected: Emotional Balance, Immune System, Respiratory System, Skin.

Aromatic Influence: Hinoki oil is believed to impart a calming[108] influence, helping to alleviate stress and anxiety[109]. It also uplifts the mind and increases spiritual awareness.

Oral Use As Dietary Supplement: None.

Safety Data: Consult with a physician before use if taking medications, pregnant, or nursing.

Blend Classification: Enhancer.

Blends With: Bergamot, clary sage, cypress, eucalyptus, floral oils, frankincense, juniper berry, resinous oils, and rosemary.

Odor: Type: Top Note (5–20% of the blend); Scent: Clean, woody, citrusy, spicy; Intensity: 2.

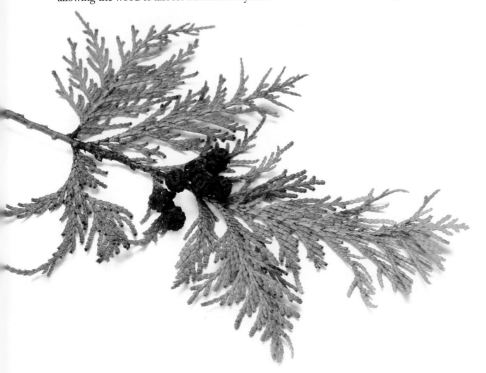

Jasmine *Jasminum officinale*

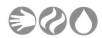

Quick Facts

Botanical Family: Oleaceae (olive)

Extraction Method: Absolute extraction from flowers

Common Primary Uses*: ⊘Hoarse Voice, ⊘Pink Eye, ⊘Sensitive Skin

Common Application Methods‡:

⊘: Can be applied neat (with no dilution) when used topically. Apply directly on area of concern or to reflex points.

⊘: Diffuse, or inhale the aroma directly.

○: Take in capsules.

Properties: Anticatarrhal, antidepressant, and antispasmodic⊕[110].

Historical Uses: Known in India as the "queen of the night" and "moonlight of the grove," women have treasured jasmine for centuries for its beautiful, aphrodisiac-like fragrance. According to Roberta Wilson, "In many religious traditions, the jasmine flower symbolizes hope, happiness, and love." Jasmine has been used for hepatitis, cirrhosis of the liver, dysentery, depression, nervousness, coughs, respiratory congestion, reproductive problems, and "to stimulate uterine contractions in pregnant women as childbirth approached." It was also used in teas, perfumes, and incense.

Other Possible Uses: This oil may help with catarrh (mucus), conjunctivitis, coughs, dysentery, eczema (when caused by emotions), frigidity, hepatitis (cirrhosis of the liver), hoarseness, labor pains, laryngitis, lethargy (abnormal drowsiness), menstrual pain and problems, muscle spasms, nervous exhaustion and tension, pain relief, respiratory conditions, sex, skin care (dry, greasy, irritated, and sensitive), sprains, and uterine disorders. Jasmine is an oil that affects the emotions; it penetrates the deepest layers of the soul, opening doors to our emotions. It produces a feeling of confidence, energy, euphoria, and optimism. It helps to reduce anxiety, apathy, depression, indifference, listlessness, and relationship dilemmas. As a cologne, it increases feelings of attractiveness.

✛ **Body System(s) Affected:** Emotional Balance, Hormonal System ⊕[111].

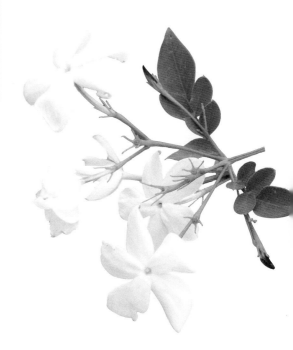

Aromatic Influence: It is very uplifting to the emotions and may help increase intuitive powers and wisdom. It may also help to promote powerful, inspirational relationships.

Oral Use As Dietary Supplement: Jasmine oil is generally regarded as safe (GRAS) for human consumption by the FDA. Dilute 1 drop oil in 1 tsp. (5 ml) honey or in ½ cup (125 ml) of beverage (e.g., soy/rice milk). Not for children under 6 years old; use with caution and in greater dilution for children 6 years old and over.

Blend Classification: Equalizer, Modifier, and Enhancer.

Blends With: Bergamot, frankincense, geranium, helichrysum, lemongrass, melissa, orange, rose, sandalwood, spearmint.

Odor: Type: Base Note (5–20% of the blend); Scent: Powerful, sweet, tenacious, floral with fruity-herbaceous undertones; Intensity: 4.

---

*See My Usage Guide section for more details. ●=Neat, ●=Dilute for Children/Sensitive Skin, ●=Dilute

Juniper Berry *Juniperus communis*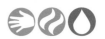

Quick Facts

Botanical Family: Cupressaceae (conifer: cypress)

Extraction Method: Steam distillation from berries and needles

Common Primary Uses*: ❍Acne, ❍Alcoholism, ❍Dermatitis/Eczema, ❍Kidney Stones, ❍Tinnitus

Common Application Methods‡:

❍: Can be applied neat (with no dilution) when used topically. Apply directly on area of concern or to reflex points.

❍: Diffuse, or inhale the aroma directly.

❍: Place 1 drop under the tongue, or take in capsules. Use with caution if pregnant or nursing.

Properties: Antiseptic, antispasmodic, astringent, cleanser, detoxifier, diuretic, stimulant, and tonic.

Historical Uses: Over the centuries, juniper has been used for physical and spiritual purification, for cleansing infections and healing wounds, for liver complaints, for embalming, for relieving arthritis and urinary tract infections, for warding off plagues, epidemics, and contagious diseases, and for headaches, kidney and bladder problems, pulmonary infections, and fevers.

Other Possible Uses: This oil may work as a detoxifier and a cleanser, which may reduce acne, dermatitis, and eczema. It may also help coughs, depression, energy, hemorrhoids, infection, increase circulation through kidneys, kidney stones, liver problems, aching muscles, nerve function and regeneration, obesity, rheumatism (promotes excretion of uric acid and toxins), ulcers, urinary infections, water retention, and wounds.

⊕ Body System(s) Affected: Digestive System, Emotional Balance, Nervous System, Skin.

Aromatic Influence: Juniper evokes feelings of health, love, and peace and may help to elevate one's spiritual awareness.

Oral Use As Dietary Supplement: Juniper berry oil is generally recognized as safe (GRAS) for human consumption by the FDA (21CFR182.20). Dilute 1 drop oil in 1 tsp. (5 ml) honey or in ½ cup (125 ml) of beverage (e.g., soy/rice milk). Not for children under 6 years old; use with caution and in greater dilution for children 6 years old and over Use with caution during pregnancy or while nursing.

Blend Classification: Equalizer.

Blends With: Bergamot, all citrus oils, cypress, geranium, lavender, melaleuca, and rosemary.

Odor: Type: Middle Note (50–80% of the blend); Scent: Sweet, balsamic, tenacious; Intensity: 3.

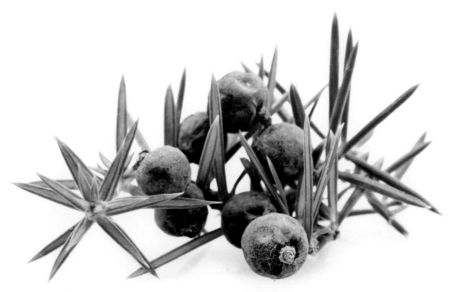

Lavender *Lavandula angustifolia*

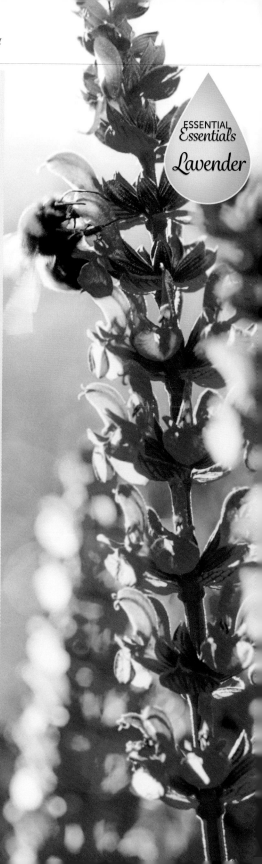

ESSENTIAL
Essentials
Lavender

Biography

Steam-distilled from the flowering tops of lavender plants, the aroma of lavender oil has been enjoyed and used to help soothe and relax for thousands of years.

Lavender is grown natively in many areas throughout the Mediterranean region of Europe, including France, Spain, Italy, and Bulgaria.

Ⓢ : Scent

- Floral
- Sweet
- Herbaceous
- Balsamic
- Woody undertones

Ⓑ : Body Systems Affected

 Cardiovascular System   Emotional Balance

 Nervous System  Skin

Top Uses

Anxiety: Add 3–5 drops lavender to an ultrasonic aromatherapy diffuser when feeling anxious.

Burns: For minor burns, gently apply 1–2 drops of lavender oil, and cover with a cloth soaked in cool water. Seek medical attention for serious burns.

Calming: Combine 5 drops ylang ylang, 6 drops lavender, and 2 drops Roman chamomile with ¼ cup (50 ml) water in a small spray bottle. Mist into the air to help calm children.

Skin Wounds: Apply 1 drop helichrysum to help stop bleeding. Add 1 drop each lavender, tea tree, and basil to a bowl of warm water. Use to wash wound.

Sleep: Add 5 drops lavender and 3 drops Roman chamomile to 2 Tbs. (25 ml) water in a small spray bottle. Spray on kids' pillows and sheets at bedtime.

Stress: Add 10 drops lavender to 1 cup (250 g) Epsom salt. Dissolve ½ cup (125 g) of the salt in warm bathwater for a relaxing bath.

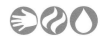

Quick Facts

Botanical Family: Labiatae (mint)

Extraction Method: Steam distillation from flowering top

Common Primary Uses*: ⊘Abuse (Healing From), ⊘⊘Agitation (Calms), ⊘Allergies, ⊘⊘Anxiety[112], ⊘Appetite Loss, ⊘⊘Arrhythmia, ⊘Atherosclerosis, ⊘Bites/Stings, ⊘Blisters, ⊘Boils, ⊘Breasts (Soothes), ⊘Burns, ⊘⊘Calming, ⊘⊘Cancer, ⊘Chicken Pox, ⊘Club Foot, ⊘Concentration, ⊘Convulsions, ⊘⊘Crying, ⊘Cuts, ⊘Dandruff, ⊘⊘ODepression, ⊘Diabetic Sores, ⊘Diaper Rash, ⊘Diuretic, ⊘Dysmenorrhea, ⊘Exhaustion, ⊘Fever, ⊘Gangrene, O⊘Gas/Flatulence, O⊘Giardia, ⊘Gnats and Midges (Repellent), ⊘⊘Grief/Sorrow, ⊘Hair (Dry), ⊘Hair (Fragile), ⊘Hair (Loss), ⊘Hay Fever, ⊘Hernia (Inguinal), ⊘Herpes Simplex, ⊘⊘Hyperactivity, ⊘Impetigo, ⊘Inflammation, ⊘⊘Insomnia, ⊘Itching, ⊘Jet Lag, ⊘Lips (Dry), ⊘Mastitis, ⊘Menopause, ⊘⊘Mental Stress, ⊘Mood Swings, ⊘Mosquito Repellent, ⊘Muscular Paralysis, ⊘⊘Pain, ⊘⊘Parasympathetic Nervous System Stimulation, ⊘Parkinson's Disease, ⊘⊘Phlebitis, ⊘⊘Physical Stress, ⊘Poison Ivy/Oak, ⊘Post Labor, ⊘⊘Postpartum Depression, ⊘Rashes, ⊘⊘Relaxation, ⊘Rheumatoid Arthritis, ⊘⊘Sedative, ⊘Seizure, ⊘Skin (Dry), ⊘Skin (Sensitive), ⊘Skin Ulcers, ⊘⊘Sleep, ⊘⊘Stress[113], ⊘Stretch Marks, ⊘Sunburn, ⊘⊘Tachycardia, ⊘Teeth Grinding, ⊘Teething Pain, ⊘⊘Tension, ⊘Thrush, ⊘Ticks, ⊘Ulcers (Leg), ⊘Varicose Ulcer, ⊘Vertigo, ⊘⊘Withdrawal, O⊘Worms, ⊘Wounds, ⊘Wrinkles

Common Application Methods‡:

⊘: Can be applied neat (with no dilution) when used topically. Apply directly on area of concern or to reflex points.

⊘: Diffuse, or inhale the aroma directly.

O: Place 1–2 drops under the tongue, or take in capsules. Can also be used in beverages or as a flavoring in cooking.

Properties: Analgesic[114], anticoagulant, anti convulsant[115], antidepressant, antifungal[116], antihistamine, anti-infectious, anti-inflammatory[117], antimicrobial[118], antimutagenic[119], antiseptic, antispasmodic, antitoxic, antitumor[120], cardiotonic, regenerative, and sedative[121].

Historical Uses: During Medieval times, people were obviously divided on the properties of lavender regarding love. Some would claim that it could keep the wearer chaste, while others claimed just the opposite—touting its aphrodisiac qualities. Its list of uses is long.

Other Possible Uses: Lavender is a universal oil that has traditionally been known to balance the body and to work wherever there is a need. If in doubt, use lavender. It may help anxiety, arthritis, asthma[122], body systems balance, bronchitis[123], bruises, carbuncles, cold sores, earaches, fainting, gallstones, relieve headaches[124], heart irregularity, reduce high blood pressure[125], hives (urticaria), hysteria, insect bites and bee stings, infection, influenza, injuries, repel insects[126], laryngitis, migraine headaches, mental clarity[127], mouth abscess, reduce mucus, nervous tension, pineal gland (activates), respiratory function, rheumatism, skin conditions (eczema, psoriasis, rashes), sprains, sunstroke, throat infections, tuberculosis, typhoid fever, and whooping cough.

Body System(s) Affected: Cardiovascular System, Emotional Balance, Nervous System, Skin.

Aromatic Influence: It promotes consciousness, health, love, peace, and a general sense of well-being. It also nurtures creativity.

Oral Use As Dietary Supplement: Lavender oil is generally recognized as safe (GRAS) for human consumption by the FDA (21CFR182.20). Dilute 1 drop oil in 1 tsp. (5 ml) honey or in ½ cup (125 ml) of beverage (e.g., soy/rice milk). Not for children under 6 years old; use with caution and in greater dilution for children years old and over.

Blend Classification: Enhancer, Modifier, and Equalizer.

Blends With: Most oils (especially citrus oils), clary sage, and geranium.

Odor: Type: Middle Note (50–80% of the blend); Scent: Floral, sweet, herbaceous, balsamic, woody undertones; Intensity: 2.

‡See Application section beginning on page 42 for more details.   ⊘=Topical, ⊘=Aromatic, O=Internal

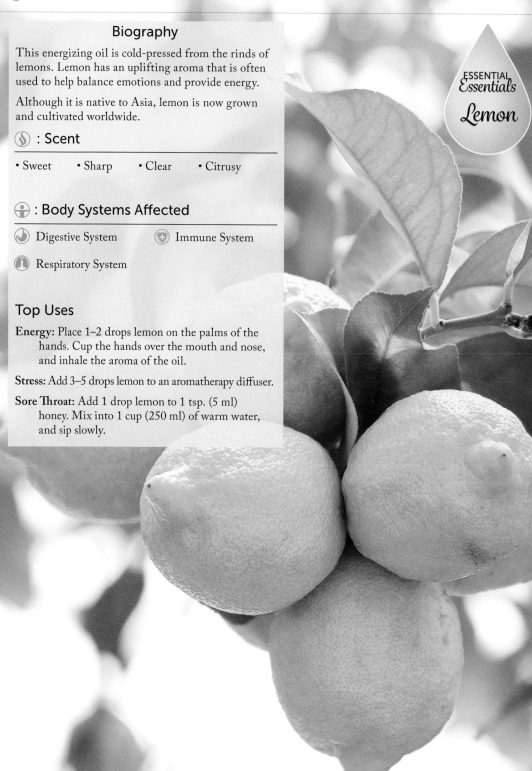

Lemon *Citrus limon*

Biography

This energizing oil is cold-pressed from the rinds of lemons. Lemon has an uplifting aroma that is often used to help balance emotions and provide energy.

Although it is native to Asia, lemon is now grown and cultivated worldwide.

Ⓢ : Scent

• Sweet   • Sharp   • Clear   • Citrusy

✛ : Body Systems Affected

Digestive System   Immune System

Respiratory System

Top Uses

Energy: Place 1–2 drops lemon on the palms of the hands. Cup the hands over the mouth and nose, and inhale the aroma of the oil.

Stress: Add 3–5 drops lemon to an aromatherapy diffuser.

Sore Throat: Add 1 drop lemon to 1 tsp. (5 ml) honey. Mix into 1 cup (250 ml) of warm water, and sip slowly.

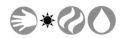

Quick Facts

Botanical Family: Rutaceae (citrus)

Extraction Method: Cold expressed from rind (requires 3,000 lemons to produce a kilo of oil)

Common Primary Uses*: ✋Air Pollution, ✋Anxiety[128], ✋☝Atherosclerosis, ☝Bites/Stings, ⭕Blood Pressure (Regulation), ✋☝Brain Injury, ☝Cold Sores, ✋☝Colds (Common), ✋Concentration[129], ☝Constipation, ✋☝⭕Depression, ☝Digestion (Sluggish), ✋☝Disinfectant, ⭕☝Dry Throat, ☝Dysentery, ☝Energizing, ☝Exhaustion, ⭕☝Fever, ✋☝Flu (Influenza), ☝Furniture Polish, ⭕☝Gout, ☝Greasy/Oily Hair, ✋☝Grief/Sorrow, ☝Gum/Grease Removal, ✋☝Hangovers, ☝Heartburn, ⭕☝Intestinal Parasites, ⭕Kidney Stones, ✋☝Lymphatic Cleansing, ☝MRSA, ✋Overeating, ✋☝Pancreatitis, ✋Physical Energy, ✋☝Postpartum Depression, ✋Purification, ✋Relaxation, ☝Skin (Tones), ✋☝Stress[130], ✋☝⭕Throat Infection, ☝Tonsillitis, ✋Uplifting, ☝Varicose Veins, ⭕☝Water Purification

Common Application Methods‡:

☝: Can be applied neat (with no dilution) when used topically. Apply directly on area of concern or to reflex points. Avoid direct sunlight or UV light for up to 12 hours after using on the skin.

✋: Diffuse, or inhale the aroma directly.

⭕: Place 1–2 drops under the tongue, or drink with a beverage. Take in capsules. Use as a flavoring in cooking.

Properties: Anticancer[131], antidepressant[132], antiseptic, antifungal[133], antioxidant[134], antiviral, astringent, invigorating, refreshing, and tonic.

Historical Uses: Lemon has been used to fight food poisoning, malaria and typhoid epidemics, and scurvy. (In fact, sources say that Christopher Columbus carried lemon seeds to America—probably just the leftovers from the fruit that was eaten during the trip.) Lemon has also been used to lower blood pressure and to help with liver problems, arthritis, and muscular aches and pains.

Other Possible Uses: This oil may be beneficial for aging[135], soothing broken capillaries, dissolving cellulite, clarity of thought, debility, digestive

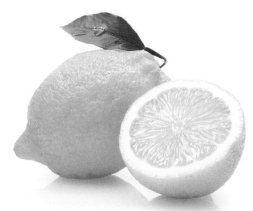

problems[136], energy, gallstones, hair (cleansing), promoting leukocyte formation, liver deficiencies in children, memory improvement, nails (strengthening and hardening), nerves[137], nervous conditions, respiratory problems, cleaning children's skin, sore throats, and promoting a sense of well-being. It works extremely well in removing gum, wood stain, oil, and grease spots. It may also brighten a pale, dull complexion by removing dead skin cells.

Body System(s) Affected: Digestive, Immune, and Respiratory Systems.

Aromatic Influence: It promotes health, healing, physical energy, and purification. Its fragrance is invigorating, enhancing, and warming.

Oral Use As Dietary Supplement: Lemon oil is generally recognized as safe (GRAS) for human consumption by the FDA (21CFR182.20). Dilute 1 drop oil in 1 tsp. (5 ml) honey or in ½ cup (125 ml) of beverage (e.g., soy/rice milk). Not for children under 6 years old; use with caution and in greater dilution for children 6 years old and over.

Safety Data: Avoid direct sunlight for up to 12 hours after use. Can cause extreme skin irritation.

Blend Classification: Modifier and Enhancer.

Blends With: Eucalyptus, fennel, frankincense, geranium, peppermint, sandalwood, and ylang ylang.

Odor: Type: Top Note (5–20% of the blend); Scent: Sweet, sharp, clear, citrusy; Intensity: 3.

Lemongrass *Cymbopogon flexuosus*

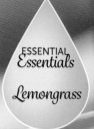

ESSENTIAL
Essentials

Lemongrass

Biography

Lemongrass oil is often used for joint and muscle pain along with its use as an insect repellent.

Lemongrass is cultivated in its native India, where the oil is steam-distilled from the plant's grass leaves.

Ⓢ : Scent

- Grassy
- Lemony
- Pungent
- Earthy
- Slightly Bitter

✚ : Body Systems Affected

🛡 Immune System 🌑 Muscles and Bones

Top Uses

Joint Injuries: Apply neat on location or reflex points on the feet. To massage on the area, combine 5–10 drops lemongrass with 1 Tbs. (15 ml) fractionated coconut oil.

Tissue Repair: Apply as a warm compress to affected area.

Insect Repellent: Combine 5 drops lavender, 5 drops lemongrass, 3 drops peppermint, and 1 drop thyme. Mixture can be placed neat on feet or added to 1 cup (250 ml) water and misted using a spray bottle.

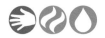

Quick Facts

Botanical Family: Gramineae (grasses)

Extraction Method: Steam distillation from leaves

Common Primary Uses*: ②Air Pollution, ②Airborne Bacteria, ⊜Carpal Tunnel Syndrome, ⊙Cholesterol⊞[138], ⊜Cramps/Charley Horses, ⊜Cystitis/Bladder Infection, ⊜Diuretic, ⊜Edema, ⊜Fleas, ⊜Frozen Shoulder, ⊙Gastritis, ⊜②Grave's Disease, ⊜②Hashimoto's Disease, ⊜Hernia (Incisional), ⊜Hernia (Inguinal), ⊜Improve Vision, ⊙⊜Lactose Intolerance, ⊜②Lymphatic Drainage, ②⊜Mental Fatigue, ⊜Muscular Dystrophy, ⊜②Paralysis, ②Purification, ⊜Retina (Strengthen), ⊜Sprains, ⊜Strain (Muscle), ⊜Tissue Repair, ⊜②Urinary Tract Infection, ⊜Varicose Veins, ⊜Whiplash (Ligaments), ⊜Wounds

Common Application Methods‡:

⊜: Can be applied neat (with no dilution), or dilute 1:1 (1 drop essential oil to 1 drop carrier oil) for children and for those with sensitive skin when using topically. Apply directly on area of concern or to reflex points.

②: Diffuse, or inhale the aroma directly.

⊙: Take in capsules. Use as a flavoring in cooking.

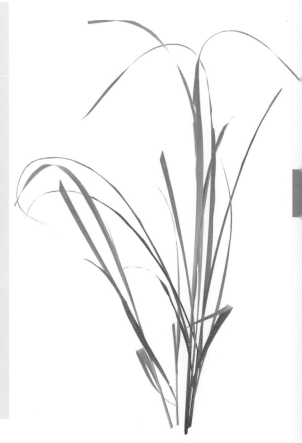

Properties: Analgesic, antibacterial⊞[139], anticancer⊞[140], anti-inflammatory⊞[141], antiseptic, insect repellent, revitalizer, sedative, tonic, and vasodilator.

Historical Uses: Lemongrass has been used for infectious illnesses and fever, as an insecticide, and as a sedative to the central nervous system.

Other Possible Uses: This oil may help with circulation, improving digestion, improving eyesight, fevers, flatulence, headaches, clearing infections, repairing ligaments, waking up the lymphatic system, getting the oxygen flowing, respiratory problems⊞[142], sore throats, tissue regeneration, and water retention.

⊕ **Body System(s) Affected:** Immune and Skeletal Systems and Muscles.

Aromatic Influence: It promotes awareness and purification.

Oral Use As Dietary Supplement: Lemongrass oil is generally recognized as safe (GRAS) for human consumption by the FDA (21CFR182.20). Dilute 1 drop oil in 1 tsp. (5 ml) honey or in ½ cup (125 ml) of beverage (e.g., soy/rice milk). Not for children under 6 years old; use with caution and in greater dilution for children 6 years old and over.

Safety Data: Can cause extreme skin irritation.

Blend Classification: Enhancer and Equalizer.

Blends With: Basil, clary sage, eucalyptus, geranium, lavender, melaleuca, and rosemary.

Odor: Type: Top Note (5–20% of the blend); Scent: Grassy, lemony, pungent, earthy, slightly bitter; Intensity: 4.

‡See Application section beginning on page 14 for more details.   ⊜=Topical, ②=Aromatic, ⊙=Internal

Lemon Myrtle *Backhousia citriodora*

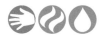

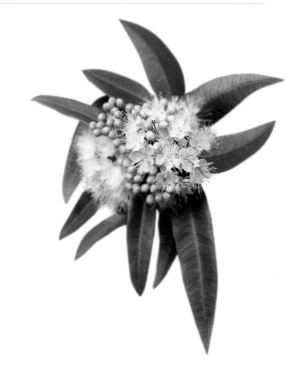

Quick Facts

Botanical Family: Myrtaceae (myrtle: shrubs and trees)

Extraction Method: Steam distillation from leaves

Common Primary Uses*: ⊙❷Antibacterial, ⊙❷Antifungal, ⊙Candida, ⊙Staph/MRSA

Common Application Methods‡:

⊙: Dilute 1:3 (1 drop essential oil to at least 3 drops carrier oil) before applying topically. Apply directly on area of concern or to reflex points.

❷: Diffuse, or inhale the aroma directly.

○: Add 1 drop to 1 cup (250 ml) of water or other beverage.

Properties: Analgesic, anxiolytic, antibacterial, antifungal, anti-inflammatory, antimicrobial, antitumor, and sedative.

Historical Uses: Dried leaves from the lemon myrtle tree have been used as food flavoring for poultry and seafood. They have also served as air fresheners in wardrobes, shoe cabinets, and vehicles. Lemon myrtle is said to smell more "lemony" than lemon. Research indicates that lemon myrtle oil has very good antibacterial activity and excellent antifungal activity, perhaps even more than Melaleuca alternifolia. Tests have also shown lemon myrtle to possess strong germicidal powers, twice that of Eucalyptus citriodora and 19.5 times that of citral alone.

Other Possible Uses: Lemon myrtle may help with viral, bacterial, and fungal infections. It has also been reported to help with sprained or torn ligaments and tendons. Due to antibacterial, antifungal, and antimicrobial actions, lemon myrtle works well as an additive to any natural cleaning product. What more agreeable way to clean than with the strong lemon scent from this oil!

⊕ **Body System(s) Affected:** Immune System, Respiratory System, Muscles and Bones.

Aromatic Influence: Lemon myrtle is elevating and refreshing.

Oral Use As Dietary Supplement: While the FDA has given no guidance on this oil, leaves from the lemon myrtle are commonly used as a spice or flavoring in Australia. Use in cooking or in beverages in small amounts (1 drop or less). Dilute 1 drop oil in 1 tsp. (5 ml) honey or in 1 cup (250 ml) of beverage (e.g., soy/rice milk). Not for children under 6 years old; use with caution and in greater dilution for children 6 years old and over.

Safety Data: Oils may irritate sensitive or damaged skin. Dilute before applying on the skin. Consult with a physician before use if taking medications (especially for diabetes), pregnant, or nursing.

Blend Classification: Enhancer and Equalizer.

Blends With: Basil, clary sage, citrus oils, eucalyptus, geranium, lavender, melaleuca, and rosemary.

Odor: Type: Top (5–20% of the blend); Scent: Lemony, crisp, sweet, slightly herbal; Intensity: 5.

---

*See My Usage Guide section for more details.   ●=Neat, ●=Dilute for Children/Sensitive Skin, ●=Dilute

Lime *Citrus aurantifolia*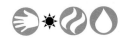

Quick Facts

Botanical Family: Rutaceae (citrus)

Extraction Method: Cold expressed from peel

Common Primary Uses*: ⬭🕸Bacterial Infections, 🜄⬭🕸Fever, ⬭Gum/Grease Removal, ⬭Skin (Revitalizing)

Common Application Methods‡:

⬭: Can be applied neat (with no dilution) when used topically. Apply directly on area of concern or to reflex points. It makes an excellent addition to bath and shower gels, body lotions, and deodorants.

🕸: Diffuse, or inhale the aroma directly.

🜄: Place 1–2 drops under the tongue, or drink with a beverage. Take in capsules. Use as a flavoring in cooking.

Properties: Antibacterial, antiseptic, antiviral, restorative, and tonic.

Historical Uses: For some time, lime was used as a remedy for dyspepsia with glycerin of pepsin. It was often used in place of lemon for fevers, infections, sore throats, colds, etc.

Other Possible Uses: This oil may be beneficial for anxiety, blood pressure, soothing broken capillaries, dissolving cellulite, improving clarity of thought, debility, energy, gallstones, hair (cleansing), promoting leukocyte formation, liver deficiencies in children, lymphatic system cleansing, memory improvement, nails (strengthening), nervous conditions, cleaning children's skin, sore throats, water and air purification, and promoting a sense of well-being. It works extremely well in removing gum, wood stain, oil, and grease spots. It may also help brighten a pale, dull complexion by removing the dead skin cells. Lime oil is capable of tightening skin and connective tissue.

Body System(s) Affected: Digestive, Immune, and Respiratory Systems.

Aromatic Influence: Lime oil has a fresh, lively fragrance that is stimulating and refreshing. It helps one overcome exhaustion, depression, and listlessness. Although unverifiable, some sources claim that inhaling the oil may stimulate the muscles around the eyes.

Oral Use As Dietary Supplement: Lime oil is generally regarded as safe (GRAS) for human consumption by the FDA. Dilute 1 drop oil in 1 tsp. (5 ml) honey or in ½ cup (125 ml) of beverage (e.g., soy/rice milk). Not for children under 6 years old; use with caution and in greater dilution for children 6 years old and over.

Safety Data: Avoid direct sunlight 12 hours after use.

Blend Classification: Enhancer and Equalizer.

Blends With: Citronella, clary sage, lavender, rosemary, other citrus oils.

Odor: Type: Top Note (5–20% of the blend); Scent: Sweet, tart, intense, lively; Intensity: 3

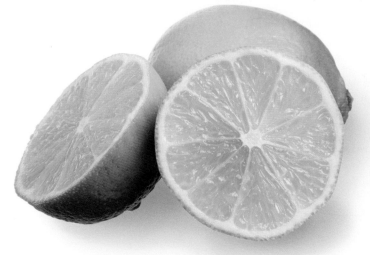

‡See Application section beginning on page 14 for more details. ⬭=Topical, 🕸=Aromatic, 🜄=Internal

Litsea *Litsea cubeba*

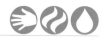

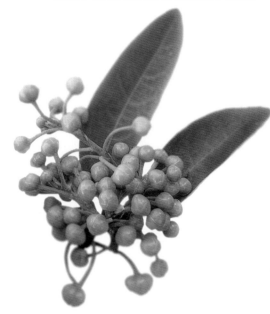

Quick Facts

Botanical Family: Lauraceae (laurel)

Extraction Method: Steam distillation from fruit

Common Primary Uses*: ◐🅐Bacterial Infections⊕[143], 🅐🅑Cleaning, 🅑🅒Energizing, ⭕Flavoring, 🅑🅒Meditation, 🅑🅒Yoga

Common Application Methods‡:

◐: Can be applied neat (with no dilution) when used topically. Apply directly on area of concern or to reflex points. Use in massage oil.

🅑: Diffuse, or inhale the aroma directly.

⭕: Place 1–2 drops in liquid, and drink as a beverage. Use as a flavoring in cooking.

Properties: Antibacterial⊕, antifungal, antiseptic, antiviral.

Historical Uses: Litsea (also known as mei (may) chang) has been used medicinally in Taiwan and China for centuries to treat pain, asthma, and digestive issues.

Other Possible Uses: This oil may also be beneficial for allergies, asthma, throat congestion, and heart arrhythmia.

Body System(s) Affected: Digestive, Immune, and Respiratory Systems.

Aromatic Influence: Litsea oil has a sweet, citrusy, floral aroma that is uplifting and energizing and may help promote feelings of balance.

Oral Use As Dietary Supplement: There is no FDA designation for *Litsea cubeba* oil at this time, but it is commonly used as a flavoring in cooking. Dilute 1 drop oil in 1 tsp. (5 ml) honey or in ½ cup (125 ml) of beverage (e.g., soy/rice milk). Not for children under 6 years old; use with caution and in greater dilution for children 6 years old and over.

Safety Data: May cause skin sensitivity. Consult with a physician before using if pregnant, nursing, or being treated for diabetes or other medical conditions.

Blend Classification: Enhancer and Equalizer.

Blends With: Lavender, rosemary, rose, petitgrain, citrus oils, ylang ylang, sandalwood, frankincense, fennel, geranium, vetiver.

Odor: Type: Middle Note (50–80% of the blend); Scent: Citrusy, floral, fresh, sweet; Intensity: 3

Magnolia *Michelia alba (Magnolia alba)*

Quick Facts

Botanical Family: Magnoliaceae

Extraction Method: Steam distillation from flowers

Common Primary Uses*: ⊘⊖Anxiety, ⊘⊖Calming, ⊖Soothing (skin)

Common Application Methods‡:

⊖: Can be applied neat (with no dilution) when used topically. Apply directly on area of concern or to reflex points.

⊘: Diffuse, or inhale the aroma directly.

Properties: Analgesic⊕¹⁴⁴, anxiolytic, antibacterial, anti-inflammatory, antimicrobial, antitumor, sedative⊕¹⁴⁵.

Historical Uses: Magnolia trees are native to Southeast Asia, and the bark of one magnolia species (*Magnolia officinalis*) is used in traditional Chinese medicine to help with digestive and respiratory issues. This variety of magnolia (*M. alba*) is believed to be a hybrid of *M. champaca* and *M. montana*.

Other Possible Uses: This oil may also be beneficial for calming, depression, and skin (cleansing and soothing).

⊕ **Body System(s) Affected:** Hormonal System, Immune System, Skin.

Aromatic Influence: benefitIt also has calming and sedating properties when inhaled.

Oral Use As Dietary Supplement: None.

Safety Data: Old or oxidized oil may irritate sensitive skin. Consult with a physician before use if taking medications, pregnant, or nursing.

Blend Classification: Enhancer and Equalizer.

Blends With: Bergamot, geranium, grapefruit, lime, marjoram, rose, sandalwood, vetiver, ylang ylang.

Odor: Type: Top to Middle (50–80% of the blend); Scent: Sweet, floral, fruity, herbal; Intensity: 2.

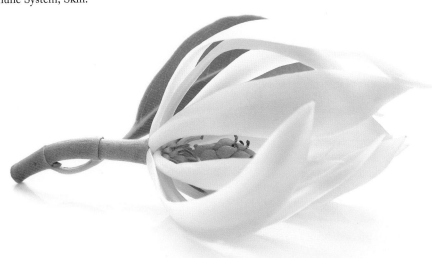

Manuka *Leptospermum scoparium*

Properties: Analgesic, antibacterial[146], antifungal, anti-infectious, antiviral, antihistamine, antiseptic, decongestant, and insecticidal.

Historical Uses: This oil has a long history of use by the Maori people for bronchitis, rheumatism, and similar conditions. Also, manuka oil has been used to treat a range of skin problems including chronic sores, ringworm, eczema, fungal infections (athlete foot and fungal nail infections), scalp itch, and dandruff. A decoction of leaves was used for urinary complaints and to reduce fever. The leaves were boiled in water and inhaled for head colds, blocked sinuses, hay fever, and even bronchitis and asthma. Leaves and bark were boiled together, and the warm liquid was rubbed on stiff backs and rheumatic joints. The leaves and young branches were put into vapor baths. The crushed leaves were applied as a poultice for many skin diseases and were directly applied to wounds and deep gashes to enhance healing and to reduce the risk of infection. The young shoots were chewed and swallowed for dysentery.

Other Possible Uses: This oil may be beneficial for abrasions, acne, bronchitis, catarrh, chafing, colds, cuts, dandruff, fungal infections, infections, insect bites and stings, muscle and joint pains, odor, rashes, scratches, skin irritations, sinusitis, sunburn, and ulcers.

Body System(s) Affected: Muscles and Bones, Respiratory System, and Skin.

Aromatic Influence: Manuka oil helps to calm sensitive nerves and to produce a feeling of well-being. Its calming aroma helps to combat stress and irritability.

Oral Use As Dietary Supplement: None.

Safety Data: Use with caution when pregnant or nursing.

Blend Classification: Enhancer and Equalizer.

Blends With: All citrus oils, cypress, eucalyptus, lavender, rosemary, and thyme.

Odor: Type: Middle Note (50–80% of the blend); Scent: Rich, fresh, woody, earthy, herbaceous; Intensity: 3.

Additional Research:

Antibacteial: Manuka oil demonstrated strong antibacterial activity against detrimental oral bacteria (Takarada et al., 2004).

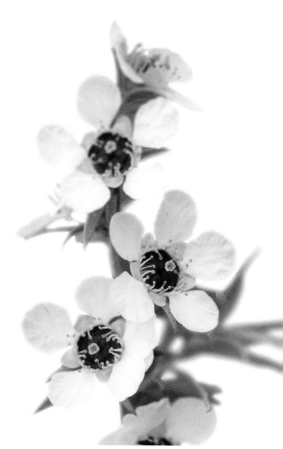

Marjoram *Origanum majorana*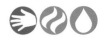

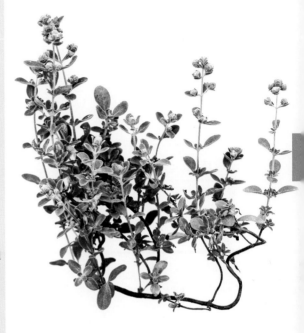

Properties: Antibacterial, anti-infectious, antiseptic, antisexual, antispasmodic, arterial vasodilator, digestive stimulant, diuretic, expectorant, sedative, and tonic.

Historical Uses: Marjoram was used to combat poisoning, fluid retention, muscle spasms, rheumatism, sprains, stiff joints, bruises, obstructions of the liver and spleen, and respiratory congestions. According to Roberta Wilson, "Those curious about their futures anointed themselves with marjoram at bedtime so that they might dream of their future mates."

Other Possible Uses: It may be relaxing and calming to the muscles that constrict and sometimes contribute to headaches. It may help anxiety, boils, bruises, burns, carbuncles, celibacy (vow not to marry), colds, cold sores, cuts, fungus and viral infections, hysteria, menstrual problems, calm the respiratory system, ringworm, shingles, shock, sores, relieve spasms, sunburns, and water retention.

⊕ Body System(s) Affected: Cardiovascular and Skeletal Systems and Muscles.

Aromatic Influence: It promotes peace and sleep.

Oral Use As Dietary Supplement: Marjoram oil is generally recognized as safe (GRAS) for human consumption by the FDA (21CFR182.20). Dilute 1 drop oil in 1 tsp. (5 ml) honey or in ½ cup (125 ml) of beverage (e.g., soy/rice milk). Not for children under 6 years old; use with caution and in greater dilution for children 6 years old and over.

Safety Data: Use with caution during pregnancy.

Blend Classification: Enhancer and Equalizer.

Blends With: Bergamot, cypress, lavender, orange, rosemary, and ylang ylang.

Odor: Type: Middle Note (50–80% of the blend); Scent: Herbaceous, green, spicy; Intensity: 3.

---

‡*See Application section beginning on page 14 for more details.*   ⊘=Topical, ⊘=Aromatic, ○=Internal

Melaleuca (Tea Tree) *Melaleuca alternifolia*

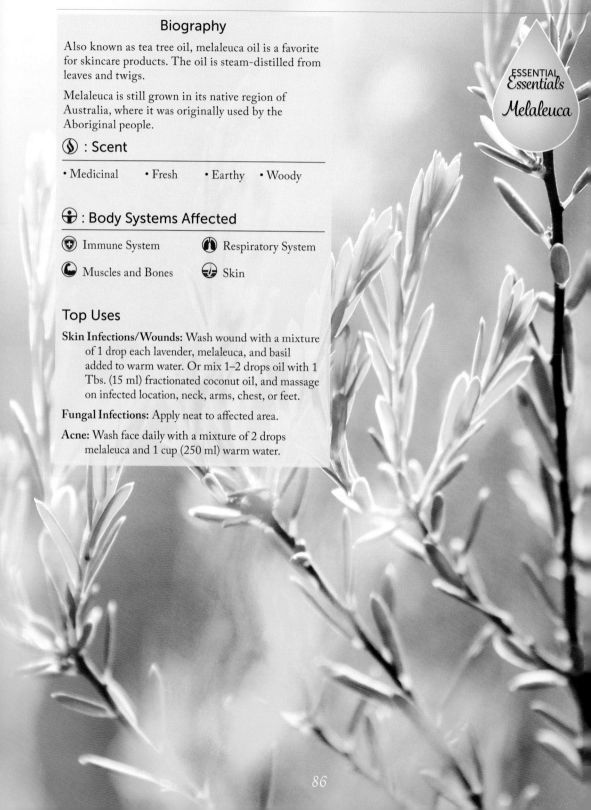

Biography

Also known as tea tree oil, melaleuca oil is a favorite for skincare products. The oil is steam-distilled from leaves and twigs.

Melaleuca is still grown in its native region of Australia, where it was originally used by the Aboriginal people.

Ⓢ : Scent

- Medicinal
- Fresh
- Earthy
- Woody

⊕ : Body Systems Affected

- Immune System
- Respiratory System
- Muscles and Bones
- Skin

Top Uses

Skin Infections/Wounds: Wash wound with a mixture of 1 drop each lavender, melaleuca, and basil added to warm water. Or mix 1–2 drops oil with 1 Tbs. (15 ml) fractionated coconut oil, and massage on infected location, neck, arms, chest, or feet.

Fungal Infections: Apply neat to affected area.

Acne: Wash face daily with a mixture of 2 drops melaleuca and 1 cup (250 ml) warm water.

ESSENTIAL
Essentials
Melaleuca

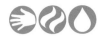

Quick Facts

Botanical Family: Myrtaceae (Myrtle: shrubs and trees)

Extraction Method: Steam distillation from leaves

Common Primary Uses*: ⬤Acne[148], ⬤Allergies, ⬤⬤Aneurysm, ⬤Athlete's Foot, ⬤Bacterial Infections, ⬤Boils[149], ⬤⬤Bronchitis, ⬤Candida, ⬤Canker Sores, ⬤Cavities, ⬤⬤Chicken Pox, ⬤Cleansing, ⬤Cold Sores, ⬤⬤Colds (Common), ⬤⬤Coughs, ⬤Cuts, ⬤Dermatitis/Eczema, ⬤Dry/Itchy Eyes, ⬤Ear Infection, ⬤Earache, ⬤⬤Flu (Influenza)[150], ⬤Fungal Infections, ⬤Gum Disease, ⬤⬤Hepatitis, ⬤Herpes Simplex, ⬤Hives, ⬤⬤Immune System (Stimulates), ⬤⬤Infected Wounds, ⬤Infection, ⬤⬤Inflammation, ⬤Jock Itch, ⬤Lice, ⬤MRSA, ⬤⬤Mumps, ⬤Nail Infection, ⬤⬤Pink Eye, ⬤Rashes, ⬤Ringworm, ⬤Rubella, ⬤Scabies, ⬤Shingles, ⬤Shock, ⬤⬤Sore Throat, ⬤Staph Infection, ⬤Sunburn, ⬤Thrush, ⬤⬤Tonsillitis, ⬤Vaginal Infection, ⬤Varicose Ulcer, ⬤⬤Viral Infections, ⬤Warts, ⬤Wounds

Common Application Methods‡:

⬤: Can be applied neat (with no dilution) when used topically. Apply directly on area of concern or to reflex points.

⬤: Diffuse, or inhale the aroma directly.

⬤: Take in capsules.

Properties: Analgesic, antibacterial[151], antifungal[152], anti-infectious, anti-inflammatory[153], antioxidant, antiparasitic, a strong antiseptic, antiviral[154], decongestant, digestive, expectorant, immune stimulant, insecticidal, neurotonic, stimulant, and tissue regenerative.

Historical Uses: The leaves of the melaleuca tree (or tea tree) have been used for centuries by the Aboriginal people of Australia to heal cuts, wounds, and skin infections. With 12 times the antiseptic power of phenol, it has some strong immune-building properties.

Other Possible Uses: This oil may help burns, digestion, hysteria, infectious diseases, mites[155], and ticks[156].

⬤ **Body System(s) Affected:** Immune, Skeletal, and Respiratory Systems, Muscles, and Skin.

Aromatic Influence: It promotes cleansing and purity.

Oral Use As Dietary Supplement: Melaleuca oil in general is approved by the FDA (21CFR172.510) for use as a Food Additive (FA) or Flavoring Agent (FL). Dilute 1 drop oil in 1 tsp. (5 ml) honey or in ½ cup (125 ml) of beverage (e.g., soy/rice milk). Not for children under 6 years old; use with caution and in greater dilution for children 6 years old and over.

Safety Data: Repeated use can possibly result in contact sensitization.

Blend Classification: Enhancer and Equalizer.

Blends With: All citrus oils, cypress, eucalyptus, lavender, rosemary, and thyme.

Odor: Type: Middle Note (50–80% of the blend); Scent: Medicinal, fresh, woody, earthy, herbaceous; Intensity: 3.

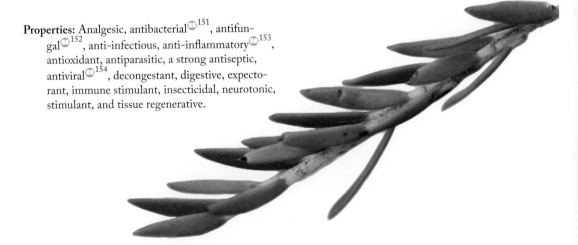

Melissa (Lemon Balm) *Melissa officinalis*

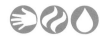

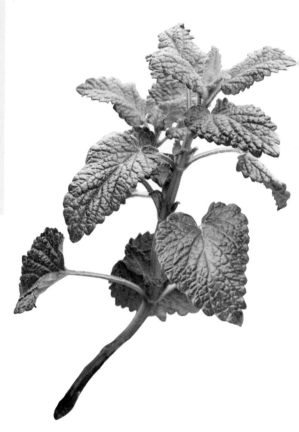

Properties: Antibacterial, antidepressant, antihistamine, antimicrobial, antispasmodic, antiviral[157], hypotensive, nervine, sedative[158], tonic, and uterine.

Historical Uses: Anciently, melissa was used for nervous disorders and many different ailments dealing with the heart or the emotions. It was also used to promote fertility. Melissa was the main ingredient in Carmelite water, distilled in France since 1611 by the Carmelite monks.

Other Possible Uses: Allergies, anxiety, asthma, bronchitis, chronic coughs, colds, cold-sore blisters[159] (apply directly three times per day), colic[160], depression, dysentery, eczema, erysipelas, fevers, heart conditions (where there is overstimulation or heat), hypertension, indigestion, inflammation[161], insect bites, insomnia, menstrual problems, migraine, nausea, nervous tension, palpitations, shock, sterility (in women), throat infections, vertigo, and vomiting. Dr. Dietrich Wabner, a professor at the Technical University of Munich, reported that a one-time application of true melissa oil led to complete remission of herpes simplex lesions. According to Robert Tisserand, "Melissa is the nearest one can find to a rejuvenator—not something which will make us young again, but which helps to cushion the effect of our mind and the world outside on our body."

⊕ Body System(s) Affected: Emotional Balance, Skin.

Aromatic Influence: Melissa has a delicate, delightful, lemony scent that is unique among essential oils, providing a wonderful support to both body and mind. It is calming and uplifting and may help to balance the emotions.

Oral Use As Dietary Supplement: Melissa oil is generally recognized as safe (GRAS) for human consumption by the FDA (21CFR182.20). Dilute 1 drop oil in 1 tsp. (5 ml) honey or in ½ cup (125 ml) of beverage (e.g., soy/rice milk). Not for children under 6 years old; use with caution and in greater dilution for children 6 years old and over.

Safety Data: Use with caution when pregnant or nursing.

Blend Classification: Enhancer, Equalizer, and Modifier.

Blends With: Geranium, lavender, and other floral and citrus oils.

Odor: Type: Middle Note (50–80% of the blend); Scent: Delicate, lemony; Intensity: 2.

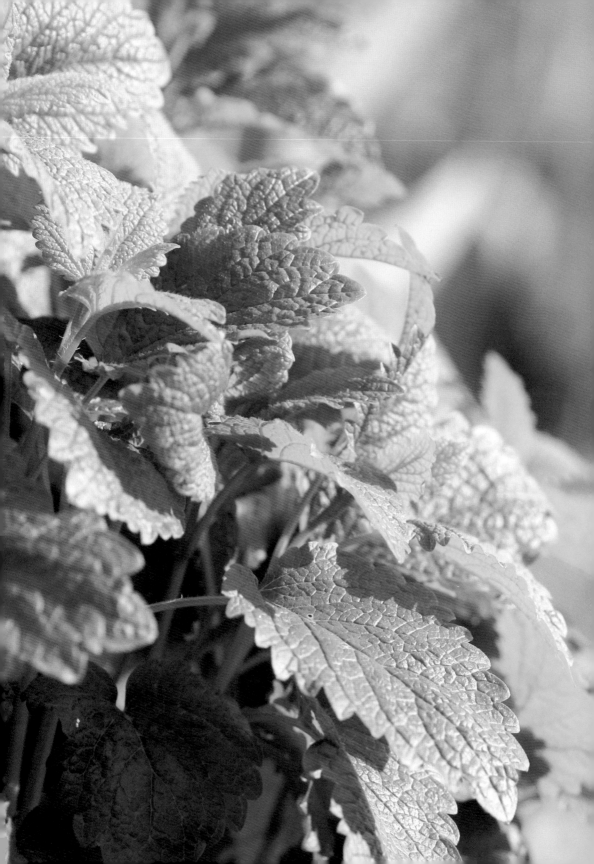

Myrrh *Commiphora myrrha*

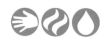

Quick Facts

Botanical Family: Burseraceae (resinous trees and shrubs)

Extraction Method: Steam distillation from gum/resin

Common Primary Uses*: 🫲🌀Cancer, 🌀Chapped/Cracked Skin, 🫲🌀Congestion, 🌀Dysentery, 🌀Gum Disease, 🫲🌀Hashimoto's Disease, 🫲🌀Hepatitis, 🫲🌀Hyperthyroidism, 🫲🌀Infection, 🫲🌀Liver Cirrhosis, 🌀Skin Ulcers, 🌀Stretch Marks, 💧🌀Ulcers (Duodenal), 🌀Weeping Wounds

Common Application Methods‡:

🫲: Can be applied neat (with no dilution) when used topically. Apply directly on area of concern or to reflex points.

🌀: Diffuse, or inhale the aroma directly.

💧: Place 1–2 drops under the tongue, or take in capsules.

Properties: Anti-infectious, anti-inflammatory 📖[162], antiseptic, antitumor 📖[163], astringent, and tonic.

Historical Uses: Myrrh was used as incense in religious rituals, in embalming, and as a cure for cancer, leprosy, and syphilis. Myrrh, mixed with coriander and honey, was used to treat herpes.

Other Possible Uses: This oil may help with appetite (increase), asthma, athlete's foot, candida, catarrh (mucus), coughs, eczema, digestion, dyspepsia (impaired digestion), flatulence (gas), fungal infection, gingivitis, hemorrhoids, mouth ulcers, decongesting the prostate gland, ringworm, sore throats, skin conditions (chapped, cracked, and inflamed)📖[164], wounds, and wrinkles.

Body System(s) Affected: Hormonal, Immune, and Nervous Systems; Skin.

Aromatic Influence: It promotes awareness and is uplifting.

Oral Use As Dietary Supplement: Myrrh oil in general is approved by the FDA (21CFR172.510) for use as a Food Additive (FA) and Flavoring Agent (FL). Dilute 1 drop oil in 1 tsp. (5 ml) honey or in ½ cup (125 ml) of beverage (e.g., soy/rice milk). Not for children under 6 years old; use with caution and in greater dilution for children 6 years old and over.

Safety Data: Use with caution during pregnancy.

Blend Classification: Modifier and Equalizer.

Blends With: Frankincense, lavender, sandalwood, and all spice oils.

Odor: Type: Base Note (5–20% of the blend); Scent: Warm, earthy, woody, balsamic; Intensity: 4.

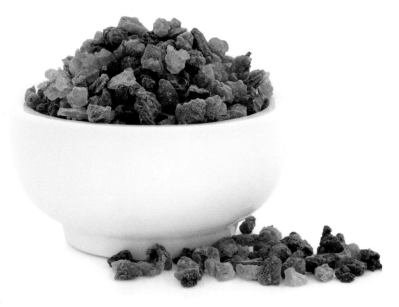

Neroli (Orange Blossom) *Citrus aurantium*

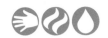

Quick Facts

Botanical Family: Rutaceae (citrus)

Extraction Method: Extracted from flowers of the bitter orange tree

Common Primary Uses*: Anxiety, Emotional Balance, Relaxing, Sensitive Skin, Stress

Common Application Methods‡:

: Can be applied neat (with no dilution) when used topically. Apply directly on area of concern or to reflex points.

: Diffuse, or inhale the aroma directly.

Properties: Antibacterial[165], antidepressant, anti-infectious, antiparasitic, antiseptic, antispasmodic, antiviral, aphrodisiac, deodorant, sedative, and tonic.

Historical Uses: Neroli has been regarded traditionally by the Egyptian people for its great attributes for healing the mind, body, and spirit. It brings everything into the focus of one and at the moment.

Other Possible Uses: This oil may help support the digestive system and may help inhibit bacteria, infections, parasites, and viruses. It may also help with anxiety, chronic diarrhea, colic, convulsions[166], depression, digestive spasms, fear, flatulence, headaches, heart (regulates rhythm), hysteria, insomnia, mature and sensitive skin, menopause[167], nervous dyspepsia, nervous tension, palpitations, PMS, poor circulation, scars, shock, stress-related conditions, stretch marks, tachycardia, thread veins, and wrinkles. In support of the skin, it works at the cell level to help shed the old skin cells and stimulate new cell growth.

Body System(s) Affected: Digestive System, Skin.

Aromatic Influence: Neroli has some powerfully soothing psychological effects. It is calming and relaxing to the body and spirit. It may also help to strengthen and stabilize the emotions and bring relief to seemingly hopeless situations. It encourages confidence, courage, joy, peace, and sensuality.

Oral Use As Dietary Supplement: Neroli oil is generally recognized as safe (GRAS) for human consumption by the FDA (21CFR182.20). Dilute 1 drop oil in 1 tsp. (5 ml) honey or in ½ cup (125 ml) of beverage (e.g., soy/rice milk). Not for children under 6 years old; use with caution and in greater dilution for children 6 years old and over. Follow label instructions, and use orally only if recommended.

Safety Data: Consult with a physician before using if pregnant or being treated for a medical condition.

Blend Classification: Equalizer, Modifier, and Personifier.

Blends With: Rose, lavender, sandalwood, jasmine, cedarwood, geranium, lemon.

Odor: Type: Middle Note (50–80% of the blend); Scent: Floral, citrusy, sweet, delicate, slightly bitter; Intensity: 3.

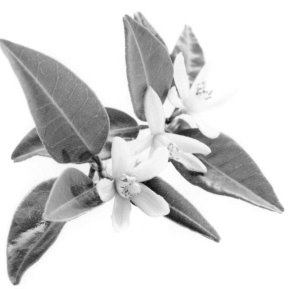

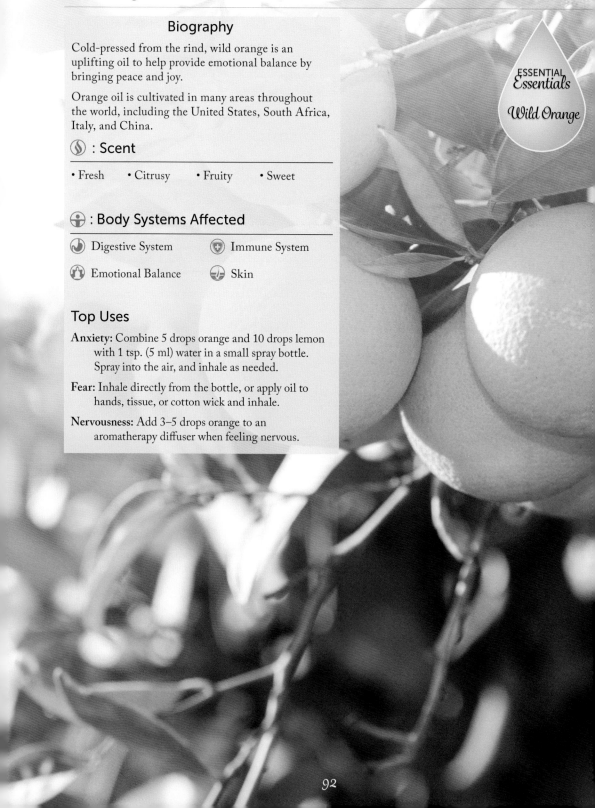

Orange *(Wild Orange) Citrus sinensis*

Biography

Cold-pressed from the rind, wild orange is an uplifting oil to help provide emotional balance by bringing peace and joy.

Orange oil is cultivated in many areas throughout the world, including the United States, South Africa, Italy, and China.

ⓢ : Scent

- Fresh
- Citrusy
- Fruity
- Sweet

⊕ : Body Systems Affected

- Digestive System
- Immune System
- Emotional Balance
- Skin

Top Uses

Anxiety: Combine 5 drops orange and 10 drops lemon with 1 tsp. (5 ml) water in a small spray bottle. Spray into the air, and inhale as needed.

Fear: Inhale directly from the bottle, or apply oil to hands, tissue, or cotton wick and inhale.

Nervousness: Add 3–5 drops orange to an aromatherapy diffuser when feeling nervous.

ESSENTIAL
Essentials

Wild Orange

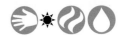

Quick Facts

Botanical Family: Rutaceae (citrus)

Extraction Method: Cold expressed from rind

Common Primary Uses*: 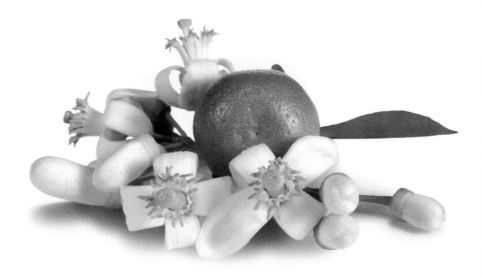Anxiety[168], Digestion (Sluggish), Fear, Heart Palpitations, Insomnia, Menopause, Nervousness, Uplifting, Withdrawal

Common Application Methods‡:

: Can be applied neat (with no dilution) when used topically. Apply directly on area of concern or to reflex points. Avoid direct sunlight for up to 12 hours after using on skin.

: Diffuse, or inhale the aroma directly.

: Place 1–2 drops under the tongue, or take in a beverage. Take in capsules. Use as a flavoring in cooking.

Properties: Anticancer[169], antidepressant, antiseptic, antispasmodic, digestive, sedative[170], and tonic.

Historical Uses: Oranges, particularly the bitter oranges, have been used for palpitation, scurvy, jaundice, bleeding, heartburn, relaxed throat, prolapse of the uterus and the anus, diarrhea, and blood in the feces.

Other Possible Uses: This oil may help appetite, bones (rickety), bronchitis, colds, colic (dilute for infants; helps them sleep), complexion (dull and oily), dermatitis, digestive system, fever, flu, lower high cholesterol, mouth ulcers, muscle soreness, obesity, sedation, tissue repair, water retention, and wrinkles.

Body System(s) Affected: Digestive and Immune Systems, Emotional Balance, Skin.

Aromatic Influence: Orange is calming and uplifting to the mind and body.

Oral Use As Dietary Supplement: Orange oil is generally recognized as safe (GRAS) for human consumption by the FDA (21CFR182.20). Dilute 1 drop oil in 1 tsp. (5 ml) honey or in ½ cup (125 ml) of beverage (e.g., soy/rice milk). Not for children under 6 years old; use with caution and in greater dilution for children 6 years old and over.

Safety Data: Avoid direct sunlight for up to 12 hours after use.

Blend Classification: Enhancer and Personifier.

Blends With: Cinnamon, frankincense, geranium, and lavender.

Odor: Type: Top Note (5–20% of the blend); Scent: Fresh, citrusy, fruity, sweet; Intensity: 1.

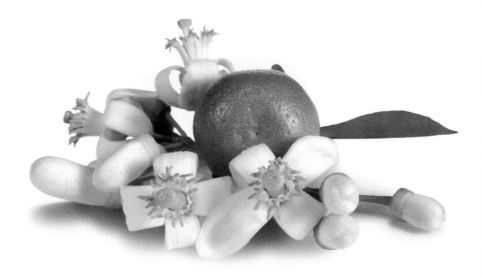

Oregano *Origanum vulgare*

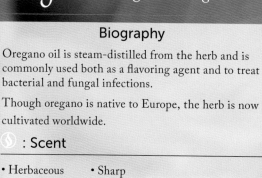

ESSENTIAL
Essentials
Oregano

Biography

Oregano oil is steam-distilled from the herb and is commonly used both as a flavoring agent and to treat bacterial and fungal infections.

Though oregano is native to Europe, the herb is now cultivated worldwide.

Ⓢ : Scent

- Herbaceous
- Sharp

✚ : Body Systems Affected

Immune System

Respiratory System

Muscles and Bones

Top Uses

Antibacterial: Mix 1 drop oregano with 3 drops carrier oil, and apply to liver area and bottoms of the feet.

Antifungal: Diffuse oregano in an aromatherapy diffuser to fight fungal infections.

Warts: For plantar warts, add 1–2 drops oregano to a few drops fractionated coconut oil. Apply 1–2 drops of mixture on location daily.

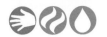

Quick Facts

Botanical Family: Labiatae

Extraction Method: Steam distillation from herb

Common Primary Uses*: 🜨🜨Athlete's Foot, 🜨Calluses, 🜨OCandida, 🜨Canker Sores, 🜨Carpal Tunnel Syndrome, 🜨Ebola Virus, 🜨🜨OFungal Infections, 🜨🜨OImmune System (Stimulates), 🜨Inflammation[171], O🜨Intestinal Parasites, 🜨MRSA, 🜨Muscle Aches, 🜨🜨Nasal Polyp, O🜨Parasites, 🜨🜨Plague, 🜨🜨Pneumonia, 🜨🜨Ringworm, 🜨OStaph Infection, 🜨OVaginal Candida, 🜨Viral Infections, 🜨Warming (Body), 🜨Warts, 🜨Whooping Cough

Common Application Methods‡:

🜨: Dilute 1:3 (1 drop essential oil to at least 3 drops carrier oil) when used topically. Dilute more heavily for children over 6 or for those with sensitive skin. Apply directly on area of concern or to reflex points.

🜨: Diffuse, or inhale the aroma directly.

O: Dilute and take in capsules. Use as a flavoring in cooking.

Properties: Antibacterial[172], antifungal[173], anti-parasitic[174], antiseptic to the respiratory system, antiviral, and immune stimulant[175].

Other Possible Uses: This oil may help colds, digestive problems, metabolic balance, obesity[176], viral and bacterial pneumonia, and strengthen vital centers.

Body System(s) Affected: Immune, Skeletal, and Respiratory Systems and Muscles.

Aromatic Influence: Strengthens one's feeling of security.

Oral Use As Dietary Supplement: Oregano oil is generally recognized as safe (GRAS) for human consumption by the FDA (21CFR182.20). Dilute 1 drop oil in 1 tsp. (5 ml) honey or in ½ cup (125 ml) of beverage (e.g., soy/rice milk). Not for children under 6 years old; use with caution and in greater dilution for children 6 years old and over.

Safety Data: Can cause extreme skin irritation.

Blend Classification: Enhancer and Equalizer.

Blends With: Basil, fennel, geranium, lemongrass, thyme, and rosemary.

Odor: Type: Middle Note (50–80% of the blend); Scent: Herbaceous, sharp; Intensity: 5.

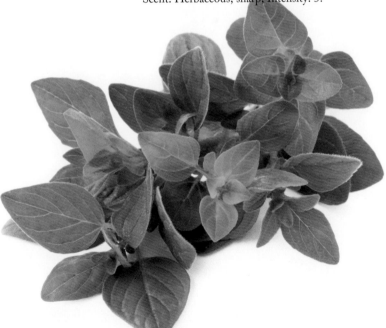

‡See Application section beginning on page 14 for more details.   🜨=Topical, 🜨=Aromatic, O=Internal

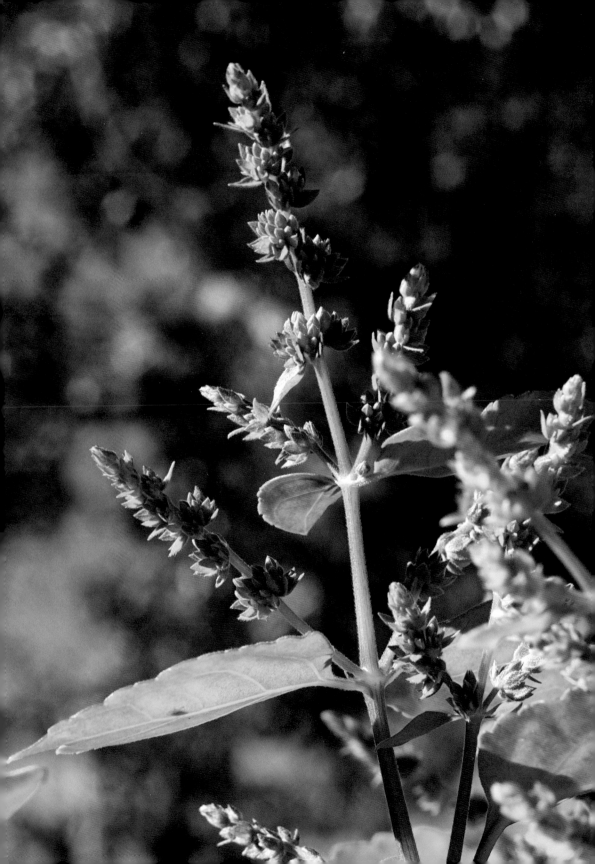

Patchouli (or Patchouly) *Pogostemon cablin*

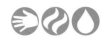

Properties: Anti-infectious, anti-inflammatory, anti-fungal, antiseptic, antitoxic, astringent, decongestant, deodorant, diuretic, insecticidal[177], stimulant (digestive), and tonic.

Historical Uses: For centuries, the Asian people used patchouli to fight infection, cool fevers, tone the skin (and entire body), and to act as an antidote for insect and snake bites. It was also used to treat colds, headaches, nausea, vomiting, diarrhea, abdominal pain, and halitosis (bad breath).

Other Possible Uses: This oil is a digester of toxic material in the body. It may also help acne, appetite (curbs), bites (insect and snake), cellulite, congestion, dandruff, depression, digestive system, relieve itching from hives, mastitis[178], skin conditions (chapped and tightens loose skin), UV radiation (protects against)[179], water retention, weeping wounds, weight reduction, and wrinkles prevention.

✴ **Body System(s) Affected:** Skin.

Aromatic Influence: It is sedating, calming[180], and relaxing—allowing it to reduce anxiety. It may have some particular influence on sex, physical energy, and money.

Oral Use As Dietary Supplement: Patchouli oil in general is approved by the FDA for use as a Food Additive (FA) and Flavoring Agent (FL). Dilute 1 drop oil in 1 tsp. (5 ml) honey or in ½ cup (125 ml) of beverage (e.g., soy/rice milk). Not for children under 6 years old; use with caution and in greater dilution for children 6 years old and over.

Blend Classification: Enhancer

Blends With: Bergamot, clary sage, frankincense, geranium, ginger, lavender, lemongrass, myrrh, pine, rosewood, sandalwood.

Odor: Type: Base Note (5–20% of the blend); Scent: Earthy, herbaceous, sweet-balsamic, rich, with woody undertones; Intensity: 4.

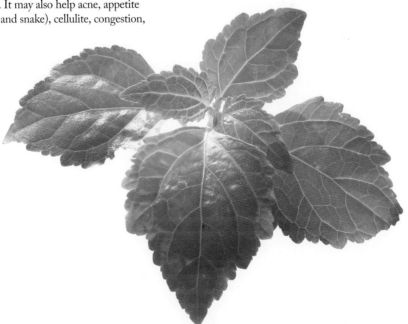

Peppermint *Mentha piperita*

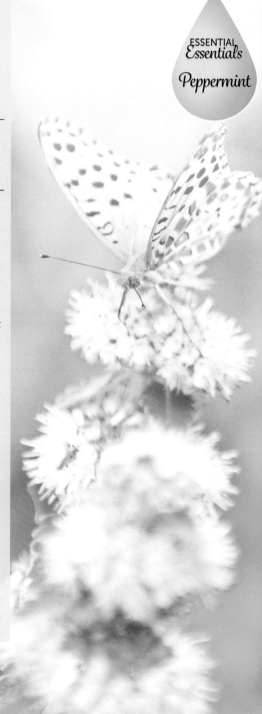

ESSENTIAL
Essentials

Peppermint

Biography

A favorite for varying concerns, peppermint oil is steam-distilled from the flowering herb.

Peppermint is grown worldwide and has been cultivated for centuries by many different peoples and cultures.

Ⓢ : Scent

- Minty
- Sharp

🜨 : Body Systems Affected

- Digestive System
- Muscles and Bones
- Nervous System
- Skin

Top Uses

Alertness/Endurance: Drop 3–4 drops peppermint on the shower floor when showering in the morning to help invigorate. Inhale the aroma of peppermint while driving to help stay alert.

Allergies: Blend 2 drops each of lavender, lemon, and peppermint oil in 1 tsp. (5 ml) fractionated coconut oil, and apply a small amount on the temples, under the nose, and on the bottoms of the feet morning and evening when dealing with seasonal allergies.

Cooling: Blend 2 drops peppermint with 2 drops eucalyptus in a bowl of cool water. Moisten a washcloth with water and use to sponge the forehead, back of neck, and feet.

Headache: Apply 1 drop each of lavender, peppermint, and frankincense to the forehead and back of the neck.

Nausea: Inhale the aroma of peppermint oil directly from the bottle.

Congestion: Drop 2 drops eucalyptus and 1 drop peppermint on the floor of the shower while showering, and inhale the vapors.

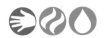

Quick Facts

Botanical Family: Labiatae (mint)

Extraction Method: Steam distillation from leaves

Common Primary Uses*: 🍃💧Alertness, 🌿🍃💧Antioxidant, 🍃💧Asthma, 🍃Autism, 🍃Bacterial Infections, 🍃💧Bell's Palsy, 🍃💧Brain Injury, 🍃💧Chronic Fatigue, 🍃Cold Sores, 🌿🍃Colon Polyps, 🍃💧Congestion, 🍃Constipation, 🍃💧Cooling (Body), 🍃Cramps/Charley Horses, 🍃🌿Crohn's Disease, 🌿🍃Diarrhea, 🍃Dysmenorrhea, 💧Endurance⚕[181], 💧Fainting, 🌿🍃💧Fever, 🍃💧🌿Flu (Influenza), 🌿🍃Gamma Radiation Exposure⚕[182], 🍃🌿Gastritis, 🍃Halitosis, 🍃💧Headaches⚕[183], 🍃Heartburn, 🍃Heatstroke, 🍃Hernia (Hiatal), 🍃Herpes Simplex, 🍃Hives, 🍃Hot Flashes, 🍃💧Huntington's Disease, 🍃💧Hypothyroidism, 🌿🍃💧Indigestion, 🌿🍃Irritable Bowel Syndrome⚕[184], 🍃Itching, 🍃Jet Lag, 🍃Lactation (Decrease Milk Production), 🍃💧Memory⚕[185], 🍃💧Migraines, 💧Motion Sickness, 🍃MRSA, 🍃💧Multiple Sclerosis, 🍃Muscle Aches, 🍃Muscle Fatigue, 🍃💧Myelin Sheath, 💧Nausea⚕[186], 🍃💧Olfactory Loss (Sense of Smell), 🍃Osteoporosis, 🍃💧Paralysis, 🍃💧Rhinitis, 🍃Scabies, 🍃Sciatica, 🍃💧Shock, 🍃💧Sinusitis, 🍃Surgical Wounds, 🍃Swollen Eyes, 🍃Tennis Elbow, 🍃🌿💧Throat Infection, 🍃💧Typhoid, 🌿🍃Ulcer (Gastric), 🍃Varicose Veins, 🌿🍃💧Vomiting

Common Application Methods‡:

🍃: Can be applied neat (with no dilution), or dilute 1:1 (1 drop essential oil to 1 drop carrier oil) for children and for those with sensitive skin when using topically. Apply directly on area of concern or to reflex points.

🌿: Diffuse, or inhale the aroma directly.

💧: Place 1–2 drops under the tongue or in a beverage. Take in capsules. Use as a flavoring in cooking.

Properties: Analgesic, antibacterial⚕[187], anticarcinogenic, anti-inflammatory⚕[188], antiseptic, antispasmodic⚕[189], antiviral⚕[190], and invigorating.

Historical Uses: For centuries, peppermint has been used to soothe digestive difficulties, freshen breath, and to relieve colic, gas, headaches, heartburn, and indigestion.

Other Possible Uses: This oil may help anger, arthritis, colic, depression, fatigue, food poisoning, hysteria, inflammation, liver problems, nerves⚕[191] (regenerate and support), rheumatism, seizures⚕[192], elevate and open sensory system, soothe and cool skin (may help keep body cooler on hot days), toothaches, tuberculosis, and add flavor to water.

Body System(s) Affected: Nervous, Digestive, Respiratory, and Skeletal Systems, Muscles, and Skin.

Aromatic Influence: It is purifying and stimulating to the conscious mind and may aid with memory and mental performance. It is cooling and may help reduce fevers.

Oral Use As Dietary Supplement: Peppermint oil is generally recognized as safe (GRAS) for human consumption by the FDA (21CFR182.20). Dilute 1 drop oil in 1 tsp. (5 ml) honey or in ½ cup (125 ml) of beverage (e.g., soy/rice milk). Not for children under 6 years old; use with caution and in greater dilution for children 6 years old and over.

Safety Data: Repeated use can possibly result in contact sensitization. Use with caution if dealing with high blood pressure. Use with caution during pregnancy.

Blend Classification: Personifier

Blends With: Basil, black pepper, cinnamon, cypress, dill, grapefruit, juniper berry, lavender, lemon, rosemary, spearmint, tea tree.

Odor: Type: Middle Note (50–80% of the blend); Scent: Minty, sharp, intense; Intensity: 5.

Petitgrain *Citrus aurantium*

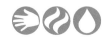

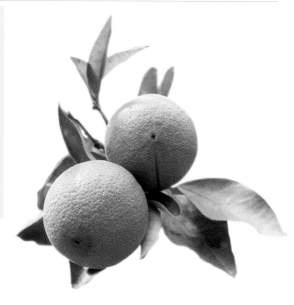

Properties: Antibacterial[193], anti-infectious, anti-inflammatory, antioxidant[194], antiseptic, antispasmodic, deodorant, and stimulant (digestive, nervous).

Historical Uses: Petitgrain (from the French term *petit grain*, meaning "small grain") derives its name from the extraction of the oil, which at one time was from the green unripe oranges when they were still about the size of a cherry. This oil is now derived from the plant's leaves. Because of its very pleasing scent, petitgrain has been used extensively in high-quality perfumes and cosmetics.

Other Possible Uses: This oil may help with acne, dyspepsia, fatigue, flatulence, greasy hair, insomnia, and excessive perspiration.

🌐 **Body System(s) Affected:** Emotional Balance.

Aromatic Influence: Petitgrain is uplifting and refreshing and helps to refresh the senses, clear confusion, reduce mental fatigue, and reduce depression. It may also help stimulate the mind, support memory, and gladden the heart.

Oral Use As Dietary Supplement: Petitgrain is generally regarded as safe (GRAS) for use in small amounts as a flavoring or additive in foods by the FDA. Dilute 1 drop oil in 1 tsp. (5 ml) honey or in ½ cup (125 ml) of beverage (e.g., soy/rice milk). Not for children under 6 years old; use with caution and in greater dilution for children 6 years old and over.

Safety Data: May cause slight skin irritation in some individuals.

Blend Classification: Enhancer, Modifier, and Personifier.

Blends With: Bergamot, clary sage, clove, geranium, jasmine, lavender, orange, and rosemary.

Odor: Type: Top Note (5–20% of the blend); Scent: Fresh, floral, citrusy, lighter in fragrance than neroli and slightly woody; Intensity: 3.

Pink Pepper *Schinus molle*

Quick Facts

Botanical Family: Anacardiaceae

Extraction Method: Steam distillation from fruit

Common Primary Uses*: 🖐️🌀Alertness, 🖐️🌀Antibacterial💧[195], 🖐️🌀Cleaning

Common Application Methods‡:

🖐️: Can be applied neat (with no dilution) when used topically. Apply directly on area of concern or to reflex points.

🌀: Diffuse, or inhale the aroma directly.

💧: Add 1 drop to 1 cup (250 ml) of water, tea, or other beverage.

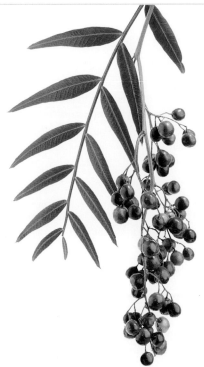

Properties: Antibacterial, antifungal, anti-inflammatory, antitumor, antiviral, antimicrobial, antispasmodic, astringent, diuretic, stimulant (digestive), and wound healing.

Historical Uses: According to Leslie Taylor, ND, "Virtually all parts of this tropical tree, including its leaves, bark, fruit, seeds, resin, and oleoresin (or balsam), have been used medicinally by indigenous peoples throughout the tropics."

Other Possible Uses: This oil may help with bronchitis, cancer💧[196], diabetes (high blood sugar), gingivitis, gonorrhea, gout, heart problems (hypertension and irregular heart beat), inflammation (general), insects (repellent)💧[197], menstrual disorders (excessive bleeding), pain relief, rheumatism, sores, swelling, tuberculosis, tumors, ulcers, urethritis, urogenital disorders, venereal diseases, warts, and wounds.

⊕ Body System(s) Affected: Immune System, Respiratory System, Skin.

Aromatic Influence: Pink pepper has a warm, spicy aroma that can help increase alertness.

Oral Use As Dietary Supplement: Pink pepper oil is generally regarded as safe (GRAS) for human consumption by the FDA. Dilute 1 drop oil in 1 tsp. (5 ml) honey or in 1 cup (250 ml) of beverage (e.g., soy/rice milk). Not for children under 6 years old; use with caution and in greater dilution for children 6 years old and over.

Safety Data: May irritate highly sensitive skin. Consult with a physician before using if taking medications, pregnant, or nursing.

Blends With: Fennel, frankincense, lavender, marjoram, rosemary, sandalwood, and other spice oils.

Odor: Type: Middle Note (50–80% of the blend); Scent: spicy, fruity, with slight woody undertone; Intensity: 3.

Roman Chamomile *Cham. nobile or Anth. nobilis*

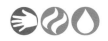

Quick Facts

Botanical Family: Compositae (daisy)

Extraction Method: Steam distillation from flowers

Common Primary Uses*: ⬤Bee/Hornet Stings, ⬤⬤Calming⬤[198], ⬤Club Foot, ⬤Dysentery, ⬤⬤Hyperactivity, ⬤⬤Insomnia, ⬤Menopause, ⬤Muscle Spasms, ⬤Neuralgia, ⬤Neuritis, ⬤⬤Parasites, ⬤Rashes, ⬤Sciatica, ⬤Shock, ⬤Skin (Dry), ⬤Sore Nipples

Common Application Methods‡:

⬤: Can be applied neat (with no dilution), or dilute 1:1 (1 drop essential oil to 1 drop carrier oil) for children and for those with sensitive skin when using topically.

⬤: Diffuse, or inhale the aroma directly.

⬤: Take in capsules.

Properties: Anti-infectious, anti-inflammatory⬤[199], antiparasitic, antispasmodic⬤[200], calming, and relaxing.

Historical Uses: It was traditionally used by the ancient Romans to give them a clear mind and to empower them with courage for their battles. According to Roberta Wilson, "Chamomile was nicknamed the 'plant's physician' because it supposedly cured any ailing plant placed near it."

Other Possible Uses: Chamomile neutralizes allergies and increases the ability of the skin to regenerate. It is a cleanser of the blood and also helps the liver to reject poisons and to discharge them. This oil may help with allergies, bruises, cuts, depression, insomnia, muscle tension, nerves (calming and promoting nerve health), restless legs, and skin conditions such as acne, boils, dermatitis, eczema, rashes, and sensitive skin. Chamomile is mild enough to use on infants and children. For centuries, mothers have used chamomile to calm crying children, ease earaches, fight fevers, soothe stomachaches and colic, and relieve toothaches and teething pain. It can safely and effectively reduce irritability and minimize nervousness in children, especially hyperactive children.

⬤ **Body System(s) Affected:** Emotional Balance, Nervous System, Skin.

Aromatic Influence: Because it is calming and relaxing, it can combat depression, insomnia⬤, and stress. It eliminates some of the emotional charge of anxiety, irritability, and nervousness. It may also be used to soothe and clear the mind, creating an atmosphere of peace and patience.

Oral Use As Dietary Supplement: Roman chamomile oil is generally recognized as safe (GRAS) for human consumption by the FDA (21CFR182.20). Dilute 1 drop oil in 1 tsp. (5 ml) honey or in ½ cup (125 ml) of beverage (e.g., soy/rice milk). Not for children under 6 years old; use with caution and in greater dilution for children 6 years old and over.

Safety Data: Can irritate sensitive skin.

Blend Classification: Personifier

Blends With: Lavender, rose, geranium, and clary sage.

Odor: Type: Middle Note (50–80% of the blend); Scent: Fresh, sweet, fruity-herbaceous, apple-like, no tenacity; Intensity: 4.

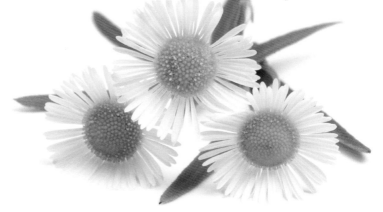

*See My Usage Guide section for more details.   ⬤=Neat, ⬤=Dilute for Children/Sensitive Skin, ⬤=Dilute

Rose Rosa damascena

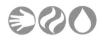

Quick Facts

Botanical Family: Rosaceae

Extraction Method: Steam distillation from flowers (a two-part process)

Common Primary Uses*: 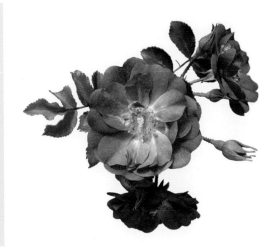Anxiety[201], Aphrodisiac, Poison Ivy/Oak, Scarring (Prevention)

Common Application Methods‡:

- : Can be applied neat (with no dilution) when used topically. Apply directly on area of concern or to reflex points.

- : Diffuse, or inhale the aroma directly.

- : Take in capsules. Use as a flavoring in cooking.

Properties: Antihemorrhagic, anti-infectious, aphrodisiac, and sedative[202].

Historical Uses: The healing properties of the rose have been utilized in medicine throughout the ages and still play an important role in the East. Rose has been used for digestive[203] and menstrual problems[204], headaches and nervous tension, liver congestion, poor circulation, fever (plague), eye infections, and skin complaints.

Other Possible Uses: This oil may help aging[205], asthma, chronic bronchitis, frigidity, gingivitis, hemorrhaging, herpes simplex, impotence, infections, lower back pain (pregnancey)[206], opioid addiction[207], prevent scarring, seizures[208], sexual debilities, skin disease, sprains, thrush, tuberculosis, ulcers, wounds, and wrinkles.

Body System(s) Affected: Emotional Balance, Skin.

Aromatic Influence: It is stimulating and elevating to the mind, creating a sense of well-being. Its beautiful fragrance is almost intoxicating and aphrodisiac-like.

Oral Use As Dietary Supplement: Rose oil is generally recognized as safe (GRAS) for human consumption by the FDA (21CFR182.20). Dilute 1 drop oil in 1 tsp. (5 ml) honey or in ½ cup (125 ml) of beverage (e.g., soy/rice milk). Not for children under 6 years old; use with caution and in greater dilution for children 6 years old and over.

Safety Data: Use with caution during pregnancy.

Blend Classification: Personifier, Enhancer, Equalizer, and Modifier

Blends With: bergamot, cedarwood, cinnamon, clary sage, clove, fennel, frankincense, geranium, jasmine, lavender, melissa, myrrh, patchouli, petitgrain, vetiver, ylang ylang.

Odor: Type: Middle to Base Notes (20–80% of the blend); Scent: Floral, spicy, rich, deep, sensual, green, honey-like; Intensity: 3.

Rosemary *Rosmarinus officinalis CT 1,8 Cineol*

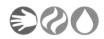

Quick Facts

Botanical Family: Labiatae (mint)

Extraction Method: Steam distillation from flowering plant

Common Primary Uses*: Addictions (Alcohol), Adenitis, Antioxidant, Arterial Vasodilator, Arthritis, Bell's Palsy, Cancer, Cellulite, Chemical Stress, Cholera, Club Foot, Constipation, Detoxification, Diabetes, Diuretic, Fainting, Fatigue, Flu (Influenza), Greasy/Oily Hair, Hair (Loss), Headaches, Inflammation, Kidney Infection, Lice, Low Blood Pressure[209], Memory, Muscular Dystrophy, Osteoarthritis, Schmidt's Syndrome, Sinusitis, Vaginal Infection, Vaginitis, Viral Hepatitis, Worms

Common Application Methods‡:

- : Can be applied neat (with no dilution), or dilute 1:1 (1 drop essential oil to 1 drop carrier oil) for children and for those with sensitive skin when used topically. Apply directly on area of concern or to reflex points. Avoid use during pregnancy.

- : Diffuse, or inhale the aroma directly.

- : Take in capsules, or place 1–2 drops under the tongue. Use as a flavoring in cooking.

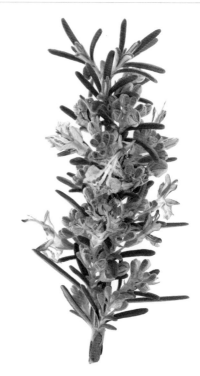

Properties: Analgesic[210], antibacterial[211], anticancer[212], anticatarrhal, antifungal[213], anti-infectious, anti-inflammatory[214], antioxidant[215], and expectorant.

Historical Uses: The rosemary plant was regarded as sacred by many civilizations. It was used as a fumigant to help drive away evil spirits and to protect against plague and infectious illness.

Other Possible Uses: This oil may help arteriosclerosis, bronchitis, chills, colds, colitis, cystitis, dyspepsia, nervous exhaustion, immune system (stimulate), otitis, palpitations, prevent respiratory infections, sour stomach, stress-related illness[216]. Note: This chemotype is said to be best used for pulmonary congestion, slow elimination, candida, chronic fatigue, and infections (especially staph and strep).

Body System(s) Affected: Immune, Respiratory, and Nervous Systems.

Aromatic Influence: Stimulates memory[217] and opens the conscious mind.

Oral Use As Dietary Supplement: Rosemary oil is generally recognized as safe (GRAS) for human consumption by the FDA (21CFR182.20). Dilute 1 drop oil in 1 tsp. (5 ml) honey or in ½ cup (125 ml) of beverage (e.g., soy/rice milk). Not for children under 6 years old; use with caution and in greater dilution for children 6 years old and over.

Safety Data: Avoid during pregnancy. Not for use by people with epilepsy. Avoid if dealing with high blood pressure.

Blend Classification: Enhancer

Blends With: Basil, frankincense, lavender, peppermint, eucalyptus, and marjoram.

Odor: Type: Middle Note (50–80% of the blend); Scent: Herbaceous, strong, camphorous, with woody-balsamic and evergreen undertones; Intensity: 3.

*See My Usage Guide section for more details.   =Neat, =Dilute for Children/Sensitive Skin, =Dilute

Sandalwood *Santalum album*

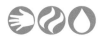

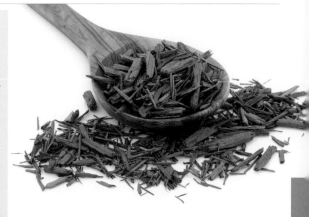

Quick Facts

Botanical Family: Santalaceae (sandalwood)

Extraction Method: Steam distillation from wood

Common Primary Uses*: 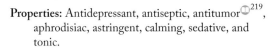Alzheimer's Disease[218], Aphrodisiac, Back Pain, Cancer, Cartilage Repair, Coma, Confusion, Exhaustion, Fear, Hair (Dry), Hiccups, Laryngitis, Lou Gehrig's Disease, Meditation, Moles, Multiple Sclerosis, Rashes, Skin (Dry), Ultraviolet Radiation, Vitiligo, Yoga

Common Application Methods‡:

- : Can be applied neat (with no dilution) when used topically. Apply directly on area of concern or to reflex points.

- : Diffuse, or inhale the aroma directly.

- : Take in capsules.

Properties: Antidepressant, antiseptic, antitumor[219], aphrodisiac, astringent, calming, sedative, and tonic.

Historical Uses: Sandalwood was traditionally used as an incense during ritual work for enhancing meditation. The Egyptians also used sandalwood for embalming.

Other Possible Uses: Sandalwood is very similar to frankincense in action. It may support the cardiovascular system and relieve symptoms associated with lumbago and the sciatic nerves. It may also be beneficial for acne, regenerating bone cartilage, catarrh, circulation (similar in action to frankincense), coughs, cystitis, depression, hiccups, lymphatic system, menstrual problems, nerves (similar in action to frankincense), nervous tension, increasing oxygen around the pineal and pituitary glands, skin infection and regeneration, and tuberculosis.

Body System(s) Affected: Emotional Balance, Muscles, Nervous and Skeletal Systems, and Skin.

Aromatic Influence: Calms, harmonizes, and balances the emotions. It may help enhance meditation.

Oral Use As Dietary Supplement: Sandalwood oil in general is approved by the FDA (21CFR172.510) for use as a Food Additive (FA) and Flavoring Agent (FL). Dilute 1 drop oil in 1 tsp. (5 ml) honey or in ½ cup (125 ml) of beverage (e.g., soy/rice milk). Not for children under 6 years old; use with caution and in greater dilution for children 6 years old and over.

Blend Classification: Modifier and Equalizer

Blends With: Cypress, frankincense, lemon, myrrh, and ylang ylang.

Odor: Type: Base Note (5–20% of the blend); Scent: Soft, woody, sweet, earthy, balsamic, tenacious; Intensity: 3.

‡See Application section beginning on page 14 for more details.   =Topical, =Aromatic, =Internal

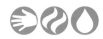

Quick Facts

Botanical Family: Pinaceae (conifer)

Extraction Method: Steam distillation from needles and twigs

Common Primary Uses*: Bronchitis, Bursitis, Cartilage Inflammation, Cleaning, Emotional Balance, Energizing, Frozen Shoulder, Furniture Polish, Massage (soothing), Muscle Fatigue, Muscle Pain, Overexercised Muscles, Relaxing, Sprains

Common Application Methods‡:

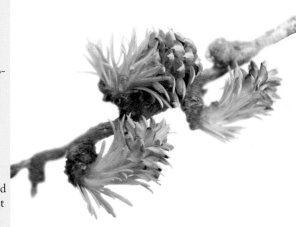

: Can be applied neat (with no dilution) when used topically. Dilute 1:1 (1 drop essential oil to at least 1 drop carrier oil) for children and for those with sensitive skin. Apply directly on area of concern or to reflex points.

: Diffuse, or inhale the aroma directly.

: Take in capsules, or take 1 drop in a beverage.

Properties: Analgesic, antiarthritic, anticatarrhal, antiseptic (pulmonary), expectorant, and stimulant.

Historical Uses: Siberian fir is found throughout the cold taiga forest in northern Eurasia and North America. Though highly regarded for its fragrant scent, the fir tree has been prized through the ages for its medicinal virtues in regards to respiratory complaints, fever, and muscular and rheumatic pain.

French Medicinal Uses: Bronchitis 220, respiratory congestion, energy.

Other Possible Uses: Fir creates the symbolic effect of an umbrella protecting the earth and bringing energy in from the universe. At night the animals in the wild lie down under the tree for the protection, recharging, and rejuvenation the trees bring them. Fir may be beneficial for reducing aches/pains from colds and the flu, fighting airborne germs/bacteria, arthritis, asthma, supporting the blood, bronchial obstructions, coughs, fevers, oxygenating the cells, rheumatism, sinusitis, and urinary tract infections.

Body System(s) Affected: Respiratory System.

Aromatic Influence: It creates a feeling of grounding, anchoring, and empowerment. It can stimulate the mind while allowing the body to relax.

Oral Use As Dietary Supplement: Siberian fir oil is approved by the FDA (21CFR172.510) for use as a Food Additive (FA) and Flavoring Agent (FL). Dilute 1 drop oil in 1 tsp. (5 ml) honey or in ½ cup (125 ml) of beverage (e.g., soy/rice milk). Not for children under 6 years old; use with caution and in greater dilution for children 6 years old and over.

Safety Data: Can irritate sensitive skin.

Blend Classification: Equalizer.

Blends With: Frankincense and lavender.

Odor: Type: Middle Notes (50–80% of the blend); Scent: Fresh, woody, earthy, sweet; Intensity: 3.

Spearmint *Mentha spicata*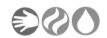

Properties: Antibacterial⊡[221], anticatarrhal, antifungal, anti-inflammatory, antiseptic, antispasmodic, hormone-like, insecticidal, and stimulant.

Historical Uses: Spearmint has been used to relieve hiccough, colic, nausea, indigestion, flatulence, headaches, sores, and scabs.

Other Possible Uses: This oil may help balance and increase metabolism, which may help burn up fats and toxins in the body. It may aid the glandular, nervous, and respiratory systems. It may also help with acne, appetite (stimulates), arthritis (pain)⊡[222], bad breath, balance, childbirth (promotes easier labor), constipation, depression, diarrhea, digestion, dry skin, eczema, fevers, headaches, intestines (soothes), kidney stones, menstruation (slow, heavy periods), migraines, nausea, sore gums, stomach (relaxes muscles), urine retention, vaginitis, weight (reduces), and bring about a feeling of well-being.

Body System(s) Affected: Digestive System, Emotional Balance.

Aromatic Influence: Its hormone-like activity may help open and release emotional blocks to bring about a feeling of balance. It acts as an antidepressant by relieving mental strain and fatigue, and by lifting one's spirits.

Oral Use As Dietary Supplement: Generally regarded as safe (GRAS) for human consumption by the FDA. Dilute 1 drop oil in 1 tsp. (5 ml) honey or in ½ cup (125 ml) of beverage (e.g., soy/rice milk). Not for children under 6 years old; use with caution and in greater dilution for children 6 years old and over.

Safety Data: Use with caution during pregnancy. Not for use on babies.

Blend Classification: Personifier

Blends With: Basil, lavender, peppermint, rosemary.

Odor: Top Note (5–20% of the blend); Scent: Minty, slightly fruity, less bright than peppermint; Intensity: 3.

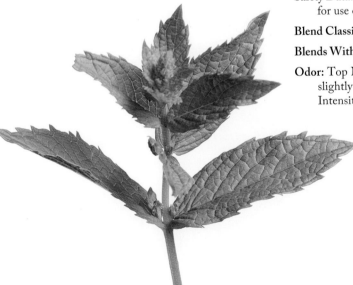

Spikenard *Nardostachys jatamansi*

Quick Facts

Botanical Family: Valerianaceae

Extraction Method: Steam distillation from rhizomes

Common Primary Uses*: ⬤Aging Skin, ⬤⬤Insomnia, ⬤⬤Nervousness, ⬤Perfume, ⬤Rashes

Common Application Methods‡:

⬤: Can be applied neat (with no dilution) when used topically. Apply directly on area of concern or to reflex points.

⬤: Diffuse, or inhale the aroma directly.

Properties: Antibacterial, antifungal, anti-inflammatory, antioxidant⬤[223], deodorant, relaxing, and skin tonic.

Historical Uses: Spikenard gets its name from the spike-shaped rhizomes (or "spikes") of the plant that the oil is distilled from. Highly prized in the Middle East during the time of Christ, spikenard is referred to several times in the Bible. Spikenard was also used in the preparation of nardinum, a scented oil of great renown during ancient times. Prized in early Egypt, it was used in a preparation called *kyphi* with other oils like saffron, juniper, myrrh, cassia, and cinnamon.

Other Possible Uses: The oil is known for helping in the treatment of allergic skin reactions, and according to Victoria Edwards, "The oil redresses the skin's physiological balance and causes permanent regeneration." Spikenard may also help with allergies, candida, flatulent indigestion, insomnia, menstrual difficulties, migraine, nausea, neurological diseases⬤, rashes, staph infections, stress, tachycardia⬤, tension, and wounds that will not heal.

🜨 **Body System(s) Affected:** Emotional Balance, Skin.

Aromatic Influence: Spikenard has an earthy, animal-like fragrance. It is balancing, soothing, and harmonizing.

Oral Use As Dietary Supplement: None.

Blend Classification: Modifier and Personifier.

Blends With: lavender, patchouli, pine, and vetiver.

Odor: Base Note (5–20% of the blend); Scent: Heavy, earthy, animal-like, similar to valerian; Intensity: 5.

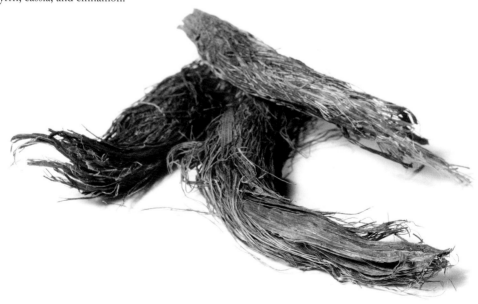

Star Anise *Illicium verum*

Quick Facts

Botanical Family: Illiciaceae

Extraction Method: Steam distillation from the fruit, seed, and leaf

Common Primary Uses*: ⬤Colic, ⬤⬤Flatulence, ⬤⬤⬤Indigestion, ⬤⬤⬤Relaxing

Common Application Methods‡:

⬤: Can be applied neat (with no dilution) when used topically. Apply directly on area of concern or to reflex points. Use in a massage oil.

⬤: Diffuse, or inhale the aroma directly.

⬤: Add 1 drop to 1 cup (250 ml) of warm water, tea, or other beverage.

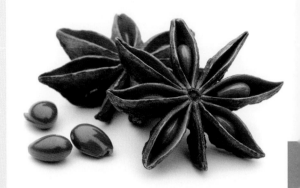

Properties: Antifungal⬤[224], antiseptic, antispasmodic, estrogen-like, diuretic, stimulant (heart), and tonic (heart).

Historical Uses: Native to Asia, star anise has been used for centuries in Chinese medicine to help with various digestive issues such as indigestion, flatulence, colic, and cramping. It has also been used to help with back pain and rheumatism.

Other Possible Uses: This oil may be beneficial for bronchitis, colitis, constipation, digestion (accelerates), diverticulitis, estrogen (increases), fertility, flatulence, hormonal imbalance, irritable bowel syndrome, menopause, parasites, PMS, prostate cancer (blend with frankincense), and respiratory system (strengthens).

Body System(s) Affected: Cardiovascular System, Digestive System, Hormonal System, Respiratory System.

Aromatic Influence: The aroma of star anise is grounding and balancing to the emotions.

Oral Use As Dietary Supplement: Star anise oil is generally regarded as safe (GRAS) for human consumption by the FDA. Dilute 1 drop oil in 1 tsp. (5 ml) honey or in ½ cup (125 ml) of beverage (e.g., soy/rice milk). Not for children under 6 years old; use with caution and in greater dilution for children 6 years old and over.

Safety Data: May irritate highly sensitive skin. Consult with a physician before use if taking medications, pregnant, or nursing.

Blends With: Bergamot, black pepper, blue tansy, fennel, ginger, juniper berry, lemongrass, patchouli, peppermint, tangerine, tarragon, and ylang ylang.

Odor: Type: Top to Middle Note (20–80% of the blend); Scent: Sweet, licorice-like, spicy, warm, slightly balsamic; Intensity: 4.

Tangerine *Citrus reticulata*

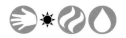

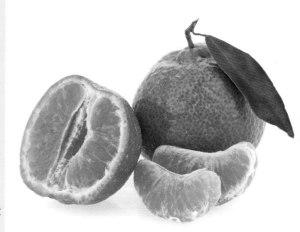

Quick Facts

Botanical Family: Rutaceae (citrus)

Extraction Method: Cold expressed from rind

Common Primary Uses*: ⭕Cooking, ✹✹Calming, ✹✹Uplifting

Common Application Methods‡:

✹: Can be applied neat (with no dilution) when used topically. Apply directly on area of concern or to reflex points. Avoid direct sunlight or UV light for up to 12 hours after using on the skin.

✹: Diffuse, or inhale the aroma directly.

⭕: Take in capsules or in a beverage. Use as a flavoring in cooking.

Properties: Anticoagulant, anti-inflammatory, laxative, and sedative.

Other Possible Uses: It may help cellulite (dissolve), circulation, constipation, diarrhea, digestive system disorders, fat digestion, dizziness, fear, flatulence, gallbladder, insomnia, intestinal spasms, irritability, limbs (tired and aching), liver problems, decongest the lymphatic system (helps to stimulate draining), obesity, parasites, sadness, the stomach (tonic), stretch marks (smooths when blended with lavender), stress, swelling, and help alleviate water retention (edema).

Body System(s) Affected: Emotional Balance, Immune System, Skin.

Aromatic Influence: Tangerine oil contains esters and aldehydes, which are sedating and calming to the nervous system. When diffused together with marjoram, tangerine can soothe emotions such as grief, anger, and shock.

Oral Use As Dietary Supplement: Tangerine oil is generally regarded as safe (GRAS) for human consumption by the FDA. Dilute 1 drop oil in 1 tsp. (5 ml) honey or in ½ cup (125 ml) of beverage (e.g., soy/rice milk). Not for children under 6 years old; use with caution and in greater dilution for children 6 years old and over.

Blend Classification: Modifier and Personifier

Blends With: Basil, bergamot, clary sage, frankincense, geranium, grapefruit, lavender, lemon, orange, and Roman chamomile.

Odor: Top Note (5–20% of the blend); Scent: Fresh, sweet, citrusy; Intensity: 3.

Thyme *Thymus vulgaris CT Thymol*

Quick Facts

Botanical Family: Labiatae (mint)

Extraction Method: Steam distillation from leaves, stems, and flowers

Common Primary Uses*: ○◔❷Antioxidant, ❷◔Asthma, ❷◔Bacterial Infections, ◔Bites/Stings, ○◔❷Blood Clots, ○◔Brain (Aging), ❷◔Bronchitis, ❷◔Colds (Common), ❷◔Croup, ◔Dermatitis/Eczema, ❷◔Fatigue, ◔Fungal Infections, ◔Greasy/Oily Hair, ◔Hair (Fragile), ◔Hair (Loss), ❷◔Mold, ◔MRSA, ○◔Parasites, ❷◔Pleurisy, ❷◔Pneumonia, ◔Prostatitis, ◔Psoriasis, ◔Radiation Wounds, ◔Sciatica, ❷◔Tuberculosis

Common Application Methods‡:

◔: Dilute 1:4 (1 drop essential oil to at least 4 drops carrier oil) when used topically. Dilute heavily for children and for those with sensitive skin. Apply directly on area of concern or to reflex points.

❷: Diffuse, or inhale the aroma directly.

○: Place 1–2 drops under the tongue, or take in capsules. Use as a flavoring in cooking.

Properties: Highly antibacterial⊕[225], antifungal⊕[226], antimicrobial⊕[227], antioxidant⊕[228], antiviral, antiseptic.

Historical Uses: It was used by the Egyptians for embalming and by the ancient Greeks to fight against infectious illnesses. It has also been used for respiratory problems, digestive complaints, the prevention and treatment of infection, dyspepsia, chronic gastritis, bronchitis, pertussis, asthma, laryngitis, tonsillitis, and enuresis in children.

Other Possible Uses: This oil is a general tonic for the nerves and stomach. It may also help with circulation, depression, digestion⊕[229], dysmenorrhea⊕[230], physical weakness after illness, flu, headaches, immunological functions, insomnia, rheumatism, urinary infections, viruses along the spine, and wounds.

⊕ Body System(s) Affected: Immune and Skeletal Systems and Muscles.

Aromatic Influence: It helps energize in times of physical weakness and stress. It has also been thought to aid concentration. It is uplifting and helps to relieve depression.

Oral Use As Dietary Supplement: Thyme oil is generally recognized as safe (GRAS) for human consumption by the FDA (21CFR182.20). Dilute 1 drop oil in 2 tsp. (10 ml) honey or in 1 cup (250 ml) of beverage (e.g., soy/rice milk). However, more dilution may be necessary due to this oil's potential for irritating mucous membranes. Not for children under 6 years old; use with caution and in greater dilution for children 6 years old and over.

Safety Data: This type of thyme oil may be somewhat irritating to the mucous membranes and dermal tissues (skin). This type of thyme should be avoided during pregnancy. Use with caution when dealing with high blood pressure.

Blend Classification: Equalizer and Enhancer.

Blends With: Bergamot, melaleuca, oregano, and rosemary.

Odor: Type: Middle Note (50–80% of the blend); Scent: Fresh, medicinal, herbaceous; Intensity: 4.

‡See Application section beginning on page 14 for more details. ◔=Topical, ❷=Aromatic, ○=Internal

111

Turmeric *Curcuma longa*

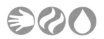

Quick Facts

Botanical Family: Zingiberaceae (ginger)

Extraction Method: Steam distillation from rhizome

Common Primary Uses*: ⬤◐❷Antioxidant, ◐❷Antibacterial, ⬤◐❷Indigestion, ⬤◐❷Neurological Diseases (Protects), ❷Skin

Common Application Methods‡:

❷: Can be applied neat (with no dilution) when used topically. Apply directly on area of concern or to reflex points.

❷: Diffuse, or inhale the aroma directly.

⬤: Add 1 drop to 1 cup (250 ml) of water, tea, or other beverage.

Properties: Analgesic, anticonvulsant, anti-inflammatory[231], antimicrobial, antimutagenic, antioxidant, antitumor, insecticidal.

Historical Uses: Native to India, the rhizome of curcumin is a bright orange-yellow color. Turmeric's unique color makes it valuable as a dye coloring, but it is also an important spice in many dishes. The herb has been used in Ayurvedic medicine for centuries to help with gastritis, jaundice, and nausea.

Other Possible Uses: Turmeric essential oil may also be beneficial for arthritis, blood clots[232], cancer, depression, epilepsy[233], joint health, neurological health[234], skin conditions (ringworm and other fungal skin conditions)[235], and pain. It may also have neuro-protective[236] properties.

⊕ **Body System(s) Affected:** Digestive System, Immune System, Skin.

Aromatic Influence: The warm, earthy aroma of turmeric is grounding to the mind and emotions, and it can help promote feelings of relaxation.

Oral Use As Dietary Supplement: Turmeric oil is generally regarded as safe (GRAS) for human consumption by the FDA. Dilute 1 drop oil in 1 tsp. (5 ml) honey or in ½ cup (125 ml) of beverage (e.g., soy/rice milk). Not for children under 6 years old; use with caution and in greater dilution for children 6 years old and over.

Safety Data: May irritate highly sensitive skin. Consult with a physician before use if taking medications (especially for diabetes), pregnant, or nursing.

Blend Classification: Personifier and Equalizer.

Blends With: Citrus oils (tangerine, in particular), ginger, pink pepper, and spice oils.

Odor: Type: Middle Note (50–80% of the blend); Scent: Warm, earthy, spicy, slightly woody; Intensity: 4.

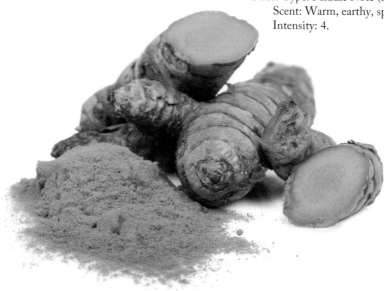

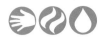

Quick Facts

Botanical Family: Gramineae (grasses)

Extraction Method: Steam distillation from roots

Common Primary Uses*: 🌿🍃ADD/ADHD, 🍃🌿Balance, 🍃🌿Termite Repellent, 🍃Vitiligo

Common Application Methods‡:

🍃: Can be applied neat (with no dilution) when used topically. Apply directly on area of concern or to reflex points. Also excellent in baths or in massage blends. A very small amount of vetiver oil is all that is needed in most applications.

🌀: Diffuse, or inhale the aroma directly.

⭘: Take in capsules.

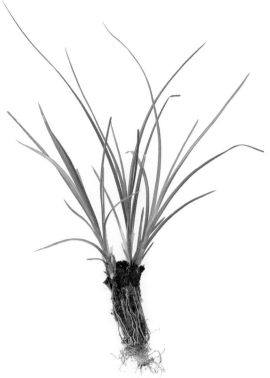

Properties: Antiseptic, antispasmodic, calming, grounding, immune stimulant, rubefacient (locally warming), sedative (nervous system), stimulant (circulatory, production of red corpuscles).

Historical Uses: The distillation of vetiver is a painstaking, labor-intensive activity. The roots and rootlets of vetiver have been used in India as a perfume since antiquity.

Other Possible Uses: Vetiver may help acne, anorexia, anxiety, arthritis, breasts (enlarge), cuts, depression (including postpartum), insomnia, muscular rheumatism, nervousness (extreme), skin care (oily, aging, tired, irritated), sprains, stress, and tuberculosis⊕[237].

🔆 **Body System(s) Affected:** Emotional Balance, Hormonal and Nervous Systems, Skin.

Aromatic Influence: Vetiver has a heavy, smoky, earthy fragrance reminiscent of patchouli with lemon-like undertones. Vetiver has been valuable for relieving stress and helping people recover from emotional traumas and shock. As a natural tranquilizer, it may help induce a restful sleep. It is known to affect the parathyroid gland.

Oral Use As Dietary Supplement: Vetiver oil in general is approved by the FDA (21CFR172.510) for use as a Food Additive (FA) and Flavoring Agent (FL). Dilute 1 drop oil in 1 tsp. (5 ml) honey or in ½ cup (125 ml) of beverage (e.g., soy/rice milk). Not for children under 6 years old; use with caution and in greater dilution for children 6 years old and over.

Safety Data: Use with caution during pregnancy.

Blends With: Clary sage, lavender, rose, sandalwood, and ylang ylang.

Odor: Type: Base Note (5–20% of the blend); Scent: Heavy, earthy, balsamic, smoky, sweet undertones; Intensity: 5.

White Fir *Abies alba*

Quick Facts

Botanical Family: Pinaceae (conifer)

Extraction Method: Steam distillation from needles

Common Primary Uses*: 🖐🌀Bronchitis, 🌀Bursitis, 🌀Cartilage Inflammation, 🖐🌀Energizing, 🌀Frozen Shoulder, 🌀Furniture Polish, 🌀Muscle Fatigue, 🌀Muscle Pain, 🌀Overexercised Muscles, 🌀Sprains

Common Application Methods‡:

🖐: Can be applied neat (with no dilution) when used topically. Dilute 1:1 (1 drop essential oil to at least 1 drop carrier oil) for children and for those with sensitive skin. Apply directly on area of concern or to reflex points.

🌀: Diffuse, or inhale the aroma directly.

⭕: Take in capsules.

Properties: Analgesic, antiarthritic, anticatarrhal, antiseptic (pulmonary), expectorant, and stimulant.

Historical Uses: The fir tree is the classic Christmas tree (short with the perfect pyramidal shape and silvery white bark). Though highly regarded for its fragrant scent, the fir tree has been prized through the ages for its medicinal virtues in regards to respiratory complaints, fever, and muscular and rheumatic pain.

Other Possible Uses: Fir creates the symbolic effect of an umbrella protecting the earth and bringing energy in from the universe. At night the animals in the wild lie down under the tree for the protection, recharging, and rejuvenation the trees bring them. Fir may be beneficial for reducing aches/pains from colds and the flu, fighting airborne germs/bacteria, arthritis, asthma, supporting the blood, bronchial obstructions, coughs, fevers, oxygenating the cells, rheumatism, sinusitis, and urinary tract infections.

🜨 Body System(s) Affected: Respiratory System.

Aromatic Influence: It creates a feeling of grounding, anchoring, and empowerment. It can stimulate the mind while allowing the body to relax.

Oral Use As Dietary Supplement: White fir oil in general is approved by the FDA (21CFR172.510) for use as a Food Additive (FA) and Flavoring Agent (FL). Dilute 1 drop oil in 1 tsp. (5 ml) honey or in ½ cup (125 ml) of beverage (e.g., soy/rice milk). Not for children under 6 years old; use with caution and in greater dilution for children 6 years old and over.

Safety Data: Can irritate sensitive skin.

Blend Classification: Equalizer.

Blends With: Frankincense and lavender.

Odor: Type: Middle Notes (50–80% of the blend); Scent: Fresh, woody, earthy, sweet; Intensity: 3.

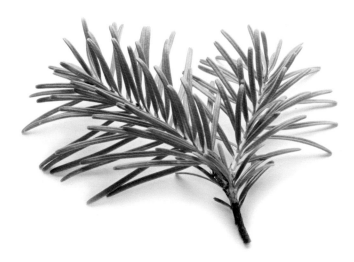

Wintergreen *Gaultheria fragrantissima or G. procumbens*

 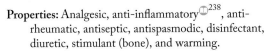
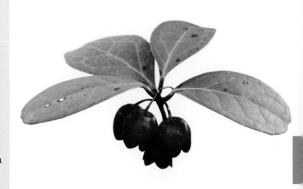

Properties: Analgesic, anti-inflammatory[238], antirheumatic, antiseptic, antispasmodic, disinfectant, diuretic, stimulant (bone), and warming.

Historical Uses: Wintergreen oil has a strong, penetrating aroma. The American Indians and early European settlers enjoyed a tea that was flavored with birch bark or wintergreen. According to Julia Lawless, "this has been translated into a preference for 'root beer' flavourings [*sic*]." A synthetic methyl salicylate is now widely used as a flavoring agent, especially in root beer, chewing gum, toothpaste, etc. In fact, the true essential oil is produced in such small quantities (compared to the very extensive uses of the synthetic methyl salicylate) that those desiring to use wintergreen essential oil for therapeutic uses should verify the source of their oil to make sure they have a true oil, not a synthetic one.

Other Possible Uses: This oil may be beneficial for acne, bladder infection, cystitis, dropsy, eczema, edema, reducing fever, gallstones, gout, infection, reducing discomfort in joints, kidney stones, draining and cleansing the lymphatic system, obesity, osteoporosis, skin diseases, ulcers, and urinary tract disorders. It is known for its ability to alleviate bone pain. It has a cortisone-like action due to the high content of methyl salicylate.

Body System(s) Affected: Skeletal System and Muscles.

Aromatic Influence: It influences, elevates, opens, and increases awareness in sensory system.

Safety Data: Avoid during pregnancy. Not for use by people with epilepsy. Some people are very allergic to methyl salicylate. Test a small area of skin first for allergies.

Blend Classification: Personifier and Enhancer.

Blends With: Basil, bergamot, cypress, geranium, lavender, lemongrass, marjoram, and peppermint.

Yarrow *Achillea millefolium*

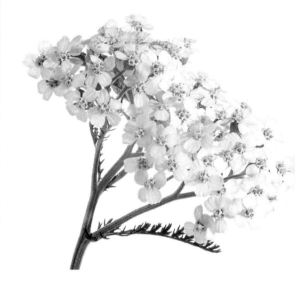

Quick Facts

Botanical Family: Compositae (daisy)

Extraction Method: Steam distillation from flowering top

Common Primary Uses*: ○⊜⊘Antioxidant⬭[239], ⊜Bleeding, ⊘Calming, ⊘Uplifting, ⊜Wounds

Common Application Methods‡:

⊜: Can be applied neat (with no dilution) when used topically. Apply directly on area of concern or to reflex points.

⊘: Diffuse, or inhale the aroma directly.

○: Add 1 drop to 1 cup (250 ml) of water, tea, or other beverage.

Properties: Anti-inflammatory, antiseptic⬭, astringent, and styptic (stops bleeding).

Historical Uses: Yarrow was used by Germanic tribes to treat battle wounds. The Chinese also considered it sacred for the harmony of the yin and yang energies within it.

Other Possible Uses: This oil may be beneficial for prostate health and hormonal balance. It may also help with acne, amenorrhea, appetite (lack of), colds, catarrh, digestion (poor), dysmenorrhea, eczema, fevers, flatulence, gastritis, gout, hair growth, headaches, hemorrhoids, hypertension, injuries, kidney stones, liver, menopause problems, neuritis, neuralgia, open leg sores, pelvic infections, prostatitis, rheumatism, scarring, sprains, stomach issues, sunburn, ulcers, urinary infections, vaginitis, varicose veins, and wounds (promotes healing).

✚ **Body System(s) Affected:** Hormonal System, Immune System, Skin.

Aromatic Influence: Balancing highs and lows, both external and internal, yarrow may allow us to have our heads in the clouds while our feet remain firm on the ground. Its balancing properties may also make it useful during meditation.

Oral Use As Dietary Supplement: Yarrow oil is approved by the FDA (21CFR172.510) for use as a Flavoring Agent (FL) in beverages. Dilute 1 drop oil in 1 tsp. (5 ml) honey or in ½ cup (125 ml) of beverage (e.g., soy/rice milk). Not for children under 6 years old; use with caution and in greater dilution for children 6 years old and over.

Safety Data: May irritate highly sensitive skin. Consult with a physician before use if taking medications, pregnant, or nursing.

Blend Classification: Personifier and Enhancer.

Blends With: Clary sage and vetiver.

Odor: Type: Middle Note (50–80% of the blend); Scent: Sharp, woody, herbaceous, with a slight floral undertone; Intensity: 4.

Ylang Ylang *Cananga odorata*

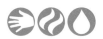

Quick Facts

Botanical Family: Annonaceae (tropical trees and shrubs—custard-apple)

Extraction Method: Steam distillation from flowers

Common Primary Uses*: ⊘⊘Aphrodisiac, ⊘⊘Arrhythmia, ⊘⊘Calming[240], ⊘Colic, ⊘⊘Crying, ⊘⊘Diabetes, ⊘Exhaustion, ⊘⊘Fear, ⊘Hair (Loss), ⊘⊘High Blood Pressure[241], ⊘⊘Hormonal Balance, ⊘⊘Hyperpnea, ⊘⊘Libido (Low), ⊘⊘Palpitations, ⊘⊘Relaxation, ⊘⊘Sedative, ⊘⊘Stress, ⊘⊘Tachycardia, ⊘⊘Tension

Common Application Methods‡:

⊘: Can be applied neat (with no dilution) when used topically. Apply directly on area of concern or to reflex points. It may be beneficial when applied over the thymus (to help stimulate the immune system).

⊘: Diffuse, or inhale the aroma directly.

⊘: Take in capsules.

Properties: Antidepressant, antiseptic, antispasmodic, sedative[242], and tonic.

Historical Uses: Interestingly enough, the original wild flowers had no fragrance. Through selection and cloning, we have this unique fragrance today. Ylang ylang has been used to cover the beds of newlywed couples on their wedding night, for skin treatments, to soothe insect bites, and in hair preparations to promote thick, shiny, lustrous hair (it is also reported to help control split ends). It has been used to treat colic, constipation, indigestion, stomachaches, and to regulate the heartbeat and respiration.

Other Possible Uses: Ylang ylang may help with rapid breathing, balancing equilibrium, frustration, balancing heart function, impotence, infection, intestinal problems, sex drive problems, shock, and skin problems.

Body System(s) Affected: Emotional Balance, Cardiovascular and Hormonal Systems.

Aromatic Influence: It influences sexual energy and enhances relationships. It may help stimulate the adrenal glands. It is calming and relaxing and may help alleviate anger.

Oral Use As Dietary Supplement: Ylang ylang oil is generally recognized as safe (GRAS) for human consumption by the FDA (21CFR182.20). Dilute 1 drop oil in 1 tsp. (5 ml) honey or in ½ cup (125 ml) of beverage (e.g., soy/rice milk). Not for children under 6 years old; use with caution and in greater dilution for children 6 years old and over.

Safety Data: Repeated use can possibly result in contact sensitization.

Blend Classification: Personifier and Modifier.

Blends With: Bergamot, geranium, grapefruit, lemon, marjoram, sandalwood, and vetiver.

Odor: Type: Middle to Base Notes (20–80% of the blend); Scent: Sweet, heavy, narcotic, cloying, tropical floral, with spicy-balsamic undertones; Intensity: 5.

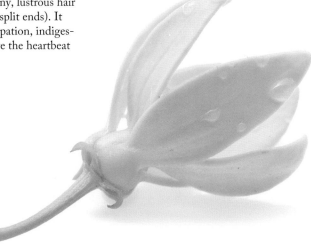

Yuzu *Citrus junos*

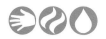

Quick Facts

Botanical Family: Rutaceae (citrus)

Extraction Method: Cold pressed from peel

Common Primary Uses*: 🌿🍃Calming ⊕243 , 🍃Warming

Common Application Methods‡:

🍃: Can be applied neat (with no dilution) when used topically. Apply directly on area of concern or to reflex points. Use in bath water.

🌀: Diffuse, or inhale the aroma directly.

💧: Add 1 drop to 1 cup (250 ml) of warm water, tea, or other beverage.

Properties: Antibacterial, calming, and warming.

Historical Uses: Yuzu fruit has been used in Japan since the 18th century in a traditional bath at winter solstice to help warm the body, improve circulation, promote healthy-looking skin, and prevent illness.

Other Possible Uses: This oil may be beneficial for acne, arthritic pain, circulation, clarity, concentration, focus, moisturizing skin, neuralgia, premenstrual syndrome, skin tone, sore throat, and sore muscles.

Body System(s) Affected: Digestive System, Immune System, Skin.

Aromatic Influence: Yuzu oil has a refreshing, citrusy aroma that is often used to help improve focus and concentration. It can also help purify the air.

Oral Use As Dietary Supplement: Citrus peel oils are generally regarded as safe (GRAS) for human consumption by the FDA. Dilute 1 drop oil in 1 tsp. (5 ml) honey or in 1 cup (250 ml) of beverage (e.g., soy/rice milk). Not for children under 6 years old; use with caution and in greater dilution for children 6 years old and over.

Safety Data: Old or oxidized oils may irritate sensitive skin. Consult with a physician before using if taking medications.

Blend Classification: Enhancer and Equalizer.

Blends With: Clary sage, lavender, neroli, rosemary, and citrus oils.

Odor: Type: Top Note (5–20% of the blend); Scent: Sweet, citrusy; Intensity: 3.

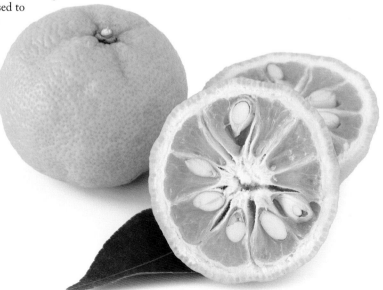

Research Endnotes

See the "Research References" in the *Appendix* for the full reference of each citation below.

Arborvitae

1   **Antibacterial:** Tsiri et al., 2009; Hudson et al., 2011.

2   **Antifungal:**Hudson et al., 2011.

3   **Anticancer Properties:** Wang et al., 2014; .Lee et al., 2013; Liu et al., 2009.

4   **Inflammation:** Han et al., 2017.

5   **Sunscreen:** Baba et al., 1998.

Basil

6   **Bronchitis:** Siurin, 1997.

7   **Antibacterial Properties:** Opalchenova et al., 2003; Berić et al., 2008.

8   **Antifungal Properties:** El-Soud et al., 2015.

9   **Antioxidant Properties:** Berić et al., 2008.

10   **Insect Repellent:** Kéita et al., 2001.

11   **Memory:** Sarahroodi et al., 2012.

Bergamot

12   **Calming:** Peng et al., 2009.

13   **Brain—Injury:** Corasaniti et al., 2007.

14   **Antifungal:** Sanguinetti et al., 2007,

15   **Inflammation:** Borgatti et al., 2011.

16   **Neuroprotective Properties:** Amantea et al., 2009.

17   **Anxiety:** Saiyudthong et al., 2011; Saiyudthong et al., 2011; Robola et al., 2017.

Birch

18   **Antiseptic Properties:** Charles et al., 2000.

Black Pepper

19   **Addiction:** Rose et al., 1994.

20   **Stimulant Properties:** Ebihara et al., 2006.

Blue Tansy

21   **Antifungal:** Greche et al., 2000.

Cardamom

22   **Inflammation:** al-Zuhair et al., 1996.

23   **Respiratory System—Lungs:** Kumari et al., 2013.

24   **Antibacterial:** Lawrence et al., 2009.

25   **Inflammation:** al-Zuhair et al., 1996.

26   **Ulcers:** Jamal et al., 2006.

Cassia

27   **Antibacterial:** Lee et al., 1998.

28   **Antifungal:** Kocevski et al., 2013.

29   **Anti-inflammatory**Sun et al., 2016.

Cedarwood

30   **Repellent:** Singh et al., 1984.

31   **Inflammation:** Tumen et al., 2013.

32   **Stroke:** Asakura et al., 2000.

Cilantro

33   **Antifungal:** Freires Ide et al., 2014.

34   **Liver—Cirrohsis:** Moustafa et al., 2012; Pandey et al., 2011.

35   **Skin:** Park et al., 2012.

Cinnamon

36   **Diabetes:** Lu, T. et al., 2012; Mishra et al., 2010; Li, R. et al., 2013; Subash et al., 2007; Ping et al., 2010.

37   **Antibacterial Properties:** Fabio et al., 2007; Filoche et al., 2005; Inouye et al., 2001; Smith-Palmer et al., 2004.

38   **Antifungal Properties:** Juglal et al., 2002; Tantaoui-Elaraki et al., 1994; Singh et al., 1995.

39   **Rheumatoid Arthritis:** Rathi et al., 2013.

Clary Sage

40   **Female-Specific Conditions—Dysmenorrhea:** Han et al., 2006; Ou et al., 2012.

41   **Antiseptic:** Sienkiewicz et al., 2015.

42   **Soothing Properties:** Pemberton et al., 2008.

Clove

43   **Blood Clots:** Saeed et al., 1994.

44   **Antibacterial Properties:** Fabio et al., 2007; Smith-Palmer et al., 2004.

45   **Antifungal Properties:** Chaieb et al., 2007; Hitokoto et al., 1980.

46   **Anti-inflammatory Properties:** Reddy et al., 1994; Halder et al., 2011.

47   **Leukemia:** Yoo et al., 2005.

48   **Antiviral Properties:** Benencia et al., 2000.

49   **Arthritis:** Grespan et al., 2012.

50   **Insect Control:** Enan, 2001.

Copaiba

51   **Acne:** da Silva et al., 2012.

52   **Antioxidant:** Dias et al., 2014.

53   **Anxiety:** Curio et al., 2009.

54   **Anti-inflammatory:** Klauke et al., 2013.

55   **Pain:** Gomes et al., 2007.

56   **Antibacterial:** Santos et al., May 2008; Bonan et al., 2015.

57   **Antioxidant:** Dias et al., 2014.

58   **Skin:** Santos et al., Nov. 2008.

59   **Anti-cancer:** Legault et al., 2007.

60   **Anxiety:** Curio et al., 2009.

Coriander

61   **Alzheimer's Disease:** Cioanca et al., 2014; Cioanca et al., 2013.

62   **Antispasmodic Properties:** Brum et al., 2001.

63   **Pain:** Taherian et al., 2012.

Cypress

64   **Antibacterial:** Selim et al., 2014.

65   **Liver—Hepatitis:** Ali et al., 2010.

Dill

66   **Cholesterol:** Bahramikia et al., 2009.

67   **Clearing Toxins:** Zheng et al., 1992.

68   **Repellent:** Lee et al., 2017.

Douglas Fir

69   **Bronchitis:** Siurin et al., 1997.

Eucalyptus

70   **Bronchitis:** Juergens et al., 1998; Siurin et al., 1997.

71   **Lice:** Choi et al., 2010; **Lice:** Greive et al., 2017.

72   **Analgesic Properties:** Liapi et al., 2007; Santos et al., 2000.

73   **Antibacterial Properties:** Charles et al., 2000.

74   **Anti-inflammatory Properties:** Santos et al., 2000; Grassmann et al., 2000.

75   **Antiviral Properties:** Schnitzler et al., 2001.

76   **Insecticidal Properties:** Enean, 2001.

‡See Application section beginning on page 14 for more details.   ◗=Topical, ◗=Aromatic, ○=Internal

77 **High Blood Pressure:** Lahlou et al., 2002.

Fennel

78 **IBS:** Portincasa et al., 2016.

79 **Antispasmodic Properties:** Ostad et al., 2001.

80 **Menopause:** Kim et al., 2012; Rahimikian et al., 2017.

81 **Colic:** Alexandrovich et al., 2003; Savino et al., 2005.

82 **PMS:** Ostad et al., 2001.

83 **Stimulating the Sympathetic Nervous System:** Haze et al., 2002.

Frankincense

84 **Arthritis:** Lima et al., 2012.

85 **Anticancer Properties:** Bhushan et al., 2007; Zou et al., 2013; Dai et al., 2013; Zhang et al., 2013, Ding et al., 2013; Li et al., 2013; Li et al., 2013, Chen et al., 2012; Li et al., 2013.

86 **Antidepressant Properties:** Moussaieff et al., 2008.

87 **Anti-inflammatory Properties:** Zhou et al., 2004; Blain et al., 2009

Geranium

88 **Antibacterial Properties:** Edwards-Jones et al., 2004; Doran et al., 2009.

89 **Anticonvulsant Properties:** Brum et al., 2001.

90 **Anti-inflammatory Properties:** Maruyama et al., 2005.

91 **Insect Repellent—Ticks:** Tabanca et al., 2013.

Ginger

92 **Nausea:** Nanthakomon et al., 2006; Vutyavanich et al., 2001; Bone et al., 1990.

93 **Arthritis:** Srivastava et al., 1992; Sharma et al., 1994.

Grapefruit

94 **Obesity:** Shen et al., 2005; Haze et al., 2010.

95 **Cancer:** Hakim et al., 2000; Vigushin et al., 1998.

96 **Sympathetic Nervous System Stimulation:** Haze et al., 2002.

97 **Anxiety:** Hozumi et al., 2017.

Green Mandarin

98 **GERD:** Sun, 2007.

99 **Skin:** d'Alessio et al., 2014.

100 **Anti-inflammatory:** Kummer et al., 2013.

101 **Antitumor:** Elegbede et al., 1984; Maltzman et al., 1989; Uedo et al., 1999.

Hawaiian Sandalwood

102 **Antitumor Properties:** Dwivedi et al., 2003; Dwivedi et al., 2005; Kaur et al., 2005.

Helichrysum

103 **Antibacterial Properties:** Chinou et al., 1996; Nostro et al., 2001.

104 **Antioxidant Properties:** Rosa et al., 2007.

105 **Antiviral Properties:** Appendino et al., 2007; Nostro et al., 2003.

Hinoki

106 **Antibacterial:** Kim et al., 2015.

107 **Anti-inflammatory:** An et al., 2013.

108 **Calming:** Chen et al., 2015.

109 **Anxiety:** Park et al., 2014.

Jasmine

110 **Antispasmodic Properties:** Lis-Balchin et al., 2002.

111 **Hormonal System:** Shrivastav et al., 1988.

Lavender

112 **Anxiety:** Lehrner et al., 2005; Cho et al., 2013; Lopez et al., 2017.

113 **Stress:** Motomura et al., 2001; Pemberton et al., 2008.

114 **Analgesic Properties:** Ghelardini et al., 1999; Olapour et al., 2013; Yazdkhasti et al., 2016.

115 **Anticonvulsant Properties:** Brum et al., 2001.

116 **Antifungal Properties:** D'Auria et al., 2005.

117 **Anti-inflammatory Properties:** Hajhashemi et al., 2003; Peana et al., 2002.

118 **Antimicrobial Properties:** Moon et al., 2006.

119 **Antimutigenic Properties:** Evandri et al., 2005.

120 **Antitumor Properties:** Lantry et al., 1997; Mills et al., 1995; Reddy et al., 1997.

121 **Sedative Properties:** Bradley et al., 2007; Buchbauer et al., 1991; Dunn et al., 1995; Guillemain et al., 1989; Itai et al., 2000; Lin et al., 2007; Shen et al., 2005; Umezu et al., 2000.

122 **Asthma:** Ueno-Iio et al., 2014.

123 **Bronchitis:** Siurin et al., 1997.

124 **Headaches:** Sasannejad et al., 2012.

125 **High Blood Pressure:** Kim et al., 2012.

126 **Insect Repellent:** Mkolo et al., 2007; van Tol et al., 2007.

127 **Mental Clarity:** Diego et al., 1998; Field et al., 2005.

Lemon

128 **Anxiety:** Ceccarelli et al., 2004.

129 **Concentration:** Ogeturk et al., 2010.

130 **Stress:** Kiecolt-Glaser et al., 2008; Komiya et al., 2006.

131 **Anticancer Properties:** Hakim et al., 2000; Vigushin et al., 1998.

132 **Antidepressant Properties:** Komori et al., 1995.

133 **Antifungal Properties:** Caccioni et al., 1998.

134 **Antioxidant Properties:** Grassmann et al., 2001.

135 **Aging:** Oboh et al., 2014; Campelo et al., 2011.

136 **Digestive Problems:** Kime et al., 2005.

137 **Nerves:** Koo et al., 2002.

Lemongrass

138 **Cholesterol:** Elson et al., 1989.

139 **Antibacterial Properties:** Doran et al., 2009; Ohno et al., 2003; Onawunmi et al., 1984.

140 **Anticancer Properties:** Carnesecchi et al., 2001; Kumar et al., 2008; Puatanachokchai et al., 2002; Sharma et al., 2009.

141 **Anti-inflammatory Properties:** Han et al., 2017.

142 **Respiratory Problems:** Inouye et al., 2001.

Litsea

143 **Antibacterial:** Su et al., 2016.

Magnolia

144 **Pain:** Peana et al., 2006.

145 **Sedative:** Linck et al., 2009.

Manuka

146 **Antibacteial:** Takarada et al., 2004.

Marjoram

147 **High Blood Pressure:** Kim et al., 2012.

See My Usage Guide section for more details.   ●=Neat, ●=Dilute for Children/Sensitive Skin, ●=Dilute

Melaleuca (Tea Tree)

148 **Acne:** Bassett et al., 1990; Enshaieh et al., 2007; Raman et al., 1995.

149 **Boils:** Feinblatt et al., 1960.

150 **Influenza:** Li et al., 2013.

151 **Antibacterial Properties:** Brady et al., 2006; Carson et al., 1995; Cox et al., 2000; Edwards-Jones et al., 2004; Ferrini et al., 2006; Hammer et al., 1996; Hammer et al., 2008; Kwieciński et al., 2009.

152 **Antifungal Properties:** Bagg et al., 2006; Banes-Marshall et al., 2001; Buck et al., 1994; Hammer et al., 2004; Mondello et al., 2006; Satchell et al., 2002; Cháfer et al., 2012.

153 **Anti-inflammatory Properties:** Brand et al., 2002; Caldefie-Chézet et al., 2006; Golab et al., 2007; Hart et al., 2000; Koh et al., 2002.

154 **Antiviral Properties:** Schnitzler et al., 2001.

155 **Mites:** Kheirkhah et al., 2007; Williamson et al., 2007.

156 **Ticks:** Iori et al., 2005.

Melissa

157 **Antiviral Properties:** Schnitzler et al., 2008.

158 **Sedative Properties:** Kennedy et al., 2006; Ballard et al., 2002.

159 **Cold-sore Blisters:** Schnitzler et al., 2008.

160 **Colic:** Savino et al., 2005.

161 **Inflammation:** Bounihi 2013.

Myrrh

162 **Anti-inflammatory Properties:** Tipton et al., 2003.

163 **Antitumor Properties:** Tan et al., 2000.

164 **Skin:** Auffray 2007.

Neroli

165 **Antibacterial:** Ammar et al., 2012.

166 Anticonvulsant: Azanchi et al., 2014.

167 **Menopause:** Choi et al., 2014.

Orange (Wild Orange)

168 **Anxiety:** Goes et al., 2012; Faturi et al., 2010; Jafarzadeh et al., 2013.

169 **Anticancer Properties:** Hakim et al., 2000; Vigushin et al., 1998.

170 **Sedative Properties:** Lehrner et al., 2000; Lehrner et al., 2005.

Oregano

171 **Inflammation:** Han et al., 2017.

172 **Antibacterial Properties:** Nostro et al., 2004; Preuss et al., 2005.

173 **Antifungal Properties:** Inouye et al., 2006; Juglal et al., 2002; Manohar et al., 2001; Tantaoui-Elaraki et al., 1994.

174 **Antiparasitic Properties:** Force et al., 2000.

175 **Immune Stimulant Properties:** Walter et al., 2004.

176 **Weight—obesity:** Cho et al., 2012.

Patchouli

177 **Insecticidal Properties:** Pavela, 2008; Zhu et al., 2003; Trongtokit et al., 2005.

178 **Pregnancy/Motherhood—Mastitis:** Li et al., 2014.

179 **UV Radiation:** Lin et al., 2014.

180 **Calming Aromatic Influence:** Haze et al., 2002.

Peppermint

181 **Endurance:** Meamarbashi et al., 2013.

182 **Gamma Radiation Exposure:** Samarth et al., 2004; Samarth et al., 2009.

183 **Headaches:** Göbel et al., 1994.

184 **Irritable Bowel Syndrome:** Cappello et al., 2007; Kline et al., 2001; Liu et al., 1997; Rees et al., 1979.

185 **Memory:** Moss et al., 2008.

186 **Nausea:** Tayarani-Najaran et al., 2013.

187 **Antibacterial Properties:** Charles et al., 2000; Imai et al., 2001; Rasooli et al., 2008; Shayegh et al., 2008.

188 **Anti-inflammatory Properties:** Adam et al., 2006; Juergens et al., 1998.

189 **Antispasmodic Properties:** Asao et al., 2003.

190 **Antiviral Properties:** Schuhmacher et al., 2003.

191 **Nerves:** Koo et al., 2001.

192 **Seizure:** Koutroumanidou et al., 2013.

Petitgrain

193 **Antibacterial:** Ellouze et al., 2012.

194 **Antioxidant:** Sarrou et al., 2013.

Pink Pepper

195 **Antibacterial:** Martins et al., 2014; Guerra-Boone et al., 2013; Gundidza, 1993.

196 **Cancer:** Lin et al., 2015, Diaz et al., 2008.

197 **Insects:** Benzi et al., 2009; Abdel-Sattar et al., 2010; Batista et al., 2016.

Roman Chamomile

198 **Anxiety and Sleep:** Cho et al., 2013.

199 **Anti-inflammatory Properties:** Safayhi et al., 1994.

200 **Antispasmodic:** Sándor et al., 2018.

Rose

201 **Anxiety:** Kheirkhah et al., 2014; Kim et al., 2011.

202 **Sedative Properties:** Umezu, 1999.

203 **Digestive System:** Sadraei et al., 2013.

204 **Female-Specific Conditions—Dysmenorrhea:** Bani et al., 2014.

205 **Brain—Aging:** Awale et al., 2011; Esfandiary et al., 2014.

206 **Lower-Back Pain:** Shirazi et al., 2016.

207 **Opioid Addiction:** Abbasi et al., 2013

208 **Seizure:** Hosseini et al., 2011; Ramezani et al., 2008.

Rosemary

209 **Blood Pressure—Low:** Fernández et al., 2014.

210 **Analgesic Properties:** González-Trujano et al., 2007.

211 **Antibacterial Properties:** Rasooli et al., 2008.

212 **Anticancer Properties:** Cheung et al., 2007; Singletary et al., 1996; Steiner et al., 2001.

213 **Antifungal Properties:** Rasooli et al., 2008.

214 **Anti-inflammatory Properties:** Takaki et al., 2008.

215 **Antioxidant Properties:** Almela et al., 2006; Moreno et al., 2006; Slamenova et al., 2002.

216 **Stress:** Aqel, 1991; Villareal et al., 2017.

217 **Memory:** Diego et al., 1998; Moss et al., 2003.

Sandalwood

218 **Alzheimer's Disease:** Jeon et al., 2011.

219 **Antitumor Properties:** Dwivedi et al., 2003; Dwivedi et al., 2005; Kaur et al., 2005.

Siberian Fir

220 **Bronchitis:** Siurin et al., 1997.

Spearmint

221 **Antibacterial Properties:** Imai et al., 2001.

222 **Arthritis:** Mahboubi, 2017.

Spikenard

223 **Antioxidant:** Maiwalanjiang et al., 2014; Maiwalanjiang et al., 2013; Maiwalanjiang et al., 2015.

Star Anise

224 **Antifungal:** Hitokoto et al., 1980; Kosalec et al., 2005.

Thyme

225 **Antibacterial Properties:** Charles et al., 2000; Fabio et al., 2007; Mohsenzadeh et al., 2007.

226 **Antifungal Properties:** Pina-Vaz et al., 2004; Tantaoui-Elaraki et al., 1994.

227 **Antimicrobial Properties:** Inouye et al., 2001.

228 **Antioxidant Properties:** Youdim et al., 1999; Youdim et al., 2000.

229 **Colon—Colitis:** Bukovska et al., 2007.

230 **Dysmenorrhea:** Salmalian et al., 2014.

Turmeric

231 **Anti-inflammatory:** Oh et al., 2014.

232 **Blood Clots:** Prakash et al., 2011.

233 **Epilepsy:** Orellana-Paucar et al., 2013.

234 **Neurological Health:** Hucklenbroich et al., 2014.

235 **Skin:** Mukda et al., 2013.

236 **Neuroprotective:** Preeti et al., 2008; Chen et al., 2018.

Vetiver

237 **Tuberculosis:** Saikia et al., 2012.

Wintergreen

238 **Anti-inflammatory Properties:** Trautmann, et al., 1991.

Yarrow

239 **Antioxidant:** Candan et al., 2003.

Ylang Ylang

240 **Calming—Sedative:** Watanabe et al., 2013.

241 **Blood Pressure:** Hongratanaworakit et al., 2004; Hongratanaworakit et al., 2006.

242 **Sedative Properties:** Moss et al., 2008.

243 **Calming:** Matsumoto et al., 2016; Matsumoto et al., 2017.

Chemical Constituents

Arborvitae

Tropolones: α-thujaplicin, β-thujaplicin (hinokitiol), & γ-thujaplicin; methyl thujate, thujic acid, β-thujaplicinol.

Basil

Alcohols (up to 65%): linalool (>55%), fenchol (>10%), cis-3-hexenol; Phenolic Ethers: methyl chavicol (or estragole—up to 47%), methyl eugenol; Oxides (up to 6%): 1,8 cineol; Esters (<7%); Monoterpenes (<2%) α & β-pinenes.

Bergamot

Monoterpenes: d-Limonene (>30%), γ-terpinene, α & β-pinenes; Esters: linalyl acetate (usually around 20%); Alcohols: linalool, geraniol, nerol, α-terpineol; Sesquiterpenes: β-caryophyllene, β-bisabolene; Furanocoumarins; Aldehydes.

Birch

Esters (99%): methyl salicylate; betulene, betulinol.

Black Pepper

Monoterpenes (up to 70%): l-limonene (<15%), δ-3-carene (<15%), β-pinene (<14%), sabinene (<10%), α-phellandrene (<9%), α-pinene (<9%), α-thujene (<4%), γ- & α-terpinene (<7%), p-cymene (<3%), myrcene (<3%), terpinolene (<2%); Sesquiterpenes (up to 60%): β-caryophyllene (up to 35%), β-selinene (<8%), β-bisabolene (<5%), α-, α-, & δ-elemenes, β-farnesene, humulene, α-copaene, α-guaiene, α- & β-cubebenes; Oxides: caryophyllene oxide (<8%); Ketones (<2%): acetophenone, hydrocarvone, piperitone; Aldehydes: piperonal; Carboxylic Acids: piperonylic acid; Furanocoumarin: α-bergamotene.

Blue Tansy

Monoterpenes (up to 55%): sabinene (<17%), myrcene (<13%), d-limonene (<10%), β-pinene (<10%), α-phellandrene (<10%), p-cymene (<8%); Ketones: camphor (<17%); Sesquiterpenes: chamazulene (up to 35%).

Cardamom

Esters (>40%): α-terpenyl acetate (30–45%), linalyl acetate (3%); Oxides: 1,8 cineol (up to 35%); Alcohols (7%): linalool, terpinen-4-ol, α-terpineol; Monoterpenes (6%): sabinene, myrcene, l-limonene; Aldehyde: geranial.

Cassia

Aldehydes: trans-cinnamaldehyde (up to 85%), benzaldehyde; Phenols (>7%): eugenol, chavicol, phenol, 2-vinylphenol; Esters: cinnamyl acetate, benzyl acetate.

Cedarwood

Sesquiterpenes: α- & β-cedrenes (up to 36%), thujopsene (up to 42%), cuparene, trans-caryophyllene; Sesquiterpene Alcohols: cedrol (up to 15%), pseudocedrol, prim-cedrol, widdrol, γ-eudesmol.

Cilantro

Aldehydes (40–50%): tetradecanal, 2-dodecenal, 13-tetradecenal, dodecanal, decanal; Alcohols (up to 40%): cyclododecanol, 1-decanol, 1-dodecanol, 1-undecanol; Phenols: eugenol; Ketones: β-ionone.

Cinnamon

Aldehydes: trans-cinnamaldehyde (<50%), hydroxycinnamaldehyde, benzaldehyde, cuminal; Phenols (up to 30%): eugenol (<30%), phenol, 2-vinylphenol; Alcohols: linalool, cinnamic alcohol, benzyl alcohol, α-terpineol, borneol; Sesquiterpenes: β-caryophyllene; Carboxylic Acids: cinnamic acid.

Clary Sage

Esters (up to 75%): linalyl acetate (20–75%); Alcohols (20%): linalool (10–20%), geraniol, α-terpineol; Sesquiterpenes (<14%): germacrene-D (up to 12%), -caryophyllene; Diterpene alcohols: sclareol (1–7%); Monoterpenes: myrcene, α- and β-pinenes, l-limonene, ocimene, terpinolene; Oxides: 1,8 cineol, linalool oxide, sclareol oxide; Ketones: α- and β-thujone; Sesquiterpene alcohols; Aldehydes; Coumarins. (More than 250 constituents.)

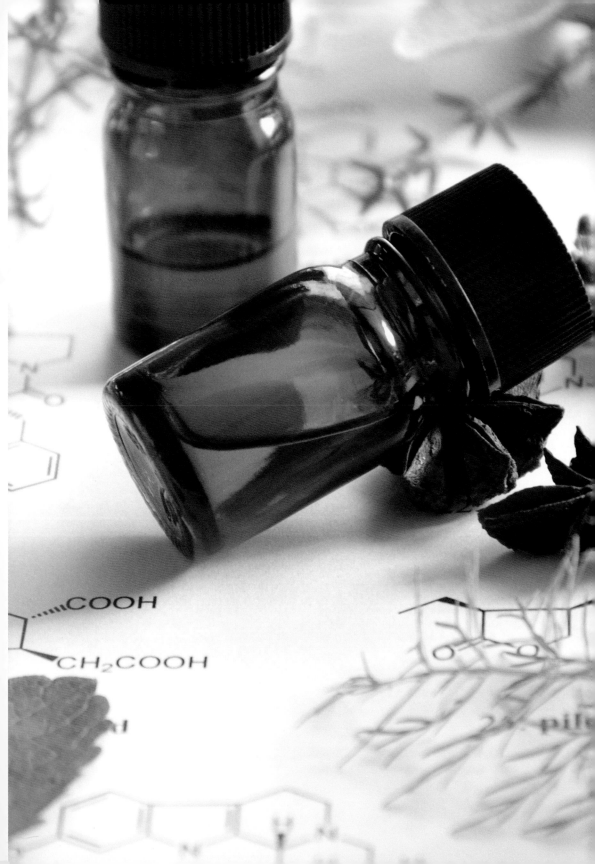

....,,,COOH

CH₂COOH

Clove

Phenols: eugenol (up to 85%), chavicol, 4-allylphenol; Esters: eugenyl acetate (up to 15%), styrallyl, benzyl, terpenyl, ethyl phenyl acetates, methyl salicylate (tr.); Sesquiterpenes (up to 14%): β-caryophyllene (<12%), humulene, α-amorphene, α-muurolene, calamenene; Oxides (<3%): caryophyllene oxide, humulene oxide; Carboxylic Acids; Ketones.

Copaiba

Sesquiterpenes (up to 90%): β-caryophyllene (up to 52%), α- & β-copaene (>15%), trans-α-bergamotene (>8%), α-cubebene, α-humulene, γ- & β-elemene, β-cubebene.

Coriander

Alcohols (up to 80%): linalool (>30%), coriandrol (<30%), geraniol, terpinen-4-ol, borneol; Monoterpenes (up to 24%): α-pinene, γ-terpinene, l-limonene, p-cymene, myrcene, camphene; Esters: geranyl acetate, linalyl acetate; Ketones: camphor, carvone; Aldehydes: decanal.

Cypress

Monoterpenes: α-pinene (>55%), δ-3-carene (<22%), l-limonene, terpinolene, sabinene, β-pinene; Sesquiterpene Alcohols: cedrol (up to 15%), cadinol; Alcohols: borneol (<9%), α-terpineol, terpinen-4-ol, linalool sabinol; Esters: α-terpinyl acetate (<5%), isovalerate, terpinen-4-yl acetate; Sesquiterpenes: δ-cadinene, α-cedrene; Diterpene Alcohols; labdanic alcohols, manool, sempervirol; Diterpene Acids; Oxides.

Dill

Monoterpenes (up to 65%): d-limonene (up to 25%), α- & β-pinenes (<30%), α- & β-phellandrenes, p-cymene; Ketones: d-carvone (<45%); Ethers (<11%).

Douglas Fir

Monoterpenes (up to 80%): α-pinene (10–20%), β-pinene (30–40%), l-limonene (<5%), δ-3-carene, camphene, terpinolene; Esters (up to 15%): bornyl acetate (<15%), geranyl acetate (<4%), bornyl & geranyl coproates; Alcohols (up to 10%): borneol, geraniol; Aldehydes: benzoicaldehyde, citrals; Ketones: camphor; Oxides: 1,8 cineol.

Eucalyptus

Oxides: 1,8 cineol (62–72%), caryophyllene oxide; Monoterpenes (up to 24%): α- & β-pinenes (<12%), l-limonene (<8%), myrcene, p-cymene; Alcohols (<19%): α-terpineol (14%), geraniol, borneol, linalool; Aldehydes (8%): myrtenal, citronellal, geranial, neral.

Fennel (Sweet)

Phenolic Ethers (up to 80%): trans-anethole (70%), methyl chavicol (or estragole) (>3%); Monoterpenes (up to 50%): trans-ocimene (<12%), l-limonene (<12%), γ-terpinene (<11%), α- & β-pinenes (<10%), p-cymene, α- & β-phellandrenes, terpiolene, myrcene, sabinene; Alcohols (up to 16%): linalool (<12%), α-fenchol (<4%); Ketones (<15%): fenchone (12%), camphor; Oxides; Phenols.

Frankincense

Monoterpenes: α-phellandrenes (up to 25%), α- & β-pinenes (<15%), α-thujene (<15%), l-limonene (<5%), sabinene (<7%), p-cymene (<10%), α-terpinene, camphene, myrcene; Sesquiterpenes (<10%): β-elemene (<5%), α-copaene; Alcohols (<10%): cis-verbenol (<5%), 4-terpineol, α-terpineol, borneol, cis-sabinol, olibanol, trans-pinocarveol, farnesol; Ketones: verbenone.

Geranium

Alcohols (up to 70%): citronellol (>32%), geraniol (<23%), linalool (<14%), nerol, γ-eudesmol, α-terpineol, menthol; Esters (up to 30%): citronellyl formate (14%), geranyl formate & acetate (<12%), other propionates, butyrates, & tiglates; Ketones: isomenthone (<8%), menthone, piperitone; Sesquiterpenes: 4-guaiadiene-6,9, α-copaene, δ- & γ-cadinenes, δ-guaiazulene, β-farnesene; Aldehydes: geranial (<6%), neral, citronellal; Monoterpenes (<5%): α- & β-pinenes, l-limonene, myrcene, ocimene; Sesquiterpene Alcohols: farnesol (<3%).

Ginger

Sesquiterpenes (up to 90%): zingiberene (up to 50%), α- & β-curcumene (<33%), β-farnesene (<20%), β-sesquiphellandrene (<9%), β- & γ-bisabolene (<7%), β-ylangene, β-elemene, α-selinene, germacrene-D; Monoterpenes: camphene (8%), β-phellandrene, l-limonene, p-cymene, α and β-pinenes, myrcene; Alcohols: nonanol (<8%), citronellol (<6%), linalool (<5%), borneol, butanol, heptanol; Sesquiterpene Alcohols:

nerolidol (<9%), zingeberol, elemol; Ketones (<6%): heptanone, acetone, 2 hexanone; Aldehydes: butanal, citronellal, geranial; Sesquiterpene Ketones: gingerone.

Grapefruit

Monoterpenes (up to 95%): d-Limonene (<92%), myrcene, α-pinene, sabinene, β-phellandrene; Tetraterpenes: β-carotene, lycopene; Aldehydes (>2%): nonanal, decanal, citral, citronellal; Furanocoumarins: aesculetin, auraptene, bergaptol; Sesquiterpene Ketones (<2%): nootketone (used to determine harvest time); Alcohols: octanol.

Green Mandarin

Monoterpenes (up to 97%): limonene (<75%), γ-terpinene (<18%); α- & β-pinenes, β-myrcene, terpinolene, p-cymene; Aldehydes: decanal, octanal; Esters: methyl n-methyl anthranilate; Alcohols: linalool, citronellol, nerol.

Hinoki

Sesquiterpene Alcohols (up to 60%): α-cadinol, T-muurolol, T-cadinol, cadin-1(10)-en-4,β-ol, β-caryophyllene alcohol; Sesquiterpenes (up to 30%): γ-cadinene, δ-cadinene, α-muurolene, β-caryophyllene, α-elemene; Monoterpenes: α-pinene, limonene.

Hawaiian Sandalwood

Sesquiterpene Alcohols (up to 98%): α- & β-santalols (up to 70%), α-bergamotol (up to 5%), cis-nuciferol, lanceol; Sesquiterpenes: α- & β-santalenes; Sesquiterpene Aldehydes: teresantalal; Carboxylic Acids: nortricycloekasantalic acid.

Helichrysum

Esters (up to 60%): neryl acetate (up to 50%), neryl propionate & butyrate (<10%); Ketones: italidione (<20%), β-diketone; Sesquiterpenes: γ-curcumene (<15%), β-caryophyllene (<5%); Monoterpenes: l-limonene (<13%), α-pinene; Alcohols: nerol (<5%), linalool (<4%), geraniol; Oxides: 1,8 cineol; Phenols: eugenol.

Jasmine

Esters (up to 50%): benzyl acetate (<28%), benzyl benzoate (<21%), methyl anthranilate, methyl jasmonate; Diterpene Alcohols: phytol (<12%), isophytol (<7%); Alcohols: linalool (<8%), benzyl alcohol, farnesol; Triterpenes: squalene (<7%); Pyrroles: indole, scatole; Ketone: cis-jasmone.

Juniper Berry

Monoterpenes (>50%): α-pinene (up to 40%), sabinene (<18%), β-myrcene (<8%), l-limonene (<6%); Sesquiterpenes (up to 30%): β-caryophyllene, α-humulene, germacrene; Esters: bornyl acetate, terpinyl acetate; Ketones: camphor, junionone, pinocamphone, thujone.

Lavender

Alcohols (up to 58%): linalool (>41%), α-terpineol, borneol, lavendulol, geraniol, nerol; Esters (approx. 50%): linalyl acetate (up to 45%), lavendulyl & geranyl acetates, α-terpenyl acetate; Monoterpenes (up to 24%): β-ocimene (<16%), d-Limonene (<5%), α- & β-pinenes, camphene, δ-3-carene; Sesquiterpenes: β-caryophyllene (<7%), χ-farnesene; Phenols: terpinen-4-ol (<6%); Aldehydes: benzaldehyde, cuminal, geranial, hexanal, myrtenal, neral; Oxides: 1,8 cineol, caryophyllene oxide, linalol oxide; Coumarins (<4%); Ketones: octanone (<3%), camphor; Lactones.

Lemon

Monoterpenes (up to 90%): d-Limonene (up to 72%), α- & β-pinenes (<30%), α- & γ-terpinenes (7–14%), sabinene, p-cymene, terpinolene, α- & β-phellandrenes; Aldehydes (up to 12%): citral, citronellal, neral, geranial, heptanal, hexanal, nonanal, octanal, undecanal; Alcohols: hexanol, octanol, nonanol, decanol, linalool, α-terpineol; Esters (<5%): geranyl acetate, neryl acetate, methyl anthranilate; Sesquiterpenes (<5%): β-bisabolene, β-caryophyllene; Tetraterpenes (<4%): β-carotene, lycopene; Phenols: terpinen-4-ol; Coumarins and Furocoumarins (<3%): umberlliferone, bergaptene, α-bergamotene, limettine, psoralen, bergamottin, bergaptol, citroptene scopoletin.

Lemon Myrtle

Aldehydes (>90%): geranial (57%), neral (37%), citronellal; Alcohols (<4%): cis- & trans-verbenol (<3%), linalool, nerol. Other trace elements include linalyl acetate, myrcene, methylheptenone, and geranic acid.

Lemongrass

Aldehydes (up to 80%): geranial (<42%), neral (<38%), farnesal (<3%), decanal; Alcohols (<15%): geraniol (<10%), α-terpineol (<3%), borneol (<2%), nerol, linalool, citronellol; Sesquiterpene Alcohols: farnesol (<13%); Esters (<11%): geranyl & linalyl acetates; Monoterpenes (<9%): myrcene (<5%), d-Limonene (<3%), β-ocimene; Sesquiterpenes: β-caryophyllene

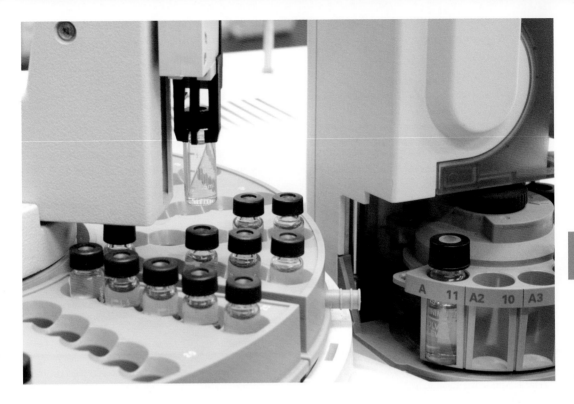

(<6%); Oxides: caryophyllene oxide (<4%); Ketones: methyl heptanone (<3%).

Lime

Monoterpenes (up to 80%): d-Limonene (<65%), α- & β-pinenes (<17%), camphene, sabinene, p-cymene, myrcene, bisabolene, dipentene, phellandrene, cadinene; Oxides (<22%): 1,8 cineol (<20%), 1,4 cineol; Aldehydes (<20%): geranial (<8%), neral (<5%), citral, citronellal, octanal, nonanal, decanal, lauric aldehyde; Alcohols (4%): α-terpineol (<2%), borneol, α-fenchol, linalool; Coumarins: limettine; Furanoids: furfural, garanoxycoumarin.

Litsea

Aldehydes (up to 75%): geranial (<42%), neral (<35%), citronellal; Monoterpenes (up to 25%): limonene (<23%), myrcene (<3%), sabinene, β-ocimene, α- & β-pinenes, camphene; Alcohols: geraniol, nerol, α-terpineol, linalool, citronellol; Esters: terpinyl acetate; Sesquiterpenes: β-caryophyllene; Ketones: 6-methyl-5-hepten-2-one.

Magnolia

Alcohols: linalool (up to 80%); Sesquiterpenes (up to 10%): β-caryophyllene, selinine, β-elemene; Monoterpenes: β-ocimene.

Manuka

Sesquiterpenes (up to 50%): trans-calamenene (<15%), Cadina-3,5-diene (<10%>), δ-cadinene (<7%), α-copaene (<7%), α- & β-selinene, α-cubebene, δ-amorphene, β-caryophyllene, aromadendrene, humulene; Cyclic Triketones (20–30%): leptospermone (<17%), iso-leptospermone (<5%), flavesone (<5%); Alcohols: linalool, geraniol; Monoterpenes: α- & β-pinenes.

Marjoram

Monoterpenes (up to 60%): α- & γ-terpinenes (<30%), sabinene (<8%), myrcene (<7%), terpinolene, ocimene, δ-3-carene, p-cymene, α- and β-pinenes, δ-cadinene, α- & β-phellandrenes, l-limonene; Alcohols (<30%): α-terpineol (<15%), cis- & trans-thujanol-4 (<12%), linalool (<8%); Phenols: terpinen-4-ol (>21%), terpinen-1-ol-3; Esters: geranyl acetate (<7%), linalyl acetate, α-terpenyl acetate; Aldehydes: citral (<6%); Sesquiterpenes (<5%): β-caryophyllene, humulene; Phenolic Ethers: trans-anethole.

Melaleuca (Tea Tree)

Monoterpenes (up to 70%): α- & γ-terpinenes (<40%), p-cymene (<12%), α- and β-pinenes (<8%), terpinolene, l-limonene, sabinene, myrcene, α-thujene; Phenols: terpinen-4-ol (<40%); Sesquiterpenes (up to 20%): α- & δ-cadinenes (<8%), aromadendrene (<7%), viridiflorene (<5%), β-caryophyllene, α-phellandrene; Oxides: 1,8 cineol (<14%), 1,4 cineol (<3%), caryophyllene oxide; Alcohols: α- & β-terpineols (<8%); Sesquiterpene Alcohols (<5%): globulol, viridiflorol.

Melissa (Lemon Balm)

Aldehydes (up to 65%): geranial (<35%), neral (<28%), citronellal (<3%), α-cyclocitral; Sesquiterpenes (<35%): β-caryophyllene (<19%), α-copaene (<5%), germacrene-D (<4%), β-bourbonene, δ- & γ-cadinenes, humulene, β-elemene; Oxides (<11%): caryophyllene oxide (<7%), 1,8 cineol (<4%); Alcohols (<7%): linalool, octen-3ol, nerol, geraniol, citronellol, isopulegol, caryophyllenol, farnesol; Esters (<7%): methyl citronellate (<5%), citronellyl, geranyl, neryl, & linalyl acetates; Ketones (<7%): methyl heptanone (<5%), farnesylacetone, octanone; Monoterpenes (<3%): cis- & trans-ocimenes, l-limonene; Sesquiterpene Alcohols: elemol, α-cadinol; Furanocoumarins: aesculetin.

Myrrh

Sesquiterpenes (up to 75%): lindestrene (up to 30%), β-, γ-, & δ-elemenes (<40%), α-copaene (<12%), β-bourbonene (<5%), muurolene, δ-cadinene, humulene, curzerene; Furanoids (<27%): methoxyfurogermacrene (<9%), furoendesmadiene (<8%), α-bergamotene (<5%), methylisopropenylfurone (<5%), furfural (<3%), furanodione (<2%), rosefuran; Ketones: (<20%): curzenone (<11%), methylisobutyl ketone (<6%), germacrone (<4%); Triterpenes (<7%): α-amyrin (<4%), α-amyrenone (<3%); Monoterpenes (<6%): ocimene, p-cymene, α-thujene, l-limonene, myrcene; Aldehydes: methylbutynal (<3%), cinnamaldehyde, cuminal; Arenes: xylene; Carboxylic Acids: acetic acid, formic acid, palmitic acid; Phenols: eugenol, cresol.

Neroli (Orange Blossom)

Alcohols (up to 53%): linalool (<44%), α-terpineol (<6%), geraniol (<3%), nerol; Sesquiterpene Alcohols (<7%): trans-nerolidol (<5%), farnesol (<2%); Monoterpenes (up to 40%); d-limonene (<18%), β-pinene (<17%), ocimene (<8%), myrcene (<4%), α-pinene, neptadecene, sabinene, camphene; Esters (>25%): linalyl acetate (<15%), methyl anthranilate (<10%), neryl & geranyl acetates; Aldehydes: decanal, benzaldehyde, vinylhexanal; Phenols: phenylethanol, benzyl alcohol; Pyrroles: indole, scatole.

Orange (Wild Orange)

Monoterpenes (up to 95%): d-Limonene (<90%), terpinolene, myrcene, α-pinene; Tetraterpenes (<8%): β-carotene (<6%), lycopene; Aldehydes (<8%): citral, decanal, citronellal, dodecanal, nonanal, octanal, α-sinensal; Alcohols (<6%): linalool, cis & trans-carveol, α-terpineol, geraniol; Ketones (<4%): 1- & d-carvone (<3%), α-ionone; Esters (<3%): citronellyl acetate, geranyl acetate, linalyl acetate, methyl anthranilate; Furanoids: auraptene, bergaptol, imperatarine; Sesquiterpene Ketones: nootkatone.

Oregano

Phenols (up to 80%): carvacrol (<75%), thymol (<5%), terpinen-4-ol; Monoterpenes (<25%): p-cymene (<10%), γ-terpinene (<9%), myrcene (<3%), α- and β-pinenes, camphene, l-limonene, α-terpinene; Sesquiterpenes (<6%): β-caryophyllene (<5%), β-bisabolene; Carboxylic Acids: rosmaric acid (<5%); Esters: linalyl acetate (<4%); Ketones: camphor, d-carvone; Alcohols: borneol, linalool, α-terpineol.

Patchouli (or Patchouly)

Sesquiterpenes (up to 63%): α-bulnesene (<20%), β-bulnesene (<16%), aromadendrene (<15%), α-gaiene (>12%), seychellene (6%), α-, β- & γ-patchoulenes (<12%), β-caryophyllene (<4%), δ-cadinene (<3%), β-gaiene, β-elemene, humulene; Sesquiterpene Alcohols (<38%): patchoulol (up to 35%), pogostol, bulnesol, guaiol, patchoulenol; Oxides (<5%): bulnesene oxide, caryophyllene oxide, guaiene oxide; Ketones: patchoulenone (<3%); Monoterpenes: α- & β-pinenes, l-limonene.

Peppermint

Phenolic Alcohols (up to 44%): menthol (<44%), piperitols; Ketones (<25%): menthone (20–30% and up to 65% if distilled in September when flowering), pulegone (<5%), piperitone (<2%), carvone, jasmone; Monoterpenes (< 15%): α and β-pinenes (<6%), l-limonene (<6%), ocimene, myrcene, p-cymene, β-phellandrene, sabinene, α-terpinene, terpinolene, camphene; Sesquiterpenes (<10%): germacrene-D (<5%),

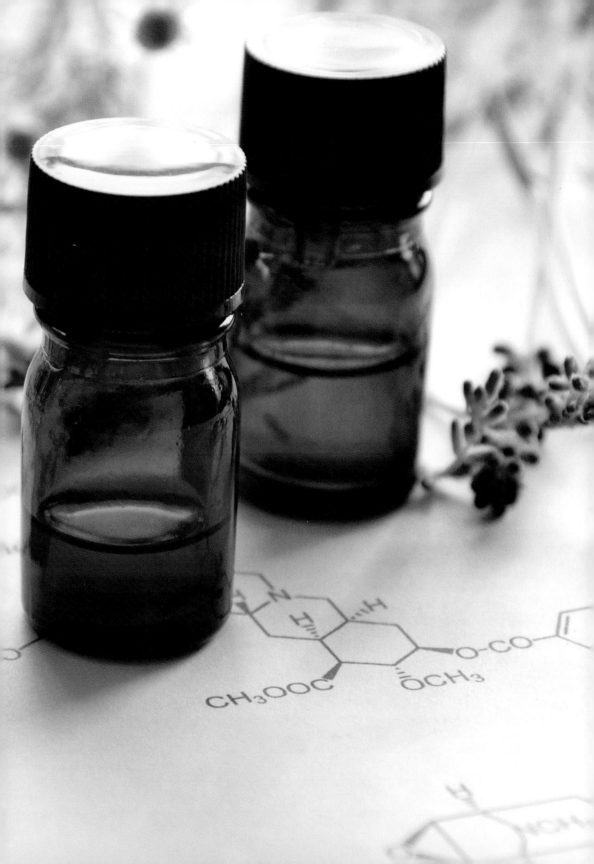

CH₃OOC ÖCH₃ O-CO

β-bourbonene, ζ-bulgarene, γ-cadinene, β-caryophyllene, β-elemene, β-farnesene, muurolene; Esters (<9%): menthyl acetate (<9%), also menthyl butyrate & isovalerate; Oxides (<9%): 1,8 cineol (<5%), piperitone oxide, caryophyllene oxide; Furanoids: menthofuran (<8%); Phenols: terpinen-4-ol (<3%); Alcohols (<3%): α-terpineol, linalool; Sesquiterpene Alcohols: viridiflorol; Furanocoumarins: aesculetin; Sulphides: mint sulfide, dimenthyl sulfide.

Petitgrain

Esters (up to 65%): linalyl acetate (<55%), geranyl acetate (<5%), neryl & α-terpenyl acetates, methyl anthranilate; Alcohols (40%): linalool (<28%), α-terpineol (<8%), geraniol (<5%), nerol, citronellol; Monoterpenes (<28%): myrcene (<6%), β-cymene (<5%), cis- & trans-ocimenes (<5%), p-cymene (<3%), β-pinene, γ-terpinene, d-limonene, phellandrene, sabinene, terpinolene; Aldehydes: decanal, geranial, neral; Phenols: thymol, terpinen-4-ol; Furanocoumarins: bergaptene, citroptene.

Pink Pepper

Monoterpenes (up to 80%): α- & β-phellandrene, limonene, myrcene, α-pinene, p-cymene; Sesquiterpenes (up to 15%): α- & β-caryophyllene, α-humulene, others; Sesquiterpinols (up to 10%): viridiflorol, spathulenol, t-cadinol, t-muurolol, elemol.

Roman Chamomile

Esters (up to 75%): isobutyl angelate (up to 25%), isoamyl methacylate (up to 25%), amyl butyrate (<15%), other angelate, butyrate, acetate, and tiglate esters; Monoterpenes (<35%): α- & β-pinenes (<20%), terpinenes, sabinene, camphene, d-Limonene, p-cymene, myrcene; Ketones: pinocarvone (14%); Sesquiterpenes (up to 12%): β-caryophyllene, chamazulene; Alcohols (>7%): trans-pinocarveol, farnesol, nerolidol.

Rose

Alcohols (up to 70%): citronellol (up to 45%), geraniol (up to 28%), nerol (<9%), linalool, borneol, α-terpineol; Monoterpenes (<25%): stearoptene (<22%), α & β-pinenes, camphene, α-terpinene, l-limonene, myrcene, p-cymene, ocimene; Alkanes (<19%): nonadecane (<15%), octadecane, eicosane, and others; Esters (<5%): geranyl, neryl, and citronellyl acetates; Phenols (<4%): eugenol, phenylethanol; Sesquiterpene Alcohols: farnesol (<2%); Oxides: rose oxide; Ketones:

α- & β-damascenone, β-ionone; Furanoids: rosefuran; Many other trace elements.

Rosemary

Oxides: 1,8 cineol (up to 55%), caryophyllene oxide, humulene oxide; Monoterpenes: α-pinene (<14%), β-pinene (<9%), camphene (<8%), l-limonene, myrcene, p-cymene, α- & β-phellandrenes, α- & γ-terpinenes; Ketones (<32%): camphor (<30%), β-thujone, verbenone, d-carvone, hexanone, heptanone; Alcohols (<20%): borneol (<12%), α-terpineol (<5%), linalool, verbenol; Sesquiterpenes (<3%): β-caryophyllene, humulene; Phenols: terpinen-4-ol; Esters: bornyl and fenchyl acetates; Acids: rosemaric acid.

Sandalwood

Sesquiterpene Alcohols: α- & β-santalols (<80%); Sesquiterpenes: α- & β-santalenes (<11%); Sesquiterpene Aldehydes: teresantalal (<3%); Carboxylic Acids: nortricycloekasantalic acid (<2%).

Siberian Fir

Monoterpenes (60–70%): camphene (<30%), α- & β-pinene (<20%), δ-3-carene (up to 12%), l-limonene (<5%), santene; Esters: bornyl acetate (up to 35%); Alcohols: borneol.

Spearmint

Ketones (up to 70%): l-carvone (<58%), dihydrocarvone (<10%), menthone (<2%), pulegone; Monoterpenes (<30%): l-limonene (<25%), myrcene (<3%), camphene, α- & β-pinenes, α-phellandrene; Alcohols (<10%): carveol (<3%), linalool, trans-thujanol-4, octanol, borneol; Sesquiterpenes (<5%): β-caryophyllene, β-bourbonene, α-elemene, β-farnesene; Esters: carvyl acetates (<4%); Oxides: 1,8 cineol (<3%); Sesquiterpene Alcohols: α-cadinol, farnesol, elemol; Phenolic Alcohols: menthol.

Spikenard

Sesquiterpenes (up to 50%): β-gurjunene (<30%), β-maalene (<9%), aristoladiene (<7%), aristolene (5%), seychellene, dihydroazulene, β-patchoulene; Monoterpenes (up to 45%): calarene (<35%), β-ionene (<8%), α- & β-pinenes, limonene, aristolene; Sesquiterpene Alcohols (<11%): patchoulol (<7%), nardol, calarenol, maaliol, valerianol; Ketones (<10%): aristolenone (<7%), β-ionone, nardostachone, valerianone (=jatamansone);

Phenolic Aldehydes: valerianal; Coumarins; Oxides: 1,8 cineol; Carboxylic Acids: jatamanshinic acid.

Star Anise

Phenolic Ethers: (E)-anethole (up to 95%), (methyl chavicol) (1–10%); Monoterpenes: limonene; Alcohols: linalool.

Tangerine

Monoterpenes (up to 95%): d-limonene (<80%), γ-terpinene (<20%), myrcene (<4%), p-cymene, α- & β-phellandrenes, β-ocimene, α- & β-pinenes, terpinolene, cadinene; Tetraterpenes (<10%): β-carotene (<6%), lycopene (<4%); Alcohols: linalool, citronellol; Aldehydes: citral, neral.

Thyme

Phenols (up to 60%): thymol (<55%), carvacrol (<10%); Monoterpenes (<54%): p-cymene (<28%), γ-terpinene (<11%), terpinolene (<6%), α-pinene (<6%), myrcene (<3%); Oxides: 1,8 cineol (<15%); Alcohols (<14%): linalool (<8%), borneol (<7%), thujanol, geraniol; Sesquiterpenes: β-caryophyllene (<8%); Carboxylic Acids: rosmaric acid (<2%), triterpenic acids (tr.); Ethers: methyl thymol (tr.), methyl carvacrol (tr.); Ketone: camphor (tr.); Also trace elements of menthone.

Turmeric

Ketones (up to 50%): turmerone, ar-turmerone, carlone; Sesquiterpenes (up to 35%): zingiberene, β-sesquiphellandrene, ar-curcumene, β-curcumene, α- & β-caryophyllene, β-bisabolene; Monoterpenes (up to 16%): α-phellandrene, turpinolene, p-cymene; Oxide: 1,8 cineole (up to 7%).

Vetiver

Sesquiterpene Alcohols (up to 42%): isovalencenol (<15%), bicyclovetiverol (<13%), khusenol (<11%), tricyclovetiverol (<4%), vetiverol, zizanol, furfurol; Sesquiterpene Ketones (<22%): α- & β-vetivones (<12%), khusimone (<6%), nootkatone (<5%); Sesquiterpenes (<4%): vitivene, tricyclovetivene, vetivazulene, β- & δ-cadinenes; Sesquiterpene Esters: vetiveryl acetate; Carboxylic Acids: benzoic, palmitic, and vetivenic acids.

White Fir

Monoterpenes (75–95%): l-limonene (34%), α-pinene (24%), camphene (21%), santene, δ-3-carene; Esters: bornyle acetate (up to 10%).

Wintergreen

Phenolic Esters: methyl salicylate (>90%); Carboxylic Acids: salicylic acid.

Yarrow

Monoterpenes (up to 65%): sabinene (<40%), α- & β-pinenes (<16%), camphene (<6%), γ-terpinene; Sesquiterpenes (<55%): chamazulene (<30%), germacrene-D (<13%), trans-β-caryophyllene, humulene, dihydroazulenes; Ketones (<30%): camphor (<18%), isoartemisia ketone (<10%), thujone; Alcohols (<10%): borneol (<9%), terpineol; Oxides (<12%): 1,8 cineol (<10%), caryophyllene oxide; Phenols: terpinen-4-ol; Esters: bornyl acetate; Lactones: achillin; Sesquiterpene Alcohols: α-cadinol.

Ylang Ylang

Sesquiterpenes (up to 55%): β-caryophyllene (<22%), germacrene-D (<20%), α-farnesene (<12%), humulene (<5%); Esters (<50%): benzyl acetate & benzoate (<25%), methyl salicylate & benzoate (<17%), farnesyl acetate (<7%), geranyl acetate (<4%), linalyl acetate; Alcohols (<45%): linalool (<40%), geraniol; Ethers: paracresyl methyl ether (<15%); Phenols (<10%): methyl p-cresol (<9%), methyl chavicol (estragole), eugenol, isoeugenol; Oxides: caryophyllene oxide (<7%); Sesquiterpene Alcohols: farnesol.

Yuzu

Monoterpenes (up to 95%): limonene (<80%), α- & γ-terpinenes (<10%), α- & β-pinenes (<5%), camphene, sabinene, β-myrcene, β-phellandrene; Alcohols (<4%): terpineol, linalool; Coumarins: limettin; Sesquiterpenes (<1%): β-farnesene.

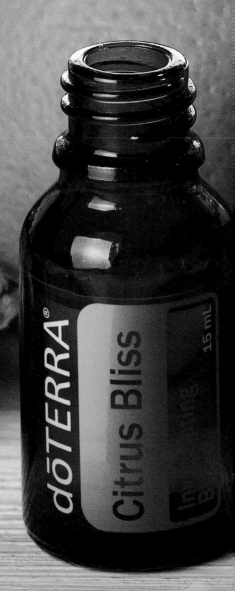

Essential Oil Blends

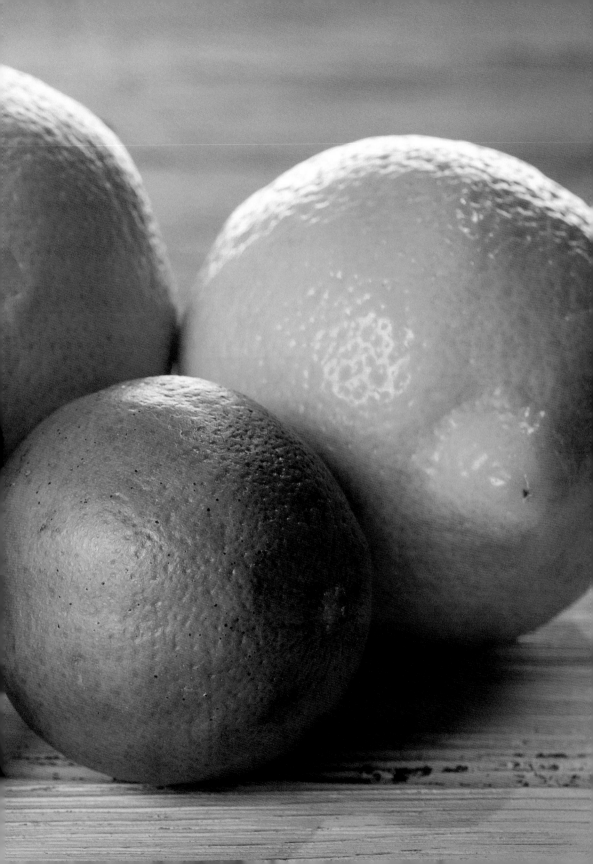

Essential Oil Blends

Note:
This section contains examples of various essential oil blends that are available commercially as well as the essential oils that each blend may contain.

For further information and research on many of the single oils contained in these blends, see the Essential Oils section of this book. Any internal use indicated for these blends is based on the use of pure, therapeutic-grade essential oils only.

Look for this symbol throughout this section for additional information on oil blends that are essential to any oils tool kit.

Symbols and Colors Used in This Section

Topical

Neat (can be used without dilution)

Aromatic

Dilute for children and those with sensitive skin

Internal

Dilute

Cleaning/Disinfecting

Body System(s) Affected

Avoid sunlight for up to 12 hours after use

See Additional Research

Avoid sunlight for up to 72 hours after use

See My Usage Guide section for more details. ●=Neat, ●=Dilute for Children/Sensitive Skin, ●=Dilute

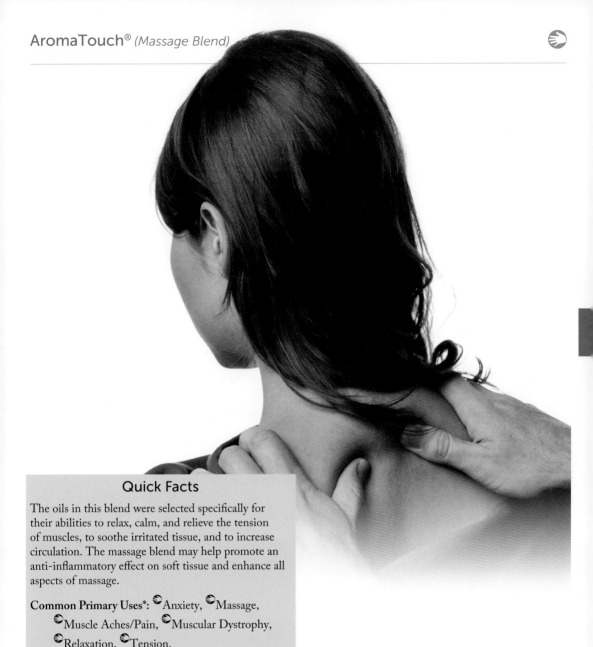

Quick Facts

The oils in this blend were selected specifically for their abilities to relax, calm, and relieve the tension of muscles, to soothe irritated tissue, and to increase circulation. The massage blend may help promote an anti-inflammatory effect on soft tissue and enhance all aspects of massage.

Common Primary Uses*: ⬛Anxiety, ⬛Massage, ⬛Muscle Aches/Pain, ⬛Muscular Dystrophy, ⬛Relaxation, ⬛Tension.

Application:

⬛: Best if applied on location for all muscles. It may also be applied over the heart or diluted with fractionated coconut oil for a full body massage. It is also beneficial when placed in bathwater.

Single Oils in This Blend:
Basil, Grapefruit, Cypress, Marjoram, Lavender, Peppermint

⬛=Topical, ⬛=Aromatic, ⬤=Internal

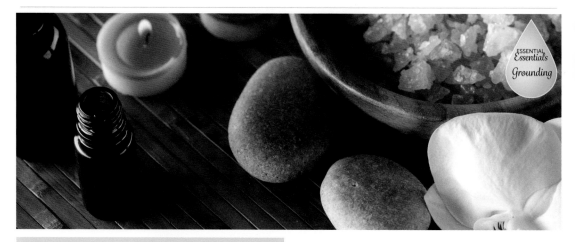

ESSENTIAL
Essentials
Grounding

Biography

The oils in this blend may help establish a feeling of calmness, peace, and relaxation. It may aid in harmonizing the various physiological systems of the body and promote tranquility and a sense of balance.

Ⓢ Aroma:

• Fresh • Sweet • Woody

⊕ Body Systems:

Ⓒ Muscles and Bones ⊕ Emotional Balance

Ⓘ Nervous System ⊕ Skin

Single Oils in This Blend:
Spruce, Ho Wood, Blue Tansy, Frankincense, German (Blue) Chamomile, Osmanthus

Top Uses

• Calming/Relaxing: Add 3 drops to 1 Tbs. (15 ml) fractionated coconut oil, and use as a soothing massage oil.

• Harmonizing/Grounding: Place 3 drops on the bottoms of the feet.

• Balancing: Diffuse in an aromatherapy diffuser.

Common Primary Uses*: Anxiety, Anxiety, Back Pain, Balance, Brain Integration, Bursitis, Coma, Confusion, Convulsions, Depression, Diabetic Sores, Energy, Fear, Grand Mal Seizure, Grief/Sorrow, Herniated Discs, Hot Flashes, Hyperactivity, Jet Lag, Lou Gehrig's Disease, Lupus, Metabolism (Balance), Mood Swings, Parkinson's Disease, Seizure

Application:

: This blend works best on the bottoms of the feet. Put six drops on bottoms of feet. Put on heart, wrists, and solar plexus from neck to thymus. To balance left and right brain, put on left fingers, and rub on right temple; or put on right fingers, and rub on left temple; or cross arms, and rub reflex points on bottoms of feet. To relieve pain along the spine, apply to reflex points on feet and on spine.

: Wear as perfume or cologne. Diffuse or inhale the aroma directly.

Carrier Oil in This Blend: Fractionated coconut oil.

Aromatic Influence: This blend of oils may help balance the body and mind. Diffuse wherever and whenever possible.

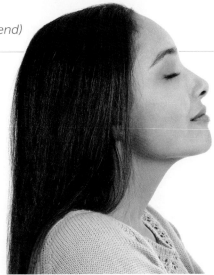
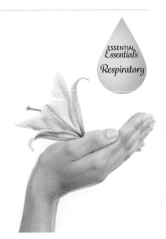

Biography

Many of the oils in this blend have been studied for their abilities to open and soothe the tissues of the respiratory system and also for their abilities to combat airborne bacteria and viruses that could be harmful to the system.

Ⓢ Aroma:

• Minty   • Fresh   • Herbaceous

⊕ Body Systems:

🫁 Respiratory System   🛡 Immune System

Single Oils in This Blend:
Laurel Leaf (Bay), Peppermint, Eucalyptus radiata, Melaleuca alternifolia, Lemon, Ravensara, Cardamom, Ravintsara

Top Uses

• Asthma/Bronchitis: Diffuse using an aromatherapy diffuser, or inhale the aroma directly from the bottle.

• Coughs: Add 8 drops to 1 tsp. (5 ml) fractionated coconut oil in a small roll-on bottle, and apply a small amount on the chest, back, and forehead.

• Congestion: Add 3–5 drops to a small bowl of hot water, and inhale the vapors.

• Sinusitis: Drop 2–3 drops on the floor of a hot shower, and inhale the aroma while showering.

Common Primary Uses*: 🄰Antiviral, 🄰Anxiety, 🄰🄱Asthma, 🄰🄱Bronchitis, 🄰🄱Congestion, 🄰🄱Cough, 🄰🄱Emphysema, 🄰🄱Influenza, 🄰🄱Mono, 🄰🄱Nasal Polyp, 🄰🄱Pneumonia, 🄰🄱Respiratory System, 🄰🄱Sinusitis, 🄰🄱Tuber-culosis

Application:

🄲: May be applied on the chest, the back, or the bottoms of the feet.

🄰: Diffuse into the air. Apply to palms of hands: cup hands over nose and mouth, and breathe deeply, or inhale the aroma of the oil directly.

Aromatic Influence: This blend of oils is excellent for opening the respiratory system when the blend is diffused or inhaled and is perfect for nighttime diffusion, allowing for restful sleep.

Safety Data: Can be irritating to sensitive skin. Dilute for young or sensitive skin.

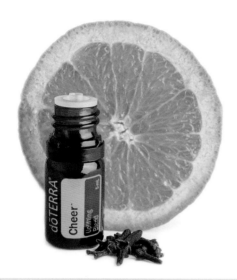

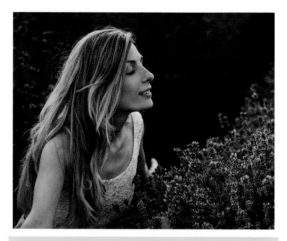

Quick Facts

This blend combines many different oils often used to help alleviate symptoms often associated with PMS, menopause, and aging.

Common Primary Uses*: Hot Flashes, Hormones (Balancing), Menopause, Menstruation, PMS

Application:

: Apply to the chest, abdomen, or back of neck as needed.

: Diffuse or inhale from the hands.

Quick Facts

This blend contains citrus and spice oils that are known to help combat feelings of gloom, distress, and disinterest, helping to cheer and uplift the mind, body, and spirit.

Common Primary Uses*: Coldness, Creativity, Depression, Grief, Joy, Positive (Feeling), Uplifting

Application:

: Diffuse or inhale the aroma directly.

: Apply on wrists, back of neck, over the heart area, or on the bottoms of the feet.

Single Oils in This Blend:
Orange, Clove, Star Anise, Lemon Myrtle, Nutmeg, Vanilla, Ginger, Cinnamon, Zdravetz

Safety Data: Repeated use can result in contact sensitization. Consult your doctor before using if you are pregnant, epileptic, or have a medical condition.

Single Oils in This Blend:
Clary Sage, Lavender, Bergamot, Roman Chamomile, Cedarwood, Ylang Ylang, Geranium, Fennel, Carrot Seed, Palmarosa, Vitex

Aromatic Influence: Helps to balance mood and calm stress and tension.

Safety Data: Repeated use may result in contact sensitization—dilute with fractionated coconut oil if this occurs. Consult your doctor before using if you are pregnant or have a medical condition.

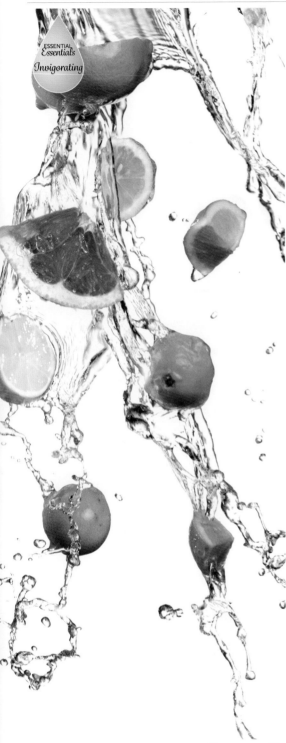

Biography

This uniquely exhilarating blend brings together all of the uplifting and stress-reducing benefits of citrus essential oils in a sweetly satisfying way. In addition to their elevating properties, many of the citrus oils in this blend have been studied for their ability to cleanse and disinfect.

Ⓢ **Aroma:**

• Citrusy • Sweet

⊕ **Body Systems:**

Ⓘ Immune System Ⓐ Emotional Balance

Single Oils in This Blend:
Orange, Lemon, Grapefruit, Mandarin, Bergamot, Tangerine, Clementine, Vanilla Bean Extract

Top Uses

• Stress: Add 5–10 drops to 1 Tbs. (15 ml) fractionated coconut oil, and use as a massage oil.

• Uplifting: Diffuse using an aromatherapy diffuser, or inhale the aroma directly from the bottle to help with anorexia and bulimia.

• Cleansing: Mix 3–5 drops with 1 cup (250 ml) of water in a bowl or bucket. Moisten a rag with this water, and use to clean countertops and other surfaces.

Common Primary Uses*: Ⓐ Calming, Ⓐ Mastitis, ⒶⒶ Depression, Ⓐ Eating Disorders, Ⓐ Sedative

Application:

Ⓢ: May be applied on the ears, heart, and wrists or may be worn as a perfume or cologne. It may be diluted with fractionated coconut oil for a full-body massage. It may also be added to water for a relaxing bath.

Ⓐ: Diffuse or inhale the aroma directly.

Ⓘ: Mixed with water, this blend can also be used to disinfect countertops and other surfaces.

Safety Data: May cause skin irritation. Avoid exposure to direct sunlight for up to 12 hours after use.

Ⓢ=Topical, Ⓐ=Aromatic, Ⓘ=Internal

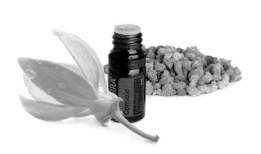

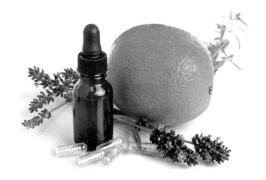

Quick Facts

This blend contains floral and tree oils that can help soothe feelings of sorrow and grief and promote uplifting feelings of peace and hope.

Common Primary Uses*: Anger, Depression, Grief/Sorrow, Happiness, Uplifting

Application:

: Diffuse or inhale the aroma directly.

: Apply on wrists, back of neck, over the heart area, or on the bottoms of the feet.

Quick Facts

The oils in this blend have been chosen for their abilities to provide antioxidant support for the cells and to promote a healthy cellular life cycle.

Common Primary Uses*: Aging, Antioxidant, Atherosclerosis, Cancer, Cellular Health, Tumors

Application:

: Dilute as needed, and apply on area of concern.

: Diffuse or inhale the aroma directly.

: Adults can take up to 8 drops internally, twice a day with food.

Single Oils in This Blend:
Frankincense, Patchouli, Ylang Ylang, Labdanum, Amyris, Sandalwood, Rose, Osmanthus

Single Oils in This Blend:
Frankincense, Orange, Litsea, Lemongrass, Thyme, Summer Savory, Clove, Niaouli

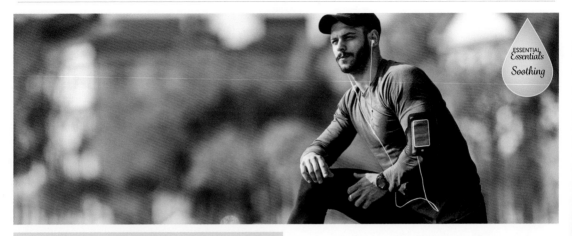

ESSENTIAL
Essentials
Soothing

Biography

This blend contains oils that are well known and are frequently studied for their abilities to soothe inflammation, alleviate pain, and reduce soreness.

Ⓢ Aroma:

- Minty • Camphoraceous • Herbaceous

⊕ Body Systems:

⚡ Nervous System   🌙 Muscles and Bones

Single Oils in This Blend:

Wintergreen, Camphor, Peppermint, Ylang Ylang, Blue Tansy, German Chamomile, Helichrysum, Osmanthus.

Top Uses

- **Arthritis:** Blend 10 drops with 1 Tbs. (15 ml) fractionated coconut oil, and massage gently on affected joints each day.

- **Back pain:** Blend 5 drops in 1 tsp. (5 ml) fractionated coconut oil, and gently massage over back to help soothe discomfort.

- **Inflammation:** Add 5 drops to 1 tsp. (5 ml) fractionated coconut oil in a small roll-on bottle, and apply on location.

- **Sore Muscles:** Add 15 drops to 1 Tbs. (15 ml) fractionated coconut oil, and use as a massage oil on sore muscles to help soothe.

Common Primary Uses*: Ⓢ Arthritis, Ⓢ Back Pain, Ⓢ Bone Pain, Ⓢ Bruises, Ⓢ Bursitis, Ⓢ Fibromyalgia, Ⓢ Inflammation, Ⓢ Joint Pain, Ⓢ Muscle Aches/Pain, Ⓢ Muscle Tension, Ⓢ Pain, Ⓢ Tension Headaches, Ⓢ Whiplash

Application:

Ⓢ: Apply as a compress on spine and on reflex points on feet. Apply on location for muscle cramps, bruises, or any other pain.

Safety Data: Repeated use may possibly result in contact sensitization. Use with caution during pregnancy.

Ⓢ=Topical, Ⓐ=Aromatic, Ⓞ=Internal

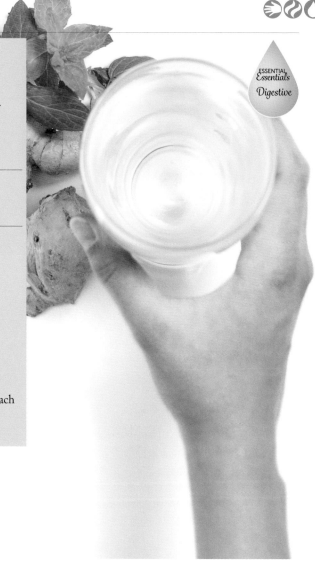

Biography

This blend may be useful for improving digestive function. The oils in this blend have been studied for their abilities in balancing the digestive system and soothing many of that system's ailments.

ⓢ Aroma:

- Minty • Anise-like
- Spicy • Sweet

⊕ Body Systems:

ⓓ Digestive System

Single Oils in This Blend:
Ginger, Peppermint, Tarragon, Fennel, Caraway, Coriander, Anise

Top Uses

- Upset Stomach/Bloating: Apply 2 drops over stomach area.
- Heartburn: Apply 1–2 drops to chest.
- Crohn's Disease: Apply 1–2 drops over the stomach and bottoms of the feet.

Common Primary Uses*: ⓢⓑBloating, ⓢⓞColitis, ⓞⓢConstipation, ⓞⓢCramps (Abdominal), ⓞⓢCrohn's Disease, ⓞⓢDiarrhea, ⓞFood Poisoning, ⓞⓢGastritis, ⓢⓞHeartburn, ⓢⓞNausea, ⓞⓢParasites, ⓢSinusitis

Application:

ⓢ: May be applied to reflex points on the feet and on the ankles. It may also be applied topically over the stomach, as a compress on the abdomen, and at the bottom of the throat (for gagging). Apply to animal paws for parasites.

ⓑ: Diffuse or inhale the aroma directly.

ⓞ: As a dietary supplement, dilute one drop in ½ cup (125 ml) of water or soy/rice milk, and sip slowly. May also be used in a retention enema for ridding the colon of parasites and for combating digestive candida.

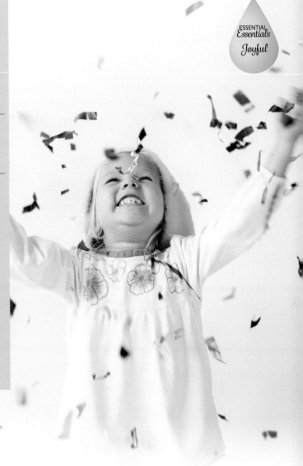

Biography

This uplifting combination of essential oils creates an energetic aroma that can help stimulate the body's chemistry when a person is feeling lethargic or sad.

ⓈAroma:

• Floral   • Woody   • Herbaceous
• Citrusy • Sweet

Body Systems:

Emotional balance

Single Oils in This Blend:
Lavandin, Lavender, Amyris, Clary Sage, Tangerine, Lemon Myrtle, Melissa, Ylang Ylang, Osmanthus, Hawaiian Sandalwood

Top Uses

• Upset Stomach/Bloating: Apply 2 drops over stomach area.

• Heartburn: Apply 1–2 drops to chest.

• Crohn's Disease: Apply 1–2 drops over the stomach and bottoms of the feet.

Common Primary Uses*: ⊘Abuse, ⊘Anxiety, ⊘Cushing's Syndrome, ⊘⊘Depression, ⊘⊘Energy, ⊘⊘Grief/Sorrow, ⊘⊘Lupus, ⊘Poison Oak/Ivy, ⊘⊘Postpartum Depression, ⊘Shock, ⊘⊘Stimulating, ⊘⊘Stress, ⊘Uplifting, ⊘Weight Loss

Application:

⊘: Rub over heart, ears, neck, thymus, temples, across brow, and on wrists. Apply on heart reflex points. Put in bathwater. Use as compress; dilute with fractionated coconut oil for a full-body massage. Place on areas of poor circulation.

⊘: Wear as perfume or cologne, especially over the heart. Put two drops on a wet cloth, and put the cloth in the dryer with washed laundry for great-smelling clothes. Diffuse or inhale the aroma directly.

Safety Data: Avoid exposure to direct sunlight for up to 12 hours after use.

⊘=Topical, ⊘=Aromatic, ○=Internal

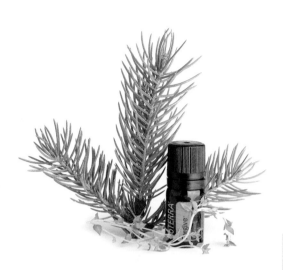

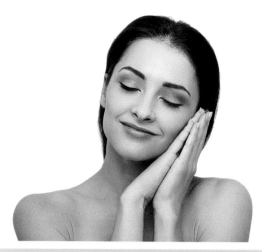

Quick Facts

This blend contains tree and herb oils that are known to help soothe feelings of anger or guilt and help promote feelings of love and forgiveness.

Common Primary Uses*: Acceptance, Anger, Blocks (Emotional), Confidence, Emotional Trauma, Grief, Guilt, Loss, Pity, Release (Emotional), Uplifting

Application:

: Diffuse or inhale the aroma directly.

: Apply on wrists, back of neck, over the heart area, or on the bottoms of the feet.

Single Oils in This Blend:
Spruce (Hemlock Spruce), Bergamot, Juniper Berry, Myrrh, Arborvitae, Nootka, Thyme, Citronella

Safety Data: Repeated use can result in contact sensitization. Consult your doctor before using if you are pregnant, epileptic, or have a medical condition.

Companion Blends: Comforting Blend, Encouraging Blend, Inspiring Blend, Reassuring Blend, Uplifting Blend.

Quick Facts

This new formulation of the Topical Blend contains oils that have been selected for their unique abilities to help protect the skin from bacterial and fungal proliferation and from other skin problems such as eczema and acne. This blend can be applied topically to infected areas.

Common Primary Uses*: Acne, Callouses, Dermatitis, Impetigo, Oily Skin

Application:

: Apply on location daily as needed.

Single Oils in This Blend:
Ho Wood, Melaleuca, Litsea Berry, Eucalyptus globulus, Geranium

Other Oils:

Black Cumin Seed Oil.

Safety Data: Repeated use may possibly result in contact sensitization. Use with caution during pregnancy.

See My Usage Guide section for more details. ●=Neat, ●=Dilute for Children/Sensitive Skin, ●=Dilute

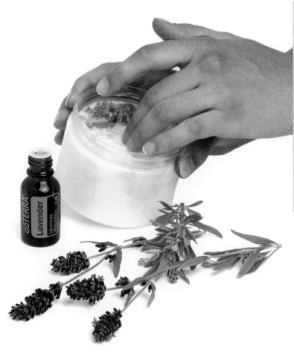

Quick Facts

This soothing blend may be useful for maintaining skin health and vitality. The oils in this blend have been studied for their abilities to help reduce inflammation, protect the skin from UV radiation, and promote healthy cellular function and proper hydration of the skin.

Common Primary Uses*: ◉Aging, ◉Chapped/Cracked Skin, ◉Dry Skin, ◉Revitalizing, ◉Wrinkles

Application:

◉: Apply directly on areas of concern. Use along with other natural skin care products.

Single Oils in This Blend:
Frankincense, Hawaiian Sandalwood, Lavender, Myrrh, Helichrysum, Rose

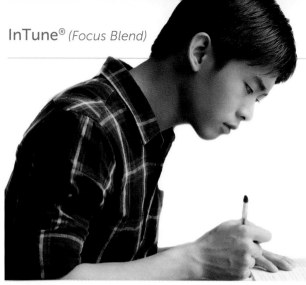

ESSENTIAL
Essentials
Focus

Biography

This blend contains oils that have been studied and used traditionally for their abilities to promote calmness, focus, and a balanced state of mind. Many of the oils in this blend contain high levels of sesquiterpenes, which have demonstrated an ability to pass the blood-brain barrier to reach the cells of the brain.

Ⓢ Aroma:

• Spicy   •Earthy   •Balsamic

⊕ Body Systems:

🜨 Hormonal system   🜨 Emotional Balance

⚡ Nervous System

Single Oils in This Blend:
Amyris (West Indian Sandalwood), Patchouli, Frankincense, Lime, Ylang Ylang, Hawaiian Sandalwood, Roman Chamomile

Top Uses

• Calming/Relaxing: Add 3 drops to 1 Tbs. (15 ml) fractionated coconut oil, and use as a soothing massage oil.

• Harmonizing/Grounding: Place 3 drops on the bottoms of the feet.

• Balancing: Diffuse in an aromatherapy diffuser.

Common Primary Uses*: 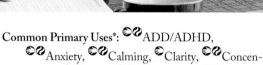ADD/ADHD, Anxiety, Calming, Clarity, Concentration, Focus, Hyperactivity, Stress

Application:

◐: Apply on back of neck and on bottoms of the feet.

◕: Diffuse or inhale the aroma directly.

Safety Data:
Repeated use may result in contact sensitization.

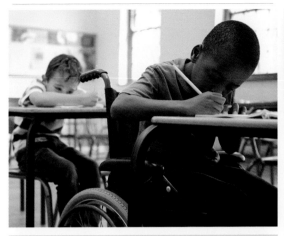

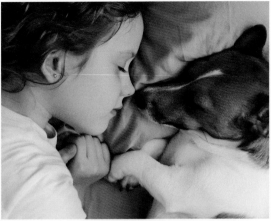

Quick Facts

Brave contains oils that are known for the ability to hesoothe anxious feelings. This blend can help promote feelings of self-worth and confidence in new and unknown situations. It is diluted in a base of fractionated coconut oil, so it is just right for young skin.

Common Primary Uses*: ◐⊘Anxiety, ◐⊘Courage, ◐⊘Uplifting

Application:

◐: Roll onto bottoms of feet, back of neck, or pulse points on wrists as needed.

⊘: Inhale the aroma directly. Roll onto a diffusing bracelet or necklace to wear throughout the day.

Single Oils in This Blend:

Orange, Amyris (West Indian Sandalwood), Osmanthus, Cinnamon Bark

Carrier Oil in This Blend: Fractionated coconut oil.

Safety Data: Keep out of reach of younger children. Consult with a physician before use if being treated for a medical condition.

Quick Facts

Calmer is designed to help soothe and promote relaxation after a busy, stressful day. It contains oils known for their calming and sedative properties. This blendcan help steady and balance the mind and emotions in preparation for a good night's sleep. It is diluted in a base of fractionated coconut oil, so it is just right for young skin.

Common Primary Uses*: ⊘◐Anger, ⊘◐Anxiety, ◐⊘Calming, ⊘◐Hyperactivity, ⊘◐Insomnia, ⊘◐Mental Fatigue, ⊘◐Mood Swings, ⊘◐Sedative, ⊘◐Sleep, ⊘◐Stress, ⊘◐Teeth Grinding, ⊘◐Tension

Application:

◐: Roll onto bottoms of feet, back of neck, chest, or pulse points on wrists as needed. Apply a small amount in palms, and then gently rub front and back of hands for a relaxing massage.

⊘: Inhale the aroma directly. Roll onto a diffusing bracelet or necklace to wear throughout the day.

Single Oils in This Blend:

Lavender, Cananga, Buddha Wood, Roman Chamomile

Carrier Oil in This Blend: Fractionated coconut oil.

Safety Data: Keep out of reach of younger children. Consult with a physician before use if being treated for a medical condition.

◐=Topical, ⊘=Aromatic, ◯=Internal

Kids: Rescuer™ (Soothing Blend)

Kids: Steady™ (Grounding Blend)

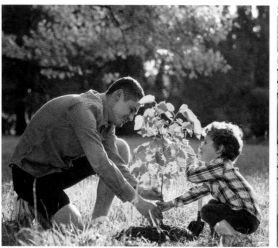

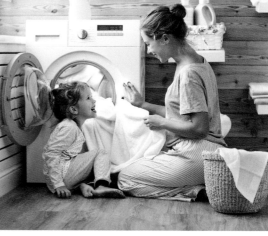

Quick Facts

Rescuer is ideal for soothing and comforting tired, achy muscles and joints at the end of a strenuous day. Oils in this blend are known for the ability to help relieve minor aches and pains. The blend is diluted in a base of fractionated coconut oil, so it is just right for young skin.

Common Primary Uses*: Back Pain, Bone Pain, Bruises, Inflammation, Joint Pain, Migraines, Muscle Aches/Pain, Muscle Tension, Pain, Stress, Tension Headache, Whiplash

Application:

: Roll onto tired or sore muscles at the end of the day or after strenuous activities. Roll onto legs to help soothe growing pains. Apply a small amount on the back, shoulders, and neck, gently massaging into tissues.

: Inhale the aroma directly. Roll onto a diffusing bracelet or necklace to wear throughout the day.

Single Oils in This Blend:

Copaiba, Lavender, Spearmint, Zanthoxylum

Carrier Oil in This Blend: Fractionated coconut oil.

Safety Data: Keep out of reach of younger children. Consult with a physician before use if being treated for a medical condition.

Quick Facts

Steady is comprised of oils known for their ability to help bring about a feeling of balance, peace, and relaxation. This blend can help focus the mind during times of distraction. It is diluted in a base of fractionated coconut oil, so it is just right for young skin.

Common Primary Uses*: ADD/ADHD, Anxiety, Balance, Brain, Confusion, Depression, Energy, Fear, Grief/Sorrow, Jet Lag, Metabolism (Balance), Mood Swings

Application:

: Roll onto bottoms of feet, back of neck, or pulse points on wrists as needed.

: Inhale the aroma directly. Roll onto a diffusing bracelet or necklace to wear throughout the day.

Single Oils in This Blend:

Amyris (West Indian Sandalwood), Balsam Fir, Coriander, Magnolia.

Carrier Oil in This Blend: Fractionated coconut oil.

Safety Data: Keep out of reach of younger children. Consult with a physician before use if being treated for a medical condition.

See My Usage Guide section for more details. =Neat, =Dilute for Children/Sensitive Skin, =Dilute

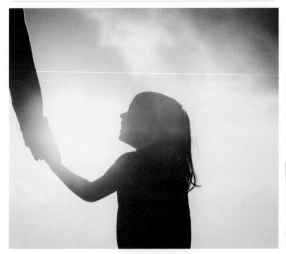

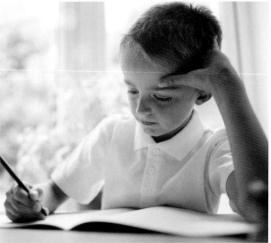

Quick Facts

Stronger is comprised of oils known to help soothe and protect the skin and body from environmental threats. This blend is diluted in a base of fractionated coconut oil, so it is just right for young skin.

Common Primary Uses*: Acne, Antibacterial, Antiseptic, Candida, Cleansing, Cuts/ Scrapes, Coughs, Insect Bites/Stings,

Application:

: Roll onto distressed or irritated skin. Apply to bottoms of feet, back of neck, or pulse points on wrists as needed.

: Inhale the aroma directly. Roll onto a diffusing bracelet or necklace to wear throughout the day.

Single Oils in This Blend:

Cedarwood, Litsea, Frankincense, Rose

Carrier Oil in This Blend: Fractionated coconut oil.

Safety Data: Keep out of reach of younger children. Consult with a physician before use if being treated for a medical condition.

Quick Facts

Thinker contains oils known for their ability to aid focus, memory, and concentration. This blend can help create a positive, nurturing atmosphere to support learning. It is diluted in a base of fractionated coconut oil, so it is just right for young skin.

Common Primary Uses*: ADD/ADHD, Alertness, Anxiety, Calming, Clarity, Concentration, Focus, Memory, Stress

Application:

: Roll onto temples, back of neck, or pulse points on wrists as needed to help maintain focus and concentration.

: Inhale the aroma directly. Roll onto a diffusing bracelet or necklace to wear throughout the day.

Single Oils in This Blend:

Vetiver, Clementine, Peppermint, Rosemary

Carrier Oil in This Blend: Fractionated coconut oil.

Safety Data: Keep out of reach of younger children. Consult with a physician before use if being treated for a medical condition.

=Topical, =Aromatic, =Internal

Quick Facts

This blend contains a combination of mint and citrus oils that can help motivate and inspire an individual to have the courage to move forward with confidence and strength.

Common Primary Uses*: Anxious Feelings, Confidence, Creativity, Defeat, Depression, Expression (Self-expression), Fear, Happiness, Positiveness, Rejection

Application:

: Diffuse or inhale the aroma directly.

: Apply on wrists, back of neck, over the heart area, or on the bottoms of the feet.

Single Oils in This Blend:
Peppermint, Clementine, Coriander, Basil, Yuzu, Melissa, Rosemary, Vanilla

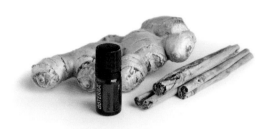

Quick Facts

This blend contains spice and herb oils that are known to help enhance passion and excitement for life.

Common Primary Uses*: Confidence, Defeat, Expression, Fear, Joy, Rejection, Uplifting, Passion

Application:

: Diffuse or inhale the aroma directly.

: Apply on wrists, back of neck, over the heart area, or on the bottoms of the feet.

Single Oils in This Blend:
Cardamom, Cinnamon, Ginger, Clove, Sandalwood, Jasmine, Vanilla, Damiana

Carrier Oil in This Blend: Fractionated coconut oil.

Safety Data: Repeated use can result in contact sensitization. Consult your doctor before using if you are pregnant, epileptic, or have a medical condition.

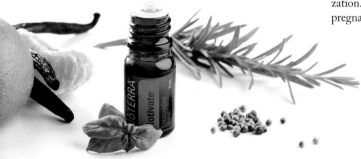

ESSENTIAL
Essentials
Protective

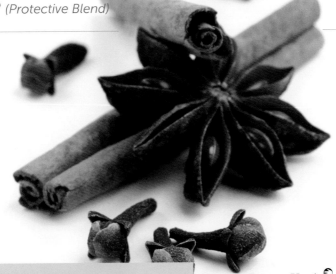

Biography

The oils in this blend have been studied for their strong abilities to kill harmful bacteria, mold, and viruses. This blend can be diffused into the air or be used to clean and purify household surfaces.

Aroma:

- Spicy
- Warm
- Citrusy
- Herbaceous

Body Systems:

Immune System

Single Oils in This Blend:

Orange, Clove Bud, Cinnamon Bark, Eucalyptus radiata, Rosemary

Top Uses

- Stress: Add 5–10 drops to 1 Tbs. (15 ml) fractionated coconut oil, and use as a massage oil.

- Uplifting: Diffuse using an aromatherapy diffuser, or inhale the aroma directly from the bottle to help with anorexia and bulimia.

- Cleansing: Mix 3–5 drops with 1 cup (250 ml) of water in a bowl or bucket. Moisten a rag with this water, and use to clean countertops and other surfaces.

Common Primary Uses*: Abscess (Oral), Air Pollution, Antibacterial, Antifungal, Antiviral, Bladder Infection, Candida, Chronic Fatigue, Cleansing, Cold Sores, Colds, Coughs, Flu, Gum Disease, Halitosis, Hypoglycemia, Infection, Lupus, Mold, Mono, MRSA, Plague, Pneumonia, Scabies, Sore Throat, Staph Infection, Warts

Application:

: Massage throat, stomach, intestines, and bottoms of feet. Dilute one drop in 15 drops of fractionated coconut oil: massage the thymus to stimulate the immune system, and massage under the arms to stimulate the lymphatic system. It is best applied to the bottoms of the feet, as it may be caustic to the skin. Dilute with fractionated coconut oil when used on sensitive/young skin.

: Diffuse or inhale the aroma directly.

Aromatic Influence: Diffuse this blend of oils periodically for 20–25 minutes at a time to help protect the body against the onset of flu, colds, and viruses.

Safety Data: Repeated use can result in extreme contact sensitization. Can cause extreme skin irritation. Use with caution during pregnancy.

=Topical, =Aromatic, =Internal

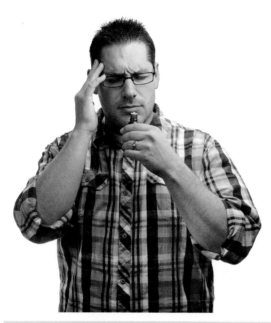

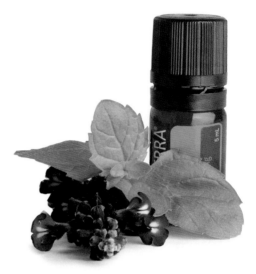

Quick Facts

The oils in this blend are known to help relieve the pain and tension associated with headaches.

Common Primary Uses*: Headaches, Migraines, Muscle Tension, Tension Headaches

Application:

: Use a roll-on applicator to apply this blend to the temples, the forehead, the back of the neck, and to the reflex areas on the hands and feet.

: Inhale the aroma directly.

Single Oils in This Blend:
Wintergreen, Lavender, Peppermint, Frankincense, Cilantro, Roman Chamomile, Marjoram, Basil, Rosemary

Safety Data: Repeated use can result in extreme contact sensitization. Can cause extreme skin irritation. Use with caution during pregnancy.

Quick Facts

This blend contains floral and mint oils that are known to help alleviate fearful, worried, and anxious feelings and replace them with peaceful contentment.

Common Primary Uses*: Anxious Feelings, Clearing (Emotional), Defeat, Depression, Fear, Guilt, Overburdened, Peace, Stress, Worried Feelings

Application:

: Diffuse or inhale the aroma directly.

: Apply on wrists, back of neck, over the heart area, or on the bottoms of the feet.

Single Oils in This Blend:
Vetiver, Lavender, Ylang Ylang, Frankincense, Clary Sage, Marjoram, Labdanum, Spearmint

Safety Data: Consult your doctor before using if you are pregnant, epileptic, or have a medical condition.

Companion Blends: Comforting Blend, Encouraging Blend, Inspiring Blend, Renewing Blend, Uplifting Blend.

*See My Usage Guide section for more details.　●=Neat, ●=Dilute for Children/Sensitive Skin, ●=Dilute

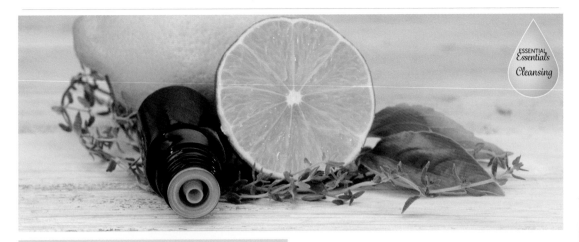

ESSENTIAL
Essentials
Cleansing

Biography

Several of the oils contained in this blend are well known and are often used to help remove odors from the air. Others have been studied for their powerful abilities to disinfect and to kill harmful microorganisms.

Ⓢ Aroma:

• Fresh   • Herbaceous   • Light

⊕ Body Systems:

⊕ Skin   ⊕ Emotional Balance

⊕ Digestive System

Single Oils in This Blend:
Lemon, Lime, Siberian Fir, Citronella, Melaleuca, Cilantro

Top Uses

• Air Cleansing: Diffuse in an aromatherapy diffuser.

• Mildew: Add 25 drops to ¼ cup (50 ml) water in a small spray bottle, and spray on surface to help neutralize mildew.

• Deodorant/Deodorizing: Add 5 drops to 1 Tbs. (15 ml) water in a small spray bottle, and spray into the air, in garbage cans, or on other surfaces needing deodorizing.

• Cleaning: Add 5 drops to a damp rag, and use to wipe down surfaces.

Common Primary Uses*: ⬡Abscess (Tooth), ⬡⬡Addictions, ⬡Airborne Bacteria, ⬡Air Pollution, ⬡Allergies, ⬡⬡Antibacterial, ⬡Boils, ⬡Bug Bites, ⬡⬡Cleansing, ⬡⬡Deodorant, ⬡⬡Deodorizing, ⬡⬡Disinfectant, ⬡Ear Infection, ⬡Infected Burns, ⬡Laundry, ⬡⬡Mice (Repel), ⬡Mildew, ⬡Skin Ulcer, ⬡Stings, ⬡Urinary Infection

Application:

⬡: Apply to reflex points on the body, ears, feet, and temples. Apply topically for infections and cleansing.

⬡: Put on cotton balls and place in air vents for an insect repellent at home or at work. Can also be added to paint to help reduce fumes. Diffuse or inhale the aroma directly.

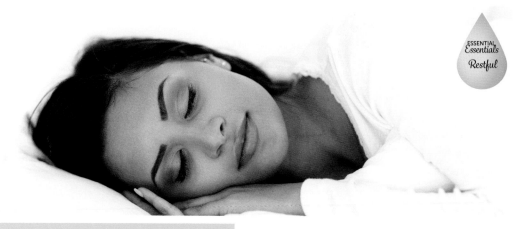

Biography

This relaxing blend contains essential oils that are often used to help calm and soothe feelings of stress, excitement, and anxiety in order to help the body have a restful sleep.

Ⓢ Aroma:

• Floral • Warm • Sweet • Herbaceous

⊕ Body Systems:

Nervous System   Emotional balance

Single Oils in This Blend:
Lavender, Ho Wood, Cedarwood, Ylang Ylang, Sweet Marjoram, Roman Chamomile, Vanilla Bean Absolute, Vetiver, Hawaiian Sandalwood.

Top Uses

• Calming: Diffuse in an aromatherapy diffuser.

• Anxiety: Apply 1 drop to the back of neck, temples, and bottoms of the feet.

• Insomnia: Add 1-2 drops to warm bathwater, and bathe before sleeping.

• Sleep: Add 15 drops to 2 Tbs. (25 ml) water in a small spray bottle. Shake, and mist a small amount on pillows and linens before sleeping.

• Mental Fatigue: Inhale the aroma directly from the bottle.

• Stress: Apply 1 drop to nape of neck, wrists, or other pulse points.

Common Primary Uses*: ADD/ADHD, Addictions, Anger, Anxiety, Calming, Hyperactivity, Insomnia, Itching, Mental Fatigue, Mood Swings, Sedative, Sleep, Stress, Teeth Grinding, Tension

Application:

: Apply under nose and to back, feet, and back of neck. Put in bathwater. Apply to navel, feet, or back of neck for insomnia.

: Wear as perfume or cologne. Diffuse or inhale the aroma directly.

*See My Usage Guide section for more details.   ●=Neat, ●=Dilute for Children/Sensitive Skin, ●=Dilute

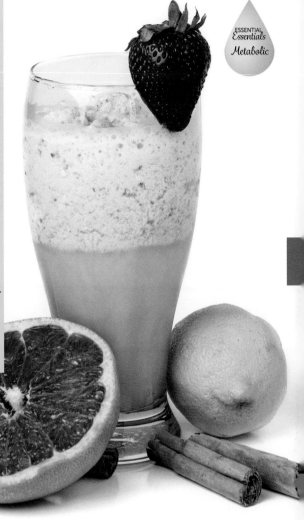

Biography

This blend is designed to help control hunger and to help limit excessive calorie intake. The oils in this blend are calming to the stomach and work to improve emotional well-being. This blend is most effective when combined with exercise and healthy eating.

Ⓢ Aroma:

• Citrusy • Sweet • Warm • Spicy

⊕ Body Systems:

Ⓓ Digestive System Ⓔ Emotional Balance

Single Oils in This Blend:
Grapefruit, Lemon, Peppermint, Ginger, Cinnamon

Top Uses

• Appetite suppressant: Add 4 drops to 2 cups (½ L) of water (or other beverage), and drink between meals throughout the day.

• Cravings: Diffuse in an aromatherapy diffuser to help reduce cravings.

Common Primary Uses*: OⓄAppetite Suppressant, OⓈCellulite, OⓄObesity, OⓄOvereating, OⓄWeight Loss

Application:

Ⓣ: Apply on wrists, bottoms of the feet, or on area of concern.

Ⓐ: Apply to palms of hands: cup hands over nose and mouth, and breathe deeply. Diffuse into the air.

Ⓘ: Add 8 drops of Slim & Sass to 2 cups (½ L) of water, and drink throughout the day between meals.

Aromatic Influence: This blend of oils is calming to the stomach and uplifting to the mind.

Safety Data: Because this blend contains citrus oils, it may increase skin photosensitivity. It is best to avoid sunlight or UV rays for 12 hours after topical application. Do not apply directly in eyes, ears, or nose. Consult your doctor before using if you are pregnant or have a medical condition.

Ⓣ=Topical, Ⓐ=Aromatic, Ⓘ=Internal

TerraShield® (Outdoor Blend)

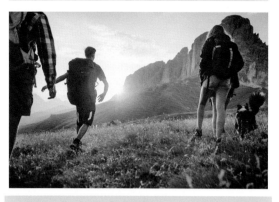

Quick Facts

This blend combines essential oils that have been proven to effectively repel biting insects and help protect the skin from UV radiation.

Common Primary Uses*: Bug/Insect Repellent

Application:

: Apply a small amount of this oil on the skin.

: Diffuse into the air, or place a few drops on ribbons and strings, and place near air vents, windows, or openings where bugs might come in.

Single Oils in This Blend:
Ylang Ylang Flower, Tamanu Seed, Nootka Wood, Cedarwood Wood, Catnip Plant, Lemon Eucalyptus Leaf, Litsea Fruit, Vanilla Bean Absolute, Arborvitae Wood.

Carrier Oil in This Blend: Fractionated coconut oil.

Aromatic Influence: It is highly repellent to many flying and crawling insects and bugs.

Whisper® (Blend for Women)

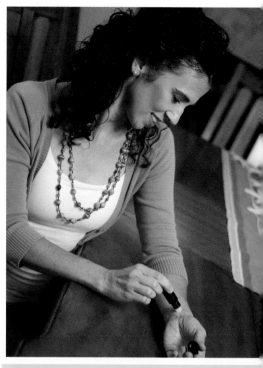

Quick Facts

This exquisite blend of oils works harmoniously with an individual's unique chemistry to create an appealing aroma—without the harmful chemicals found in many of today's perfumes.

Common Primary Uses*: Aphrodisiac, Frigidity, Hormonal Balance

Application:

: Add 5–6 drops to 1 Tbs. (15 ml) fractionated coconut oil for use in massage.

: Diffuse or wear as a perfume.

Single Oils in This Blend:
Patchouli, Bergamot, Hawaiian Sandalwood, Rose, Jasmine, Cinnamon Bark, Vetiver, Ylang Ylang, Labdanum, Cocoa Bean Extract, Vanilla Bean Extract

Carrier Oil in This Blend: Fractionated coconut oil.

---

*See My Usage Guide section for more details.   ●=Neat, ●=Dilute for Children/Sensitive Skin, ●=Dilute

Yarrow Pom™ *(Active Botanical Nutritive)*

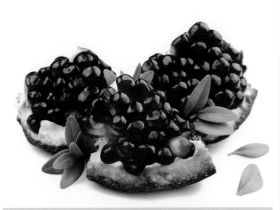

Quick Facts

This unique formulation combines the skin benefits of yarrow essential oil with the powerful antioxidant and cellular health properties of pomegranate seed oil. Pomegranate seed oil has been studied for its abilities to help lessen insulin resistence and reduce weight gain, as well as for its anti-inflammatory, antioxidant, and anti-tumoral properties.

Common Primary Uses*: ⭕Aging, ⭕Antioxidant, ⭕⯂Cancer, ⭕Cellular Health, ⭕Diabetes, ⭕Obesity, ⯂⭕Skin (Healing).

Application:

⯂: Apply on area of concern.

🌀: Inhale the aroma directly. Or apply to a diffusing bracelet or necklace to wear throughout the day.

⭕: Take 1–2 drops daily in a capsule or in 1 cup (250 ml) of beverage.

Single Oil in This Blend:

Yarrow

Carrier Oil in This Blend:

Pomegranate Seed Oil

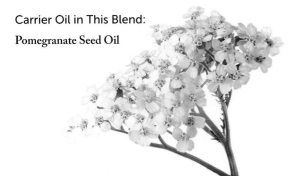

Yoga: Align *(Centering Blend)*

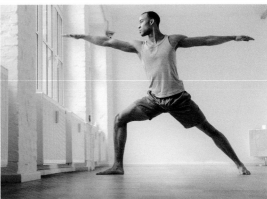

Quick Facts

This blend is designed to help bring order to the chaos that surrounds our daily lives, bringing alignment, focus, trust, purpose, and understanding to what matters most.

Common Primary Uses*: ⯂🌀Focus, ⯂🌀Yoga

Application:

⯂: Apply to the wrists, heart area, and back of neck. Apply on reflex points on the hands and feet.

🌀: Diffuse, or inhale from the hands.

Single Oils in This Blend:

Bergamot, Coriander, Marjoram, Peppermint, Geranium, Basil, Rose, Jasmine

Aromatic Influence: Helps to uplift and motivate the mind and emotions, while still keeping one centered and focused.

⯂=Topical, 🌀=Aromatic, ⭕=Internal

Quick Facts

This blend is designed to help ground and anchor the mind and emotions to help promote a sense of courage, calmness, and assurance, allowing one a firm base from which to move onward with life.

Common Primary Uses*: Calming, Centering, Yoga

Application:

: Apply on the heart, ankles, bottoms of the feet, and the base of the spine.

: Diffuse, or inhale from the hands.

Single Oils in This Blend:

Lavender, Cedarwood, Frankincense, Cinnamon, Sandalwood, Black Pepper, Patchouli.

Aromatic Influence: Helps to uplift and motivate the mind and emotions, while still keeping one centered and focused.

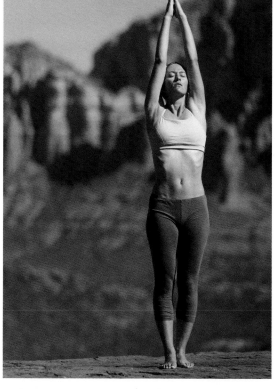

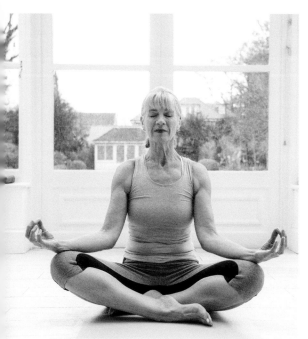

Quick Facts

This blend helps promote feelings of inspiration and joy, helping one to arise and move beyond opposition and challenges in life.

Common Primary Uses*: Inspiration, Joy, Yoga

Application:

: Apply to the wrists, heart area, and back of neck. Apply on reflex points on the hands and feet.

: Diffuse, or inhale from the hands. Wear as perfume or on aromatherapy jewelry.

Single Oils in This Blend:

Lemon, Grapefruit, Siberian Fir, Osmanthus, Melissa

Aromatic Influence: Helps to uplift and inspire the mind and emotions, promoting feelings of strength, confidence, and courage to move forward and achieve.

See My Usage Guide section for more details.   ●=Neat, ●=Dilute for Children/Sensitive Skin, ●=Dilute

Zendocrine® *(Detoxification Blend)*

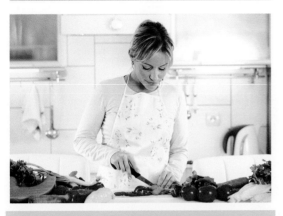

Quick Facts

This blend contains oils that have been studied for their abilities to help support organ cleansing and healthy tissue function.

Common Primary Uses*: ○◖Endocrine Support, ○◖Hormonal Balance

Application:

◖: Massage on bottoms of feet.

◿: Diffuse or inhale the aroma directly.

○: Take 3–5 drops of the Detoxification Blend in capsules either alone or with a Detoxification Complex supplement capsule up to once a day.

Single Oils in This Blend:
Rosemary, Cilantro, Juniper Berry, Tangerine, Geranium

Essential Supplements

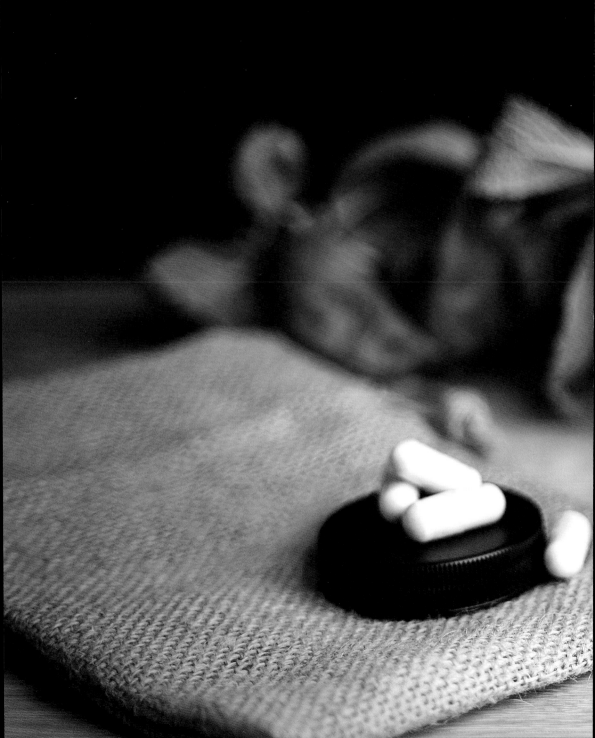

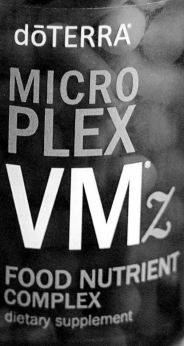

Essential Oil–Inspired Wellness Supplements

This section contains various essential oil–inspired supplements that are available commercially and the essential ingredients that each supplement contains.

For further information and research on many of the single oils contained in these supplements, see the Essential Oils section of this book.

a2z Chewable™

Chewable Multivitamin

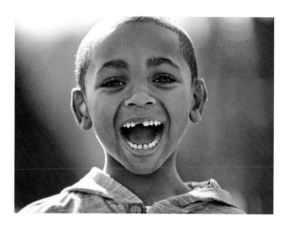

This supplement is a complete daily nutrient supplement for children and for those who have a hard time swallowing pills.

Key Ingredients:

−Vitamin and Mineral Complex:

Vitamin A (natural alpha and beta carotene), Vitamin C (from acerola cherry fruit extract), Vitamin D$_3$ (as cholecalciferol), Vitamin E (as d-alpha tocopheryl acetate and mixed tocopherols), Thiamin/Vitamin B1 (as thiamine HCl), Riboflavin/Vitamin B2, Niacin/Vitamin B3 (as niacinamide), Vitamin B6 (as pyridoxine HCl), Folic Acid, Vitamin B12 (as methylcobalamin), Biotin, Pantothenic Acid/Vitamin B5 (as d-calcium pantothenate), Calcium (as calcium amino acid chelate), Iron (iron amino acid chelate), Iodine (from potassium iodide), Magnesium (as magnesium amino acid chelate), Zinc (as zinc amino acid chelate), Copper (as copper amino acid chelate), Manganese (as manganese amino acid chelate), Potassium (as potassium glycinate), Choline (as choline bitartrate), Inositol.

−Superfood Blend:

Pineapple (Bromelain Protease Enzymes), Pomegranate Extract (Ellagic Acid), Lemon Bioflavonoids, Spirulina, Sunflower Oil, Others: Rice Bran, Beet Greens, Broccoli, Brown Rice, Carrot, Mango, Cranberry, Rose Hips, Spinach.

−Cellular Vitality Complex Blend:

Tomato Fruit Extract (Lycopene), Grape Seed Extract (Proanthocyanidins), Marigold Flower Extract (Lutein).

Alpha CRS+®

Cellular Vitality Complex

Alpha CRS+ contains important ingredients that may help to increase cellular health, vitality, and energy.

Key Ingredients:

Boswellia serrata Extract (beta-Boswellic Acids), Scuttelaria Root Extract (Baicalin), Milk Thistle Extract (Silymarin), Pineapple Extract (Bromelain Protease Enzymes), *Polygonum cuspidatum* Extract (Resveratrol), Green Tea Leaf Extract, Pomegranate Fruit Extract (Ellagic Acid), Turmeric Root Extract (Curcumin), Grape Seed Extract (Proanthocyanidins), Sesame Seed Extract, Pine Bark Extract, Acetyl-L-Carnitine, Alpha Lipoic Acid, Coenzyme Q(10), Quercetin, Ginkgo Biloba Leaf Extract, Tummy Taming Blend.

Bone Nutrient Lifetime Complex

This supplement combines bioavailable vitamins and minerals that have demonstrated a role in promoting bone health and in preventing age- and nutritional-related calcium loss and bone demineralization.

Key Ingredients:

Vitamin C (as magnesium ascorbate), Vitamin D-2 (as ergocalciferol) and Vitamin D-3 (as cholacalciferol), Biotin (as d-biotin), Calcium (as coral calcium), Magnesium (as magnesium chelate), Zinc (as yeast), Copper (as yeast), Manganese (as yeast), Boron (as yeast).

Breathe® Respiratory Drops

Respiratory Lozenge Drops

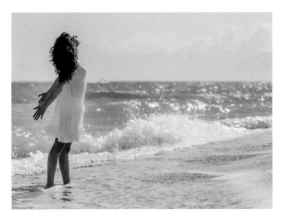

These drops combine many essential oils that are often used and studied for their abilities to help support the respiratory system.

Key Ingredients:

Lemon Essential Oil, Peppermint Essential Oil, *Eucalyptus radiata* Essential Oil, Thyme Essential Oil, Melissa Essential Oil, Cardamom Essential Oil.

Copaiba Softgels

These unique softgels contain copaiba essential oil in a base of olive oil. Copaiba oil contains high levels of beta-caryophyllene, which has been studied for its ability to affect one of the two cannibinoid receptors in the body. Cannabinoid receptors—found throughout the body—are involved in a variety of physiological processes, including appetite, pain sensation, mood, and memory. The two known cannabinoid receptors are CB1 and CB2. When activated, both CB1 and CB2 help with inflammation, pain, and mood. The difference is that activation of the CB1 receptor (which is activated by marijuana) also creates a psychoactive high in the body, while activation of the CB2 receptor does not cause any psychoactive effects. Beta-caryophyllene activates only the CB2 receptor, allowing it to powerfully affect inflammation, pain, and mood, without any psychoactive side-effects (Klauke et al., 2013; Fine et al., 2013; Cheng et al., 2014; Alberti et al., 2017).

Key Ingredients:

Copaiba Essential Oil

DDR Prime® Softgels

Essential Oil Cellular Complex

The oils in this essential oil blend have been chosen for their abilities to provide antioxidant support for the cells and to promote a healthy cellular life cycle.

Key Ingredients:

Frankincense, Orange, Litsea, Lemongrass, Thyme, Summer Savory *(Satureja hortensis)*, Clove, Niaouli *(Melaleuca quinquenervia)*.

Deep Blue Polyphenol Complex®

Soothing Polyphenol Complex

Like Deep Blue, this polyphenol nutritional supplement provides natural support for aching muscles, sore joints, and other occasional discomforts. The polyphenols, found in green tea, resveratrol, grape juice, and pomegranate juice, provide antioxidant power.

Key Ingredients:

Frankincense *(Boswellia serrata)* Gum Resin Extract, Turmeric Root Extract (Curcumin), Green Tea Leaf Extract, Pomegranate *(Punica granatum)* Fruit Extract, Grape *(Vitis vinifera)* Seed Extract:, Resveratrol (from *Polygonum cuspidatum* Extract), Tummy Taming Blend.

DigestTab®

Digestive Calcium Tablets

DigestTab combines the acid-neutralizing benefits of calcium carbonate with an infusion of essential oils that have been studied for their abilities to soothe digestive symptoms and support the digestive system.

Key Ingredients:

Calcium Carbonate, Ginger Essential Oil, Peppermint Essential Oil, Tarragon Essential Oil, Fennel Essential Oil, Caraway Essential Oil, Coriander Essential Oil, Anise Essential Oil.

DigestZen® Softgels

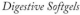

Digestive Softgels

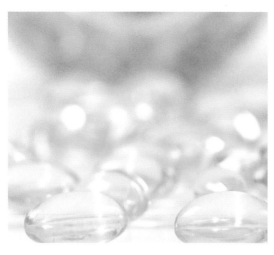

DigestZen Softgels are a convenient way to take the DigestZen, which contains oils that have been studied for their abilities to soothe digestive symptoms and support the digestion system.

Key Ingredients:

Ginger, Peppermint, Tarragon, Fennel, Caraway, Coriander, Anise.

DigestZen Terrazyme®

Digestive Enzyme Complex

This supplement blends food-derived enzymes and mineral cofactors that can aid in the digestion and absorption of critical nutrients that are lacking in many of today's diets.

Key Ingredients:

Protease (Aspergillus), Papain (Papaya), Amylase (Aspergillus), Lactase (Aspergillus), Lipase (Rhizopus), Alpha Galactosidase (Aspergillus), Cellulase (Trichoderma), Sucrase (Saccharomyces), Betaine HCL, Glucoamylase (Aspergillus), Anti-gluten Enzyme Blend (Aspergillus), Tummy Taming Blend, Companion Supplements.

GX Assist®

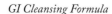

GI Cleansing Formula

GX Assist blends essential oils with caprylic acid to help support the gastrointestinal tract in eliminating pathogens.

Key Ingredients

Oregano Essential Oil, Melaleuca Essential Oil, Lemon Essential Oil, Lemongrass Essential Oil, Peppermint Essential Oil, Thyme Essential Oil, Caprylic Acid.

IQ Mega®

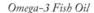

Omega-3 Fish Oil

Omega-3 Fish Oil provides all of the essential fatty acid benefits from fish oil without the fishy taste. It should be molecularly filtered to remove the fish aroma and naturally flavored with orange essential oil for a great taste even kids will love.

Key Ingredients:

Fish Oil Concentrate (EPA, DHA), Vitamin D, Vitamin E (as natural mixed tocopherols), Vitamin C (as ascorbyl palmitate), Orange Essential Oil.

Microplex VMz®

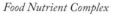

Food Nutrient Complex

This multivitamin combines natural vitamins and minerals with a complex of whole-food nutrients and minerals that are bound to a glycoprotein matrix to help enhance their bioavailability. These nutrients help support healthy cell, tissue, and system function. Additionally, this supplement contains a whole-food blend and a patented enzyme assimilation system to help further enhance nutrient bioavailability.

Key Ingredients:

Vitamin A (as a & b carotene and retinyl palmitate), vitamin C (as calcium ascorbate and magnesium ascorbate), vitamon D3 (as cholecaliferol), vitamin E (as natural mixed tocopherols and tocotrienols), vitamin K (as glycoprotein matrix), thiamin (as glycoprotein matrix), riboflavin (as glycoprotein matrix), niacin (as glycoprotein matrix), vitamin B6 (as glycoprotein matrix), folate (as natural lemon (citrus limon) peel extract, oregen FA), Vitamin B12 (as glycoprotein matrix), biotin (as glycoprotein matrix), pantothenic acid (as glycoprotein matrix), calcium (as malate dimacal, natural coral, and ascorbate), iron (as bis-glycinate chelate) ferrochel, iodine (from kelp (*Laminaria digitata*) stem and leaf powder), Magnesium (as dimagnesium malate and ascorbate), Zinc (as bis-glycinate chelate), Selenium (as glycinate and selenomethionine), Copper (as bis-glycinate chelate), Manganese (as bis-glycinate chelate), Chromium (as nicotinate glycinate chelate), Polyphenol Blend, Whole-Food Blend, Tummy Taming Blend.

Mito2Max®

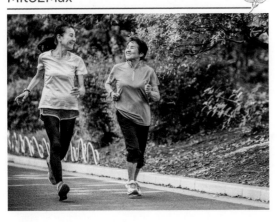

Energy & Stamina Complex

This multi-nutrient supplement would be a natural alternative to unhealthy energy drinks to support stamina and increase cellular health, vitality, and energy.

Key Ingredients:

Acetyl-L-Carnitine HCL, Alpha Lipoic Acid, Coenzyme Q(10), Lychee (*Litchi chinensis*) Fruit Extract, Green Tea (*Camellia sinensis*) Leaf Polyphenol Extract, Quercetin (from *Sophorae japonica* Bud), Cordyceps (*Cordyceps sinensis*) Mycelium, Ginseng (*Panax quinquefolius*) Root Extract, Ashwagandha (*Withania somnifera*) Root Extract.

On Guard® Protecting Throat Drops

Protective Throat Drops

These drops offer the relief of a throat drop, soothing dry and scratchy throats, combined with the immune-protectant power of the essential oils that make up On Guard.

Key Ingredients:

Orange Essential Oil, Clove Bud Essential Oil, Cinnamon Bark Essential Oil, *Eucalyptus radiata* Essential Oil, Rosemary Essential Oil, Cassia Essential Oil, Myrrh Essential Oil.

On Guard®+ Softgels

Protective Softgels

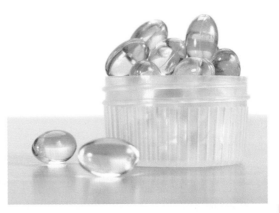

Combines the power of On Guard with black pepper, oregano, and melissa essential oils to help support the immune system.

Key Ingredients:

Orange Essential Oil, Clove Bud Essential Oil, Black Pepper Essential Oil, Cinnamon Bark Essential Oil, *Eucalyptus radiata* Essential Oil, Oregano Essential Oil, Rosemary Essential Oil, Melissa Essential Oil.

PB Assist®+

Probiotic Defense Formula

This supplement blends six strains of probiotic intestinal flora that can help support healthy colonies of friendly microflora in the digestive tract. These probiotics are recommended to be taken using a special double-coated capsule that protects the flora as they pass through the stomach.

Key Ingredients:

Lactobacillus acidophilus, Bifidobacterium lactis, Lactobacillus salivarious, Lactobacillus casei, Bifidobacterium bifidum, Bifidobacterium longum, Fructo-Oligosaccharide (FOS).

PB Assist® Jr

Probiotic Powder

This supplement blends 6 strains of probiotic intestinal flora that can help support healthy colonies of friendly microflora in the digestive tract. These strains have been studied for their abilities to help support healthy digestion and to help protect against harmful infections that are common in childhood. These probiotics are recommended to be taken using a special micro-encapsulation that protects the flora as they pass through the stomach.

Key Ingredients:

Lactobacillus rhamnosus, Lactobacillus salivarius, Lactobacillus plantarum LP01 and LP02, Bifidobacterium breve, Bifidobacterium lactis, Fructo-Oligosaccharide (FOS).

Phytoestrogen Lifetime Complex

Phytoestrogen Complex

This complex may help women maintain a healthy estrogen balance with a potent blend of phytoestrogens (plant-derived estrogen-mimicking compounds) from soy, pomegranate, and flax seeds.

Key Ingredients:

Soy Extract (64% isoflavones with a minimum 50% genistein), Flax Seed Extract (40% lignan), Pomegranate Extract (40% ellagic acid).

Safety Data: If pregnant, lactating, or experiencing any health conditions, consult a physician before using.

Serenity™ Restful Complex Softgels

This unique supplement combines the powerful sedative and anti-anxiety effects of lavender essential oil and l-theanine with melissa, passionflower, and German chamomile extracts to help calm, soothe, and prepare the body and mind to enter a relaxed state of sleep.

Key Ingredients:

Lavender Essential Oil, L-Theanine (Green Tea Extract), Lemon Balm (Melissa) Extract, Passionflower (Passiflora incarnata) Extract, German Chamomile Extract.

Slim & Sassy® Control™ Bars

Appetite Suppressant Bars

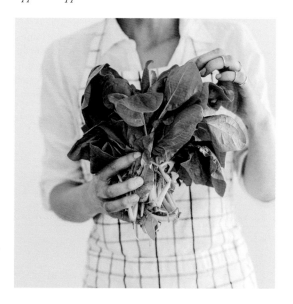

Slim & Sassy Control Bars are filled with natural ingredients to help manage weight, hunger, and well-being. One of the key ingredients found in these bars is a spinach leaf extract that has been shown to significantly reduce appetite for up to 6 hours. Slim & Sassy Control Bars can be used for weight management when combined with a healthy lifestyle, exercise, and a balanced nutrition.

Key Ingredients:

Organic Brown Rice Syrup and Honey, Yogurt, Spinach (Spinacia oleracea) Leaf Extract, High Oleic Sunflower Oil, Whey Protein Crisp, Gluten-Free Rolled Oats, Almonds, Sunflower Seeds, Raisins, Organic Flax Meal, Sesame Seeds, Chia Seeds, Tocopherols

Slim & Sassy® Control™ Instant Drink Mix

Appetite Suppressant Drink Mix

This powdered drink mix combines the action of Slim & Sassy with natural ingredients to help manage weight, hunger, and well-being. One of the key ingredients found in this drink mix is a spinach leaf extract that has been shown to significantly reduce appetite for up to 6 hours. This drink mix can be used for weight management when combined with a healthy lifestyle, exercise, and balanced nutrition. The drink mix can be mixed in water, a trim shake, or a favorite beverage.

Key Ingredients:

Spinach (*Spinacia oleracea*) Leaf Extract, Ground Flax (*Linum usitatissimum*) Seed Powder, Grapefruit Essential Oil, Lemon Essential Oil, Peppermint Essential Oil, Ginger Essential Oil, Cinnamon Essential Oil, Potato (*Solanum tuberosum*) Tuber Extract.

Slim & Sassy® TrimShake

Trim Shake

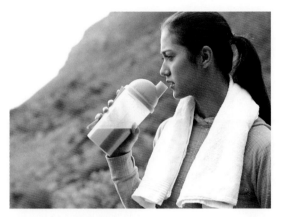

Choose a high-fiber, high-protein meal alternative drink powder with a low glycemic index and low calories. These shakes should contain extracts from the ashwagandha plant (*Withania somnifera*) that have shown potential to decrease blood serum levels of cortisol (Abedon, 2008) and to reduce stress (Archana et al., 1999; Bhattacharya et al., 1987). Cortisol—a hormone created by the adrenal glands—is released into the blood as the result of stress or anxiety, and it also plays a role in the body's sleep/wake cycle. When an individual is exposed to constant or chronic stress, levels of cortisol remain elevated in the body, disrupting the body's ability to relax and its ability to sleep naturally. Chronic stress and abnormally elevated cortisol levels have also been associated with increased cravings and with increased levels of obesity and abdominal weight (De Vriendt et al., 2009; Wallerius et al., 2003).

Key Ingredients:

Protein Blend, Potato Protein Extract, Fiber Blend, Ashwagandha (*Withania somnifera*) Root and Leaf Extracts, Stevia, Vitamins and Minerals: Key vitamins and minerals are listed below:

Calcium (dicalcium phosphate), Magnesium (magnesium oxide), Vitamin C (ascorbic acid), Vitamin E (vitamin E acetate), Vitamin B7 (biotin), Vitamin B3 (niacinamide), Iodine (potassium iodide), Zinc (zinc oxide), Vitamin A (vitamin A acetate), Copper (copper gluconate), Vitamin B5 (D-calcium pantothenate), Vitamin D3, Vitamin B6 (pyridoxine hydrochloride), Vitamin B2 (riboflavin), Vitamin B1 (thiamine mononitrate), Vitamin B12, Folic acid.

Slim & Sassy® V Shake

Vegan Trim Shake

Slim & Sassy V Shake has the same high fiber and high protein content, the ashwagandha root and leaf extracts, and the potato protein extracts found in the regular Trim Shakes—but with natural, vegan-friendly options.

Key Ingredients:

Protein Blend, Potato Protein Extract, Fiber Blend, Ashwagandha (*Withania somnifera*) Root and Leaf Extracts, Stevia.

TerraGreens®

Fruit & Veggie Drink Mix

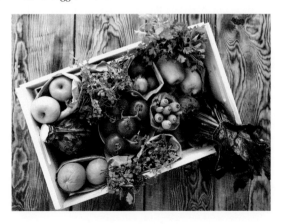

TerraGreens consist of a wide assortment of fruits and vegetables known to contain high levels of vitamins, minerals, and other important nutrients that are often missing from the diet of the average person. This drink mix can help boost overall nutrient levels in the average diet, helping to support the body in maintaining optimal health.

Key Ingredients:

Kale, Collard Greens, Dandelion Greens, Wheat Grass, Barley Grass, Guava, Acerola Cherry, Goji Berry, Lemon Essential Oil, Ginger Essential Oil.

TriEase® Softgels

Seasonal Blend Softgels

These softgels combine three powerful essential oils that have been studied for their abilities to help the body respond appropriately to symptoms related to seasonal allergies.

Key Ingredients:

Lemon Essential Oil, Lavender Essential Oil, Peppermint Essential Oil.

vEO Mega®

Vegan Essential Oil Omega Complex

This supplement is a vegan-friendly blend of essential fatty acids that is particularly high in beneficial omega-3 fatty acids. It also includes the potent antioxidant astaxanthin and a unique essential oil blend that helps enhance the benefits of the essential fatty acids.

Key Ingredients:

Algae Oil (DHA), Flaxseed Oil (ALA), Inca Inchi Seed Oil (ALA), Astaxanthin, Lutein, Lycopene, Zeaxanthin, Alpha & Beta Carotene, Borage Seed Oil (GLA), Cranberry Seed Oil (ALA), Pomegranate Seed Oil (CLNA), Pumpkin Seed Oil, Grape Seed Oil, Vitamin D (cholecalciferol), Vitamin E (d-alpha & mixed tocopherols), Clove Bud Essential Oil, Frankincense Essential Oil, Thyme Essential Oil, Cumin Essential Oil, Orange Essential Oil, Peppermint Essential Oil, Ginger Essential Oil, Caraway Seed Essential Oil, German Chamomile Essential Oil.

xEO Mega®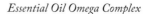

Essential Oil Omega Complex

This complex is a blend of essential fatty acids. It includes essential fatty acids from both marine and land sources, the potent antioxidant astaxanthin, and an essential oil blend that helps enhance the benefits of the essential fatty acids.

Key Ingredients:

Fish Oil (as Anchovy, Sardine, and Mackerel) and Calamari Oil Concentrates (EPA, DHA, and other Omega-3s), *Echium plantagineum* Seed Oil (ALA, SDA, and GLA), Pomegranate Seed Oil, Astaxanthin, Lutein (from Marigold Flower), Zeaxanthin (from Marigold Flower), Lycopene (from Tomato Fruit), Vitamin A (as alpha and beta carotene), Vitamin D_3 (as natural cholecalciferol), Vitamin E (d-alpha & natural mixed tocopherols), Clove Essential Oil, Frankincense Essential Oil, Thyme Essential Oil, Cumin Essential Oil, Orange Essential Oil, Peppermint Essential Oil, Ginger Essential Oil, Caraway Essential Oil, German Chamomile Essential Oil.

Zendocrine® Detoxification Complex

Detoxification Complex

This supplement is a blend of whole food–based nutrients that may help promote healthy endocrine gland functions and the filtering of toxins by the body's systems.

Key Ingredients:

Psyllium Seed Husk Powder, Barberry Leaf, Turkish Rhubarb Stem, Kelp, Milk Thistle Seed (Silymarin), Osha Root, Safflower Petals, Acacia Gum Bark, Burdock Root, Clove Bud, Dandelion Root (Inulin), Garlic Fruit, Marshmallow Root, Red Clover Leaf (Isoflavones), Enzyme Assimilation System.

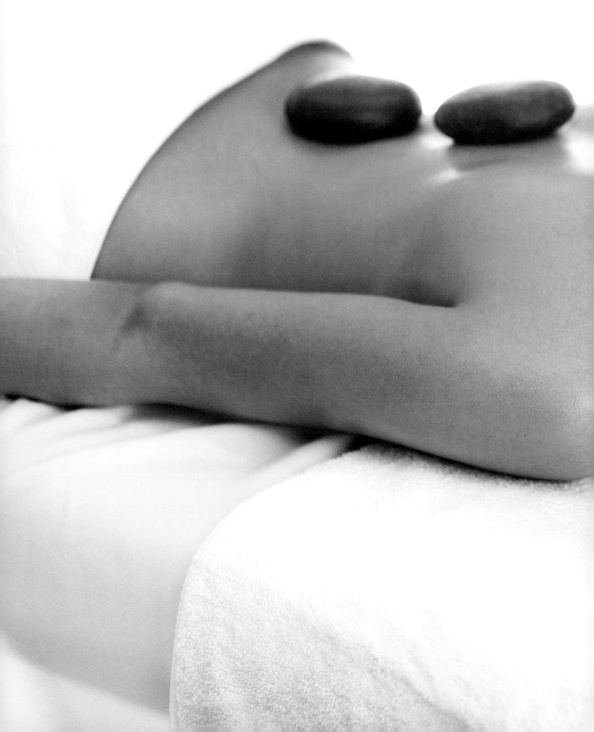

Personal Care and Spa

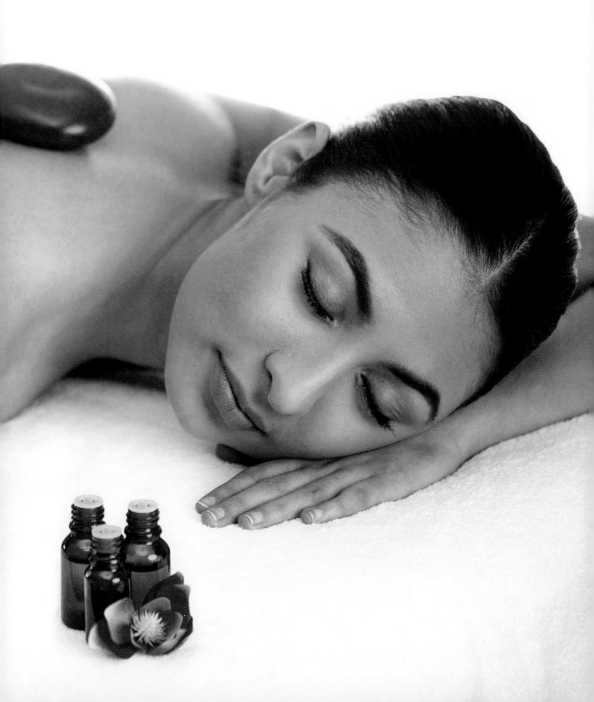

Personal Care and Spa

This section contains examples of various types of essential oil–inspired personal care and spa formulations that are available commercially as well as the key ingredients that each type of product contains. See the Essential Oils and the Essential Oil Blends sections of this book for more information on the single essential oil and blend suggestions indicated here.

Anti-Aging Eye Cream

Eye Cream

This unique cream targets fine lines and wrinkles that appear around the eyes and helps the skin in that area maintain a full, youthful appearance.

Key Ingredients:

Frankincense Essential Oil, Ylang Ylang Essential Oil, Blue Tansy Essential Oil, Meadowfoam Seed Oil, Pullulan, Red Algae Extract, Bukachiol.

Anti-Aging Moisturizer

Anti-Aging Moisturizer combines several ingredients that have been studied for their abilities to combat many of the visible signs of aging by reducing wrinkles and fine lines and improving skin elasticity and tone.

Key Ingredients:

Lavender Essential Oil, Jasmine Essential Oil, Geranium Essential Oil, Frankincense Essential Oil, Palmitoyl Oligopeptides and Tetrapeptide-7 (Matrikine Messaging), Sodium Hyaluronate (Patented Hyaluronic Acid Spherulites), Grapeseed Oil, Summer Snowflake Bulb Extract, Acetyl Octapeptide-3 (Proprietary Octapeptide), Vitamin Blend.

Baby: Diaper Rash Cream

This gentle cream safely and effectively creates a natural barrier to protect a baby's sensitive skin. It soothes and relieves diaper rash while moisturizing the skin.

Key Ingredients:

Lavender Essential Oil, Carrot Seed Essential Oil, Melaleuca Essential Oil, Non-Nano Zinc Oxide, Muyao Shea Butter.

Baby: Hair and Body Wash

This unique baby washcontains natural ingredients that are gentle on a baby's delicate skin. It has a soft, delicate aroma that is soothing to babies and children of all ages.

Key Ingredients:

Lavender Essential Oil, Roman Chamomile Essential Oil, Vanilla Extract, Muyao Shea Butter.

Baby: Lotion

This unique lotion combines natural ingredients to help moisturize baby's skin. It contains the soft, gentle aroma of lavender and Roman chamomile essential oils blended with a hint of vanilla.

Key Ingredients:

Lavender Essential Oil, Roman Chamomile Essential Oil, Vanilla Extract, Muyao Shea Butter, Coconut Oil, Apple Fruit Extract.

Bightening Gel

Skin Brightening Gel

Bightening Gel combines ingredients that have been studied for their abilities to promote even pigmentation and tone in the skin and to help lessen the appearance of dark spots associated with aging.

Key Ingredients:

Bergamot Essential Oil, Juniper Essential Oil, Melissa Essential Oil, Daisy Extract, Ginger Root Extract, Vitamin C.

Breathe® Vapor Stick

Respiratory Vapor Stick

This handy stick combines many essential oils that are often used and studied for their abilities to help support the respiratory system in an easy-to-apply solid stick.

Key Ingredients:

Lemon Essential Oil, Peppermint Essential Oil, *Eucalyptus globulus* Essential Oil, Thyme Essential Oil, Melissa Essential Oil, Cardamom Essential Oil.

Citrus Bliss® Hand Lotion

Invigorating Blend Hand & Body Lotion

This lotion offers the same natural benefits of the regular Hand & Body Lotion, plus the added benefits of Citrus Bliss.

Key Ingredients:

Citrus Bliss: This blend contains essential oils of orange, lemon, grapefruit, mandarin, bergamot, tangerine, and clementine, with vanilla bean extract. *See Hand & Body Lotion for other suggested ingredients and research.*

Citrus Bliss® Invigorating Bath Bar

Invigorating Bath Bar

This invigorating soap combines the skin protecting abilities of sunflower, safflower, palm, coconut, and jojoba oils with naturally exfoliating oatmeal kernels and the stimulating aroma of Citrus Bliss.

Key Ingredients:

Citrus Bliss, Oatmeal (*Avena sativa*) Kernel, Sodium Cocoate (Saponified Coconut Oil, Sodium Safflowerate (Saponified Safflower Oil).

Correct-X®

Essential Ointment

This all natural ointment harnesses the healing power of essential oils to help soothe skin irritations and enhance the natural process of healing.

Key Ingredients:

Frankincense Essential Oil, Helichrysum Essential Oil, Melaleuca Essential Oil, Cedarwood Essential Oil, Lavender Essential Oil, Bisabolol, Jojoba Oil, Phellodendron Amurense Bark Extract.

Deep Blue® Rub

Soothing Rub

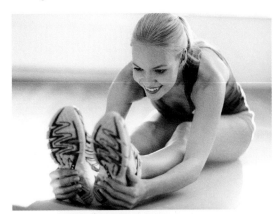

This massage and sports cream contains Deep Blue. This blend is comprised of oils that have been studied for their abilities to help reduce muscle, joint, and bone pain and inflammation. Additionally, this moisturizing cream contains ingredients known to stimulate sensations of warmth and coolness to help soothe tissue soreness and stiffness.

Key Ingredients:

Wintergreen Essential Oil, Camphor Essential Oil, Peppermint Essential Oil, Blue Tansy Essential Oil, Ylang Ylang Essential Oil, German Chamomile Essential Oil, Helichrysum Essential Oil, Osmanthus Essential Oil, *Eucalyptus globulus* Essential Oil, Menthol, *Capsicum frutescens* Fruit Extract.

Detoxifying Mud Mask

This natural earth mask combines the cleansing properties of copper, kaolin, and bentonite with skin-nourishing botanicals and natural essential oils that help purify, nourish, and soothe the skin.

Key Ingredients:

Juniper Berry Essential Oil, Grapefruit Essential Oil, Myrrh Essential Oil, Natural Earth Clay, *Butyrospermum parkii* (Shea) Butter, *Lens esculenta* (Lentil) Seed Extract, Malachite Extract.

Exfoliating Body Scrub

This natural body scrub combines exquisite vegetable oils that help nourish and soothe the skin with stimulating, uplifting essential oils.

Key Ingredients:

Orange Essential Oil, Grapefruit Essential Oil, Ginger Essential Oil, Sweet Almond Oil, Sunflower Seed Oil, Macadamia Nut Oil, Kukui Nut Oil.

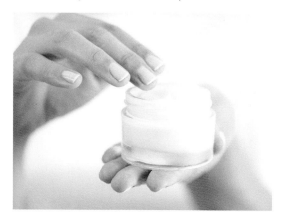

Facial Cleanser

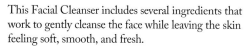

This Facial Cleanser includes several ingredients that work to gently cleanse the face while leaving the skin feeling soft, smooth, and fresh.

Key Ingredients:

Melaleuca Essential Oil, Peppermint Essential Oil, Yucca Root Extract, Soapbark Extract, Macadamia Seed Oil, Sodium PCA, Vitamin E.

Hand & Body Lotion

This lotion blends several ingredients that have been studied for their unique moisturizing and skin-protecting abilities with natural, botanical ingredients. It should be formulated so that you can mix in your desired essential oil or blend to create your own custom lotion for many different uses.

Key Ingredients:

Sunflower Seed Oil, Coconut Oil, Macadamia Seed Oil, Murumura Seed Butter, Cupuacu (Theobroma) Seed Butter, Inca Inchi Seed Oil, *Olea europaea* (Olive) Fruit Unsaponifiables, Jojoba Oil, *Bellis perennis* (Daisy) Flower Extract.

HD Clear® Facial Lotion

Topical Facial Lotion

This clearing facial lotion will help to remove skin blemishes while providing lasting moisture for the skin. Using the power of essential oils, this lotion helps relieve acne and other skin blemishes.

Key Ingredients:

Melaleuca Essential Oil, Eucalyptus Essential Oil, Geranium Essential Oil, Ho Wood Essential Oil, Litsea Essential Oil, Vitamin B$_3$, Amino Acids, Black Cumin Seed Oil, Chaulmoogra Oil, Magnolia, Manuka, White Willow Bark.

HD Clear® Foaming Face Wash

Topical Face Wash

HD Clear Foaming Face Wash blends several ingredients that have been studied for their abilities to help clarify the skin and to create a hostile environment for detrimental skin bacteria.

Key Ingredients:

Rosewood Essential Oil, Melaleuca Essential Oil, *Eucalyptus globulus* Essential Oil, Geranium Essential Oil, Lemongrass Essential Oil, Black Cumin Seed Oil, Ho Wood Essential Oil, Litsea Essential Oil, White Willow Bark Extract, *Glycyrrhiza inflata* Root Extract, *Candida bombicola* Ferment, Vitamin A.

Healthy Hold Glaze

Hair Glaze

Healthy Hold Glaze combines several ingredients that have been studied for their abilities to provide a heat-activated flexible hold for hair without chemical build up, while helping to protect and strengthen the hair on the molecular level.

Key Ingredients:

Lavender Essential Oil, Peppermint Essential Oil, Marjoram Essential Oil, Cedarwood Essential Oil, Lavandin Essential Oil, Rosemary Essential Oil, Niaouli (*Melaleuca quinquenervia*) Essential Oil, Eucalyptus (*E. globulus*) Essential Oil, Tangerine Essential Oil.

Hydrating Body Mist with Beautiful

Hydrating Body Mist with Beautiful combines moisturizing vegetable oils along with the Beautiful essential oil blend to help promote healthy, clear, youthful looking skin.

Key Ingredients:

Lime Essential Oil, Osmanthus Essential Oil, Bergamot Essential Oil, Frankincense Essential Oil, Coconut Oil, Sunflower Seed Oil, Passion Fruit Seed Oil, Avocado Oil.

Hydrating Cream

Hydrating Cream combines essential oils known for their abilities to soothe and balance the skin's natural moisture levels with a complex of signaling molecules that have been studied for their abilities to help promote the production of collagen and other intracellular matrix proteins that are crucial for fuller, smoother-appearing skin.

Key Ingredients:

Lavender Essential Oil, Geranium Essential Oil, Frankincense Essential Oil, Lactococcus Ferment Lysate, *Laminaria digitata* Extract, Mugwort Extract, *Theobroma cacao* (Cocoa) Seed Butter.

Invigorating Scrub

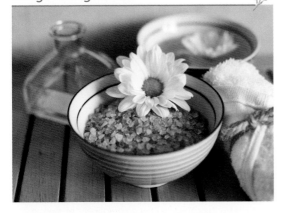

Invigorating Scrub combines fragrant and nourishing essential oils, vegetable extracts, and other natural incredients known for their ability to exfoliate and polish skin.

Key Ingredients:

Grapefruit Essential Oil, Peppermint Essential Oil, Jojoba Beads (Hydrogenated Jojoba Oil), Mandarin Orange Extract, Jasmine Flower and Leaf Extract, Greater Burdock Root Extract.

Lip Balm

Help hydrate and soothe lips with these natural moisturizing lip balms.

Key Ingredients:

Original Blend:

> Orange Essential Oil, Peppermint Essential Oil.

Tropical Blend:

> Lime Essential Oil, Clementine Essential Oil, Ylang Ylang Essential Oil.

Herbal Blend:

> Spearmint Essential Oil, Marjoram Essential Oil, Lemon Verbena Essential Oil.

Coconut Oil, Moringa Oil, Kukui Nut Oil.

Moisturizing Bath Bar

This unique soap combines the moisturizing abilities of palm, coconut, and jojoba oils with aloe leaf juice and the stimulating aroma of bergamot and grapefruit essential oils.

Key Ingredients:

Bergamot Essential Oil, Grapefruit Essential Oil, Sodium Cocoate (Saponified Coconut Oil), Vegetable Glycerin, Jojoba Oil, Aloe Leaf Juice.

Natural Deodorant

This natural deodorant combines the natural deodorizing and antibacterial properties of cypress, melaleuca, bergamot, and cedarwood essential oils in a base of beeswax, coconut oil, shea butter, and cornstarch.

Key Ingredients:

Beeswax, Coconut Oil, Shea Butter, Cypress Essential Oil, Melaleuca Essential Oil, Bergamot Essential Oil, Cedarwood Essential Oil.

On Guard® Cleaner Concentrate

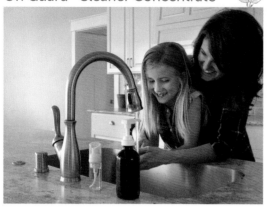

This natural cleaner combines the protective benefits of On Guard with plant-based ingredients to create a tough, yet safe and non-toxic, multi-purpose household cleaner.

Key Ingredients:

On Guard: contains orange, clove bud, cinnamon bark, *Eucalyptus radiata*, and rosemary essential oils.

On Guard® Foaming Hand Wash

Protective Hand Wash

On Guard Foaming Hand Wash combines several essential oils into a healthy, all-natural hand soap that is gentle enough for even those with sensitive skin to use. It leaves hands feeling clean, soft, and fresh while it protects against harmful microorganisms.

Key Ingredients:

Sweet Orange Essential Oil, Clove Bud Essential Oil, Cinnamon Bark Essential Oil, Rosemary Oil,

On Guard® Laundry Detergent

Protective Laundry Detergent

This detergent combines the natural antiseptic properties of the oils contained in On Guard with naturally based surfactants, enzymes, and stabilizers.

Key Ingredients:

On Guard: contains orange, clove bud, cinnamon bark, *Eucalyptus radiata*, and rosemary essential oils, **Naturally Sourced Enzymes, Natural Surfactants, Natural Corn-Based Enzyme Stabilizer.**

On Guard® Mouthwash

Protective Mouthwash

This natural mouthwash formulation offers the protective benefits of On Guard enhanced with peppermint, wintergreen, and myrrh essential oils.

Key Ingredients:

On Guard, Wintergreen Essential Oil, Myrrh Essential Oil, Peppermint Essential Oil, Miswak Extract, Monk Fruit Extract, Natural Xylitol.

On Guard® Natural Whitening Toothpaste

Protective Toothpaste

This natural toothpaste formulation offers the protective benefits of On Guard along with peppermint, wintergreen, and myrrh essential oils.

Key Ingredients:

On Guard: contains orange, clove bud, cinnamon bark, *Eucalyptus radiata*, and rosemary essential oils;

Myrrh Essential Oi, Peppermint Essential Oil, Calcium Hydroxyapatite, Natural Xylitol, Hydrated Silica.

Pore Reducing Toner

Skin Toner

This toner includes ingredients that have been studied for their abilities to help reduce the visible size of pores while eliminating skin irritation and stress.

Key Ingredients:

Lavender Essential Oil, Ylang Ylang Essential Oil, German Chamomile Essential Oil, Aloe Leaf Juice, Watermelon Fruit Extract, Apple Fruit Extract, Lentil Seed and Fruit Extracts, Witch Hazel.

Protecting Shampoo

Protecting Shampoo blends ingredients that have been studied for their abilities to cleanse and protect hair, especially hair that has been chemically treated or heat styled. This shampoo combines the benefits of essential oils with natural sugar beet derivatives and oat peptides to naturally protect, repair, and condition damaged hair—and to protect hair against future damage.

Key Ingredients:

Sugar Beet Derivative (Betaine), Oat Peptides, Emulsion of Silica, Orange Essential Oil, Lime Essential Oil.

Refreshing Body Wash

This natural body wash contains several ingredients that work to gently cleanse the skin while leaving it feeling soft, smooth, and refreshed.

Key Ingredients:

Grapefruit Essential Oil, Bergamot Essential Oil, Cedarwood Essential Oi, Sodium Methyl Oleoyl Taurate.

Replenishing Body Butter

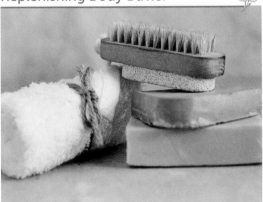

This body butter combines natural ingredients that help to moisturize and soothe trouble areas of the skin that take the most abuse, such as the elbows, feet, and hands.

Key Ingredients:

Orange Essential Oil, Douglas Fir Essential Oil, Frankincense Essential Oil, Shea Butter, Avocado Oil, Cocoa Seed Butter, Jojoba Oil.

Reveal Facial System

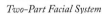

Two-Part Facial System

The Reveal Facial System consists of a two-part spa-grade facial care system that combines ingredients that have been studied for their abilities to help exfoliate and polish the skin and then deliver protein-building peptides to help maintain fuller, more radiant skin.

Key Ingredients:

Pumpkin Fruit Enzyme, Acetyl Hexapeptide-8, Ceramide 2, Palmitoyl Oligopeptide and Palmitoyl Tripeptide-38 (Matrikine Messaging), Orange Essential Oil, Lime Essential Oil.

Root to Tip Serum

Hair Serum

Root to Tip Serum combines beneficial essential oils with Moroccan argan oil to nourish, protect, moisturize, and revitalize the hair and scalp.

Key Ingredients:

Argan (*Argania spinosa*) Oil, Lavender Essential Oil, Peppermint Essential Oil, Marjoram Essential Oil, Cedarwood Essential Oil, Lavandin Essential Oil, Rosemary Essential Oil, Niaouli (*Melaleuca quinquenervia*) Essential Oil, Eucalyptus (*E. globulus*) Essential Oil.

Rose Hand Lotion

Rose Hand & Body Lotion

This lotion offers the same natural benefits of the regular Hand & Body Lotion, plus the added benefits of rose essential oil.

Key Ingredients:

Rose Essential Oil.

see Hand & Body Lotion for other suggested ingredients and research.

Serenity Bath Bar

Calming/Restful Bar

This soothing soap combines the skin protecting abilities of sunflower, safflower, palm, coconut, and jojoba oils with the moisturizing properties of shea butter and the calming aroma of Serenity.

Key Ingredients:

Serenity, Sodium Cocoate (Saponified Coconut Oil), Aloe Leaf Juice.

Smoothing Conditioner

This conditioner combines several ingredients known for their ability to help restore luminosity, shine, fullness, and overall health to hair. This formulation is designed to help smooth the outside layer of the hair strands, reducing mechanical damage caused by friction. This conditioner combines the benefits of essential oils with natural botanical extracts to naturally condition and repair damaged hair and to protect hair against future damage.

Key Ingredients:

Botanical Extracts, Lavender Essential Oil, Peppermint Essential Oil, Marjoram Essential Oil, Cedarwood Essential Oil, Lavandin Essential Oil, Rosemary Essential Oil, Niaouli (*Melaleuca quinquenervia*) Essential Oil, Eucalyptus (*E. globulus*) Essential Oil.

Tightening Serum

Skin Tightening Serum

Tightening Serum combines ingredients that have been studied for their abilities to hydrate and tighten the skin in order to reduce the appearance of fine lines and wrinkles.

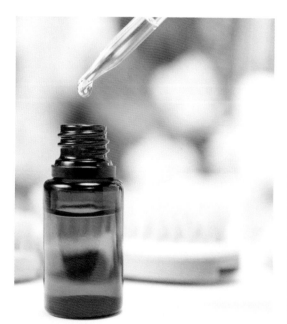

Key Ingredients:

Frankincense Essential Oil, Sandalwood Essential Oil, Myrrh Essential Oil, *Acacia senegal* and Hydrolyzed Rhizobian Gums (Rhizobian & Acacia Gum Extracts), Perfluorodecalin (Proprietary Perfluorocarbon), *Fagus sylvatica* Bud Extract (Beech Tree Bud Extract), Betaine.

Veráge™ Cleanser

Youthful Skin Cleanser

This natural gel cleanser will reduce the appearance of skin aging by hydrating, nourishing, and smoothing the skin. To help produce a glowing youthful complexion, use this cleanser to remove makeup and dirt, deeply clean pores, and energize skin.

Key Ingredients:

Orange Essential Oil, Basil Essential Oil, Melaleuca Essential Oil, Amino Acids and Lipids, Coconut Oil, Olive Oil.

Veráge™ Immortelle Hydrating Serum

Youthful Hydrating Serum

This anti-aging hydrating serum combines the action of Immortelle with other natural ingredients to reduce the appearance of skin aging. By emulating the natural micronutrients of the skin this serum renews the youthful properties associated with healthy skin, such as firmness, elasticity, and hydration.

Key Ingredients:

Frankincense Essential Oil, Hawaiian Sandalwood Essential Oil, Lavender Essential Oil, Myrrh Essential Oil, Helichrysum Essential Oil, Rose Essential Oil, Lipids, Olive Oil, Jojoba Oil, Macadamia Oil.

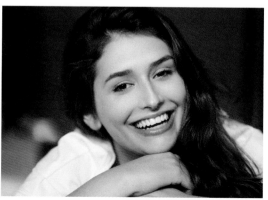

Veráge™ Moisturizer

Youthful Moisturizing Lotion

This moisturizing facial lotion is ideal for all skin types and provides hydration as well as skin nourishment. As the lotion hydrates deeply it helps to reduce wrinkles and smooth the skin.

Key Ingredients:

Jasmine Essential Oil, Geranium Essential Oil, Sea Buckthorn Berry Essential Oil, Juniper Berry Essential Oil, Rice Bran Oil, Shea Butter, Phellodendron Amurense Bark Extract.

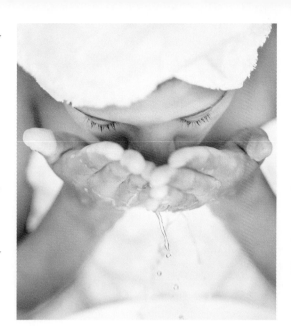

Veráge™ Toner

Youthful Skin Toner

This nourishing skin toner will reduce the appearance of skin aging by tightening, toning, and smoothing the skin. To help produce a youthful complexion, use this toner to increase skin glow, tone, and texture, and tighten pores.

Key Ingredients:

Ylang Ylang Essential Oil, Coriander Essential Oil, Cypress Essential Oil, Palmarosa Essential Oil, Witch Hazel, Aloe.

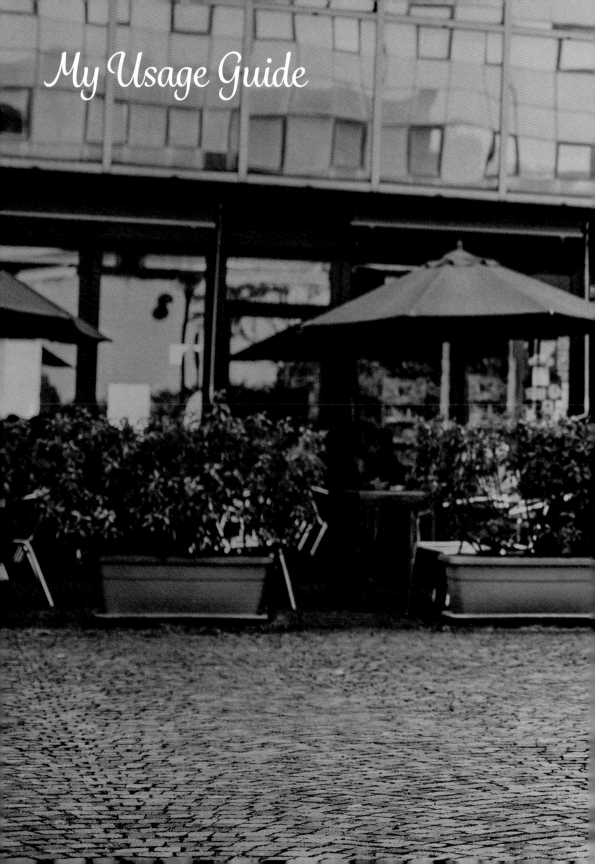

My Usage Guide

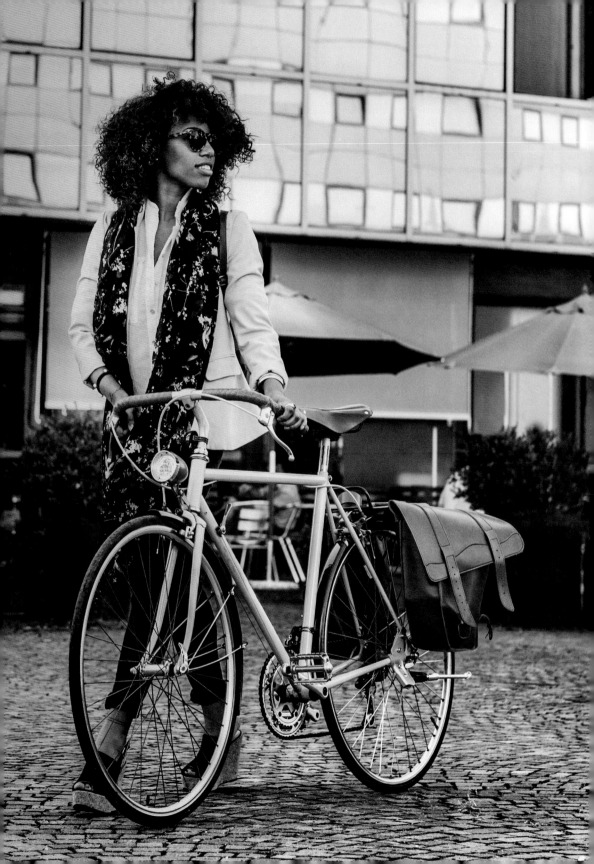

My Usage Guide: How to Use This Section

This section is a compilation of many different health conditions and the various essential oils, blends, and supplements that are commonly used and recommended for each condition.

Example Entry:

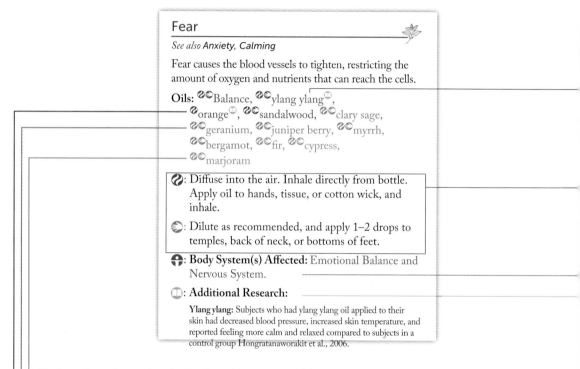

Fear

*See also **Anxiety, Calming***

Fear causes the blood vessels to tighten, restricting the amount of oxygen and nutrients that can reach the cells.

Oils: Balance, ylang ylang, orange, sandalwood, clary sage, geranium, juniper berry, myrrh, bergamot, fir, cypress, marjoram

- Diffuse into the air. Inhale directly from bottle. Apply oil to hands, tissue, or cotton wick, and inhale.
- Dilute as recommended, and apply 1–2 drops to temples, back of neck, or bottoms of feet.
- **Body System(s) Affected:** Emotional Balance and Nervous System.
- **Additional Research:**

Ylang ylang: Subjects who had ylang ylang oil applied to their skin had decreased blood pressure, increased skin temperature, and reported feeling more calm and relaxed compared to subjects in a control group Hongratanaworakit et al., 2006.

Under each **condition**, the oils, blends, and supplements have been grouped as:

- Primary Recommendations: Try these oils, blends, or supplements first.

- Secondary Recommendations: Try these oils or blends second. Supplements listed as secondary recommendations may be useful for general nutritional support of the body systems involved in prevention or healing from a specific condition.

- Other Recommendations : Oils, blends, and supplements that may also help, depending on the underlying cause.

The criteria for grouping within these categories include the recommendations of experts within the field of essential oils, supporting scientific research studies, historical uses of the oils and the herbs and plants they are derived from, and more recent French medicinal uses for the oils. However, since each individual may have different underlying causes for his or her specific condition, what may work for one individual may be different than what works for another.

Also listed under each condition are recommendations for how to use or apply these oils or supplements for that particular condition. The three main application and usage methods are aromatic, topical, and internal. The recommended methods are indicated next to each oil as a small ✪ for Aromatic, ◐ for Topical, and ◯ for Internal.

✪: Aromatic means that the oils are breathed or inhaled through the mouth and nose. This could include breathing the aroma of the oil directly from the bottle or breathing in oil that has been applied to the hands or to another material such as a tissue or cotton wick. It could also mean breathing the vapor or mist of an oil that has been diffused or sprayed into the surrounding air.

◐: Topical means that the oils are applied directly onto the skin, hair, or other surface of the body. This can be through direct application of the oils to the skin or by using the oils in massages, baths, or within a cream, lotion, or soap. While some oils can be applied neat (without dilution), others may need to be diluted before topical application, especially for young or sensitive skin. Refer to the Single Essential Oils section of this book or the Dilution Reference Chart (following these notes) for recommended dilutions for the oils listed in this book.

◯: Internal means that the oils or supplements are taken orally. This can be done either by adding the oil to a food or beverage that is then consumed, placing a drop of oil under the tongue, or by swallowing a capsule that has the essential oil or supplement inside.

For more information on specific ways essential oils can be applied or used, see the Science and Application of Essential Oils section in this book.

The large ✪, ◐, or ◯ listed near the bottom of each entry refers to recommended application methods specific for that condition.

⊕: Listed with each entry are the main body systems primarily affected by each health condition. For more information on all of the oils and products discussed within this book and which body systems they primarily affect, see Appendix A: Body Systems Chart.

⬭: For many conditions listed in this section there is also additional supporting research.

Many entries also include **definitions** of conditions and terms (listed directly underneath the topic), **subtopics** related to that condition, and even **recipes or blends** that can be used for that condition.

Example Entry:

Below are some additional things to keep in mind as you use and apply the essential oils, blends, and supplements listed in this section.

Oils: ◐melaleuca, ✪◐oregano◯, ◐peppermint, ◐thyme, ◐geranium, ◐lavender

Blend 1: Combine 2 drops lavender, 2 drops melaleuca, and 2 drops thyme. Apply 1–2 drops on ringworm three times a day for 10 days. Then mix 30 drops melaleuca with 2 Tbs. (25 ml) fractionated coconut oil, and use daily until ringworm is gone.

—Thrush:

Thrush is another name for oral candidiasis (*see Candida above*). Thrush results in uncomfortable or painful white or yellow patches in the mouth.

Oils: ◐melaleuca◯, ◐lavender, ◐eucalyptus, ◐marjoram, ◐thyme

My Usage Guide: Dilution Reference Chart—Oils

Single Oil Name	Recommended Dilution		
	Adults	Child/Sensitive	Expectant Mother
Arborvitae	●	●◇	✕
Basil	●	●◇	✕
Bergamot	●✽	●✽✽	●✽✽
Birch	●	●◇	✕
Black Pepper	●◇◇◇	▽	▽
Blue Tansy	●	●◇	●◇◇
Cardamom	●	●	●
Cassia	●◇◇◇◇	▽	✕
Cedarwood	●	●◇◇	▽
Cilantro	●	●	●
Cinnamon	●◇◇◇	▽	✕
Clary Sage	●	●	▽
Clove	●◇	●◇◇◇◇	▽
Copaiba	●	●◇	●
Coriander	●	●	●
Cypress	●	●	▽
Dill	●	●	●
Douglas Fir	●	●◇	●◇◇
Eucalyptus	●	●◇	●
Fennel	●	●◇	▽
Frankincense	●	●	●
Geranium	●	●◇	●
Ginger	●✽	●◇	●
Grapefruit	●	●	●
Green Mandarin	●✽	●✽	●✽
Hawaiian Sandalwood	●	●	●
Helichrysum	●	●	●
Hinoki	●	●◇	●◇
Jasmine	●	●	●
Juniper Berry	●	●◇	●
Lavender	●	●	●
Lemon	●✽	●✽	●✽
Lemon Myrtle	●◇◇◇	●◇◇◇◇	●◇◇◇
Lemongrass	●	●◇	●◇
Lime	●✽	●◇✽	●✽
Litsea	●	●◇	●◇
Magnolia	●	●◇	●◇
Manuka	●	●	●◇
Marjoram	●	●◇	▽
Melaleuca	●	●	●

Single Oil Name	Recommended Dilution		
	Adults	Child/Sensitive	Expectant Mother
Melissa	●	●	▽
Myrrh	●	●	▽
Neroli	●	●	●◇◇
Orange	●✽	●✽	●✽
Oregano	●◇◇◇◇	▽	▽
Patchouli	●	●◇	●◇
Patchouli	●	●	●
Peppermint	●	●◇	▽
Pink Pepper	●	●◇	●◇
Petitgrain	●	●◇	●
Roman Chamomile	●	●◇	●
Rose	●	●	●
Rosemary	●	●◇	✕
Sandalwood	●	●	●
Siberian Fir	●	●◇	●◇
Spearmint	●	●◇	▽
Spikenard	●	●	●
Star Anise	●	●◇	▽
Thyme	●◇◇◇◇	▽	✕
Turmeric	●	●◇	▽
Vetiver	●	●	▽
White Fir	●	●◇	●◇
Wintergreen	●	●◇	✕
Yarrow	●	●◇	●◇
Ylang Ylang	●	●	●
Yuzu	●✽	●◇✽	●✽

Primary Recommendations • Secondary Recommendations • Other Recommendations

Oil Blend Name	Recommended Dilution		
	Adults	Child/Sensitive	Expectant Mother
AromaTouch	●	●	●
Balance	●	●	●
Brave	●	●	●
Breathe	●	●:○	●
Calmer	●	●	●
Cheer	●	●:○	●:○
Citrus Bliss	●✳	●✳	●✳
ClaryCalm	●	●:○	▽
Console	●	●	●
DDR Prime	●	●:○	▽
Deep Blue	●	●:○	●
DigestZen	●	●	▽
Elevation	●✳	●✳	●✳
Forgive	●	●:○	●:○
HD Clear	●	●	▽
Immortelle	●	●	▽
InTune	●	●:○	●:○
Motivate	●	●:○	●:○
On Guard	●	●:○	▽
Passion	●	●:○	●:○
PastTense	●	●:○	▽
Peace	●	●	●
Purify	●	●	●
Rescuer	●	●	●
Serenity	●	●	●
Slim & Sassy	●✳	●:○✳	▽
Steady	●	●	●
Stronger	●	●	●
TerraShield	●	●	●
Thinker	●	●	●
Whisper	●	●	●
Yarrow Pom	●	●:○	●:○
Yoga Blends	●	●:○	●:○
Zendocrine	●:○	●:○○○○	▽

 Can be used neat (without dilution)

 For ratios like this, the first drop represents the proportion of essential oil to use, and the second drop represents the proportion of carrier oil (such as fractionated coconut oil) to use. For this ratio, you would blend 1 part essential oil with 1 part carrier oil before applying.

 Use with extreme caution and dilute heavily

 Avoid

 Avoid sunlight for up to 12 hours after use

 Avoid sunlight for up to 72 hours after use

⊜=Topical, ⊘=Aromatic, ○=Internal

Additional Notes on Using Essential Oils

— If essential oils get into your eyes by accident or if they burn the skin a little, do not try to remove the oils with water. This will only drive the oils deeper into the tissue. It is best to dilute the essential oils on location with a pure vegetable oil (such as fractionated coconut oil).

— The FDA has approved some essential oils generically for internal use and given them the following designations: GRAS (Generally Recognized As Safe for human consumption), FA (Food Additive), or FL (Flavoring agent). *These designations are listed under Oral Use As Dietary Supplement for each single oil in the Single Essential Oils section of this book.*

— Using some oils such as lemon, orange, grapefruit, bergamot, etc., before or during exposure to direct sunlight or UV rays (tanning beds, for example) may cause a rash, pigmentation, or even severe burns. Please see the safety information under each oil in the Essential Oils chapter of this book for further information; then either dilute these oils and test a small area, or avoid their use altogether.

— Caution should be used with oils such as clary sage and fennel during pregnancy. These oils contain active constituents with hormone-like activity and could possibly stimulate adverse reactions in the mother, although there are no recorded cases in humans.

— Particular care should be taken when using cassia, cinnamon, lemongrass, oregano, and thyme, as they are some of the strongest and most caustic oils. It is best to dilute them with a pure vegetable oil.

— When a blend or recipe is listed in this section, rather than mix the oils together, it may be more beneficial to layer the oils: that is, apply a drop or two of one oil, rub it in, and then apply another oil. If dilution is necessary, a pure vegetable oil can be applied on top. Effectiveness is in the layering.

— Less is often better: use 1–3 drops of oil and no more than 6 drops at a time. Stir, and rub on in a clockwise direction.

— When applying oils to infants and small children, dilute 1–2 drops pure essential oil with 1–3 tsp. (5–15 ml) of a pure vegetable oil (such as fractionated coconut oil). If the oils are used in the bath, always use a bath gel base as a dispersing agent for the oils. See *Children and Infants* in this section for more information about the recommended list of oils for babies and children.

— The body absorbs oils the fastest through inhalation (breathing) and second fastest through application to the feet or ears. Layering oils can increase the rate of absorption.

— The life expectancy of a cell is 120 days (4 months). When cells divide, they make duplicate cells. If the cell is diseased, new diseased cells will be made. When we stop the mutation of the diseased cells (create healthy cells), we stop the disease. Essential oils have the ability to penetrate and carry nutrients through the cell membrane to the nucleus and improve the health of the cell.

— *Use extreme caution when diffusing cassia or cinnamon,* as they may burn the nostrils if you put your nose directly next to the nebulizer of the diffuser where the mist is coming out.

— When traveling by air, you should always have your oils hand-checked. X-ray machines may interfere with the frequency of the oils.

— Keep oils away from the light and heat—although they seem to do fine in temperatures up to 90° F (30° C). If stored properly in a cool, dark environment, they can maintain their maximum potency for many years.

Symbols and Colors Used in This Section

● Primary Recommendations	⊜ Topical
● Secondary Recommendations	❷ Aromatic
● Other Recommendations	⬤ Internal
✛ Body System(s) Affected	❸ Cleaning/Disinfecting
▥ See Additional Research	

Primary Recommendations • Secondary Recommendations • Other Recommendations

My Usage Guide

ADD/ADHD

Attention deficit disorder or attention deficit/hyper-activity disorder is a psychological condition characterized by inattentiveness, restlessness, and difficulty concentrating. Although most individuals exhibit all of these symptoms at some point, ADD is characterized by a frequency and duration of these symptoms that are inappropriate to an individual's age.

> *Simple Solutions—ADD/ADHD:* Combine 3 drops lavender and 3 drops basil on a natural stone or unglazed clay pendant, and wear throughout the day.

Oils: InTune, Steady, Thinker, Serenity, Calmer, vetiver, lavender

Blend 1: Combine equal parts lavender and basil. Diffuse, or apply 1–3 drops on the crown of the head.

: Diffuse into the air. Inhale oil directly from the bottle, or applied to a tissue or cotton wick.

: Dilute as recommended, and apply 1–3 drops on the bottoms of the feet and/or on the spine.

: **Body System(s) Affected:** Nervous System and Emotional Balance.

AIDS/HIV

*See also **Antiviral***

Acquired immune deficiency syndrome (AIDS) is a disease of the human immune system. AIDS progressively inhibits the effectiveness of the immune system, leaving the human body susceptible to both infections and tumors. AIDS is caused by the human immuno-deficiency virus (HIV), which is acquired by direct contact of the bloodstream or mucous membrane with a bodily fluid (such as blood, breast milk, vaginal fluid, semen, and preseminal fluid) containing HIV.

Oils: helichrysum, On Guard, lemon, bergamot, Balance

: Diffuse into the air. Inhale oil applied to a tissue or cotton wick.

: Dilute as recommended, and apply 1–3 drops on the bottoms of the feet and/or on the spine.

: **Body System(s) Affected:** Immune System.

Additional Research:

Helichrysum: Appendino et al., 2007; **Bergamot:** Balestrieri et al., 2011.

Abscess

*See **Oral Conditions: Abscess***

Abuse

Abuse is the harmful treatment or use of something or someone. Abuse has many different forms: physical, sexual, verbal, spiritual, psychological, etc. Abuse in all of its forms often has long-lasting negative effects on the person or thing abused.

Oils: Elevation, lavender, melissa, sandalwood

: Apply oil topically over the heart, rub on each ear, and then cup hands and inhale deeply to help release negative emotions associated with abuse.

: **Body System(s) Affected:** Emotional Balance.

Acne

Acne is a skin condition, generally of the face, commonly found in adolescents and young adults. Acne is characterized by red, irritating blemishes (pimples) on the skin. Most commonly, acne is found on the oil-producing parts of the body such as the face, chest, back, upper arms, and back of neck. Acne is a blockage of a skin pore by dead skin cells, tiny hairs, and oil secreted by the sebaceous glands located near the hair follicles in the face, neck, and back. This blockage occurs deep within the skin. Acne is not currently believed to be caused by dirt on the face or by eating certain foods, and research has indicated that over-scrubbing the face may actually make acne worse.

> *Simple Solutions—Acne:* Add 2 drops melaleuca to 1 cup (250 ml) warm water, and use water to gently wash face once a day.

Oils: HD Clear, melaleuca, juniper berry, copaiba, manuka, Stronger, lavender, cedarwood, petitgrain, geranium, sandalwood, thyme, vetiver, lemon, lemongrass, marjoram, patchouli

=Topical, =Aromatic, O=Internal

Other Products: ⊘HD Clear Foaming Face Wash and ⊘HD Clear Facial Lotion

—Infectious:

Oils: ⊘HD Clear, ⊘melaleuca⊕, ⊘clove

Other Products: ⊘HD Clear Foaming Face Wash and ⊘HD Clear Facial Lotion

⊜: Dilute as recommended, and apply one of the above oils on location. Place about 10 drops of oil in a 1–2 oz. spray bottle filled with water, and mist your face several times per day.

⊕: **Body System(s) Affected:** Skin.

⊡: **Additional Research:**

Melaleuca: Raman et al., 1995; Enshaieh et al., 2007; Bassett et al., 1990.

Addictions

Addiction is an obsession, compulsion, or extreme psychological dependence that interferes with an individual's ability or desire to function normally. Common addictions include drugs, alcohol, coffee, tobacco, sugar, video games, work, gambling, money, explicit images, compulsive overeating, etc.

> *Simple Solutions—Addictions:* Diffuse grapefruit oil using an aromatherapy diffuser to help calm and soothe withdrawal symptoms.

—Alcohol:

Oils: ⊜⊘rosemary, ⊜⊘Purify, ⊜⊘Serenity, ⊜⊘juniper berry, ⊜⊘helichrysum, ⊜⊘lavender, ⊜⊘orange

—Drugs:

Oils: ⊜⊘Purify, ⊜⊘Serenity, ⊜⊘grapefruit (withdrawal)⊕, ⊜⊘lavender, ⊜⊘basil, ⊜⊘eucalyptus, ⊜⊘marjoram, ⊜orange, ⊜sandalwood, ⊘Roman chamomile, ⊜wintergreen

—Opioid Addiction:

Opioid addiction has become an increasingly significant problem throughout the world due to the increasing availability of natural and synthetic opioids. As of 2016, opioid overdose was among the top causes of death in individuals under the age of 50 in the United States.

Oils: ⊜⊘Serenity, ⊜⊘rose (withdrawal)⊕, ⊜⊘grapefruit (withdrawal), ⊜⊘lavender, ⊜⊘basil, ⊜orange, ⊜sandalwood, ⊘Roman chamomile

—Smoking:

Oils: ⊘black pepper, ⊘clove, or ⊘On Guard on tongue

—Sugar:

Oils: ⊜Purify, ⊜Serenity

—Technology:

When someone has a technology addiction, he or she increasingly practices a frequent and obsessive technology-related behavior despite negative consequences. Technology addictions can include online gaming, shopping, researching, and social media use, among other things.

Oils: ⊜Serenity, ⊜⊘lavender, ⊜⊘grapefruit

—Withdrawal:

Oils: ⊜⊘lavender, ⊜⊘grapefruit, ⊜⊘orange, ⊜⊘sandalwood, ⊜⊘marjoram

—Work:

Oils: ⊘lavender, ⊘basil, ⊘marjoram, ⊘geranium

⊘: Diffuse into the air. Inhale the aroma of the oil directly.

⊜: Dilute as recommended, and apply to temples or to reflex points.

⊕: **Body System(s) Affected:** Emotional Balance.

⊡: **Additional Research:**

Grapefruit and Orange: Yun, 2014; Black Pepper: Rose et al., 1994.

Addison's Disease

See Adrenal Glands: Addison's Disease

Adenitis

Adenitis is an acute or chronic inflammation of the lymph glands or lymph nodes.

> *Simple Solutions—Adenitis:* Dilute 2 drops rosemary in 1 tsp. (5 ml) fractionated coconut oil, and apply over lymph nodes daily.

Oils: ⊜rosemary

⊜: Dilute as recommended, and apply on location.

⊕: **Body System(s) Affected:** Immune System.

Adrenal Glands

The adrenal glands are two small glands located on top of the kidneys. The inner part of the adrenal gland, called the medulla, is responsible for producing adrenalin, a hormone that helps control blood pressure, heart rate, and sweating. The outer part of the adrenal gland, called the cortex, is responsible for producing corticosteroids, hormones that help control metabolism and help regulate inflammation, water levels, and levels of electrolytes such as sodium and potassium. An imbalance in adrenal function can lead to problems such as Addison's disease (a lack of adrenal hormones in the body due to suppressed adrenal functioning) or Cushing's syndrome (an over-abundance of corticosteroids, typically due to over-active adrenal functioning).

Oils: ⬭basil, ⬭rosemary, ⬭clove, ⬭Elevation

Other Products: ⵔAlpha CRS+, ⵔMicroplex VMz, ⵔa2z Chewable, ⵔxEO Mega or vEO Mega, ⵔIQ Mega

—Addison's Disease:

Addison's disease is a condition where the function of the adrenal glands is either severely limited or completely shut down in their ability to produce hormones. This is most often caused by an autoimmune disorder where the body's own immune system attacks the cells in the adrenal glands, but it can also be caused by cancer, tuberculosis, or other diseases. The loss of hormones from the adrenal cortex can cause extreme dehydration due to fluid loss and low levels of sodium. Early symptoms can include tiredness, dizziness when standing up, thirst, weight loss, and dark patches of pigmentation appearing on the skin. If untreated, this disease can eventually lead to kidney failure, shock, and death.

Oils: ⬭Elevation

Other Products: ⵔMicroplex VMz, ⵔAlpha CRS+ (for cellular support), ⵔa2z Chewable, ⵔxEO Mega or vEO Mega, ⵔIQ Mega

—Cushing's Syndrome:

Cushing's syndrome is a condition where there is an over-abundance of corticosteroids (such as cortisol) in the body, typically caused by an over-production of these steroids by the adrenal glands. This over-production in the adrenal glands can be caused by a growth in the adrenal glands or by a tumor in the pituitary gland leading to the production of too much corticotropin (the hormone that stimulates production of corticosteroids in the adrenal gland). This syndrome can also be caused by taking artificial cortisone or cortisone-like substances. Symptoms of excessive corticosteroids include weight gain, muscle loss, and weakness, bruising, and osteoporosis.

Oils: ⬭Elevation, ⬭lemon, ⬭basil, ⬭On Guard

Other Products: ⵔMicroplex VMz, ⵔAlpha CRS+ (for cellular support), ⵔa2z Chewable, ⵔxEO Mega or vEO Mega, ⵔIQ Mega

—Schmidt's Syndrome *(Polyglandular Deficiency Syndrome (or Autoimmune Polyendocrine Syndrome) Type 2):*

This syndrome refers specifically to an autoimmune disorder that causes Addison's disease as well as decreased thyroid function. See ***Addison's Disease*** (above) and ***Thyroid: Hypothyroidism*** for oils and products to help support the adrenal glands and thyroid.

Stimulate glands: ⬭basil, ⬭rosemary, ⬭clove, ⬭geranium

Strengthen glands: ⬭peppermint

⬭: Apply as a warm compress over kidney area. Dilute as recommended, and apply on location or on reflex points on the feet.

ⵔ: Take capsules as directed on package.

✛: Body System(s) Affected: Endocrine System.

Aging

*See also **Alzheimer's Disease, Antioxidant, Cells, Female-Specific Conditions: Menopause, Hair: Loss**, and **Skin: Wrinkles** for other age-related issues.*

Simple Solutions—Aging: Diffuse lemon oil for 15 minutes daily to help promote memory.

Oils: ⵔDDR Prime, ⬭Immortelle, ⵔYarrow Pom, ⵔlemon⬭, ⬭frankincense, ⬭sandalwood

Other Products: ⬭Anti-Aging Moisturizer, ⬭Veráge Cleanser, ⬭Youthful Pore Reducing Toner, ⬭Veráge Immortelle Hydrating Serum, ⬭Veráge Moisturizer, ⬭Facial Cleanser, ⬭Invigorating Scrub, ⬭Pore Reducing Toner, ⬭Skin Serum. ⵔMito2Max, ⵔAlpha CRS+, ⵔxEO Mega or vEO Mega, ⵔIQ Mega, ⵔMicroplex VMz, ⵔPB Assist+

ⵔ: Take oil with food, or take capsules as directed on package.

⬭: Dilute as recommended, and apply to skin. Combine with carrier oil, and massage into skin.

⬰: Diffuse, or inhale from a tissue or cotton wick.

⬭=Topical, ⬰=Aromatic, ⵔ=Internal

: Body System(s) Affected: Skin and Nervous System.

: Additional Research:

Lemon: Oboh et al., 2014; Campelo et al., 2011.

Agitation

See Calming

Airborne Bacteria

See Antibacterial

Air Pollution

Air Pollution is the presence in the atmosphere of chemicals, biological material, or other matter that can potentially harm humans, the environment, or other living organisms.

> *Simple Solutions—Air Cleansing:* Diffuse Purify in an aromatherapy diffuser.

Oils: ⊘Purify, ⊘On Guard, ⊘lemon, ⊘lemongrass, ⊘peppermint, ⊘rosemary, ⊘eucalyptus, ⊘cypress, ⊘grapefruit

—Disinfectants:

Oils: ⊘Purify, ⊘lemon, ⊘eucalyptus, ⊘clove, ⊘grapefruit, ⊘peppermint, ⊘wintergreen

Blend 1: Combine lemongrass and geranium oil, and diffuse into the air⊕.

: Diffuse into the air.

: Body System(s) Affected: Respiratory System.

: Additional Research:

Blend 1: Doran et al., 2009.

Alcoholism

See Addictions: Alcohol

Alertness

Alertness is the state of being watchful or paying close attention. It includes being prepared to react quickly to danger, emergencies, or any other situation.

> *Simple Solutions—Alertness:* Drop 3–4 drops of peppermint oil on the shower floor when showering in the morning to help invigorate.
> Inhale the aroma of peppermint while driving to help stay alert.

Oils: ⊘⊜peppermint⊕, ⊜⊘Thinker, ⊘ylang ylang⊕, ⊘⊜lemon, ⊘⊜pink pepper, ⊘⊜basil, ⊘⊜rosemary

: Diffuse into the air. Inhale oil applied to a tissue or cotton wick.

: Dilute as recommended, and apply to the temples and bottoms of the feet.

: Body System(s) Affected: Nervous System.

: Additional Research:

Peppermint: Moss et al., 2008; Ylang ylang: Hongratanaworakit et al., 2004.

Allergies

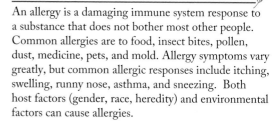

An allergy is a damaging immune system response to a substance that does not bother most other people. Common allergies are to food, insect bites, pollen, dust, medicine, pets, and mold. Allergy symptoms vary greatly, but common allergic responses include itching, swelling, runny nose, asthma, and sneezing. Both host factors (gender, race, heredity) and environmental factors can cause allergies.

> *Simple Solutions—Allergies:* Blend 2 drops each of lavender, lemon, and peppermint oil in 1 tsp. (5 ml) fractionated coconut oil, and apply a small amount on the temples, under the nose, and on the bottoms of the feet morning and evening when dealing with seasonal allergies.

Oils: ⊜melaleuca⊕, O⊜lavender⊕, O⊜lemon⊕, O⊘peppermint⊕, ⊜Roman chamomile, ⊜⊘melissa, ⊜⊘patchouli, ⊘⊜blue tansy, ⊜eucalyptus, ⊜spikenard (skin)

Other Products: OTriEase Softgels, OBreathe Respiratory Drops, ⊜Breathe Vapor Stick, OMicroplex VMz, OAlpha CRS+, Oa2z Chewable

—Coughing:

Oils: ⊘⊜Purify

—Hay Fever

Oils: ⊜lavender⊕, ⊘eucalyptus, ⊘rose, ⊜peppermint

Recipe 1: Apply 1 drop of peppermint on the base of the neck 2 times a day. Tap the thymus (located just below the notch in the neck) with pointer fingers. Diffuse peppermint.

Recipe 2: For allergy rashes and skin sensitivity, apply 3 drops lavender, 6 drops Roman chamomile, 2 drops myrrh, and 1 drop peppermint on location.

🝱: Dilute as recommended, and apply to sinuses and to bottoms of feet.

🝱: Diffuse into the air. Inhale oil applied to a tissue or cotton wick.

🝱: **Body System(s) Affected:** Respiratory System and Immune System.

🝱: **Additional Research:**

Melaleuca: Brand et al., 2002; Brand et al., 2002; Koh et al., 2002; **Lavender:** Kim et al., 1999; **Lemon:** Ferrara et al., 2012; **Peppermint:** Juergens et al., 1998.

Alzheimer's Disease

See also **Brain, Memory**

Alzheimer's is a progressive and fatal disease that attacks and kills brain cells, causing a loss of memory and other intellectual capacities. Alzheimer's is most commonly diagnosed in individuals over the age of 65. As the disease progresses, sufferers often experience mood swings, long-term memory loss, confusion, irritability, aggression, and a decreased ability to communicate.

Simple Solutions—Alzheimer's: Diffuse a blend of 1 part coriander and 2 parts lemon using an aromatherapy diffuser for 15 minutes daily.

Oils: 🝱coriander🝱, 🝱lemon🝱, 🝱cinnamon🝱, 🝱spikenard

Supplements: 🝱Mito2Max, 🝱Alpha CRS+🝱

—Blood-Brain Barrier:

Studies have shown that sesquiterpenes can pass the blood-brain barrier. Oils high in sesquiterpenes include sandalwood, ginger, myrrh, vetiver, ylang ylang, and frankincense.

Oils: 🝱frankincense, 🝱sandalwood🝱

🝱: Take oils in capsules. Take supplements as directed on package.

🝱: Diffuse oils into the air.

🝱: Dilute as recommended, and apply over brain stem area on back of neck.

🝱: **Body System(s) Affected:** Nervous System.

🝱: **Additional Research:**

Coriander: Cioanca et al., 2014; Cioanca et al., 2013; **Lemon:** Oboh et al., 2014; **Alpha CRS+:** Yang et al., 2005; Park et al., 2008; **Sandalwood:** Jeon et al., 2011; **Cinnamon:** Frydman-Marom et al., 2011.

Amnesia

See **Memory**

Analgesic

See **Pain**

Aneurysm

See also **Blood**

An aneurysm is a swelling or dilation of a blood vessel in the area of a weakened blood vessel wall.

Simple Solutions—Aneurysm: Diffuse a blend of 5 drops frankincense, 1 drop helichrysum, and 1 drop cypress in an aromatherapy diffuser.

Oils: 🝱cypress, 🝱melaleuca, 🝱clary sage, 🝱helichrysum, 🝱frankincense

Herbs: Cayenne pepper, garlic, hawthorn berry

🝱: Dilute as recommended, and apply to temples, heart, and reflex points for heart on the feet.

🝱: Diffuse into the air. Inhale oil applied to a tissue or cotton wick.

🝱: **Body System(s) Affected:** Cardiovascular System.

Anger

See **Calming**

Angina

See **Cardiovascular System: Angina**

Animals

Only 1–2 drops of oil are necessary on most animals, as they respond more quickly to the oils than do humans. Fractionated coconut oil can be added to extend the oil over larger areas and to heavily dilute the essential oil for use on smaller animals, especially cats.

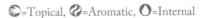
🝱=Topical, 🝱=Aromatic, 🝱=Internal

—Bleeding:

Oils: ⬭helichrysum, ⬭geranium

—Bones (Pain):

Oils: ⬭wintergreen, ⬭Deep Blue, ⬭lemongrass

—Calm:

Oils: ⬭⬭Serenity, ⬭⬭lavender, ⬭⬭Citrus Bliss

—Cancer, Skin

Oils: ⬭sandalwood⬭, ⬭frankincense

—Cats:

> Valerie Worwood says that you can treat a cat
> like you would a child (see **Children/Infants**).
> Dilute oils heavily with carrier oil. *Avoid mela-*
> *leuca, and use oils with extreme caution.*

—Colds and Coughs:

Oils: ⬭eucalyptus, ⬭melaleuca (not for cats). Apply on
fur or stomach.

—Cows:

Oils: For scours, use 5 drops ⬭DigestZen on stomach
(dilute with fractionated coconut oil to cover a
larger area). Repeat 2 hours later.

—Dogs:

—Anxiety/Nervousness

Oils: ⬭Serenity, ⬭lavender, ⬭Balance. Rub
1–2 drops between hands, and apply to
muzzle, between toes, on tops of feet for
the dog to smell, and on edges of ears.

—Arthritis:

Oils: ⬭frankincense⬭

Blend 1: Blend equal parts rosemary, lavender,
and ginger. Dilute with fractionated coconut
oil, and apply topically on affected joints.

—Bone Injury:

Oils: ⬭wintergreen

—Dermatitis:

Oils: ⬭melaleuca⬭. Note: Some adverse
effects have been reported with the use of
larger amounts of melaleuca oil on some
species of dogs. Contact a veterinarian
before using melaleuca on a dog. For
smaller dogs, use only a small amount of
oil, heavily diluted.

—Heart Problems:

Oils: ⬭peppermint (on paws), ⬭On Guard
(apply on back with warm compress)

—Sleep:

Oils: ⬭lavender (on paws), ⬭Serenity (on
stomach)

—Stroke:

Oils: ⬭frankincense (on brain stem/back of
neck), ⬭Balance (on each paw)

—Ticks and Bug Bites:

Oils: ⬭Purify (drop directly on tick, or dilute
and apply to wound)

—Travel Sickness:

Oils: ⬭peppermint (dilute, and rub
on stomach)

—Earache:

Blend 2: Combine 1 drop melaleuca, 1 drop lavender, and 1 drop Roman chamomile in 1 tsp. (5
ml) fractionated coconut oil. Apply 1–2 drops to
inside and outside of ear.

—Ear Infections:

Oils: ⬭Purify. Dip cotton swab in oil, and apply to
inside and front of ear.

—Fleas:

Oils: ⬭lemongrass, ⬭eucalyptus. Add 1–2 drops of oil
to shampoo.

—Horses:

—Anxiety/Nervousness

Oils: ⬭Serenity. Rub 1–2 drops between
hands, and apply to nose, knees, tongue,
and front of chest.

—Hoof Rot:

Blend 3: Combine 1 drop Roman chamomile,
1 drop thyme, and 1 drop melissa in 1
tsp. (5 ml) fractionated coconut oil, and
apply on location.

—Infection:

Oils: ⬭On Guard

—Leg Fractures:

Oils: ⬭ginger. Dilute oil, and apply oil to leg
with a hot compress wrapped around
the leg. Massage leg after the fracture
is healed with a blend of ⬭rosemary

Primary Recommendations • Secondary Recommendations • Other Recommendations

and 🍃thyme diluted with fractionated coconut oil. This may strengthen the ligaments and prevent calcification.

– Muscle Tissue

Oils: Apply equal parts 🍃lemongrass and 🍃lavender on location, and wrap to help regenerate torn muscle tissue.

– Wounds:

Oils: 🍃helichrysum

— Parasites:

Oils: 🍃lavender, 🍃DigestZen, 🍃cedarwood. Rub on paws to help release parasites.

🍃: Apply as directed above. Dilute as recommended, and apply on location.

🌀: Diffuse into the air.

⬜: **Additional Research:**

Sandalwood: Dwivedi et al., 1997; Dwivedi et al., 2003; Dwivedi et al., 2005; Dwivedi et al., 2006; Banerjee et al., 1993; Arasada et al., 2008; **Frankincense:** Fan et al., 2008; **Melaleuca:** Reichling et al., 2004; **Lime, Lavender, Marjoram, Oregano, Peppermint, Helichrysum:** Nardoni et al., 2014; **Oregano:** Mugnaini et al., 2012.

Anorexia

See Eating Disorders: Anorexia

Antibacterial

See also Disinfectant

The term antibacterial refers to anything that kills bacteria or that limits its ability to grow or reproduce.

Simple Solutions—Antibacterial: Add 5 drops of On Guard to a damp rag, and use to wipe down surfaces.

Oils: 🅞🍃On Guard, 🍃melaleuca⬜, 🍃🌀thyme⬜, 🍃🌀cinnamon⬜, 🍃🌀Stronger, 🍃peppermint⬜, 🌀🍃Purify, litsea⬜, pink pepper⬜, 🍃lemon myrtle, 🍃🌀lime, 🍃🌀lemongrass⬜, 🍃helichrysum⬜, 🍃🌀geranium⬜, 🍃rosemary⬜, 🍃🌀clove, 🍃oregano⬜, 🍃🌀turmeric, 🌀Breathe, 🍃cypress⬜, 🍃arborvitae⬜, 🍃cedarwood, 🍃basil, 🍃cassia⬜, 🍃🌀lemon, 🍃eucalyptus, 🍃grapefruit, 🍃marjoram, 🍃clary sage, 🍃lavender⬜, 🍃frankincense, 🍃juniper berry

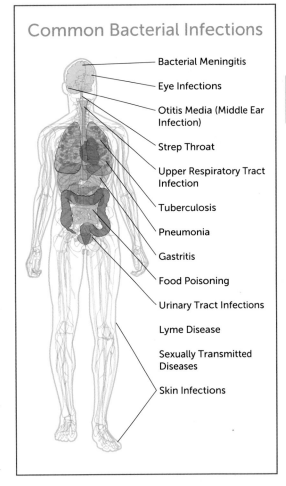

Common Bacterial Infections

- Bacterial Meningitis
- Eye Infections
- Otitis Media (Middle Ear Infection)
- Strep Throat
- Upper Respiratory Tract Infection
- Tuberculosis
- Pneumonia
- Gastritis
- Food Poisoning
- Urinary Tract Infections
- Lyme Disease
- Sexually Transmitted Diseases
- Skin Infections

Blend 1: For an antibiotic blend, place 12 drops of On Guard, 6 drops oregano, and 2 drops frankincense in a size "00" capsule, and ingest every 4–8 hours.

Other Products: 🅞On Guard+ Softgels, 🍃On Guard Foaming Hand Wash & 🍃Correct-X to help eliminate bacteria on the skin, 🍃On Guard Cleaner Concentrate to help eliminate bacteria from household surfaces, 🅞PB Assist+, 🅞PB Assist Jr, 🅞GX Assist to help support the intestinal tract against harmful bacteria.

— Airborne Bacteria:

Oils: 🌀cinnamon⬜, 🌀lemongrass⬜, 🌀geranium⬜, 🌀On Guard, 🌀Purify, 🍃🌀Stronger, 🌀oregano

— Cleansing:

Oils: Purify

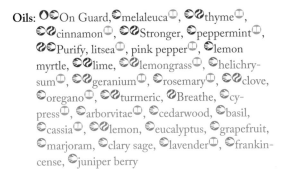

🍃=Topical, 🌀=Aromatic, 🅞=Internal

—MRSA (Methicillin Resistant *Staphylococcus aureus*):

Oils: ⊘melaleuca▢, ⊘oregano▢, ⊘geranium▢, ⊘On Guard, ⊘frankincense, ⊘peppermint▢, ⊘lemon myrtle, ⊘lemon, ⊘thyme, ⊘cinnamon, ⊘clove, ⊘eucalyptus, ⊘lemongrass, ⊘orange, ⊘grape-fruit, ⊘lavender

Recipe 1: Place 2–5 drops each of oregano, On Guard, and frankincense (followed by lemon and peppermint) on bottoms of feet every 2 hours.

—Staph (*Staphylococcus aureus*) Infection:

Oils: O⊘On Guard, O⊘melaleuca▢, ⊘oregano▢, ⊘helichrysum▢, ⊘thyme▢, ⊘geranium▢, ⊘Purify, ⊘lavender **Note:** peppermint may make a staph infection more painful.

Other Products: OOn Guard+ Softgels

⊘: Dilute as recommended, and apply on location. Dilute and apply to liver area and bottoms of the feet. Use hand wash as directed on packaging.

O: Place 1–2 drops of oil under the tongue, or place oils in empty capsules and swallow. Take supplements as directed.

⊘: Diffuse into the air. Combine a few drops in a small spray bottle with distilled water, and spray into the air.

⊕: **Body System(s) Affected:** Immune System.

⊕ **Additional Research:**

  Melaleuca: Cox et al., 2000; Feinblatt et al., 1960; Hammer et al., 2008; Shapiro et al., 1994; Filoche et al., 2005; Brady et al., 2006; Carson et al., 1995; Edwards-Jones et al., 2004; Ferrini et al., 2006; Kwieciński et al., 2009; Loughlin et al., 2008; **Thyme:** Shapiro et al., 1994; Filoche et al., 2005; Inouye et al., 2001; Mohsenzadeh et al., 2007; Inouye et al., 2001; **Cinnamon:** Filoche et al., 2005; Inouye et al., 2001; **Peppermint:** Shapiro et al., 1994; Imai et al., 2001; Rasooli et al., 2008; **Litsea:** Su et al., 2016; **Pink Pepper:** Martins et al., 2014; Guerra-Boone et al., 2013; Gundidza, 1993; **Lemongrass:** Inouye et al., 2001; Doran et al., 2009; Ohno et al., 2003; **Helichrysum:** Chinou et al., 1996; Nostro et al., 2001; **Geranium:** Edwards-Jones et al., 2004; Doran et al., 2009; **Rosemary:** Rasooli et al., 2008; **Oregano:** Nostro et al., 2004; **Cypress:** Selim et al., 2014; **Cassia:** Lee et al., 1998; **Arborvitae:** Hudson et al., 2011; **Lavender:** Yap et al., 2014.

Anticatarrhal

See Congestion: Catarrh

Anticoagulant

See Blood: Clots

Antidepressant

See Depression

Antifungal

Fungi are a broad range of organisms such as yeast, mold, and mushrooms. While many fungi are safe and beneficial, some create mycotoxins, which are chemicals that can be toxic to plants, animals, and humans. Examples of fungi that can be detrimental to humans include black mold, *Candida*, and ringworm.

> *Simple Solutions—Antifungal:* Diffuse On Guard in an aromatherapy diffuser.

> *Simple Solutions—Antifungal:* Mix 20 drops On Guard with ¼ cup (50 ml) water in a small spray bottle, spray on surfaces, and wipe down.

> *Simple Solutions—Nails:* Apply melaleuca oil to toenails to help keep a clean appearance.

Oils: ⊘melaleuca▢, ⊘⊘Ooregano▢, ⊘thyme▢, ⊘⊘cinnamon▢, ⊘clove▢, ⊘⊘On Guard, ⊘arborvitae▢, ⊘lavender▢, ⊘peppermint▢, ⊘rosemary▢, ⊘lemon▢, ⊘turmeric▢, ⊘⊘Stronger, ⊘spikenard, ⊘lemon myrtle, ⊘Purify, ⊘⊘blue tansy, ⊘⊘patchouli, ⊘lemongrass, ⊘pink pepper, ⊘juniper berry, ⊘geranium

Other Products: ⊘On Guard Foaming Hand Wash, ⊘On Guard Cleaner Concentrate, OPB Assist+, OPB Assist Jr, OGX Assist

—Athlete's Foot:

  Athlete's foot (tinea pedis) is a fungal infection that develops on the skin of the feet. This infection causes itching, redness, and scaling of the skin, and in severe cases it can cause painful blistering or cracking of the skin.

> *Simple Solutions—Athlete's Foot:* Mix 25 drops melaleuca with 2 Tbs. (15 g) cornstarch, and sprinkle a small amount in shoes each night.

Oils: ⊘melaleuca▢, ⊘⊘oregano▢, ⊘turmeric▢, ⊘cypress, ⊘thyme, ⊘geranium, ⊘lavender

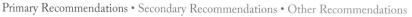

—Candida:

Candida refers to a genus of yeast that are normally found in the digestive tract and on the skin of humans. These yeast are typically symbiotically beneficial to humans. However, several species of *Candida*, most commonly *Candida albicans*, can cause infections such as vaginal candidiasis or thrush (oral candidiasis) that cause localized itching, soreness, and redness *(see* **Vaginal: Candida** *for further application methods)*. In immune system–compromised individuals, these infection-causing species of *Candida* can spread further, leading to serious, life-threatening complications.

Oils: ⬢melaleuca⬒, ⬢⬤oregano⬒, ⬢clove⬒, ⬢On Guard, ⬢⬤Stronger, ⬢⬤peppermint⬒, ⬢thyme⬒, ⬢dill⬒, ⬢cilantro⬒, ⬢lavender⬒, ⬢lemon myrtle, ⬢eucalyptus, ⬢rosemary, ⬢spikenard, ⬢⬤DigestZen

—Mold:

Mold are a type of microscopic multi-cellular fungi that grow together to form filaments. Mold is found throughout the world and can survive in extreme conditions. While most mold does not adversely affect humans, an over-abundance of mold spores can cause allergies or other problems within the respiratory system. Additionally, some types of mold produce toxins that can be harmful to humans or to animals.

Oils: ⬤On Guard, ⬤⬢clove⬒, ⬤⬢thyme⬒, ⬤⬢cinnamon⬒, ⬤⬢oregano⬒, ⬤⬢rosemary⬒, ⬤Purify

—Ringworm:

Ringworm (or tinea) is a fungal infection of the skin that can cause itching, redness, and scaling of the skin. The name comes from the ring-shaped patches that often form on the skin.

Oils: ⬢melaleuca, ⬤⬢oregano⬒, ⬢turmeric⬒, ⬢peppermint, ⬢thyme, ⬢bergamot⬒, ⬢geranium, ⬢lavender

Blend 1: Combine 2 drops lavender, 2 drops melaleuca, and 2 drops thyme. Apply 1–2 drops on ringworm three times a day for 10 days. Then mix 30 drops melaleuca with 2 Tbs. (25 ml) fractionated coconut oil, and use daily until ringworm is gone.

—Thrush:

Thrush is another name for oral candidiasis *(see* **Candida** *above)*. Thrush results in uncomfortable or painful white or yellow patches in the mouth.

Oils: ⬢melaleuca⬒, ⬢lavender, ⬢eucalyptus, ⬢marjoram, ⬢thyme

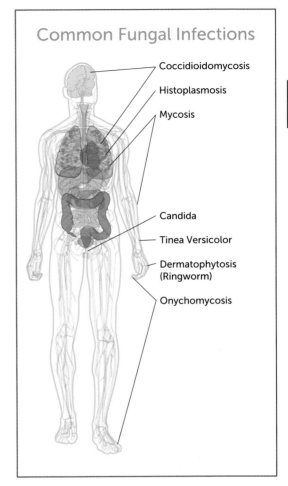

Common Fungal Infections

- Coccidioidomycosis
- Histoplasmosis
- Mycosis
- Candida
- Tinea Versicolor
- Dermatophytosis (Ringworm)
- Onychomycosis

⬢: Dilute as recommended, and apply on location. Apply as a warm compress over affected area.

⬤: Diffuse into the air.

◯: Take capsules as directed on package.

⬢: **Body System(s) Affected: Immune System.**

▭: **Additional Research:**

Melaleuca: Bagg et al., 2006; Banes-Marshall et al., 2001; Cox et al., 2000; D'Auria et al., 2001; Hammer et al., 2004; Mondello et al., 2006; Vazquez et al., 2000; Satchell et al., 2002; Cháfer et al., 2012; **Oregano:** Juglal et al., 2002; Inouye et al., 2006; Manohar et al., 2001; Tantaoui-Elaraki et al., 1994; **Thyme:** Tantaoui-Elaraki et al., 1994; Pina-Vaz et al., 2004; Hitokoto et al., 1980; **Cinnamon:** Juglal et al., 2002; Tantaoui-Elaraki et al., 1994; Singh et al., 1995; **Clove:** Juglal et al., 2002; Hitokoto et al., 1980; Chaieb et al., 2007; **Arborvitae:** Hudson et al., 2011; **Lavender:** Behnam et al., 2006; D'Auria et al., 2005; **Dill:** Chen et al., 2014; **Cilantro:** Freires Ide et al., 2014; **Peppermint:** Mimica-Dukić et al., 2003; **Bergamot:** Sanguinetti et al., 2007; **Rosemary:** Rasooli et al., 2008; **Lemon:** Caccioni et al., 1998; **Turmeric:** Mukda et al., 2013; **Cassia:** Kocevski et al., 2013.

⬢=Topical, ⬤=Aromatic, ◯=Internal

Antihemorrhaging

See **Blood: Hemorrhaging**

Antihistamine

See **Allergies**

Anti-Infectious

See **Infection, Antibacterial, Antiviral, Antifungal**

Anti-Inflammatory

See **Inflammation**

Antimicrobial

See **Antibacterial, Antifungal, Antiviral**

Antioxidant

As part of its normal metabolic processes, the body uses and creates oxidative molecules, each capable of transferring electrons to itself from other molecules or substances. This type of reaction can create molecules known as free radicals (Davies, 1995). If left unchecked in the body, these free radicals can bind or react with different molecular structures, altering their abilities to function normally. Under normal, healthy conditions, the body's own systems are able to create or metabolize enough antioxidant materials to neutralize the ability of these oxidative molecules to create free radicals. But when the body comes under stress—including physical stress, psychological stress, poor nutrition, or disease— the amount of oxidative molecules being produced can increase, and the delicate balance between oxidative molecules and antioxidants can be thrown off, potentially overwhelming the body's own antioxidant mechanisms. This "oxidative stress" (Sies, 1997) creates a condition optimal for the formation of many free radicals, which in turn can potentially cause enough damage to the cell's normal structures to cause cell death, mutation, or loss of its ability to function normally within the body (Rhee, 2006; Vertuani et al., 2004).

> *Simple Solutions—Antioxidant:* Add 2 drops clove to olive oil in an empty capsule, and swallow.

Oils: ⭕DDR Prime, 🌢🍃clove⬜, ⭕🌢🍃thyme⬜, 🌢🍃rosemary⬜, ⭕Yarrow Pom, 🌢🍃pep-permint⬜, ⭕🌢🍃yarrow⬜, 🌢🍃melaleuca⬜, 🌢🍃helichrysum⬜, 🍃copaiba⬜, ⭕🌢🍃turmeric, 🌢🍃Purify, 🌢🍃On Guard, 🌢🍃Breathe, 🌢🍃Deep Blue, 🍃cinnamon, 🌢🍃frankincense, 🌢🍃oregano⬜, 🌢🍃Roman chamomile, 🌢🍃petitgrain, 🌢🍃spikenard

Other Products: ⭕Alpha CRS+ or ⭕a2z Chewable, which contains polyphenols that act as powerful antioxidants, such as quercetin⬜, epigallocatechin gallate⬜, ellagic acid⬜, resveratrol⬜, baicalin⬜, and others⬜. ⭕Mito2Max. ⭕TerraGreens for a whole food source of essential nutrients and antioxidants.

⭕: Take capsules as directed. Use oils recommended as flavoring agents in cooking. Place 1–3 drops of oil in an empty capsule, and ingest it as a dietary supplement.

🌢: Diffuse into the air. Inhale directly from bottle. Apply oil to hands, tissue, or cotton wick, and inhale.

🍃: Dilute as recommended, and apply on the skin and reflex points on the feet. Dilute in a carrier oil, and massage into the skin. Apply as a hot compress.

☘: **Body System(s) Affected:** Immune System.

📖: **Additional Research:**

Clove: Chaieb et al., 2007; Wei et al., 2007; **Thyme:** Vigo et al., 2004; Youdim et al., 1999; Youdim et al., 2000; **Rosemary:** Almela et al., 2006; Cheung et al., 2007; Moreno et al., 2006; Siurin, 1997; **Peppermint:** Mimica-Dukić et al., 2003; Samarth et al., 2006; Samarth et al., 2009; **Yarrow:** Candan et al., 2003; **Melaleuca:** Caldefie-Chézet et al., 2006; Caldefie-Chézet et al., 2004; **Copaiba:** Dias et al., 2014; **Helichrysum:** Rosa et al., 2007; **Oregano:** Asensio et al., 2011; **Quercetin:** Boots et al., 2008; **Epigallocatechin gallate:** Tuzcu et al., 2008; Sriram et al., 2008; **Ellagic acid:** Bagchi et al., 1993; **Resveratrol:** Chakraborty et al., 2008; **Baicalin:** Jung et al., 2008; **Other Polyphenols:** Roy et al., 2002; Maatta-Riihinet et al., 2005; Bao et al., 2008.

Antiparasitic

See **Parasites**

Antirheumatic

See **Arthritis: Rheumatoid Arthritis**

Antiseptic

See **Antibacterial, Antifungal, Antiviral**

Antiviral

The term "antiviral" refers to something that is able to inhibit or stop the development, function, or replication of an infection-causing virus.

> *Simple Solutions—Cold Sores:* Combine 4 tsp. (5 g) beeswax pellets, 1 Tbs. (10 g) cocoa butter, and 3 Tbs. (45 ml) jojoba oil, and melt in the microwave (30 seconds at a time, stirring in between) or in a double boiler. Cool slightly, and add 5 drops melissa, 5 drops peppermint, and 5 drops helichrysum essential oil. Pour in small jars or lip balm containers, and allow to cool completely. Apply a small amount of balm on cold sores as needed.

Oils: helichrysum, melaleuca, clove, On Guard, melissa, Breathe, lime, cinnamon, lemon, oregano, peppermint, eucalyptus, thyme, orange, grapefruit, clary sage, juniper berry, myrrh, pink pepper, geranium, lavender, sandalwood, rosemary, cypress

Other Products: On Guard+ Softgels, On Guard Foaming Hand Wash to help protect against skin-borne microorganisms, On Guard Cleaner Concentrate to help eliminate microorganisms from household surfaces. On Guard Protecting Throat Drops to soothe irritated and sore throats. Alpha CRS+, a2z Chewable, xEO Mega or vEO Mega, IQ Mega, Microplex VMz to help support the immune system.

—Airborne Viruses:

Oils: On Guard

—Ebola Virus:

Oils: cinnamon, oregano

—Epstein-Barr Virus:

Oils: On Guard

—Herpes Simplex:

Oils: peppermint, clove, helichrysum, melaleuca, lavender, eucalyptus, cypress, lemon

—HIV: *See also AIDS*

Oils: helichrysum, On Guard, lemon, Balance

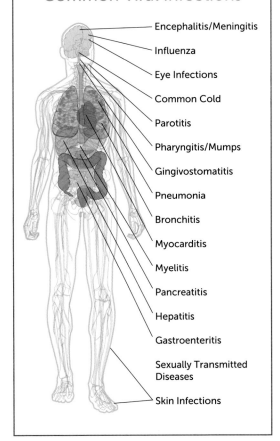

Common Viral Infections

- Encephalitis/Meningitis
- Influenza
- Eye Infections
- Common Cold
- Parotitis
- Pharyngitis/Mumps
- Gingivostomatitis
- Pneumonia
- Bronchitis
- Myocarditis
- Myelitis
- Pancreatitis
- Hepatitis
- Gastroenteritis
- Sexually Transmitted Diseases
- Skin Infections

—Respiratory:

Oils: eucalyptus, On Guard

—Spine:

Blend 1: 5 drops oregano and 5 drops thyme. Apply to bottoms of feet and along the spine.

: Dilute as recommended, and apply on location or to reflex points on the bottoms of the feet. Use hand wash as directed on packaging.

: Diffuse into the air. Inhale oil applied to a tissue or cotton wick.

: Take capsules as directed on package.

: **Body System(s) Affected:** Immune System.

: **Additional Research:**

Helichrysum: Appendino et al., 2007; Nostro et al., 2003; **Melaleuca:** Schnitzler et al., 2001; **Clove:** Benencia et al., 2000; **Melissa:** Schnitzler et al., 2008; **Peppermint:** Schuhmacher et al., 2003; **Eucalyptus:** Schnitzler et al., 2001; **Menthol, thymol, methyl salicylate, and eucalyptol:** Meiller et al., 2005.

=Topical, =Aromatic, =Internal

Anxiety

Anxiety is the body's way of preparing itself to deal with a threat or to deal with future stressful events. While this response is normal and happens as part of the body's natural response to stress, this response can also happen at inappropriate times or too frequently, as in the case of anxiety disorders. Anxiety can include both physical and mental symptoms such as fear, nervousness, nausea, sweating, increased blood pressure and heart rate, feelings of apprehension or dread, difficulty concentrating, irritability, restlessness, panic attacks, and many others.

> *Simple Solutions—Anxiety:* Diffuse lavender in an aromatherapy diffuser when feeling anxious.

> *Simple Solutions—Anxiety:* Combine 5 drops orange and 10 drops lemon with 1 tsp. (5 ml) water in a small spray bottle, and spray into the air and inhale as needed.

Oils: lavender, orange, lemon, copaiba, rose, magnolia, Peace, InTune, Serenity, Calmer, Brave, Steady, Thinker, Motivate, AromaTouch, Elevation, Balance (on back of neck) and Breathe (on chest), neroli, blue tansy, ylang ylang, melissa, frankincense, sandalwood, cedarwood, juniper berry, Citrus Bliss, bergamot, geranium, lime, clary sage, basil, cypress, marjoram, Douglas fir

Other Products: Therapeutic Bath Salts. Add 1–2 drops of essential oil to ¼ cup (50 g) bath salts, and dissolve in warm bathwater for an anxiety-relieving bath.

- Diffuse into the air. Inhale directly from bottle. Apply oil to hands, tissue, or cotton wick, and inhale.

- Place 1–2 drops in 1 Tbs. (15 ml) fractionated coconut oil, and massage into the skin. Dilute as recommended, and apply to back of neck, temples, or reflex points on feet. Add 1–2 drops to ¼ cup (50 g) bath salts, and dissolve in warm bathwater.

- **Body System(s) Affected:** Nervous System and Emotional Balance.

- **Additional Research:**

  Lavender: Bradley et al., 2007; Dimpfel et al., 2004; Dunn et al., 1995; Itai et al., 2000; Umezu, 2000; Lehrner et al., 2005; **Lavender and Roman Chamomile:** Cho et al., 2013; **Orange:**

Lehrner et al., 2005; Carvalho-Freitas et al., 2002; Lehrner et al., 2000; Jafarzadeh et al., 2013; Goes et al., 2012; Faturi et al., 2010; **Lemon:** Komiya et al., 2006; **Copaiba:** Curio et al., 2009; **Rose:** Kheirkhah et al., 2014; Kim et al., 2011; **Melissa:** Kennedy et al., 2006; **Bergamot:** Saiyudthong et al., 2011; **Clary Sage:** Gross et al., 2013; **Cassia:** Jung et al., 2012; **Cypress:** Park et al., 2014; **Aromatherapy Massage:** Wilkinson et al., 2007; **Carvacrol in thyme and oregano:** Melo et al., 2010.

Apathy

See Depression

Aphrodisiac

An aphrodisiac is a substance used to stimulate feelings of love or sexual desire. Many books of aromatherapy tout the aphrodisiac qualities of a number of oils. Perhaps an aphrodisiac to one individual may not be to another. The most important factor is to find an oil that brings balance to the mind and body. A balanced individual is more likely to extend love.

> *Simple Solutions—Aphrodisiac:* Blend 2 Tbs. (25 ml) jojoba oil with 10 drops ylang ylang, 6 drops patchouli, 5 drops clove, 6 drops orange, and 2 drops clary sage.

> *Simple Solutions—Aphrodisiac:* Dissolve 2 drops ylang ylang, 2 drops clary sage, 1 drop lemongrass, and 2 drops sandalwood in 2 tsp. (10 ml) of pure grain (or perfumer's) alcohol. Combine with water in a 1 oz. spray bottle. Mist into the air and on bed linens.

Oils: sandalwood, ylang ylang, rose, jasmine, Whisper, cinnamon, ginger, clary sage

- Diffuse into the air. Dissolve 2–3 drops in 2 tsp. (10 ml) pure grain or perfumer's alcohol, combine with distilled water in a 1–2 oz. spray bottle, and spray into the air or on clothes or bed linens.

- Dilute as recommended and wear on temples, neck, or wrists as a perfume or cologne. Combine 3–5 drops of your desired essential oil with 1 Tbs. (15 ml) fractionated coconut oil to use as a massage oil. Combine 1–2 drops with ¼ cup (50 g) Therapeutic Bath Salts, and dissolve in warm bathwater for a romantic bath.

- **Body System(s) Affected:** Emotional Balance.

Appetite

Appetite is the body's desire to eat, expressed as hunger. Appetite is important in regulating food intake to provide the body with the necessary nutrients to sustain life and maintain energy.

> *Simple Solutions—Appetite:* Diffuse grapefruit in an aromatherapy diffuser to help quell cravings.

—Loss of Appetite:

Oils: ⊘lavender▢, ⊘ginger, ⊘lemon, ⊘orange

—Suppressant:

Oils: O⊘Slim & Sassy, ⊘grapefruit▢

Other Products: OSlim & Sassy TrimShakes

O: Add 8 drops of Slim & Sassy to 2 cups (½ L) of water, and drink throughout the day between meals. Drink Trim or V Shake 1–2 times a day as a meal alternative.

⊘: Diffuse into the air. Inhale oil applied to a tissue or cotton wick.

⊕: **Body System(s) Affected:** Digestive System, Nervous System, and Endocrine System.

▢: **Additional Research:**

Lavender: Shen et al., 2005; Grapefruit: Shen et al., 2005.

Arteries

See also **Blood, Cardiovascular System**

Arteries are the vessels of the circulatory system that function to carry blood away from the heart.

—Arterial Vasodilator:

A vasodilator is a substance that causes a blood vessel to dilate (increase in diameter) through the relaxation of the endothelial cells lining the vessel walls. This gives the blood more room to flow and lowers blood pressure.

Oils: ⊖eucalyptus▢, ⊖rosemary▢, ⊖marjoram

—Atherosclerosis:

Atherosclerosis is a hardening of the arteries due to a build-up of plaques along the arterial wall.

Oils: ⊖⊘lemon▢, ⊘lavender▢, ⊖rosemary, ⊖ginger, ⊖cedarwood, ⊖thyme, ⊖juniper berry, ⊖wintergreen

⊖: Dilute as recommended, and apply to carotid arteries in neck, over heart, and reflex points on the feet.

⊘: Diffuse into the air. Inhale directly from bottle. Apply oil to hands, tissue, or cotton wick, and inhale.

⊕: **Body System(s) Affected:** Cardiovascular System

▢: **Additional Research:**

Eucalyptus: Lahlou et al., 2002; Rosemary: Lahlou et al., 2002; Lemon: Grassmann et al., 2001; Lavender: Nikolaevski et al., 1990.

Arthritis

See also **Inflammation, Joints**

Arthritis is the painful swelling, inflammation, and stiffness of the joints.

> *Simple Solutions—Arthritis:* Blend 3 drops frankincense, 4 drops peppermint, and 2 drops marjoram with 1 Tbs. (15 ml) fractionated coconut oil. Massage gently on affected joints each day. If desired, 10 drops Deep Blue may be substituted for the above oils.

Oils: ⊖⊘frankincense▢, ⊖⊘rosemary▢, ⊖⊘marjoram▢, ⊖Deep Blue, ⊖⊘manuka, ⊖⊘eucalyptus▢, ⊖⊘fir, ⊖⊘peppermint▢, ⊖⊘lavender▢, ⊖⊘cypress, ⊖⊘juniper berry, ⊖⊘ginger, ⊖⊘Roman chamomile, ⊖⊘helichrysum, ⊖⊘cedarwood, ⊖⊘wintergreen, ⊖⊘basil, ⊖⊘clove▢

Blend 1: Combine equal parts wintergreen and Deep Blue. Apply on location.

Other Products: OAlpha CRS+▢

—Arthritic Pain:

Oils: ⊖Deep Blue, ⊖wintergreen, ⊖ginger

—Osteoarthritis:

Osteoarthritis is a degenerative arthritis where the cartilage that provides lubrication between the bones in a joint begins to break down, becoming rough and uneven. This causes the bones in the joint to wear and create rough deposits that can become extremely painful.

Oils: ⊖rosemary, ⊖marjoram, ⊖Deep Blue, ⊖geranium, ⊖wintergreen, ⊖thyme, ⊖basil, ⊖lavender, ⊖eucalyptus

Other Products: OAlpha CRS+

—Rheumatoid Arthritis:

Rheumatoid arthritis is arthritis caused by inflammation within the joint, causing pain and possibly causing the joint to degenerate.

⊖=Topical, ⊘=Aromatic, O=Internal

Oils: marjoram, lavender, cypress, Deep Blue, geranium, bergamot, clove, ginger, manuka, lemon, rosemary, wintergreen, cinnamon, eucalyptus, oregano (chronic), peppermint, Roman chamomile, thyme

Other Products: O Alpha CRS+

: Dilute as recommended, and apply on location. Apply as a warm compress over affected area. Dilute 1–2 drops in 1 Tbs. (15 ml) fractionated coconut oil, and use as a massage oil. Add 1–2 drops to ¼ cup (50 g) Therapeutic Bath Salts, and dissolve in warm bathwater for a soaking bath.

: Diffuse into the air.

: **Body System(s) Affected:** Muscles and Skeletal System.

: **Additional Research:**

Frankincense: Fan et al., 2005; Rosemary: Kim et al., 2005; Marjoram: Kim et al., 2005; Eucalyptus: Kim et al., 2005; Peppermint: Kim et al., 2005; Lavender: Kim et al., 2005; Alpha CRS+: Morinobu et al., 2008; Clove: Sharma et al., 1994; Ginger: Sharma et al., 1994; Eugenol Found in Cassia, Cinnamon, and Clove : Grespan et al., 2012; Cinnamon: Rathi et al., 2013; Coriander: Nair et al., 2012.

Asthma

Asthma is a disease that causes the lung's airways to narrow, making it difficult to breathe. Episodes (or attacks) of asthma can be triggered by any number of things, including smoke, pollution, dust mites, and other allergens. Asthma causes reoccurring periods of tightness in the chest, coughing, shortness of breath, and wheezing.

> *Simple Solutions—Asthma:* Gently massage 2 drops lavender on chest.

Oils: eucalyptus, frankincense, peppermint, thyme, Breathe, Douglas fir, oregano, lemon, myrrh, lavender, geranium, cypress, clary sage, ylang ylang, rose, helichrysum, marjoram, rosemary

—Attack

Oils: Breathe, eucalyptus, frankincense (calming), lavender, marjoram

: Diffuse into the air. Inhale directly from bottle. Apply oil to hands, tissue, or cotton wick, and inhale.

: Dilute as recommended and apply to the chest, throat, or back. Add 2–3 drops to 1 Tbs. (15 ml) fractionated coconut oil, and massage onto chest, shoulders, and back.

: **Body System(s) Affected:** Respiratory System.

: **Additional Research:**

Eucalyptus: Vigo et al., 2004; Juergens et al., 1998; Peppermint: Juergens et al., 1998; Lavender: Ueno-Iio et al., 2014; Laurel Leaf (Bay Leaf) in Breathe: Lee, T. et al., 2013.

Athlete's Foot
See Antifungal: Athlete's Foot

Attention Deficit Disorder
See ADD/ADHD

Autism

Autism is a developmental disorder that impairs the normal development of communication, sociality, and human interaction.

—Reduce Anxiety/Fear: *See also Anxiety*

Oils: geranium, clary sage, bergamot

—Stimulate the Senses: *See also Stimulating*

Oils: peppermint, basil, lemon, rosemary

: Add 1–2 drops to 1 Tbs. (15 ml) fractionated coconut oil, and massage into skin.

: **Body System(s) Affected:** Nervous System.

Comments: Only apply these oils when the autistic child is willing and open to receive them. If the experience is forced or negative, the autistic child will associate these oils with a negative experience when used again.

Auto-Immune Diseases
See Grave's Disease, Hashimoto's Disease, Lupus

Awake
See Alertness, Jet Lag

Babies
See Children and Infants

Oils: ⬭Deep Blue, ⬭Balance, ⬭Rescuer, ⬭cypress, ⬭eucalyptus, ⬭geranium, ⬭lavender, ⬭Roman chamomile, ⬭oregano, ⬭peppermint, ⬭rosemary, ⬭juniper berry, ⬭thyme

> *Simple Solutions—Backache:* Combine 3 drops peppermint with 1 drop wintergreen in 1 tsp. (5 ml) fractionated coconut oil. Gently massage on lower back to help soothe muscle aches.

Spine

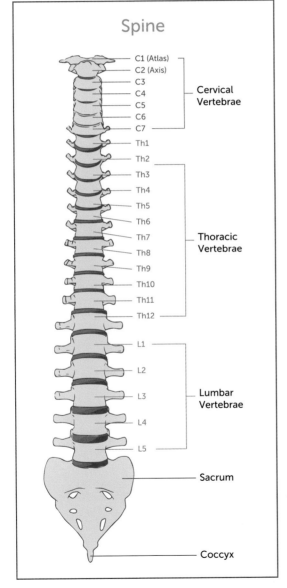

- C1 (Atlas)
- C2 (Axis)
- C3
- C4 — Cervical Vertebrae
- C5
- C6
- C7
- Th1
- Th2
- Th3
- Th4
- Th5
- Th6
- Th7 — Thoracic Vertebrae
- Th8
- Th9
- Th10
- Th11
- Th12
- L1
- L2
- L3 — Lumbar Vertebrae
- L4
- L5
- Sacrum
- Coccyx

—Calcified Spine

Calcification occurs when calcium builds up in tissue and causes the tissue to harden. As people age, calcification can cause the ligaments of the spine to thicken and harden, making the spinal canal narrow and creating pressure on the spinal nerve.

Oils: ⬭Deep Blue, ⬭geranium, ⬭rosemary

—Deteriorating Spine:

Deteriorating disc disease occurs as people age and their spinal discs begin to deteriorate. As deterioration progresses, movement becomes restricted, and pain in the neck and back increases. Although most commonly associated with aging, disc deterioration can be caused by back injuries as well.

Oils: ⬭Deep Blue

—Herniated Discs:

In between the bones of the spine are cushioning discs that keep the spine flexible and act as shock absorbers. A herniated disc is caused when one of the discs of the spine is damaged and either bulges or breaks open. When the herniated disc presses on a nerve, it causes pain in the buttock, thigh, and calf. Herniated discs can be caused by spinal injuries or by the wear and tear that come with age as the discs begin to dry out

Oils: ⬭Deep Blue, ⬭Balance (3 drops on location), ⬭peppermint, ⬭cypress (strengthens blood capillary walls, improves circulation, anti-inflammatory)

—Lumbago/Lower Back Pain:

Oils: ⬭sandalwood, ⬭Deep Blue

—Muscular Fatigue:

Oils: ⬭clary sage, ⬭marjoram, ⬭lavender, ⬭rosemary

—Pain:

Oils: ⬭Balance, ⬭Deep Blue, ⬭Rescuer

Blend 1: Combine 5–10 drops each of lavender, eucalyptus, and ginger, and apply 2–3 drops on location or as a warm compress.

Blend 2: Combine 5–10 drops each of peppermint, rosemary, and basil, and apply 2–3 drops on location or as a warm compress.

—Stiffness:

Oils: ⬭marjoram, ⬭Balance

—Viruses Along Spine:

Oils: ⬭oregano, ⬭eucalyptus

⬭=Topical, ⬭=Aromatic, ⬭=Internal

⟳: Dilute as recommended, and apply along the spine, on affected muscles, or on reflex points on the feet. Dilute 1–3 drops in 1 Tbs. (15 ml) fractionated coconut oil, and massage into muscles on the back or along the spine. Apply as a warm compress over affected area.

☉: Body System(s) Affected: Muscles and Skeletal System.

Bacteria

See Antibacterial

Balance

Oils: ⟳🍃Balance, ⟳🍃Steady, ⟳🍃frankincense, ⟳🍃vetiver, ⟳🍃ylang ylang, 🍃☉cedarwood

—Electrical Energies:

Oils: 🍃Balance, 🍃frankincense

Application Methods:

⟳: Dilute as recommended, and apply on location. Apply 3–6 drops of Balance to the bottom of each foot, and, if desired, apply some to the neck and shoulders. Hold the palm of each hand to the bottom of each corresponding foot (left to left and right to right) for 5–15 minutes to help balance electrical energies.

🌀: Diffuse into the air.

☉: Body System(s) Affected: Emotional Balance.

Baldness

See Hair: Loss

Bath

Using essential oils in the bath can be a wonderful way to receive and possibly enhance the benefits of the oils.

Oils: 🍃lavender, 🍃geranium, 🍃Roman chamomile, 🍃ylang ylang

Some common ways to use essential oils in the bath include the following:

Direct: Add 1–3 drops of oil directly to bathwater while the bath is filling. Oils will be drawn to your skin quickly from the top of the water, so use non-irritating oils such as lavender, ylang ylang, etc., or dilute the oil with fractionated coconut oil to safe topical application dilutions.

Bath Gel: To disperse the oil throughout the bathwater, add 5–10 drops of your favorite essential oil to 1 Tbs. (15 ml) of unscented bath and shower gel.

Bath Salts: For a relaxing mineral bath, add 1–5 drops of your desired essential oil to ¼–½ cup (50–125 g) of Therapeutic Bath Salts or Epsom salt; mix well. Dissolve salt in warm bathwater while the tub is filling.

☉: Body System(s) Affected: Skin.

Bed Wetting

See Bladder: Bed Wetting

Bell's Palsy

See Nervous System: Bell's Palsy

Birthing

See Pregnancy/Motherhood

Bites/Stings

See also Insects/Bugs: Repellent

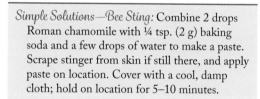

Simple Solutions—Bee Sting: Combine 2 drops Roman chamomile with ¼ tsp. (2 g) baking soda and a few drops of water to make a paste. Scrape stinger from skin if still there, and apply paste on location. Cover with a cool, damp cloth; hold on location for 5–10 minutes.

Oils: 🍃thyme, 🍃basil, 🍃lemon, 🍃cinnamon, 🍃lavender

—Allergic:

Oils: 🍃Purify

—Bees and Hornets

Oils: 🍃Roman chamomile, 🍃basil, 🍃Purify, 🍃lavender, 🍃lemongrass, 🍃lemon, 🍃peppermint, 🍃thyme

Recipe 1: Remove the stinger, and apply a cold compress of Roman chamomile to the area for several hours or for as long as possible.

—Gnats and Midges:

Oils: 🍃lavender

Recipe 2: Mix 3 drops thyme in 1 tsp. (5 ml) cider vinegar or lemon juice. Apply to bites to stop irritation.

—Mosquitoes:

Oils: 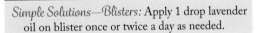lavender, 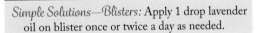helichrysum

—Snakes:

Oils: 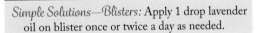basil

—Spiders:

Oils: 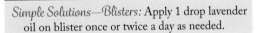basil, 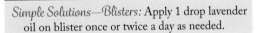Purify (with melaleuca), 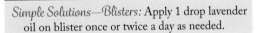lavender, 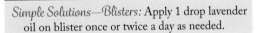lemongrass, 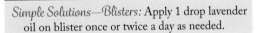lemon, 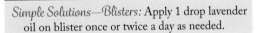peppermint, 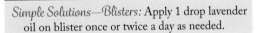thyme

Recipe 3: Mix 3 drops lavender and 2 drops Roman chamomile with 1 tsp. (5 ml) alcohol. Apply to area 3 times per day.

—Ticks:

Oils: After getting the tick out, apply 1 drop lavender every 5 minutes for 30 minutes.

Removing Ticks:

Do not apply mineral oil, Vaseline, or anything else to remove the tick, as this may cause it to inject the spirochetes into the wound.

Be sure to remove the entire tick. Get as close to the mouth as possible, and firmly tug on the tick until it releases its grip. Don't twist. If available, use a magnifying glass to make sure that you have removed the entire tick.

Save the tick in a jar, and label it with the date, where you were bitten on your body, and the location or address where you were bitten for proper identification by your doctor, especially if you develop any symptoms.

Do not handle the tick.

Wash hands immediately.

Check the site of the bite occasionally to see if any rash develops. If it does, seek medical advice promptly.

—Wasps:

Recipe 4: Combine 1 drop basil, 2 drops Roman chamomile, 2 drops lavender, and 1 tsp. (5 ml) apple cider vinegar. Apply to area 3 times a day.

●: Dilute as recommended, and apply on location.

●: **Body System(s) Affected:** Skin.

Bladder

See also **Urinary Tract**

The urinary bladder is a hollow organ that collects urine before it is disposed by urination. The bladder sits on the pelvic floor.

Simple Solutions—Bed Wetting: Combine 5 drops cypress and 3 drops ylang ylang with 2 Tbs. (25 ml) water in a small spray bottle. Mist on pillow and sheets just before bedtime.

—Bed Wetting and Incontinence:

Oils: 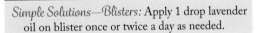cypress (rub on abdomen at bedtime), 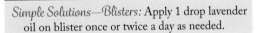ylang ylang.

—Cystitis/Infection:

Oils: 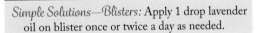lemongrass, ●●On Guard, 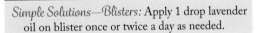sandalwood, 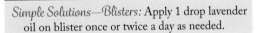juniper berry, 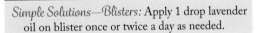thyme, 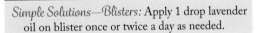cedarwood, 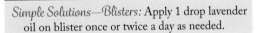basil, 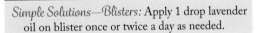cinnamon, 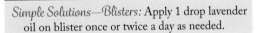clove, 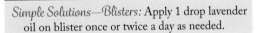eucalyptus, 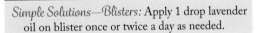frankincense, 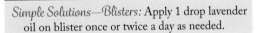lavender, 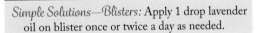bergamot, 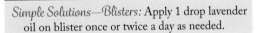fennel, 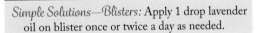marjoram, 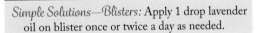oregano

Other Products: ●On Guard+ Softgels

●: Dilute as recommended, and apply on abdomen and on reflex points on the feet. Add 1–2 drops to warm bathwater; bathe for 10–15 minutes.

●: Add 1 drop to 1 cup (250 ml) juice or water; drink three times a day.

●: **Body System(s) Affected:** Digestive System.

●: **Additional Research:**

Ylang ylang: (Kim et al., 2003).

Bleeding

See **Blood: Bleeding**

Blister

Simple Solutions—Blisters: Apply 1 drop lavender oil on blister once or twice a day as needed.

Oils: 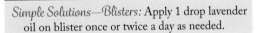lavender

●: Apply oil to blister as often as needed.

Bloating

See **Digestive System: Bloating**

Blood

Blood is the fluid inside the body that transports oxygen and nutrients to the cells and carries waste away from the cells. It also transports cells involved in the immune and inflammatory response, hormones and other chemical

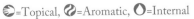
●=Topical, ●=Aromatic, ●=Internal

messengers that regulate the body's functions, and platelets that help facilitate the blood clotting necessary to repair damaged blood vessels. Blood is primarily composed of plasma (water with dissolved nutrients, minerals, and carbon dioxide) that carries red blood cells (the most numerous type of cells in blood, responsible for transporting oxygen), white blood cells (cells involved in the immune system and immune response), and platelet cells. Blood is circulated in the body by the pumping action of the heart propelling blood through various blood vessels. Proper and healthy circulation and function of blood throughout the body is critical for health and even for the sustaining of life.

> *Simple Solutions—Bleeding:* Add 3 drops helichrysum to ½ cup (125 ml) cool water in a bowl. Dampen a small rag in the mixture. Apply on bleeding area and apply pressure to help stop.

—Blood Pressure

Oils: ⭕lemon (will regulate pressure—either raise or lower as necessary), lime

–High (hypertension)

Oils: ylang ylang, marjoram, eucalyptus, lavender, clove, clary sage, lemon, wintergreen **Note:** Avoid rosemary, thyme, and possibly peppermint.

Bath 1: Place 3 drops ylang ylang and 3 drops marjoram in bathwater, and bathe in the evening twice a week.

Blend 1: Combine 10 drops ylang ylang, 5 drops marjoram, and 5 drops cypress in 2 Tbs. (25 ml) fractionated coconut oil. Rub over heart and reflex points on left foot and hand.

Blend 2: Combine 5 drops geranium, 8 drops lemongrass, and 3 drops lavender in 2 Tbs. (25 ml) fractionated coconut oil. Rub over heart and reflex points on left foot and hand.

–Low

Oils: rosemary, blue tansy

🌀: Diffuse into the air. Inhale the aroma directly.

⭕: Place 1–2 drops of oil under the tongue or place 1–3 drops of oil in an empty capsule; ingest up to 3 times per day.

💧: Dilute as recommended, and apply on location, on reflex points on feet and hands, and over heart.

—Bleeding (stops):

Oils: helichrysum, geranium, yarrow, rose

💧: Dilute as recommended, and apply on location.

—Broken Blood Vessels

Oils: helichrysum, grapefruit

💧: Dilute as recommended, and apply on location, on reflex points on feet and hands, and over heart.

—Cholesterol:

Cholesterol is a soft, waxy substance found in the bloodstream and in all of the body's cells. The body requires some cholesterol to function properly, but high levels of cholesterol narrow and block the arteries and increase the risk of heart disease.

Oils: helichrysum

💧: Dilute as recommended, and apply on reflex points on feet and hands, and over heart.

—Circulation: *See Cardiovascular System*

—Cleansing

Oils: helichrysum, geranium, Roman chamomile

💧: Dilute as recommended, and apply on reflex points on feet and hands, and over heart.

—Clots:

Blood clots occur as a natural bodily defense to repair damaged blood vessels and to keep the body from losing excessive amounts of blood. However, clotting can become dangerous if an internal blood clot breaks loose in the circulatory system and blocks the flow of blood to vital organs.

Oils: clove, fennel, thyme, grapefruit

⭕: Place 1–2 drops of oil under the tongue or place 1–3 drops of oil in an empty capsule; ingest up to 3 times per day.

💧: Dilute as recommended, and apply on location, on reflex points on feet and hands, and over heart.

🌀: Diffuse into the air. Inhale the aroma directly.

—Hemorrhaging:

Hemorrhaging is excessive or uncontrollable blood loss.

Oils: helichrysum, ylang ylang, rose

💧: Dilute as recommended, and apply on location.

—High Blood Sugar: *See Diabetes*

Primary Recommendations • Secondary Recommendations • Other Recommendations

—Low Blood Sugar:

The term "blood sugar" refers to the amount of glucose in the bloodstream. When the blood glucose drops below its normal level, this is called "low blood sugar" or "hypoglycemia." Since glucose is such an important source of energy for the body, low blood sugar can result in light-headedness, hunger, shakiness, weakness, confusion, nervousness, difficulty speaking, and anxiety.

Oils: ⬡On Guard, ⬡cinnamon, ⬡clove, ⬡thyme

Other Products: ⬤On Guard+ Softgels

⬡: Dilute as recommended, and apply on location, on reflex points on feet and hands, and over heart.

—Stimulates Blood Cell Production

Oils: ⬤⬡peppermint⬡, ⬤⬡lemon

⬤: Place 1–2 drops of oil under the tongue or place 1–3 drops of oil in an empty capsule; ingest up to 3 times per day. Take supplement as directed.

⬡: Dilute as recommended, and apply on location, on reflex points on feet and hands, and over heart.

—Vessels: *See Arteries, Capillaries, Veins*

⬤: **Body System(s) Affected:** Cardiovascular System.

⬤: **Additional Research:**

Ylang ylang: Hongratanaworakit et al., 2006; Hongratanaworakit et al., 2004; **Ylang ylang, lavender, marjoram:** Kim et al., 2012; **Marjoram:** Lahlou et al., 2002; **Eucalyptus:** Lahlou et al., 2002; **Rosemary:** Fernández et al., 2014; **Clove:** Saeed et al., 1994; **Fennel:** Tognolini et al., 2007; **Peppermint:** Samarth et al., 2004.

Body Systems

See Cardiovascular System, Digestive System, Endocrine System, Lymphatic System, Muscles/Connective Tissue, Skeletal System, Nervous System, Respiratory System, Skin

Boils

See also Antibacterial

A boil is a skin infection that forms in a hair follicle or oil gland. The boil starts as a red, tender lump that after a few days forms a white or yellow point in the center as it fills with pus. Boils commonly occur on the face, neck, armpits, buttock, and shoulders and can be very painful.

> *Simple Solutions—Boils:* Add 5 drops melaleuca oil and 2 drops lavender to 2 cups (½ L) clean hot water in a bowl. Soak a clean washcloth with the solution, and use to wash infected area twice a day.

Oils: ⬡melaleuca⬡, ⬡lavender, ⬡Purify, ⬡lemongrass, ⬡lemon, ⬡frankincense, ⬡clary sage

⬡: Dilute as recommended, and apply on location.

⬤: **Body System(s) Affected:** Skin and Immune System.

⬤: **Additional Research:**
Melaleuca: (Feinblatt, 1960).

Bones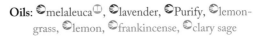

See Skeletal System

Bowel

See Digestive System

Brain

The brain is the central part of the nervous system. It is responsible for processing sensory stimuli and for directing appropriate behavioral responses to each stimulus, or set of stimuli. The brain also stores memories and is the center of thought.

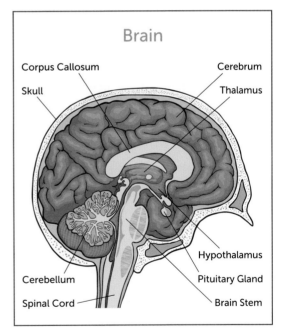

Brain

- Corpus Callosum
- Skull
- Cerebrum
- Thalamus
- Cerebellum
- Spinal Cord
- Hypothalamus
- Pituitary Gland
- Brain Stem

Oils: ⬡lavender⬡, ⬤lemon⬡, ⬡lemongrass, ⬡clary sage, ⬡cypress, ⬡geranium

Other Products: ⬤xEO Mega or vEO Mega or ⬤IQ Mega for omega-3 fatty acids essential for proper

⬡=Topical, ⬡=Aromatic, ⬤=Internal

brain function, **O**Microplex VMz for vitamins and minerals critical for brain health.

⊘: Diffuse into the air. Inhale directly from bottle. Apply oil to hands, tissue, or cotton wick, and inhale.

⊜: Dilute as recommended, and rub onto the brain stem area, back of neck, temples, behind ears down to jaw, or on reflex points on the feet. Apply as a cold compress.

◐: Take capsules as directed on package. Place 1–2 drops of oil under the tongue; or place 1–2 drops of oil in an empty capsule and swallow the capsule.

—Activates Right Brain

Oils: ⊘⊜geranium, ⊘⊜grapefruit, ⊘⊜helichrysum, ⊘⊜wintergreen, ⊘⊜Roman chamomile

⊘: Diffuse into the air. Inhale directly from bottle. Apply oil to hands, tissue, or cotton wick, and inhale.

⊜: Dilute as recommended, and rub onto the brain stem area, or on reflex points on the feet.

—Aging:

Oils: **O**⊜thyme, ⊘⊜frankincense, myrrh, rose

◐: Place 1–2 drops of oil under the tongue or place 1–2 drops of oil in an empty capsule; swallow capsule.

⊜: Dilute as recommended, and rub onto the brain stem area, back of neck, temples, behind ears down to jaw, or on reflex points on the feet.

—Broken Blood Vessels: *See Blood: Broken Blood Vessels*

—Concentration: *See Concentration*

—Concussion:

A concussion is a type of brain injury that causes temporary or permanent impairment in the brain's functioning. Concussions most commonly occur as a result of a blow to the head. Concussion symptoms include headaches, dizziness, blurred vision, vomiting, disorientation, difficulty focusing attention, ringing in the ears, selective memory loss, etc.

Oils: ⊘⊜frankincense, ⊜cypress

⊘: Diffuse into the air. Inhale directly from bottle. Apply oil to hands, tissue, or cotton wick, and inhale.

⊜: Dilute as recommended, and rub onto the brain stem area, back of neck, temples, behind ears down to jaw, or on reflex points on the feet. Apply as a cold compress.

—Injury

Oils: ⊘⊜frankincense, ⊘⊜bergamot, ⊘⊜peppermint, ⊘⊜lemon, ⊘⊜Balance, ⊘⊜lemongrass

⊘: Diffuse into the air. Inhale the aroma of the oil directly.

⊜: Dilute as recommended, and rub onto the brain stem area, back of neck, temples, behind ears down to jaw, or on reflex points on the feet.

—Integration

Oils: ⊘⊜Balance, ⊘⊜Steady, ⊘⊜helichrysum, ⊘⊜geranium, ⊘⊜clary sage, ⊘⊜cypress, ⊘⊜lemongrass

⊘: Diffuse into the air. Inhale the aroma of the oil directly.

⊜: Dilute as recommended, and rub onto the brain stem area, back of neck, temples, behind ears down to jaw, or on reflex points on the feet.

—Learning and Memory: *See Memory*

—Mental Fatigue:

Oils: ⊘⊜frankincense

—Myelin Sheath:

The myelin sheath is an insulating layer of protein and fatty substances that forms around nerves (including those in the brain), increasing the speed of nerve impulses. Damage to the myelin sheath interrupts these nerve impulses and can cause diseases such as multiple sclerosis, peripheral neuropathy, central pontine myelinolysis, and other neurological diseases.

Oils: ⊘⊜peppermint, ⊘⊜frankincense, ⊘⊜lemongrass, ⊘⊜juniper berry, ⊘⊜Balance, ⊜⊜geranium

Other Products: OxEO Mega or vEO Mega or **O**IQ Mega, which contains the omega-3 fatty acid DHA that helps support the myelin sheath

⊘: Diffuse into the air. Inhale directly from bottle. Apply oil to hands, tissue, or cotton wick, and inhale.

⊜: Apply as a cool compress over the brain stem area, back of neck, temples, behind ears down to jaw, or on reflex points on the feet.

—Oxygenate:

Oils: ⊜eucalyptus, ⊜rosemary, ⊘⊜helichrysum, ⊘⊜sandalwood, ⊜marjoram

Recipe 1: Place 3 drops each of helichrysum and sandalwood on the back of the neck, on the temples, and behind the ears down to the jaw once or twice a day.

⊘: Diffuse into the air. Inhale the aroma directly.

⊜: Dilute as recommended, and rub onto the brain stem area, back of neck, temples, behind ears down to jaw, or on reflex points on the feet.

⊕: **Body System(s) Affected:** Nervous System.

—Stroke: *See Stroke*

—Tumor: *See Cancer: Brain*

⊡: **Additional Research:**

Lavender: Fielt et al., 2005; Diego et al., 1998; **Lemon:** Fukumoto et al., 2006; Koo et al., 2002; **Thyme:** Youdim et al., 2000; **Rose:** Awale et al., 2011; **Myrrh:** Xu et al., 2011; **Frankincense:** Moussaieff et al., 2008; **Bergamot:** Amantea et al., 2009; Corasaniti et al., 2007; Kuwahata et al., 2013; **Peppermint:** Koo et al., 2001; **Eucalyptus:** Nasel et al., 1994; **Rosemary:** Nasel et al., 1994; **Marjoram:** Nasel et al., 1994; (-) -Linalool found in basil, bergamot, cinnamon, clary sage, coriander, cypress, eucalyptus, fennel sweet , geranium, ginger, helichrysum, jasmine, lavender, lemon, lemongrass, lime, marjoram, oregano, peppermint, rosemary, tangerine, thyme, wild orange, and ylang ylang essential oils : Batista et al., 2010.

Breast

See also Cancer: Breast. For issues related to lactation and motherhood, see Pregnancy/Motherhood

Oils: ⊜clary sage, ⊜geranium, ⊜lemongrass, ⊜fennel, ⊜cypress, ⊜vetiver

—Enlarge and Firm:

Oils: ⊜clary sage

⊜: Dilute as recommended, and apply on location or on reflex points on feet.

⊕: **Body System(s) Affected:** Endocrine System.

Breathing

See Respiratory System: Breathing

Bronchitis

See also Antibacterial, Antifungal, Antiviral, Congestion, Inflammation, Respiratory System

Bronchitis is the inflammation of the bronchi (the tubes that lead from the trachea to the lungs). Symptoms include coughing, breathlessness, and thick phlegm.

> *Simple Solutions—Bronchitis:* Apply 2 drops of eucalyptus on the chest.

Oils: ⊘⊜eucalyptus⊡, ⊘⊜thyme⊡, ⊘⊜fir, ⊘⊜basil, ⊘⊜Breathe, ⊘⊜Douglas fir, ⊘⊜manuka, ⊘⊜On Guard, ⊘⊜clary sage, ⊘⊜cypress, ⊘⊜cedarwood, ⊘⊜melaleuca, ⊘⊜marjoram, ⊘⊜peppermint, ⊘⊜rosemary, ⊘⊜wintergreen, ⊘⊜myrrh, ⊘⊜clove, ⊘⊜frankincense, ⊘⊜ginger, ⊘⊜lavender, ⊘⊜lemon, ⊘⊜sandalwood, ⊘⊜bergamot

—Chronic

Oils: ⊘⊜eucalyptus, ⊘⊜oregano, ⊘⊜sandalwood

—Children

Oils: ⊘⊜eucalyptus, ⊘⊜melaleuca, ⊘⊜lavender, ⊘⊜Roman chamomile, ⊘⊜rosemary

—Clear Mucus:

Oils: ⊘⊜sandalwood, ⊘⊜thyme, ⊘⊜bergamot, ⊘⊜On Guard

⊘: Diffuse into the air. Inhale directly from bottle. Apply oil to hands, tissue, or cotton wick, and inhale.

⊜: Dilute as recommended, and apply to chest, sinuses, neck, or reflex points on the feet. Add 2–3 drops to water; gargle.

⊕: **Body System(s) Affected:** Respiratory System.

⊡: **Additional Research:**

Eucalyptus: Vigo et al., 2004; Lu et al., 2004; Juergens et al., 1998; Thyme: Vigo et al., 2004.

Bruises

See also Capillaries

A bruise is an injury to tissue that results in blood capillaries breaking and spilling blood into the tissue. This can cause swelling, soreness, and a visible discoloration when the bruise is near the skin.

> *Simple Solutions—Bruises:* Add 5 drops helichrysum to 1 tsp. (5 ml) fractionated coconut oil in a small roll-on bottle, and apply over the bruised area.

Oils: ⊜helichrysum, ⊜geranium, ⊜fennel, ⊜Deep Blue (for pain), ⊜Rescuer, ⊜On Guard, ⊜lavender

⊜: Dilute as recommended, and apply 1–2 drops on location.

⊕: **Body System(s) Affected:** Skin and Cardiovascular System.

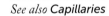

⊜=Topical, ⊘=Aromatic, ○=Internal

Bugs

See *Insects/Bugs*

Bulimia

See *Eating Disorders: Bulimia*

Bunions

See *Bursitis: Bunion*

Burns

A burn is an injury to tissue caused by heat, chemicals, or radiation. The tissue most often affected by burns is the skin. Minor burns can cause redness and pain over a small area and do not break the skin. For minor heat burns, immediately immerse the affected skin in cool water to stop the heat from causing more damage to the tissue. More serious burns that involve areas of the body larger than the palm of the hand or that involve blistering, swelling, intense pain that lasts for more than a day, or visible skin damage should be attended to by a medical professional. Skin damaged by burns is more prone to developing infection as it cannot act as a barrier against invading microorganisms.

> *Simple Solutions—Burns:* For minor burns, gently apply 1–2 drops of lavender oil, and cover with a cloth soaked in cool water. If the burn covers large areas of the body, is blistering, or has visible skin damage, seek immediate medical attention.

Oils: lavender, geranium, melaleuca, peppermint, helichrysum, Roman chamomile

Other Products: Microplex VMz to help replace minerals depleted from the skin and tissues surrounding a burn.

—Infected:

Oils: Purify

—Pain:

Oils: lavender

—Healing:

Oils: lavender

Blend 1: Blend together 1 drop geranium and 1 drop helichrysum; apply on location.

—Peeling:

Oils: lavender

—Sunburn:

> *Simple Solutions—Sunburn:* Mix 10 drops lavender oil with ¼ cup (50 ml) cool water in a small spray bottle. Shake well, and spray on location to help soothe.

Oils: lavender, melaleuca, Roman chamomile, manuka

Recipe 1: Place 10 drops lavender in a 4 oz. misting spray bottle filled with distilled water. Shake well, and spray on location to aid with pain and healing.

—Sun Screen:

Oils: helichrysum

: Dilute as recommended, and apply on location. Add 2–3 drops oil to 2 Tbs. (25 ml) water in a spray bottle; shake well, and mist on location.

: **Body System(s) Affected:** Skin.

Bursitis

Bursitis is the inflammation of the fluid-filled sack located close to joints that provides lubrication for tendons, skin, and ligaments rubbing against the bone. Bursitis is caused by infection, injury, or diseases such as arthritis and gout. Bursitis causes tenderness and pain which can limit movement.

> *Simple Solutions—Bursitis:* Apply 1 drop cypress oil on location. Alternate holding a hot and cold damp rag over the area every 5 minutes for 20 minutes total.

Oils: Balance, fir, basil, cypress, Deep Blue, ginger, Roman chamomile, marjoram, juniper berry, wintergreen

Recipe 1: Apply 1–3 drops each of Balance, fir, and basil on location. Alternate cold and hot packs (10 min. cold and then 15 min. hot) until pain subsides.

Recipe 2: Apply 6 drops marjoram on shoulders and arms, and wait 6 minutes. Then apply 3 drops of wintergreen, and wait 6 minutes. Then apply 3 drops cypress.

—Bunion:

A bunion is bursitis of the big toe. It is often caused by constrictive shoes that force the big toe to point inward and the base of the big toe to jut outward. This misplacement can irritate the bursa at the base of the toe and cause it to become inflamed, causing further irritation.

Oils: ⬒cypress, ⬒juniper berry

⬒: Dilute as recommended, and apply 1–2 drops on location.

✛: **Body System(s) Affected:** Immune and Skeletal Systems and Muscles.

Callouses

*See **Skin: Callouses***

Calming

*See also **Anxiety***

> *Simple Solutions—Calming:* Diffuse Serenity in an aromatherapy diffuser.

> *Simple Solutions—Calming:* Combine 5 drops ylang ylang, 6 drops lavender, and 2 drops Roman chamomile with ¼ cup (50 ml) water in a small spray bottle. Mist into the air to help calm children.

Oils: ⬒⬒lavender⬓, ⬒⬒InTune, ⬒⬒ylang ylang⬓, ⬒⬒melissa⬓, ⬒⬒Serenity, ⬒⬒Calmer, ⬒⬒Thinker, ⬒⬒cedarwood, ⬒⬒yuzu⬓, ⬒⬒blue tansy, ⬒⬒hinoki⬓, ⬒⬒magnolia, ⬒⬒Anchor, ⬒⬒green mandarin, ⬒yarrow, ⬒Citrus Bliss, ⬒⬒myrrh, ⬒⬒juniper berry

—Agitation:

Oils: ⬒⬒lavender⬓, ylang ylang⬓, ⬒⬒geranium⬓, ⬒⬒bergamot, ⬒⬒Serenity, ⬒⬒sandalwood, ⬒⬒cedarwood, ⬒⬒Balance, ⬒⬒marjoram, ⬒⬒myrrh, ⬒⬒clary sage, ⬒⬒rose, ⬒⬒frankincense, ⬒⬒Elevation

—Anger:

Oils: ⬒⬒Serenity, ⬒⬒lavender, ⬒⬒ylang ylang, ⬒⬒Balance, ⬒⬒Elevation, ⬒⬒bergamot, ⬒⬒geranium, ⬒⬒cedarwood, ⬒⬒frankincense, ⬒⬒sandalwood, ⬒⬒cypress, ⬒⬒lemon, ⬒⬒myrrh, ⬒⬒marjoram, ⬒⬒helichrysum, ⬒⬒rose, ⬒⬒orange

—Hyperactivity:

Oils: ⬒⬒InTune, ⬒⬒lavender⬓, ⬒⬒Calmer, ⬒⬒Serenity, ⬒⬒Balance, ⬒⬒Thinker, ⬒⬒Roman chamomile, ⬒Citrus Bliss

—Sedative:

Oils: ⬒⬒lavender⬓, ⬒⬒Serenity, ⬒⬒Calmer, ⬒Citrus Bliss, ⬒⬒bergamot⬓, ⬒⬒ylang ylang⬓, ⬒⬒cedarwood, ⬒⬒geranium, ⬒⬒vetiver, ⬒⬒juniper berry, ⬒⬒frankincense, ⬒⬒sandalwood, ⬒⬒orange, ⬒⬒rose, ⬒⬒lemongrass, ⬒⬒clary sage, ⬒⬒marjoram

⬒: Diffuse into the air. Inhale directly from bottle. Apply oil to hands, tissue, or cotton wick, and inhale.

⬒: Dilute as recommended, and apply 1–2 drops to back of neck, temples, chest, shoulders, back, or reflex points on the feet. Place 1–2 drops in 1 Tbs. (15 ml) fractionated coconut oil, and massage into the back, shoulders, neck, or arms.

✛: **Body System(s) Affected:** Emotional Balance.

⬚: **Additional Research:**

Lavender: Huang et al., 2008; Lin et al., 2007; Lehrner et al., 2000; Buchbauer et al., 1991; Guillemain et al., 1989; Brum et al., 2001; **Ylang ylang:** Moss et al., 2008; Hongratanaworakit et al., 2006; Watanabe et al., 2013; **Melissa:** Ballard et al., 2002; **Geranium:** Umezo et al., 2008; **Yuzu:** Matsumoto et al., 2016; Matsumoto et al., 2017; **Hinoki:** Chen et al., 2015; **Bergamot:** Peng et al., 2009.

Cancer

Cancer can be any of many different conditions where the body's cells duplicate and grow uncontrollably, invade healthy tissues, and possibly spread throughout the body. It is estimated that 95% of cancers result from damage to DNA during a person's lifetime rather than from a pre-existing genetic condition (American Cancer Society, 2008). The most important factor leading to this DNA damage is DNA mutation. DNA mutation can be caused by radiation, environmental chemicals we take into our bodies, free radical damage, or DNA copying or division errors. If the body is working properly, it can correct these mutations either by repairing the DNA or by causing the mutated cell to die. When the DNA mutation is severe enough that it allows the cell to bypass these controls, however, the mutated DNA can be copied to new cells that continue to replicate and create more and more new cells uncontrollably, leading to a cancerous growth within an individual.

Oils: ⬒⬒⬒frankincense⬓, ⬒⬒⬒sandalwood⬓, ⬒⬒lavender⬓, ⬒DDR Prime, ⬒⬒arborvitae⬓, ⬒⬒Yarrow Pom, ⬒⬒⬒rosemary⬓, ⬒⬒⬒lemongrass⬓, ⬒⬒⬒clove⬓, ⬒⬒basil⬓, ⬒⬒⬒geranium⬓, ⬒⬒⬒clary sage⬓, ⬒citrus oils⬓, ⬒rose

⬒=Topical, ⬒=Aromatic, ⬒=Internal

Other Products: ⚪Alpha CRS+ contains multiple nutrients that have been studied for their abilities to combat different types of cancer, including polyphenols (such as resveratrol⚪, baicalin⚪, EGCG⚪, quercetin⚪, ellagic acid⚪, and catechin⚪) and coenzyme Q10. ⚪xEO Mega or vEO Mega or ⚪IQ Mega and ⚪Microplex VMz to help support cellular and immune function.

Note: Healthcare professionals are emphatic about avoiding heavy massage when working with cancer patients. Light massage may be used—but never over the trauma area.

—Bone:

Oils: 🌿frankincense

—Brain:

Oils: 🌿frankincense⚪, 🌿myrrh⚪, 🌿clove

Recipe 1: Combine 15 drops frankincense, 6 drops clove, and 1 Tbs. (15 ml) fractionated coconut oil. Massage lightly on spine every day. Diffuse 15 drops frankincense and 6 drops clove for 30 minutes, three times a day.

Recipe 2: Diffuse frankincense, and massage the brain stem area lightly with frankincense neat.

—Breast:

Oils: 🌿rosemary⚪, 🌿lavender⚪, 🌿frankincense⚪, 🌿arborvitae⚪, ⚪Yarrow Pom, 🌿clary sage⚪, 🌿clove, 🌿basil⚪, 🌿sandalwood, 🌿oregano, 🌿lemongrass, 🌿marjoram

—Cervical:

Oils: 🌿frankincense, 🌿geranium, 🌿fir, 🌿cypress, 🌿clove, 🌿lavender, 🌿lemon

—Colon:

Oils: ⚪🌿lavender⚪, 🌿geranium⚪, 🌿frankincense, 🌿arborvitae⚪, 🌿lemongrass⚪

—Leukemia:

Oils: 🌿frankincense⚪, 🌿lemongrass⚪, 🌿rosemary⚪, 🌿clary sage⚪, 🌿clove⚪

—Liver:

Oils: 🌿frankincense⚪, 🌿lemongrass⚪, 🌿lavender⚪, 🌿rosemary⚪

—Lung:

Oils: 🌿frankincense⚪ (apply to chest, or mix 15 drops with 1 tsp. (5 ml) fractionated coconut oil for nightly rectal retention enema), 🌿lavender⚪

—Prostate

Oils: 🌿frankincense (blend 15 drops with 1 tsp. (5 ml) fractionated coconut oil for nightly rectal retention enema), 🌿arborvitae⚪, ⚪Yarrow Pom

—Skin/Melanoma:

Oils: 🌿⚪Hawaiian sandalwood⚪, 🌿arborvitae⚪, 🌿frankincense, ⚪citrus oils⚪

—Throat:

Oils: 🌿frankincense, 🌿lavender

—Uterine:

Oils: 🌿geranium, 🌿frankincense

🌿: Dilute as recommended, and apply 1–5 drops on location and on reflex points on the feet and hands. Apply as a warm compress over affected area.

🌀: Diffuse into the air. Inhale oil directly or applied to hands, tissue, or a cotton wick.

⚪: Take capsules as recommended on package. Place 1–2 drops of oil under the tongue or add 1–3 drops of oil in an empty capsule; swallow capsule. Repeat up to twice daily as needed.

⊕: **Body System(s) Affected:** Immune System.

⚪: **Additional Research:**

Frankincense: Hunan et al., 1999; Bhushan et al., 2007; Zou et al, 2013; Dai et al, 2013; Zhang et al., 2013; Ding et al., 2013; Li et al, 2013; Li et al., 2013; Chen et al., 2012; Li et al., 2013; Hostanska et al., 2002; Li et al., 2013; Yu et al., 2011; Dai et al., 2013; Chen et al., 2012; Zhang et al., 2013; **Sandalwood:** Banerjee et al., 1993; Kaur et al., 2005; Dwivedi et al., 2006; Dwivedi et al., 2005; Dwivedi et al., 2003; Dwivedi et al., 1997; Arasada et al., 2008; Santha et al., 2015; **Lavender:** Evandri et al., 2005; Katdare et al., 1997; Reddy et al., 1997; Lantry et al., 1997; Mills et al., 1995; **Arborvitae:** Wang et al., 2014; Lee et al., 2013; Liu et al., 2009; **Rosemary:** Singletary et al., 1996; Cheung et al., 2007; Steiner et al., 2001; Debersac et al., 2001; **Lemongrass:** Dudai et al., 2005; Sharma et al., 2009; Carnesecchi et al., 2001; Kumar et al., 2008; Puatanachokchai et al., 2002; **Clove:** Legault et al., 2007; **Clary Sage:** Noori et al., 2013; **Basil:** Al-Ali et al., 2013; Berić et al., 2008; **Geranium:** Carnesecchi et al., 2001; **Clary Sage:** Dimas et al., 1999; **Clove:** Yoo et al., 2005; **Citrus oils:** Hakim et al., 2000; **Resveratrol:** Jang et al., 1997; Lee et al., 2008; Schlachterman et al., 2008; **Baicalin:** Zhou et al., 2008; Franek et al., 2005; Miocinovic et al., 2005; **EGCG:** Hazgui et al., 2008; Shankar et al., 2008; **Quercetin:** Schlachterman et al., 2008; Paliwal et al., 2005; Aalinkeel et al., 2008; Bobe et al., 2008; Nothlings et al., 2007; Cui et al., 2008; **Ellagic acid:** Mandal et al., 1990; **Catechin:** Schlachterman et al., 2008; Bobe et al., 2008; Nothlings et al., 2007; Cui et al., 2008; **Myrrh:** Tan et al., 2000; **Geranium:** Carnesecchi et al., 2001; **Hawaiian Sandalwood:** Kaur et al., 2005; Dwivedi et al., 2006; Dwivedi et al., 2005; Dwivedi et al., 2003; Dwivedi et al., 1997; Arasada et al., 2008.

Primary Recommendations • Secondary Recommendations • Other Recommendations

Candida

See Antifungal: Candida

Canker Sores

Canker sores are small, round sores that develop in the mouth, typically inside the lips and cheeks or on the tongue.

> *Simple Solutions—Canker Sores:* Combine 1 drop melaleuca with ½ tsp. (2.5 ml) olive oil 1 tsp. (5 g) baking soda. Apply a small amount on location.

Oils: melaleuca, oregano, On Guard, Roman chamomile, myrrh

🜨: Dilute as recommended, and apply 1 drop on location.

✚: **Body System(s) Affected:** Skin.

Capillaries

Capillaries are the small, thin blood vessels that allow the exchange of oxygen and other nutrients from the blood to cells throughout the body and allow the exchange of carbon dioxide and other waste materials from these tissues back to the blood. The capillaries connect the arteries (that carry blood away from the heart) and veins (that carry blood back to the heart).

—Broken Capillaries:

Oils: geranium, cypress, oregano, thyme, Roman chamomile

Blend 1: Apply 1 drop lavender and 1 drop Roman chamomile on location.

🜨: Dilute as recommended, and apply 1–2 drops on location.

✚: **Body System(s) Affected:** Cardiovascular System.

Carbuncles

See Boils

Cardiovascular System

The cardiovascular (or circulatory) system is the system responsible for transporting blood to the various tissues throughout the body. It is comprised of the heart and blood vessels such as arteries, veins, and capillaries.

Oils: orange, cypress, cinnamon, copaiba, sandalwood, thyme, neroli

Other Products: O Alpha CRS+ and O a2z Chewable contain several polyphenols (including proanthocyanidin polyphenols from grape seed, the polyphenols EGCG, and ellagic acid) and coenzyme Q10, which have been found to have beneficial cardiovascular effects.

🜨: Dilute oils as recommended, and apply oils to carotid arteries, heart, feet, under left ring finger, above elbow, behind ring toe on left foot, and to reflex points on the feet. Add 1–2 drops to bathwater for a bath. Add 1–2 drops to 1 Tbs. (15 ml) fractionated coconut oil for massage oil, and massage on location or on chest, neck, or feet.

🜁: Diffuse into the air. Inhale oil applied to hands, tissue, or cotton wick.

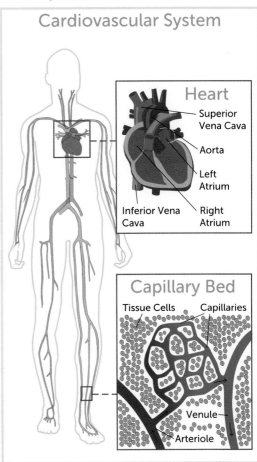

Cardiovascular System

Heart
- Superior Vena Cava
- Aorta
- Left Atrium
- Inferior Vena Cava
- Right Atrium

Capillary Bed
- Tissue Cells
- Capillaries
- Venule
- Arteriole

🜨=Topical, 🜁=Aromatic, O=Internal

—**Angina:**

Angina is pain in the chest due to a lack of blood flow to the heart. Angina is felt as a squeezing, tightening, aching, or pressure in the chest. The pain can also extend to the arms, back, jaw, neck, and teeth.

Oils: ⊛ginger, ⊛orange (for false angina)

⊙: Massage gently onto chest and feet, and apply on carotid artery.

⊘: Diffuse into the air.

—**Arrhythmia:**

Arrhythmia is any abnormal heart rhythm. *See also Palpitations and Tachycardia below.*

Oils: ⊛ylang ylang⊙, ⊛lavender, ⊛Deep Blue, ⊛neroli

⊘: Diffuse into the air. Inhale the aroma.

⊙: Dilute oils as recommended, and apply oils to carotid arteries, heart, feet, under left ring finger, above elbow, behind ring toe on left foot, and to reflex points on the feet.

—**Atherosclerosis:**

Atherosclerosis is a hardening of the arteries due to a buildup of plaques (called atheromas) along the arterial wall.

Oils: ○⊛lemon⊙, ⊛lavender⊙, ○⊛melissa⊙, ○⊛dill⊙, ○DDR Prime, ⊛rosemary, ⊛ginger, ⊛thyme, ⊛wintergreen

⊘: Diffuse into the air.

◐: Take 1–2 drops under the tongue or in a capsule or with water.

⊙: Massage gently onto chest and feet, and apply on carotid artery.

—**Blood Pressure:** *See Blood: Blood Pressure*

—**Cardiotonic:**

Oils: ⊛lavender, ⊛thyme

⊙: Dilute oils as recommended, and apply oils to carotid arteries, heart, feet, under left ring finger, above elbow, behind ring toe on left foot, and to reflex points on the feet.

⊘: Diffuse into the air. Inhale the aroma.

—**Circulation:**

Oils: ⊛cypress, ⊛copaiba, ⊛thyme, ⊛peppermint, ⊛clary sage, ⊛wintergreen, ⊛Citrus Bliss, ⊛rosemary, ⊛geranium, ⊛cinnamon, ⊛helichrysum, ⊛neroli, ⊛Serenity, ⊛basil

⊙: Add 1–2 drops to 1 Tbs. (15 ml) fractionated coconut oil for massage oil, and massage on location or on chest, neck, or feet.

⊘: Diffuse into the air. Inhale the aroma.

—**Heart:**

Oils: ⊛ylang ylang, ⊛marjoram ⊛geranium, ⊛cypress, ⊛Balance, ⊛ginger, ⊛lavender, ⊛rosemary, ⊛Deep Blue

⊙: Dilute oils as recommended, and apply oils to carotid arteries, heart, feet, under left ring finger, above elbow, behind ring toe on left foot, and to reflex points on the feet.

⊘: Diffuse into the air. Inhale the aroma.

—**Heart Tissue**

Oils: ⊛marjoram, ⊛lavender, ⊛peppermint, ⊛rosemary, ⊛cinnamon, ⊛rose

⊙: Dilute oils as recommended, and apply oils to carotid arteries, heart, feet, under left ring finger, above elbow, behind ring toe on left foot, and to reflex points on the feet.

⊘: Diffuse into the air. Inhale the aroma.

—**High Cholesterol:** *See Cholesterol*

—**Hypertension:** *See Blood: Blood Pressure*

—**Palpitations:**

Palpitations are rapid and forceful contractions of the heart.

Oils: ⊛ylang ylang, ⊛orange, ⊛lavender, ⊛melissa, ⊛peppermint

⊙: Dilute oils as recommended, and apply oils to carotid arteries, heart, feet, under left ring finger, above elbow, behind ring toe on left foot, and to reflex points on the feet.

⊘: Diffuse into the air. Inhale the aroma.

—**Phlebitis:**

Phlebitis is the inflammation of a superficial vein, typically in the legs or groin area. Wearing support hose or a compression bandage over the affected area can help aid in healing.

Oils: ⊛helichrysum, ⊛lavender, ⊛cypress, ⊛geranium, ⊛grapefruit, ⊛Balance

: Add 1–2 drops to 1 Tbs. (15 ml) fractionated coconut oil for massage oil, and gently massage on location or on feet.

: Diffuse into the air. Inhale the aroma.

—Prolapsed Mitral Valve:

Oils: marjoram

: Dilute oils as recommended, and apply oils to carotid arteries, heart, feet, under left ring finger, above elbow, behind ring toe on left foot, and to reflex points on the feet.

: Diffuse into the air. Inhale the aroma.

—Tachycardia:

Tachycardia is an abnormally rapid resting heart rate, indicating a possible over-working of the heart.

Oils: lavender, ylang ylang, orange, spikenard, neroli

: Dilute oils as recommended, and apply oils to carotid arteries, heart, feet, under left ring finger, above elbow, behind ring toe on left foot, and to reflex points on the feet.

: Diffuse into the air. Inhale the aroma.

: **Body System(s) Affected:** Cardiovascular System.

: **Additional Research:**

Thyme: Youdim et al., 1999; **Grape seed:** Bagchi et al., 2003; **EGCG:** Basu et al., 2007; Brown et al., 2008; Devika et al., 2008; **Ellagic acid:** Anderson et al., 2001; Chang et al., 2008; Yu et al., 2005; **Coenzyme Q10:** Tiano et al., 2007; Belardinelli et al., 2006; Kuettner et al., 2005; Belardinelli et al., 2005; **Ylang ylang:** Hongratanaworakit et al., 2004; **Lemon:** Grassmann et al., 2001; **Lavender:** Nikolaevski et al., 1990; **Melissa:** Jun et al., 2012; **Dill:** Bahramikia et al., 2009; **Basil:** Fathiazad et al., 2012.

Carpal Tunnel Syndrome

Carpal tunnel syndrome is a painful condition of the hand, wrist, and fingers. This condition is caused by inflamed carpal ligaments in the wrist causing pressure on the median nerve. The carpal ligaments can become inflamed due to one of many possible factors: wrist trauma or injury, fluid retention, work stress, or certain strenuous wrist activities. Symptoms include tingling or numbness of the fingers and hand, pain starting in the wrist and extending to the arm or shoulder or to the palms or fingers, a general sense of weakness, and difficulty grasping small objects.

Simple Solutions—CTS: Blend 3 drops basil, 3 drops marjoram, 2 drops lemongrass, and 2 drops cypress with 1 Tbs. (15 ml) fractionated coconut oil. Massage a small amount gently into the arm from the shoulder to the fingertips.

Oils: frankincense, basil, marjoram, lemongrass, oregano, cypress, eucalyptus, lavender

Recipe 1: Apply 1 drop basil and 1 drop marjoram on the shoulder, and massage oils into the skin. Then apply 1 drop lemongrass on the wrist and 1 drop oregano on the rotator cuff in the shoulder, and massage into the skin. Next apply 1 drop marjoram and 1 drop cypress on the wrists and 1 drop cypress on the neck down to the shoulder, and massage into the skin. Lastly, apply peppermint from the shoulder down the arm to the wrist and then out to the tips of each finger, and massage into the skin.

: Dilute oils as recommended, and apply oils on area of concern. Add 1–2 drops to 1 Tbs. (15 ml) fractionated coconut oil for massage oil, and massage on location.

: **Body System(s) Affected:** Immune and Skeletal Systems.

Cartilage

See Skeletal System: Cartilage, Muscles/Connective Tissue: Cartilage Injury

Cataracts

See Eyes: Cataracts

Catarrh

See Congestion: Catarrh

Cavities

See Oral Conditions: Cavities

Cells

Oils: DDR Prime, Yarrow Pom

Other Products: Alpha CRS+, Microplex VMz and a2z Chewable for antioxidant support to help protect cells and DNA and for necessary nutrients, Mito2Max for cellular energy support,

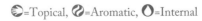 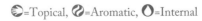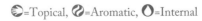

and ^{O}xEO Mega or vEO Mega or ^{O}IQ Mega for omega-3 fatty acids necessary for cellular health

—DNA & Mutation:

DNA is the genetic material of the cell. DNA contains all of the codes that enable the cell to build the materials needed for proper structure and function. Mutation of DNA can lead to cell death or to cancer.

—Antimutagenic Oils:

Oils: 🌿🍃peppermint🌼, 🌿🍃lavender🌼, 🌿🍃rosemary🌼, 🌿🍃basil🌼, 🌿🍃fennel🌼

○: Take 3–5 drops in an empty capsule, or with food and beverage. Take up to twice per day as needed.

🥄: Dilute oils as recommended, and apply oils on area of concern. Add 1–2 drops to 1 Tbs. (15 ml) fractionated coconut oil for massage oil, and massage on location.

🌀: Diffuse into the air. Inhale oil applied to hands, tissue, or cotton wick.

📖: **Additional Research:**

Peppermint: Romero-Jiménez et al., 2005; **Lavender:** Evandri et al., 2005; **Rosemary:** Slamenova et al., 2002; **Basil:** Berić et al., 2008; **Fennel:** Tripathi et al., 2013.

Cellulite

See also **Weight**

Cellulite refers to deposits of fat under the skin of the thighs, abdomen, and buttocks that cause the skin to appear dimpled.

> *Simple Solutions—Cellulite:* Combine 5 drops grapefruit with 1 tsp. (5 ml) jojoba oil in a small roll-on container, and apply on location.

Oils: ○🍃Slim & Sassy, 🍃grapefruit, 🍃rosemary, 🍃basil, 🍃orange, 🍃lemon, 🍃lime, 🍃cypress, 🍃juniper berry, 🍃lavender, 🍃oregano, 🍃fennel, 🍃geranium

Recipe 1: Add 5 drops grapefruit and 5 drops lemon to 1 gallon (4 L) drinking water. Adjust to taste, and drink throughout the day.

○: Add 8 drops of Slim & Sassy to 2 cups (½ L) of water, and drink throughout the day between meals.

🥄: Dilute as recommended, and apply 1–2 drops on location. Add 1–2 drops to 1 Tbs. (15 ml) fractionated coconut oil, and massage on location.

🧬: **Body System(s) Affected:** Skin and Digestive System.

Charley Horse

See **Muscles/Connective Tissue: Cramps/Charley Horses**

Chemicals

See **Detoxification**

Chilblains

See also **Inflammation, Lupus**

Chilblains are inflammatory swelling, itching, redness, or blisters that appear on hands and feet from exposure to cold. They usually appear seasonally with cold weather and clear up in 1–3 weeks, especially if the weather gets warmer. Chilblains may also be associated with other conditions, such as lupus.

> *Simple Solutions—Chilblains:* Combine 3 drops frankincense and 2 drops cypress with 1/2 cup (250 g) Epsom salt, and dissolve in warm (not hot) bathwater. Soak the affected area for 20–30 minutes.

Oils: 🍃frankincense, 🍃myrrh, 🍃Deep Blue, 🍃lavender, 🍃eucalyptus, 🍃cypress, 🍃rosemary, 🍃copaiba

🥄: Dilute as recommended, and apply 1–2 drops on location. Add 1–2 drops to 1 tsp. (5 ml) fractionated coconut oil in a roll-on vial, and apply on location.

🧬: **Body System(s) Affected:** Skin, Muscles and Bones.

Childbirth

See **Pregnancy/Motherhood**

Childhood Diseases

See also **Antiviral, Antibacterial**

—Chicken Pox: *See also* **Shingles**

Chicken pox is a common childhood illness caused by the virus varicella zoster. Symptoms of chicken pox include mild fever, weakness, and a rash. The rash appears as red spots that form into blisters that eventually burst and then crust over. Chicken pox can occur between 10 and 21 days

---

after contact with the virus and is contagious up to 5 days before and 5 days after the rash appears. Chicken pox is highly contagious and can be contracted by anyone, but it is most common in children under the age of 15.

> *Simple Solutions—Chicken Pox:* Combine 10 drops lavender and 10 drops Roman chamomile with ½ cup (125 ml) calamine lotion. Mix and apply a small amount twice a day over affected areas.

Oils: ◐lavender, ◐◉melaleuca, ◐Roman chamomile, ◐eucalyptus, ◉lemon, ◉bergamot

Recipe 1: Add 2 drops lavender to 1 cup (200 g) baking soda. Dissolve in warm bathwater, and bathe to help relieve itching.

—Measles:

Measles is a viral infection of the respiratory system that causes coughing, runny nose, red eyes, fever, and a rash on the skin.

> *Simple Solutions—Measles:* Diffuse eucalyptus radiata in an aromatherapy diffuser.

Oils: ◉◐eucalyptus○, ◉◐melaleuca, ◉◐lavender

—Mumps:

Mumps is a viral infection that causes fever, chills, headache, and painful swelling of the saliva glands.

> *Simple Solutions—Mumps:* Apply 1 drop melaleuca on swollen glands once a day.

Oils: ◐◉melaleuca, ◐lavender, ◉lemon

—Rubella (German Measles):

Rubella, or German measles, is a viral infection that causes rash, fever, runny nose, and joint pain.

Oils: ◐melaleuca, ◐lavender

—Whooping Cough:

Whooping cough, or pertussis, is a bacterial infection that causes cold-like symptoms, followed by severe coughing fits.

> *Simple Solutions—Whooping Cough:* Mix 2 drops each of cinnamon, hyssop, and thyme, and place in a water-misting aromatherapy diffuser. Run once or twice a day for 15 minutes. Use only 1 drop of each for very young children.

Oils: ◐oregano, ◐◉basil, ◐◉thyme, ◐clary sage, ◐cypress, ◐lavender, ◐Roman chamomile, ◐grapefruit, ◉eucalyptus, ◉melaleuca, ◉peppermint, ◉rose

◓: Dilute as recommended, and apply on location or on chest, neck, back, or reflex points on the feet. Add 1–2 drops to 4 cups (1 L) warm water, and use water for a sponge bath.

◐: Diffuse into the air. Diffuse other antiviral oils such as lemon as well. *See Antiviral.*

◓: **Body System(s) Affected:** Immune System.

Children and Infants

When using essential oils on children and infants, it is always best to dilute the pure essential oil with a carrier oil. For older children, dilute 1–2 drops essential oil in ½–1 tsp. (2–5 ml) of carrier oil. For newborns and infants, dilute 1–2 drops in 2 Tbs. (25 ml) of carrier oil. If the oils are used in a bath, always use a bath gel base as a dispersing agent for the essential oils.

Keep the oils out of children's reach. If an oil is ever ingested, give the child an oil-soluble liquid such as milk, cream, or half-and-half. Then call your local poison control center, or seek emergency medical attention. A few drops of pure essential oil shouldn't be life-threatening, but it is best to take these precautions.

Several oils that are generally considered safe for children include cypress, frankincense, geranium, ginger, lavender, lemon☀, marjoram, melaleuca, orange☀, rosemary▽, sandalwood, thyme, and ylang ylang.

☀: These oils are photosensitive; always dilute, and do not use when skin will be exposed soon to direct sunlight.

▽: This oil should never be used undiluted on infants or children.

Oils: ◐◉Brave, ◐◉Calmer, ◐◉Rescuer, ◐◉Steady, ◐◉Stronger, ◐◉Thinker

Other Products: ◐Baby Hair and Body Wash, ◐Baby Lotion, ◐Diaper Rash Cream

—Colic:

Colic is any extended period of crying and fussiness that occurs frequently in an infant. While the exact cause is not known, it has been speculated that the cause may be from indigestion, the buildup of gas, lactose intolerance, or a lack of needed probiotic bacteria in the intestines.

◐=Topical, ◉=Aromatic, ○=Internal

Simple Solutions—Colic: Blend 1 drop each of Roman chamomile, lavender, and geranium with 2 Tbs. (25 ml) almond oil. Apply a small amount on the stomach and back.

Oils: fennel, star anise, marjoram, bergamot, ylang ylang, ginger, Roman chamomile, rosemary, melissa

: Dilute 1–2 drops of oil in 2 Tbs. (25 ml) fractionated coconut oil, and massage a small amount of this blend gently on stomach and back.

—Common Cold: *See Antiviral*

A cold is a viral infection that causes a stuffy or runny nose, congestion, cough, and sneezing.

Simple Solutions—Colds: Diffuse thyme oil using an aromatherapy diffuser.

Oils: thyme, lemon, cedarwood, Stronger, sandalwood, rosemary, rose

: Dilute 1–2 drops of oil in 2 Tbs. (25 ml) fractionated coconut oil, and massage a little on neck and chest.

: Diffuse into the air.

—Constipation:

Constipation is when feces becomes too hard and dry to expel easily from the body.

Oils: rosemary, ginger, orange

: Dilute 1–2 drops of oil in 2 Tbs. (25 ml) fractionated coconut oil, and massage on stomach and feet.

—Cradle Cap:

Cradle cap is a scaling of the skin on the head that commonly occurs in young infants. The scaling is yellowish in color and often disappears by the time the infant is a few months old.

Simple Solutions—Cradle Cap: Blend 2 drops geranium with 2 Tbs. (25 ml) olive oil. Apply a small amount on the head no more than once per day as needed.

Recipe 1: Combine 2 Tbs. (25 ml) almond oil with 1 drop lemon and 1 drop geranium. Apply a small amount of this blend on the head.

—Croup:

Croup is a viral respiratory infection that causes inflammation of the area around the larynx (voice box) and a distinctive-sounding cough. Often,

taking an infant or child outside to breathe cool night air can help open the restricted airways, as can humidity.

Oils: marjoram, thyme, Stronger, sandalwood

: Diffuse into the air.

: Dilute 1–2 drops in 2 Tbs. (25 ml) fractionated coconut oil, and massage on chest and neck.

—Crying:

Oils: ylang ylang, lavender, Roman chamomile, Brave, Calmer, geranium, cypress, frankincense

: Diffuse into the air.

: Dilute 1–2 drops in 2 Tbs. (25 ml) fractionated coconut oil. Massage.

—Diaper Rash:

Diaper rash is a red rash of the skin in the diaper area caused by prolonged skin exposure to the moisture and different pH of urine and feces. Often, more frequent bathing of the area and diaper changes will help alleviate the rash.

Simple Solutions—Diaper Rash: Blend 1 drop Roman chamomile, 1 drop lavender, and 1 tsp. (5 ml) fractionated coconut oil in a small roll-on bottle. Apply on location.

Oils: lavender

Other Products: Diaper Rash Cream

Blend 2: Combine 1 drop Roman chamomile and 1 drop lavender with 1 tsp. (5 ml) fractionated coconut oil, and apply on location.

: Dilute 1–2 drops in 2 Tbs. (25 ml) fractionated coconut oil, and apply a small amount of this mixture on location.

—Digestion (sluggish):

Oils: lemon, orange

: Dilute 1–2 drops in 2 Tbs. (25 ml) fractionated coconut oil, and massage a small amount on feet and stomach.

—Dry Skin:

Oils: sandalwood

Other Products: Baby Hair and Body Wash, Baby Lotion

🜄: Dilute 1–2 drops in 2 Tbs. (25 ml) fractionated coconut oil, and apply a small amount on location.

—Earache:

Oils: 🜄melaleuca, 🜄🜁Stronger, 🜄Roman chamomile, 🜄lavender, 🜄thyme

Blend 3: Combine 2 Tbs. (25 ml) fractionated coconut oil with 2 drops lavender, 1 drop Roman chamomile, and 1 drop melaleuca. Put a drop on a cotton ball or cotton swab, and apply in ear, behind the ear, and on reflex points on the feet.

🜄: Dilute 1–2 drops in 2 Tbs. (25 ml) fractionated coconut oil, and apply a small amount behind the ear. Place a drop on a cotton ball, and place in the ear.

—Fever:

Oils: 🜄lavender, 🜁peppermint, 🜄🜁Stronger

🜄: Dilute 1–2 drops in 2 Tbs. (25 ml) fractionated coconut oil, and massage a small amount on the neck, feet, behind ears, and on back.

🜁: Diffuse into the air.

—Flu:

Flu, or influenza, is a viral infection that affects the respiratory system. Symptoms may include coughing, sneezing, fever, runny nose, congestion, muscle aches, nausea, and vomiting.

Oils: 🜄🜁cypress, 🜄🜁lemon, 🜄🜁Stronger

🜄: Dilute 1 drop oil in an unscented bath gel, and use for a bath.

🜁: Diffuse into the air.

—Hyperactive: *See Calming, ADD/ADHD*

—Jaundice:

Jaundice is a condition where the liver cannot clear the pigment bilirubin quickly enough from the blood, causing the blood to deposit the bilirubin into the skin and whites of the eyes, turning them a yellowish color.

Oils: 🜄geranium, 🜄lemon, 🜄rosemary

🜄: Dilute 1–2 drops in 2 Tbs. (25 ml) fractionated coconut oil, and massage a small amount on the liver area and on the reflex points on the feet.

—Premature:

Since premature babies have very thin and sensitive skin, it is best to avoid the use of essential oils.

—Rashes:

Oils: 🜄lavender, 🜄Roman chamomile, 🜄sandalwood

Other Products: 🜄Baby Lotion

🜄: Dilute 1–2 drops in 2 Tbs. (25 ml) fractionated coconut oil, and apply a small amount on location.

—Teeth Grinding:

Oils: 🜄lavender, 🜄🜁Calmer, 🜄🜁Serenity

🜄: Dilute 1–2 drops in 2 Tbs. (25 ml) fractionated coconut oil, and massage a small amount on the feet.

🜁: Diffuse into the air.

—Tonsillitis:

Tonsillitis is inflammation of the tonsils, two lymph-filled tissues located at the back of the mouth that help provide immune support. These may become inflamed due to a bacterial or viral infection.

Oils: 🜄melaleuca, 🜄lemon, 🜄🜁Stronger, 🜄Roman chamomile, 🜄lavender, 🜄ginger

🜄: Dilute 1–2 drops in 2 Tbs. (25 ml) fractionated coconut oil, and apply a small amount to tonsils and lymph nodes.

—Thrush: *See also Antifungal*

Thrush is an oral fungal infection caused by *Candida albicans*. It causes painful white-colored areas to appear in the mouth.

Oils: 🜄melaleuca⬭, 🜄🜁Stronger, 🜄lavender⬭, 🜄thyme⬭, 🜄lemon, 🜄geranium

🜄: Dilute 1–2 drops in 2 Tbs. (25 ml) fractionated coconut oil, and apply a small amount on location.

⬭: **Additional Research:**

Fennel: Alexandrovich et al., 2003; **Fennel and melissa:** Savino et al., 2005; **Rosemary:** Kim et al., 2005; **Melaleuca:** Bagg et al., 2006; Banes-Marshall et al., 2001; **Lavender:** D'Auria et al., 2005; **Thyme:** Pina-Vaz et al., 2004.

Chills

See Fever, Warming Oils

Cholera

Cholera is a potentially severe bacterial infection of the intestines by the *Vibrio cholerae* bacteria. This infection can cause severe diarrhea, leading to dehydration that can cause low blood pressure, shock, or death. Rehydration with an oral rehydration solution is the most

🜄=Topical, 🜁=Aromatic, ⬭=Internal

effective way to prevent dehydration. If no commercially prepared oral rehydration solution is available, a solution made from 1 tsp. (5 g) salt, 8 tsp. (35 g) sugar, and 4 cups (1 L) clean water (with some mashed fresh banana, if available, to add potassium) can work in an emergency.

> *Simple Solutions—Cholera:* Add 1 drop rosemary to 1 tsp. (5 ml) fractionated coconut oil, and apply on the stomach twice a day.

Oils: ⊘rosemary, ⊘clove

⊜: Dilute as recommended, and apply to stomach and on reflex points on the feet.

⊕: **Body System(s) Affected:** Immune System and Digestive System.

Cholesterol

Cholesterol is an important lipid that comprises part of the cell membrane and myelin sheath and that plays a role in nerve cell function. It is created by the body and can be found in many foods we eat. An imbalance of certain types of cholesterol in the blood has been theorized to play a role in the formation of plaques in the arteries (atherosclerosis).

> *Simple Solutions—Cholesterol:* Add 5 drops lemongrass and 5 drops dill to 2 Tbs. (25 ml) olive oil in a small dropper bottle. Massage over stomach and bottoms of feet daily. Add a small amount of this blend to a capsule, and swallow.

Oils: ○lemongrass▢, ⊘clary sage, ⊘helichrysum, ○⊜dill▢, ⊘lavender▢, ○⊜juniper berry▢

⊜: Dilute as recommended, and apply to liver area and reflex points on the feet.

○: Place 1–2 drops in a capsule, and swallow.

⊘: Diffuse into the air.

⊕: **Body System(s) Affected:** Cardiovascular System.

▢: **Additional Research:**

> Lemongrass: Elson et al., 1989; **Dill:** Bahramikia et al., 2009; **Lavender:** Nikolaevski et al., 1990; **Juniper Berry:** Gumral et al., 2013; **Camphene found in coriander, frankincense, ginger, lavender, lime, peppermint, roman chamomile, rose, rosemary, spearmint, fir :** Vallianou et al., 2011.

Chronic Fatigue

Chronic fatigue syndrome refers to a set of debilitating symptoms that may include prolonged periods of

fatigue that are not alleviated by rest, difficulty concentrating, muscle and joint pain, headaches, and sore throats that cannot be explained by any other known medical condition. While the exact cause of chronic fatigue syndrome is not known, some have theorized that it is caused by a virus (such as the Epstein-Barr virus) left in the body after an illness.

> *Simple Solutions—Chronic Fatigue:* Combine 3 drops peppermint with 1 cup (250 g) Epsom salt. Dissolve ½ cup (125 g) in warm bathwater for a soothing bath.

Oils: ⊜⊘On Guard, ⊜⊘peppermint, ⊜⊘basil, ⊜⊘lemongrass, ○⊜DigestZen, ⊜⊘rosemary, ⊜⊘lavender

Other Products: ○Mito2Max, ○Alpha CRS+ or ○a2z Chewable to help support healthy cellular energy levels. ○xEO Mega or vEO Mega or ○IQ Mega, and ○Microplex VMz to help supply necessary nutrients to support cell and immune function.

⊜: Dilute as recommended, and apply 1–2 drops to sore muscles or joints, to the back, or to the feet. Add 1–2 drops to warm bathwater for a bath.

○: Take capsules as directed on package. Add 1–2 drops of oil to an empty capsule; swallow.

⊘: Diffuse into the air. Inhale directly from bottle. Apply oil to hands, tissue, or cotton wick, and inhale.

⊕: **Body System(s) Affected:** Immune System, Nervous System, and Emotional Balance.

Cigarettes

See Addictions: Smoking

Circulatory System

See Cardiovascular System

Cirrhosis

See Liver: Cirrhosis

Cleansing

See also Housecleaning

Oils: ⊜⊘Purify, ⊜⊘On Guard, ⊜⊘Stronger, ⊘melaleuca

Other Products: ⊖On Guard Foaming Hand Wash to cleanse hands and protect against harmful microorganisms.

—Cuts:

Oils: ⊖lavender, ⊖melaleuca, ⊖Stronger,

—Master Cleanse or Lemonade Diet:

Combine 2 Tbs. (25 ml) fresh lemon or lime juice (approximately ½ lemon), 2 Tbs. (25 ml) grade B maple syrup, and ¹/₁₀ tsp. (150 mg) cayenne pepper (or to taste) with 1¼ cups (300 ml) distilled water. In case of diabetes, use black strap molasses instead of the maple syrup. Drink 6–12 glasses of this mixture daily, with an herbal laxative tea taken first thing in the morning and just before retiring at night. Refer to the booklet *The Master Cleanser* for more specifics and for suggestions of how to come off of this cleanse.

⊖: Dilute as recommended, and apply on location. Dilute 1–3 drops in 1 Tbs. (15 ml) fractionated coconut oil, and use as massage oil. Use hand wash as directed on packaging.

⊘: Diffuse into the air.

Colds

See also Antiviral, Coughs, Congestion

A cold is a viral infection that causes a stuffy or runny nose, congestion, cough, sore throat, or sneezing.

Simple Solutions—Colds: Blend 5 drops lemon and 5 drops thyme in 1 Tbs. (15 ml) jojoba oil. Apply a small amount to the throat, forehead, chest, and back of neck 2–3 times per day.

Oils: ⊘⊖thyme, ⊘⊖lemon, ⊘⊖On Guard, ⊘⊖melaleuca, ⊘⊖hinoki, ⊘⊖sandalwood, ⊘eucalyptus, ⊘⊖rosemary, ⊘⊖lime, ⊘⊖peppermint (for nasal congestion), ⊘⊖Breathe (for respiratory congestion), ⊘⊖Douglas fir, ⊖ginger, ⊘⊖copaiba, ⊘⊖basil, ⊘⊖lavender, ⊘Oorange, ⊘⊖oregano

Other Products: OBreathe Respiratory Drops, ⊘⊘Breathe Vapor Stick, OOn Guard+ Softgels. OMicroplex VMz for nutrients essential to support cellular and immune system health.

Recipe 1: When you first notice a sore throat, apply a tiny amount of melaleuca to the tip of the tongue, and then swallow. Repeat this a few times every 5–10 minutes. Then massage a couple of drops on the back of the neck.

⊖: Dilute as recommended, and apply 1–2 drops to throat, temples, forehead, back of neck, sinus area, below the nose, chest, or reflex points on the feet.

⊘: Diffuse into the air. Place 1–2 drops in a bowl of hot water, and inhale the vapors. Inhale directly from bottle. Apply oil to hands, tissue, or cotton wick, and inhale.

O: Take capsules as directed on package. Place 1–2 drops of oil under the tongue or place 1–2 drops of oil in an empty capsule, and swallow.

⊕: **Body System(s) Affected:** Immune System.

Cold Sores

See also Antiviral, Herpes Simplex

Cold sores are blisters or sores in the mouth area caused by an infection of the herpes simplex virus.

Simple Solutions—Cold Sores: Combine 4 tsp. (6 g) beeswax pellets, 1 Tbs. (10 g) cocoa butter, and 3 Tbs. (45 ml) jojoba oil, and melt in the microwave (30 seconds at a time, stirring in between) or in a double boiler. Cool slightly, and add 5 drops melissa, 5 drops peppermint, and 5 drops helichrysum essential oil. Pour into small jars or lip balm containers, and allow to cool completely. Apply a small amount of balm on cold sores as needed.

Oils: ⊖melaleuca⊕, ⊖melissa⊕, ⊖peppermint⊕, ⊖lemon, ⊖On Guard, ⊖geranium, ⊖lavender, ⊖bergamot

⊖: Dilute as recommended, and apply 1–2 drops on location.

⊕: **Body System(s) Affected:** Immune System and Skin.

⊡: **Additional Research:**

Melaleuca: Schnitzler et al., 2001; **Melissa:** Schnitzler et al., 2008; **Peppermint:** Schuhmacher et al., 2003.

Colic

See Children and Infants: Colic

Colitis

See Colon: Colitis

⊖=Topical, ⊘=Aromatic, O=Internal

Colon

See also Cancer: Colon, Digestive System

The colon, or large intestine, is the last part of the digestive system. Its function is to extract water and vitamins created by friendly bacterial flora from the material moving through the digestive system.

Oils: 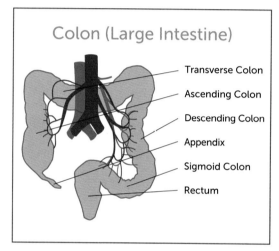DigestZen, peppermint

Other Products: PB Assist+ or PB Assist Jr to help restore friendly flora to the intestinal wall. GX Assist to help the digestive system eliminate pathogens. DigestZen Softgels to help support healthy digestion. Zendocrine Detoxification Complex to help support healthy colon functioning.

—**Cancer:** *See Cancer: Colon*

Colon (Large Intestine)

- Transverse Colon
- Ascending Colon
- Descending Colon
- Appendix
- Sigmoid Colon
- Rectum

—**Colitis:**

Colitis is inflammation of the large intestine or colon. The exact cause is not known but may involve an auto-immune response. Symptoms can include abdominal pain, tenderness, frequent need to expel stools, diarrhea, and possibly bloody stools and fever in the case of ulcerative colitis.

Oils: DigestZen, helichrysum, peppermint, thyme, oregano, rosemary, clove

Other Products: DigestZen Softgels to help support healthy digestion.

—**Diverticulitis:**

Diverticulitis is the inflammation of a diverticula (a small balloon-like sac that sometimes forms along the wall of the large intestine, especially in older individuals), typically due to infection. It causes pain in the abdomen and tenderness on the lower-left-hand part of the stomach.

Oils: cinnamon, lavender

—**Polyps:** *See also Cancer: Colon*

Polyps are tumors that arise from the bowel surface and protrude into the inside of the colon. Most polyps eventually transform into malignant cancer tumors.

Oils: peppermint

: Dilute as recommended, and apply 1–2 drops on lower abdomen or on reflex points on the feet. Use 1–2 drops in warm bathwater for a bath.

: Take capsule as directed on package. Place 1–2 drops in an empty capsule; swallow.

: Diffuse into the air. Inhale directly from bottle. Apply oil to hands, tissue, or cotton wick, and inhale.

: **Body System(s) Affected:** Digestive System.

: **Additional Research:**

Peppermint: Juergens et al., 1998; **Rosemary:** Minaiyan et al., 2011; **Thyme and Oregano:** Bukovska et al., 2007.

Coma

Simple Solutions—Coma: Alternate applying 1 drop frankincense or 1 drop bergamot to the back of the neck just below the skull once a day.

Oils: frankincense, Balance, sandalwood, cypress, peppermint

: Dilute as recommended, and massage 1–2 drops on the brain stem area, mastoids (behind ears), temples, and bottoms of feet.

: **Body System(s) Affected:** Nervous System.

Complexion

See Skin

Concentration (Poor)

Simple Solutions—Concentration: Apply 5 drops InTune to a natural stone or unglazed clay pendant, and wear throughout the day.

Oils: 🔄🌀InTune, 🔄🌀Thinker, 🌀lavender🔲, 🌀lemon🔲, 🌀Douglas fir, 🌀petitgrain, 🌀peppermint, 🌀orange, 🌀cedarwood, 🌀cypress, 🌀juniper berry, 🌀eucalyptus, 🌀rosemary, 🌀sandalwood, 🌀ylang ylang

Other Products: OxEO Mega or vEO Mega or OIQ Mega, which contains omega-3 fatty acids necessary for proper brain cell function.

🔄: Apply on back of neck and bottoms of feet.

🌀: Diffuse into the air. Apply, and inhale from hands, tissue, or cotton wick.

⭕: Take capsules as directed on package.

🔗: **Body System(s) Affected:** Emotional Balance.

🔲: **Additional Research:**

Lavender: Field et al., 2005; Diego et al., 1998; **Lemon:** Ogeturk et al., 2010.

Concussion

See Brain: Concussion

Confusion

Simple Solutions—Confusion: Inhale the aroma of frankincense directly from the bottle.

Oils: 🔄🌀InTune, 🌀frankincense, 🌀sandalwood, 🌀Balance, 🔄🌀Steady, 🌀rosemary, 🌀peppermint, 🌀juniper berry, 🌀marjoram, 🌀cedarwood, 🌀basil, 🌀ylang ylang, 🌀fir, 🌀thyme, 🌀geranium, 🌀rose, 🌀ginger

🔄: Apply on back of neck and bottoms of feet.

🌀: Diffuse into the air. Inhale directly from bottle. Apply oil to hands, tissue, or cotton wick, and inhale.

🔗: **Body System(s) Affected:** Emotional Balance.

Congestion

Congestion is the blockage of the nasal passages, sinuses, or upper respiratory tract due to inflamed tissues and blood vessels or to an increased output of mucus. Congestion can make it difficult to breathe freely and can sometimes cause pain.

Simple Solutions—Chest & Throat: Combine 6 Tbs. (75 g) coconut oil and 1.5 Tbs. (7 g) beeswax pellets, and melt in a microwave (30 seconds at a time, stirring in between) or double boiler. Let cool slightly, and add 20 drops eucalyptus, 15 drops lemon, and 20 drops peppermint. Pour into small jars or salve containers, and allow to cool completely. Apply a small amount of salve on the chest and throat as needed.

Simple Solutions—Congestion: Diffuse Breathe in an aromatherapy diffuser.

Simple Solutions—Congestion: Drop 2 drops eucalyptus and 1 drop peppermint on the floor of the shower while showering, and inhale the vapors.

Oils: 🔄🌀eucalyptus🔲, 🔄🌀peppermint, 🔄🌀Breathe, 🌀🔄Douglas fir, 🌀cinnamon, 🔄🌀juniper berry, 🔄🌀cypress, 🔄🌀melaleuca, 🔄🌀cedarwood, 🔄🌀cardamom, 🔄🌀ginger, 🔄🌀rosemary, 🔄🌀fennel, 🔄🌀citrus oils, 🔄🌀patchouli

—Catarrh:

Catarrh refers to the secretion of mucus and white blood cells from the mucous membranes in the sinuses and nasal passages in response to an infection.

Oils: 🔄🌀cypress, 🔄🌀helichrysum, 🔄🌀Breathe, 🔄🌀On Guard, 🔄🌀eucalyptus, 🔄🌀Douglas fir, 🔄🌀frankincense, 🔄🌀myrrh, 🔄🌀rosemary, 🔄🌀ginger

—Expectorant:

An expectorant is an agent that helps dissolve thick mucus in the trachea, bronchi, or lungs for easier elimination.

Oils: 🌀🔄eucalyptus🔲, 🌀🔄marjoram, 🌀🔄frankincense, 🌀🔄helichrysum, 🌀🔄cardamom

—Mucus:

Mucus is the substance produced by epithelial cells to coat the mucous membranes in the respiratory tract, digestive tract, and reproductive system. Mucus plays an important role in helping to protect these surfaces from different substances or from microorganisms they come in contact with. When one of these surfaces becomes infected or inflamed, an excess of mucus is often produced. An excess of mucus can lead to difficulty breathing in the sinuses, nasal passages,

🔄=Topical, 🌀=Aromatic, ⭕=Internal

or respiratory tract. For oils to help combat an excess of mucus, see the entries above.

Oils: ⬭◯DigestZen (with ginger—helps digest old mucus)

⬭: Dilute 1–2 drops in 1 Tbs. (15 ml) fractionated coconut oil, and massage on chest, neck, back, and feet.

⬭: Diffuse into the air. Place 1–2 drops in a bowl of hot water, and inhale the vapor. Inhale directly from bottle. Apply oil to hands, tissue, or cotton wick, and inhale.

◯: Add 1–2 drops of each oil to an empty capsule; swallow.

⬭: **Body System(s) Affected:** Respiratory System.

⬭: **Additional Research:**

Eucalyptus: (Lu et al., 2004).

Conjunctivitis

See *Eyes: Pink Eye*

Connective Tissue

See *Skeletal System: Cartilage, Muscles/Connective Tissue*

Constipation

See *Digestive System: Constipation*

Convulsions

See *Seizure: Convulsions*

Cooling Oils

Typically, oils that are high in aldehydes and esters can produce a cooling effect when applied topically or diffused.

> *Simple Solutions—Congestion:* Diffuse Breathe in an aromatherapy diffuser.

Oils: ⬭⬭peppermint, ⬭⬭eucalyptus, ⬭⬭melaleuca, ⬭⬭lavender, ⬭⬭Roman chamomile, ⬭⬭citrus oils

⬭: Dilute as recommended, and apply 1–2 drops on location. Add 1–2 drops to bathwater, and bathe. Add 1–2 drops to basin of cool water, and sponge over skin.

⬭: Diffuse into the air.

⬭: **Body System(s) Affected:** Skin.

Corns

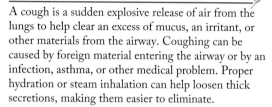

See *Foot: Corns*

Coughs

A cough is a sudden explosive release of air from the lungs to help clear an excess of mucus, an irritant, or other materials from the airway. Coughing can be caused by foreign material entering the airway or by an infection, asthma, or other medical problem. Proper hydration or steam inhalation can help loosen thick secretions, making them easier to eliminate.

> *Simple Solutions—Cough:* Mix 1 drop eucalyptus and 1 drop lemon with 1 Tbs. (15 ml) honey. Mix about ⅓ of the honey mixture with 1 cup (250 ml) warm water, and drink slowly.

> *Simple Solutions—Cough:* Diffuse Breathe in an aromatherapy diffuser.

> *Simple Solutions—Cough:* Combine 1 drop each eucalyptus, melaleuca, and lemon with 1 tsp. (5 ml) jojoba oil, and apply over chest and back.

Oils: ⬭⬭Breathe, ⬭⬭melaleuca, ⬭⬭eucalyptus, ⬭⬭Douglas fir, ⬭⬭frankincense, ⬭⬭On Guard, ⬭⬭cardamom, ⬭⬭Stronger, ⬭⬭peppermint, ⬭⬭fir, ⬭⬭juniper berry, ⬭⬭cedarwood, ⬭⬭sandalwood, ⬭⬭thyme, ⬭⬭myrrh, ⬭⬭ginger

Other Products: ⬭⬭Breathe Vapor Stick, ◯Breathe Respiratory Drops, ◯On Guard+ Softgels. ◯On Guard Protecting Throat Drops to soothe irritated and sore throats.

—**Allergy:**

Oils: ⬭Purify

—**Severe:**

Oils: ⬭⬭frankincense

⬭: Diffuse into the air. Use throat drops as directed on package.

⬭: Dilute as recommended, and apply 1–2 drops on the throat and chest.

◯: Take supplements as directed on packaging.

Primary Recommendations • Secondary Recommendations • Other Recommendations

Body System(s) Affected: Respiratory System.

Cradle Cap

See Children and Infants: Cradle Cap

Cramps

See Digestive System: Cramps, Female-Specific Conditions: Menstruation, Muscles/Connective Tissue: Cramps/Charley Horses

Crohn's Disease

Crohn's disease is a chronic inflammation of part of the intestinal wall, thought to be caused by an over-active immune response. It can cause abdominal pain, diarrhea, nausea, and loss of appetite.

> *Simple Solutions—Crohn's Disease:* Apply 1–2 drops of DigestZen over the stomach and bottoms of the feet.

Oils: 🜂❂peppermint🜊, 🜂❂DigestZen, ❂basil

🜂: Add 1–2 drops of oil to an empty capsule; swallow.

🜂: Dilute as recommended and apply on stomach and feet.

 Body System(s) Affected: Digestive System.

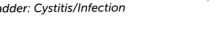 **Additional Research:**

> **Peppermint:** (Adam et al., 2006).

Cuts

See also Wounds, Antibacterial, Blood: Bleeding

> *Simple Solutions—Cuts:* Apply 1 drop of helichrysum on cut to help stop bleeding. Add 1 drop each of lavender, melaleuca, and basil to a bowl of warm water, and use the water to wash the area around the cut.

Oils: ❂helichrysum, ❂lavender, ❂melaleuca, ❂basil🜊, ❂On Guard, ❂❂Stronger, ❂hinoki, ❂Roman chamomile, ❂cypress

🜂: Dilute as recommended, and apply 1–2 drops on location.

 Body System(s) Affected: Skin.

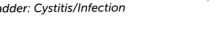 **Additional Research:**

> **Basil:** (Orafidiya et al., 2003).

Cystitis

See Bladder: Cystitis/Infection

Dandruff

See Hair: Dandruff

Decongestant

See Congestion

Degenerative Disease

A degenerative disease is a disease where the affected tissues or organs are damaged due to internal mechanisms rather than infection. Quite a few different diseases can be categorized as degenerative diseases, including Alzheimer's disease, cancer, Parkinson's disease, atherosclerosis, diabetes, osteoporosis, rheumatoid arthritis, and many others. To mitigate degenerative diseases, support the cells and tissues through proper nutrition, reducing stress, exercising regularly, and eliminating toxins. See specific conditions in this guide for oils and other products that can support the body for each condition.

Delivery

See Pregnancy/Motherhood: Delivery

Dental Infection

See Oral Conditions

Deodorant

> *Simple Solutions—Deodorant:* Melt 1 Tbs. (5 g) beeswax pellets and 3 Tbs. (40 g) coconut oil in a microwave (30 seconds at a time, stirring in between) or in a double boiler. Stir in ¼ cup (30 g) cornstarch, ¼ cup (50 g) baking soda, and 5 drops vitamin E oil. Add 5 drops melaleuca and 5 drops lavender. Pour into empty deodorant containers, and allow to cool and harden. Apply once or twice a day as needed.

🜂=Topical, ❂=Aromatic, 🜂=Internal

Oils: ⬡Purify, ⬡melaleuca, ⬡lavender, ⬡geranium, ⬡eucalyptus, ⬡cedarwood, ⬡cypress, ⬡Elevation, ⬡Serenity, ⬡Breathe, ⬡Whisper, ⬡spikenard

Other Products: ⬡Natural Deodorant

⬡: Apply deodorant under the arms. Dilute oils as recommended, and apply 1–2 drops on the skin. Dilute 2–3 drops in 1 Tbs. (15 ml) fractionated coconut oil, and apply under the arms. Add 2–3 drops to ½ cup (65 g) cornstarch and ¼ cup (50 g) baking soda, and apply under the arms, on the feet, or on other areas of the body.

⬡: **Body System(s) Affected:** Skin.

Deodorizing

Oils: ⬡Purify, ⬡peppermint, ⬡cedarwood, ⬡clary sage

⬡: Diffuse into the air. Dissolve 8–10 drops in 1 tsp. (5 ml) perfumer's or pure grain alcohol (such as vodka), and combine with distilled water in a 1 oz. spray bottle. Spray into the air or on affected surface.

Depression

Depression is a disorder marked by excessive sadness, energy loss, feelings of worthlessness, irritableness, sudden weight loss or gain, trouble sleeping, and loss of interest in activities normally enjoyed. These symptoms can continue for weeks or months if not treated and can destroy an individual's quality of life.

> *Simple Solutions—Depression:* Inhale lemon oil directly from the bottle for a quick pick-me-up.

Oils: ⬡⬡⬡lemon⬡, ⬡⬡frankincense⬡, ⬡⬡Motivate, ⬡⬡Cheer, ⬡⬡InTune, ⬡⬡Console, ⬡⬡⬡lavender⬡, ⬡⬡bergamot⬡, ⬡⬡petitgrain, ⬡⬡Elevation, ⬡⬡Balance, ⬡⬡Steady, ⬡⬡Peace, ⬡⬡Citrus Bliss⬡, ⬡⬡melissa, ⬡⬡clary sage⬡, ⬡⬡rosemary⬡, ⬡⬡ylang ylang⬡, ⬡⬡grapefruit⬡, ⬡⬡Serenity, ⬡⬡⬡lime, ⬡⬡geranium, ⬡⬡ginger, ⬡juniper berry, ⬡⬡basil, ⬡⬡sandalwood, ⬡⬡⬡patchouli

—**Postpartum Depression:** *See Pregnancy/Motherhood: Postpartum Depression*

—**Sedatives:**

Oils: ⬡⬡lavender⬡, ⬡⬡ylang ylang, ⬡⬡petitgrain, ⬡⬡melissa⬡, ⬡⬡Roman chamomile,

⬡⬡sandalwood, ⬡⬡cedarwood, ⬡⬡rose, ⬡⬡clary sage, ⬡⬡cypress, ⬡⬡juniper berry, ⬡⬡frankincense, ⬡⬡bergamot, ⬡⬡marjoram

⬡: Diffuse into the air. Inhale directly from bottle. Apply oil to hands, tissue, or cotton wick, and inhale.

⬡: Dilute as recommended, and apply 1–2 drops to temple or forehead. Add 5–10 drops to 1 Tbs. (15 ml) fractionated coconut oil, and use as massage oil. Add 1–3 drops to warm bathwater, and bathe.

⬡: Add 1–2 drops to 1 cup (250 ml) distilled water or ½ cup (125 ml) rice or almond milk, and drink. Add 1–2 drops to empty capsule, and swallow.

⬡: **Body System(s) Affected:** Nervous System.

⬡: **Additional Research:**

Lemon: Komiya et al., 2006; Komori et al., 1995; Komori et al., 1995; **Frankincense:** Moussaieff et al., 2008; **Lavender:** Kim et al., 2005; Lee et al., 2006; Guillemain et al., 1989; Buchbauer et al., 1991; Huang et al., 2008; Lin et al., 2007; **Bergamot:** Komori et al., 1995; **Citrus Bliss:** Komori et al., 1995; **Clary sage:** Seol et al., 2010; **Rosemary:** Machado et al., 2013; **Ylang ylang:** Hongratanaworakit et al., 2006; **Grapefruit:** Komori et al., 1995; **Melissa:** Ballard et al., 2002.

Dermatitis

See Skin: Dermatitis/Eczema

Despair

See Depression

Detoxification

Detoxification is the act of clearing toxins out of the body. These toxins may be addictive drugs, alcohol, or any other harmful substance.

Oils: ⬡helichrysum, ⬡rosemary⬡, ⬡juniper berry, ⬡coriander⬡

⬡: Dilute as recommended, and apply to liver area, intestines, and reflex points on the feet.

⬡: **Additional Research:**

Rosemary: Debersac et al., 2001; **Coriander:** Velaga et al., 2014.

Diabetes

Diabetes is a disease characterized by the body's inability to properly produce or use the hormone insulin. Insulin, produced in the pancreas, helps regulate the level of sugars in the blood, as well as the conversion

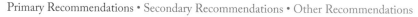

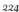

of starches and sugar into the energy necessary for life. Common diabetes symptoms include a frequent need to drink and urinate, blurred vision, mental fatigue, and possibly weight gain (depending on the type). Over time, diabetes can lead to additional complications, such as strokes, heart disease, kidney failure, and even the necessity of removing a limb.

Oils: ⬤◉cinnamon◯, ⬤◉◉rosemary◯, ◉◉geranium, ⬤◉◉basil◯, ⬤Yarrow Pom, ◉◉ylang ylang, ◉◉eucalyptus, ⬤◉◉On Guard, ◉◉cypress, ◉juniper berry, ⬤◉dill◯, ⬤◉cassia◯, ◉◉ginger, ◉◉fennel, ◉◉lavender

Blend 1: Combine 8 drops clove, 8 drops cinnamon, 15 drops rosemary, and 10 drops thyme with ¼ cup (50 ml) fractionated coconut oil. Put on feet and over pancreas.

Blend 2: Combine 5 drops cinnamon and 5 drops cypress. Rub on feet and pancreas.

Other Products: ⬤On Guard+ Softgels

—Pancreas Support:

Oils: ◉cinnamon◯, ◉geranium

—Sores (Diabetic):

Those suffering from diabetes have to be especially careful about sores of any kind, especially those on the feet and hands. Diabetes decreases blood flow, so wounds heal much slower. Many who suffer from diabetes experience decreased sensation in their hands and feet, making it more difficult to even notice an injury right away. Even a small sore left untreated can turn into an ulcer, ultimately making amputation necessary.

Oils: ◉lavender, ◉Balance

⬤: Place 1–2 drops of oil under the tongue or place 1–2 drops in empty capsule and swallow. Take supplements as directed on packaging.

◉: Dilute as recommended, and apply on back, chest, feet, and over pancreas.

◉: Diffuse into the air.

◉: **Body System(s) Affected:** Endocrine System.

◯: **Additional Research:**

Cinnamon: Lu, T. et al., 2012; Mishra et al., 2010; Subash et al., 2007; Ping et al., 2010; Li, R. et al., 2013; **Rosemary:** Bakirel et al., 2008; **Basil:** Agrawal et al., 1996; **Melissa:** Chung et al., 2010; **Dill:** Takahashi et al., 2013; **Helichrysum and Grapefruit:** da la Garza et al., 2013; **Cassia:** Lee, 2002; **D-Limonene found in lime, lemon, bergamot, dill, grapefruit, lavender, lemongrass, Roman chamomile, tangerine, and wild orange essential oils :** Jing et al., 2013.

Diaper Rash

*See **Children and Infants: Diaper Rash***

Diarrhea

*See **Digestive System: Diarrhea***

Digestive System

The human digestive system is the series of organs and glands that process food. The digestive system breaks down food, absorbs nutrients for the body to use as fuel, and excretes as bowel movements the part that cannot be broken down.

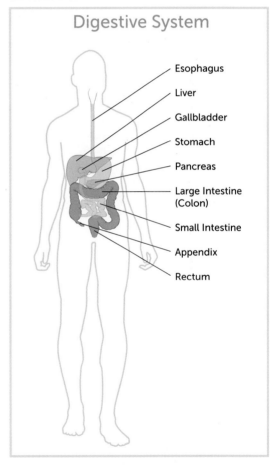

Digestive System

- Esophagus
- Liver
- Gallbladder
- Stomach
- Pancreas
- Large Intestine (Colon)
- Small Intestine
- Appendix
- Rectum

Oils: ⬤◉◉peppermint◯, ⬤◉◉ginger◯, ◉◉lemongrass (purifies)◯, ⬤◉◉DigestZen, ⬤◉◉fennel, ⬤◉◉turmeric, ⬤◉◉wintergreen◯, ⬤◉◉marjoram (stimulates), ⬤◉◉oregano◯, ⬤◉◉rosemary◯, ◉◉clary sage, ◉⬤copaiba, ◉neroli,

◉=Topical, ◉=Aromatic, ⬤=Internal

◐◲◱cardamom, ◐◲◱grapefruit, ◐◲◱basil, ◐◲◱lemon◲, ◲◱cinnamon, ◐◲◱clove, ◲◱juniper berry, ◐◲◱orange, ◐◲◱bergamot

Regimen 1: Use ◐GX Assist for 10 days to help support the digestive system in eliminating pathogenic microorganisms, followed by ◐PB Assist+ or ◐PB Assist Jr for 5 days to help rebuild friendly flora to aid digestion and prevent pathogenic bacteria.

Other Products: ◐DigestZen Softgels to help support healthy digestion. ◐DigestZen Terrazyme for healthy digestion, enzymatic function, and cellular metabolism. ◐Alpha CRS+, ◐xEO Mega or vEO Mega, ◐IQ Mega, ◐Microplex VMz, ◐a2z Chewable to provide essential nutrients, vitamins, and minerals for digestive system cellular support.

◐: Take capsules as directed on package. Add 1–2 drops of oil to 2 cups (½ L) of water, and drink. Add oils as flavoring to food. Place 1–2 drops of oil in an empty capsule, and swallow.

◱: Dilute oil as recommended, and apply 1–2 drops on stomach or reflex points on feet. Dilute 1–2 drops in 1 Tbs. (15 ml) fractionated coconut oil, and massage over abdomen and lower back. Apply as a warm compress over affected area.

◲: Diffuse into the air. *See Negative Ions* for oils that produce negative ions when diffused to help stimulate the digestive system. Inhale oil directly or applied to hands, tissue, or cotton wick.

—Bloating:

Bloating is an abnormal swelling, increase in diameter, or feeling of fullness and tightness in the abdominal area as gas and liquid are trapped inside. Common causes of bloating can include overeating, menstruation, constipation, food allergies, and irritable bowel syndrome.

Simple Solutions—Bloating: Combine 5 drops fennel with 1 tsp. (5 ml) fractionated coconut oil in a small roll-on bottle, and apply on stomach once or twice a day as needed.

Oils: ◱◲DigestZen

Other Products: ◐DigestTab, ◐DigestZen Softgels

◱: Dilute as recommended, and apply to stomach and to reflex points on the feet.

◲: Diffuse into the air.

—Constipation:

Constipation is a condition characterized by infrequent or difficult bowel movements. A person is considered constipated if he or she has fewer than three bowel movements a week or if the stools are hard and difficult to expel. Common causes of constipation include a lack of fiber, dehydration, ignoring the urge to have a bowel movement, depression, medications, large dairy intake, stress, and abuse of laxatives.

Simple Solutions—Constipation: Combine 1 drop each of rosemary, lemon, and peppermint with 1 tsp. (5 ml) fractionated coconut oil, and massage gently on stomach and back.

Oils: ◱rosemary◲, ◱lemon◲, ◱peppermint◲, ◱marjoram, ◱DigestZen, ◱ginger, ◱fennel, ◱orange, ◱◲copaiba, ◱rose, ◱juniper berry, ◱sandalwood

Other Products: ◐DigestZen Softgels to help support healthy digestion.

◱: Dilute as recommended, and apply oils on abdomen. Add 1–2 drops to 1 Tbs. (15 ml) fractionated coconut oil, and massage onto abdomen.

◐: Take capsules as directed.

—Cramps (Abdominal):

Cramps are sudden, involuntary muscle contractions that often cause severe pain. Abdominal cramps are commonly caused by stress, menstruation, mild food poisoning, and *Irritable Bowel Syndrome (below)*.

Oils: ◐◱DigestZen, ◐◱basil, ◱clary sage

Other Products: ◐DigestZen Softgels to help support healthy digestion.

Recipe 1: Flavor water with 5 drops DigestZen, and drink for stomach pains and cramps.

◐: Place 3 drops DigestZen and 3 drops basil in an empty capsule; swallow. Take capsules as directed.

◱: Dilute as recommended, and massage oil onto abdomen over area of pain.

—Diarrhea:

Diarrhea is an abnormal increase in the frequency of bowel movements, marked by loose, watery stools. Diarrhea is defined as more than three bowel movements a day. Cases of diarrhea that last more than two days can become a serious problem and cause dehydration. Rehydration with an oral rehydration solution is the most effective way to prevent dehydration. If no commercially prepared oral rehydration solution is available, a solution made from 1 tsp. (5 g) salt, 8 tsp. (35 g) sugar, and 4 cups (1 L) clean water (with some mashed fresh banana, if available, to add potassium) can work in an emergency. Diarrhea is usually caused by a viral, parasitic, or bacterial infection.

Simple Solutions—Diarrhea: Blend 3 drops peppermint and 2 drops fennel with 1 tsp. (5 ml) fractionated coconut oil in a small roll-on bottle, and apply over stomach as needed.

Oils: O◐peppermint, O◐ginger, ◐geranium, O◐DigestZen, ◐orange, ◐patchouli, ◐melaleuca, ◐sandalwood, ◐copaiba, ◐lavender, ◐Roman chamomile, ◐cypress, ◐eucalyptusm, ◐neroli

Other Products: ODigestZen Softgels to help support healthy digestion.

–Children:

Oils: ◐geranium, ◐ginger, ◐sandalwood

O: Place 1–2 drops in an empty capsule, and swallow. Take supplement as directed.

◐: Dilute as recommended, and apply 1–2 drops on abdomen. Apply as a warm compress over affected area.

—Gas/Flatulence:

Simple Solutions—Gas/Flatulence: Combine 5 drops fennel with 1 tsp. (5 ml) fractionated coconut oil in a small roll-on bottle, and apply on stomach once or twice a day as needed.

Oils: O◐lavender, O◐ginger, O◐star anise, ◐peppermint, O◐cardamom, ◐eucalyptus, ◐bergamot, ◐myrrh, ◐juniper berry, ◑◐petitgrain, ◐neroli, ◐copaiba, ◐rosemary

Other Products: ODigestTab, ODigestZen Softgels to help support healthy digestion.

O: Place 1–2 drops in an empty capsule, and swallow. Take supplement as directed.

◐: Dilute as recommended, and apply 1–2 drops on stomach, abdomen, or reflex points on the feet

—Gastritis: *See also Inflammation*

Gastritis is inflammation of the stomach lining.

Oils: O◐DigestZen, O◐peppermint, Olemongrass◐, ◐Ofennel

Other Products: ODigestZen Softgels to help support healthy digestion.

O: Add 1 drop of oil to rice or almond milk; take as a supplement. Place 1–2 drops in an empty capsule; swallow capsule. Take supplement as directed.

◐: Dilute as recommended, and apply 1–2 drops on stomach. Apply as a warm compress over stomach.

—GERD (Gastroesophageal Reflux Disease):

Gastroesophageal reflux disease (GERD) is a digestive disease that causes stomach acid to frequently flow back into the tube connecting the mouth and stomach (esophagus). This backwash (acid reflux) can irritate the lining of the esophagus.

Oils: Olemon◐, Ogreen mandarin◐

—Giardia:

Giardia are parasites that infect the gastrointestinal tract of humans and animals. The form of *Giardia* that affects humans causes severe diarrhea. *See Diarrhea above* for information on rehydration.

Oils: O◐lavender◐

O: Place 1–2 drops in an empty capsule; swallow capsule.

◐: Dilute as recommended, and apply 1–2 drops on abdomen or reflex points on the feet.

—Heartburn:

Heartburn is a painful burning sensation in the chest or throat. It occurs as a result of backed up stomach acid in the esophagus. Heartburn is often brought on by certain foods, medication, pregnancy, and alcohol.

Simple Solutions—Heartburn/Indigestion: Add 1 drop peppermint to 1 tsp. (5 ml) honey. Dissolve in 1 cup (250 ml) warm water, and drink slowly.

Oils: ◐lemon, ◐peppermint, ◐ODigestZen

Blend 1: Blend 2 drops lemon, 2 drops peppermint, and 3 drops sandalwood in 1 Tbs. (15 ml) fractionated coconut oil. Apply to breast bone in a clockwise motion using the palm of the hand. Apply to reflex points on the feet.

Other Products: ODigestTab, ODigestZen Softgels to help support healthy digestion.

◐: Dilute as recommended, and apply 1–2 drops to chest.

◐=Topical, ◑=Aromatic, O=Internal

○: Add 1 drop of oil to rice or almond milk; take as a supplement. Place 1–2 drops in an empty capsule; swallow capsule. Take supplement as directed.

—Indigestion:

The term "indigestion" is used to describe abdominal discomfort felt after a meal. Symptoms of indigestion include belching, bloating, nausea, heartburn, a feeling of fullness, and general abdominal discomfort. Indigestion can be caused by overeating or eating too fast, alcoholic or carbonated drinks, particular foods, etc.

Oils: ○◔◑peppermint, ○◔◑ginger, ○◔star anise, ○◔◑turmeric, ○◔DigestZen, ◔◑lavender, ◔◑orange, ○◔◑lime, ◔◑thyme, ◔◑myrrh, ◔◑grapefruit, ◔◑petitgrain, ◔neroli

Other Products: ○DigestZen Softgels to help support healthy digestion. ○DigestTab, ○DigestZen Terrazyme for healthy digestion, enzymatic function, and cellular metabolism.

○: Add 1–2 drops of oil to 1 cup (250 ml) of almond or rice milk; drink. Place 1–2 drops of oil in an empty capsule; swallow capsule. Take capsules as directed on package.

◔: Dilute oil as recommended, and apply 1–2 drops on stomach or reflex points on feet. Dilute 1–2 drops in 1 Tbs. (15 ml) fractionated coconut oil, and massage over abdomen and lower back. Apply as a warm compress over stomach area.

◑: Diffuse into the air.

—Intestines:

The intestines are the largest organs in the digestive track. The intestines include the small intestine, which begins just below the stomach and is responsible for digesting and absorbing nutrients from the food, and the large intestine, which begins at the end of the small intestine and is responsible for reabsorbing water and some vitamins before the undigested food and waste is eliminated.

Oils: ◔○basil, ◔○marjoram, ◔○ginger, ◔○rose◔, ◔○rosemary

Other Products: ○GX Assist to help the digestive system eliminate pathogens. ○PB Assist+ or ○PB Assist Jr to provide friendly intestinal flora to aid digestion and help prevent pathogenic bacteria. ○DigestZen Terrazyme for healthy digestion, enzymatic function, and cellular metabolism.

◔: Dilute oil as recommended, and apply 1–2 drops on stomach or reflex points on feet. Dilute 1–2 drops in 1 Tbs. (15 ml) fractionated coconut oil, and massage over abdomen and lower back. Apply as a warm compress over affected area.

○: Take capsules as directed on package. Add 1–2 drops of oil to 2 cups (½ L) of water; drink. Add oils as flavoring to food. Place 1–2 drops of oil in a capsule, and swallow.

—Intestinal Parasites:
See Parasites: Intestinal

—Irritable Bowel Syndrome:

Irritable bowel syndrome is an intestinal disorder characterized by reoccurring diarrhea, bloating, gas, constipation, cramping, and abdominal pain. Irritable bowel syndrome is one of the most commonly diagnosed disorders by doctors.

Oils: ○◔peppermint◔, ○◔DigestZen

○: Add 2 drops of each oil to 1 cup (250 ml) distilled water, and drink 1–2 times per day. Place 2 drops of each oil in an empty capsule; swallow capsule.

◔: Dilute 1–2 drops in 1 Tbs. (15 ml) fractionated coconut oil, and apply over the abdomen with a hot compress.

—Nausea/Upset Stomach:

Oils: ◔○DigestZen, ○◔ginger◔, ◔◑peppermint, ◔lavender, ◔◑ClaryCalm, ◔clove

Other Products: ○DigestZen Softgels to help support healthy digestion.

○: Place 1–2 drops in an empty capsule; swallow capsule. Place 1 drop in 1 cup (250 ml) rice or almond milk, and drink. Take supplement as directed.

◔: Dilute as recommended, and apply behind ears, on stomach, or on reflex points on the feet.

◑: Diffuse into the air. Inhale directly from bottle. Apply oil to hands, tissue, or cotton wick, and inhale.

—Parasites: *See Parasites*

—Stomach:

The stomach is the organ mainly responsible for breaking food apart using strong acids. It is located below the esophagus and before the intestines.

Oils: ○◔basil, ○◔peppermint, ○lemongrass◔, ○◔ginger, ○◔DigestZen

Other Products: ○DigestZen Softgels to help support healthy digestion.

○: Place 1–2 drops in an empty capsule, and swallow. Take supplement as directed.

◐: Dilute as recommended, and apply 1–2 drops on stomach, abdomen, or reflex points on the feet

—Ulcers: *See Ulcers*

⊕: **Body System(s) Affected:** Digestive System.

⊞: **Additional Research:**

Peppermint: Adam et al., 2006; Asao et al., 2003; Kim et al., 2005; Rees et al., 1979; Liu et al., 1997; Kline et al., 2001; Capello et al., 2007; May et al., 1996; **Ginger:** Nanthakomon et al., 2006; Vutyavanich et al., 2001; Bone et al., 1990; **Lemongrass:** Ohno et al., 2003; **Lemon/Green Mandarin:** Sun, 2007; **Wintergreen:** Trautmann et al., 1991; **Oregano:** Force et al., 2000; **Rosemary:** Kim et al., 2005; **Lemon:** Kim et al., 2005; **Lavender:** Moon et al., 2006; **Rose:** Sadraei et al., 2013.

Disinfectant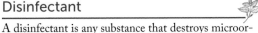

A disinfectant is any substance that destroys microorganisms on non-living surfaces.

Oils: ◐⊘lemon, ◐⊘Purify, ◐⊘grapefruit, ⊘lemongrass○, ⊘geranium○

Other Products: On Guard Foaming Hand Wash to cleanse hands and protect against harmful microorganisms.

Blend 1: Add 10 drops lavender, 20 drops thyme, 5 drops eucalyptus, and 5 drops oregano to a large bowl of water. Use to disinfect small areas.

◐: Add 1–2 drops of oil to a wet cloth, and use to wipe down counters and other surfaces. Use hand wash as directed on packaging.

⊘: Diffuse into the air.

⊕: **Body System(s) Affected:** Immune System and Skin.

⊞: **Additional Research:**

Lemongrass: Doran et al., 2009; **Geranium:** Doran et al., 2009.

Diuretic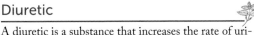

A diuretic is a substance that increases the rate of urination and fluid elimination from the body.

Oils: ◐lemongrass, ◐rosemary, ◐cedarwood, ◐lavender, ◐patchouli, ◐grapefruit, ◐cypress, ◐fennel, ◐orange, ◐lemon, ◐oregano, ◐juniper berry, ◐marjoram

◐: Dilute as recommended, and apply oils to kidney area on back and to bottoms of feet.

⊕: **Body System(s) Affected:** Digestive System.

Diverticulitis

See Colon: Diverticulitis

Dysentery

*See also **Antibacterial, Digestive System: Diarrhea***

Dysentery is severe, frequent diarrhea, often with blood or mucus, that occurs due to infection by bacteria or amoeba. Dysentery can be fatal due to dehydration if left untreated. *See Digestive System: Diarrhea* for information on rehydrating the body.

> *Simple Solutions—Dysentery:* Blend 3 drops peppermint and 2 drops myrrh with 1 tsp. (5 ml) fractionated coconut oil, and apply on stomach. Use rehydration solution (see above), and seek medical attention.

Oils: ◐myrrh, ◐eucalyptus, ◐lemon, ◐Roman chamomile, ◐cypress, ◐clove (amoebic), ◐melissa

◐: Dilute as recommended, and apply on abdomen and on bottoms of feet.

⊕: **Body System(s) Affected:** Digestive System.

Dyspepsia

*See **Digestive System: Indigestion***

Ears

Oils: ◐⊘helichrysum, ◐⊘Purify, ◐⊘eucalyptus, ◐⊘melaleuca, ◐juniper berry, ◐⊘geranium, ◐⊘Balance, ◐⊘marjoram

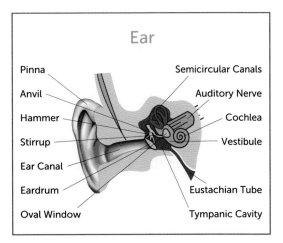

Ear

Pinna
Anvil
Hammer
Stirrup
Ear Canal
Eardrum
Oval Window

Semicircular Canals
Auditory Nerve
Cochlea
Vestibule
Eustachian Tube
Tympanic Cavity

◐=Topical, ⊘=Aromatic, ○=Internal

—Earache:

> *Simple Solutions—Earache:* Add 1 drop each of basil and melaleuca to a cotton ball. Hold the cotton over the ear canal (not in the ear canal) for 30 minutes.

Oils: basil, melaleuca, helichrysum

—Hearing in a Tunnel:

Oils: Purify

—Infection:

Oils: melaleuca, Purify, lavender

—Inflammation:

Oils: eucalyptus

—Tinnitus:

Tinnitus is a ringing or other audible noise in the ears caused by ear infection, wax buildup, or a block in the eustachian tube.

> *Simple Solutions—Tinnitus:* Add 1 drop helichrysum to a cotton ball. Hold the cotton over the ear canal (not in the ear canal) for 30 minutes.

Oils: helichrysum, juniper berry

- Caution: Never put oils directly into the ear canal. Dilute as recommended, and apply 1–2 drops on surface of the ear and behind the ear on the mastoid bone. Apply 1 drop oil to small cotton ball, and place over opening to ear canal (do not press into the ear canal). Place 1 drop oil on cotton swab, and swab around the ear canal.

- Diffuse into the air.

- **Body System(s) Affected:** Skin, Immune System, Nervous System, and Respiratory System.

Eating Disorders

> *Simple Solutions—Eating Disorders:* Diffuse grapefruit in an aromatherapy diffuser to help soothe the mind when feeling withdrawals from food or compulsive behaviors.

—Anorexia:

Anorexia is a psychological disorder where a person becomes obsessed with body size and weight, often depriving him or herself of food to avoid gaining weight.

Oils: grapefruit, Citrus Bliss

- : Diffuse into the air. Inhale directly from bottle. Apply oil to hands, tissue, or cotton wick, and inhale.

—Bulimia:

Bulimia is a disorder categorized by periods of overeating, or binging, followed by periods of self-induced vomiting, fasting, or abuse of laxatives and diuretics to purge the body of the food or to compensate for the overeating.

Oils: grapefruit, Citrus Bliss

- : Diffuse into the air. Inhale directly from bottle. Apply oil to hands, tissue, or cotton wick, and inhale.

—Overeating:

Overeating is eating too much food for the body. It can include binging (eating so much at one time that the stomach is overly filled and uncomfortable or painful) or chronic overeating (eating more than the body needs over a long period of time). Consistently overeating can lead to obesity and other health problems.

Oils: Slim & Sassy, grapefruit, lemon, peppermint, ginger

Other Products: Slim & Sassy TrimShakes

- : Add 8 drops of Slim & Sassy to 2 cups (½ L) of water, and drink throughout the day between meals. Drink Trim or V Shake 1–2 times per day as a meal alternative.

- : Diffuse into the air. Inhale directly from bottle. Apply oil to hands, tissue, or cotton wick, and inhale.

- **Body System(s) Affected:** Nervous System, Digestive System, and Emotional Balance.

- **Additional Research:**

  Grapefruit: Shen et al., 2005; **Lemon:** Shen et al., 2005.

Eczema

See Skin: Dermatitis/Eczema

Edema

See also Allergies, Diuretic, Inflammation

Edema is swelling caused by the abnormal accumulation of fluids in a tissue or body cavity. This can be caused by an allergic reaction, inflammation, injury, or as a signal of problems with the heart, liver, or kidneys.

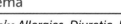

Primary Recommendations • Secondary Recommendations • Other Recommendations

Oils: ⊘grapefruit, ⊘lemongrass, ⊘cypress, ⊘geranium, ⊘rosemary, ⊘cedarwood, ⊘juniper berry

⊖: Dilute as recommended, and apply 1–2 drops on location.

◐: Add 1–2 drops to 1 cup (250 ml) of water, and drink every 3 hours.

⊕: **Body System(s) Affected:** Cardiovascular System, Endocrine System, and Immune System.

Elbow

See Joints: Tennis Elbow

Emergency Oils

The following oils are recommended to have on hand in case of an emergency:

Clove: Use as an analgesic (for topical pain relief) and a drawing salve (to pull toxins/infection from the body). Good for acne, constipation, headaches, nausea, and toothaches.

Frankincense: Enhances effect of any other oil. It facilitates clarity of mind, accelerates all skin recovery issues, and reduces anxiety and mental and physical fatigue. Reduces hyperactivity, impatience, irritability, and restlessness. Helps with focus and concentration.

Lavender: Use for agitation, bruises, burns (can mix with melaleuca), leg cramps, herpes, heart irregularities, hives, insect bites, neuropathy, pain (inside and out), bee stings, sprains, sunburn (combine with frankincense), and sunstroke. Relieves insomnia, depression, and PMS and is a natural antihistamine (asthma or allergies).

Lemon: Use for arthritis, colds, constipation, coughs, cuts, sluggishness, sore throats, sunburn, and wounds. It lifts the spirits and reduces stress and fatigue. Internally it counteracts acidity, calms an upset stomach, and encourages elimination.

Lemongrass: Use for sore and cramping muscles and charley horses (with peppermint; drink lots of water). Apply to bottoms of feet in winter to warm them.

Melaleuca: Use for bug bites, colds, coughs, cuts, deodorant, eczema, fungus, infections (ear, nose, or throat), microbes (internally), psoriasis, rough hands, slivers (combine with clove to draw them out), sore throats, and wounds.

Oregano: Use as heavy-duty antibiotic (internally with olive oil or coconut oil in capsules or topically on bottoms of feet—follow up with lavender and peppermint). Also for fungal infections and for reducing pain and inflammation of arthritis, backache, bursitis, carpal tunnel syndrome, rheumatism, and sciatica. Always dilute.

Peppermint: Use as an analgesic (for topical pain relief, bumps, and bruises). Can also be used for circulation, fever, headache, indigestion, motion sickness, nausea, nerve problems, or vomiting.

AromaTouch: Use for relaxation and stress relief. It is soothing and anti-inflammatory and enhances massage.

Breathe: Use for allergies, anxiety, asthma, bronchitis, congestion, colds, coughs, flu, and respiratory distress.

Deep Blue: Use for pain relief. Works well in cases of arthritis, bruises, carpal tunnel, headaches, inflammation, joint pain, migraines, muscle pain, sprains, and rheumatism. Follow with peppermint to enhance effects.

DigestZen: Use for all digestion issues such as bloating, congestion, constipation, diarrhea, food poisoning (internal), heartburn, indigestion, motion sickness, nausea, and stomachache. Also works well on diaper rash.

On Guard: Use to disinfect all surfaces. It eliminates mold and viruses and helps to boost the immune system (bottoms of feet or internally; use daily).

Purify: Use for airborne pathogens, cuts, germs (on any surface), insect bites, itches (all types and varieties), and wounds. Also boosts the immune system.

TerraShield: Deters all flying insects and ticks from human bodies and pets.

Emotions

See also Anxiety, Calming, Depression, Fear, Grief/Sorrow, Stress: Emotional Stress, Uplifting

To put it simply, emotions are the way we currently feel. These feelings come in response to what we see, smell, hear, feel, taste, think, or have experienced and can affect our future thoughts and behavior. While much is still being discovered about the complex psychological and physiological processes involved in emotions, researchers have discovered that emotions involve many different systems in the body, including the brain, the sensory system, the endocrine/hormonal system, the autonomic nervous system, the immune

⊖=Topical, ⊘=Aromatic, ◐=Internal

system, and the release or inhibition of neurotransmitters (such as dopamine) in the brain. Recent research has also begun to uncover compelling evidence that various essential oils and their components have the ability to affect each one of these systems, making the use of essential oils an intriguing tool for helping to balance emotions in the human body.

Oils: Console, Motivate, Passion, Peace, Forgive, Cheer, AromaTouch, Balance, Citrus Bliss, Elevation, Serenity, ClaryCalm, Whisper, Zendocrine, cypress, geranium, lavender, rose, orange, peppermint, neroli

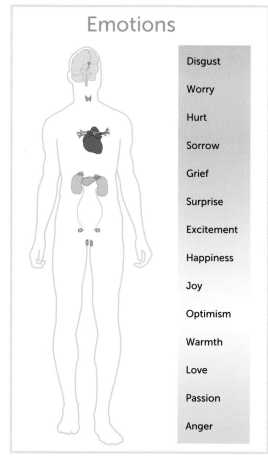

Emotions

Disgust

Worry

Hurt

Sorrow

Grief

Surprise

Excitement

Happiness

Joy

Optimism

Warmth

Love

Passion

Anger

—Acceptance:

Oils: Forgive, Elevation

—Alertness: *See also Alertness*

Oils: peppermint, ylang ylang, black pepper, juniper berry, cinnamon

—Anger:

Oils: Serenity, Forgive, lavender, Console, InTune, ylang ylang, melissa, Elevation, Balance, helichrysum

—Anxious: *See also Anxiety*

Oils: Peace, lavender, orange, lemon, neroli, InTune, Serenity, Motivate, AromaTouch, Elevation, Balance (on back of neck), Breathe (on chest)

—Balance:

Oils: Balance, AromaTouch, Citrus Bliss, geranium, juniper berry, lavender, neroli, orange, sandalwood, vetiver

—Blocks:

Oils: Forgive, cypress, frankincense, helichrysum, sandalwood, Balance

—Clearing:

Oils: Elevation, Peace, juniper berry, Balance

—Coldness:

Oils: Cheer, myrrh, ylang ylang

—Concentration: *See also Concentration*

Oils: InTune, Arise, lavender, lemon, peppermint, neroli

—Confidence:

Oils: Elevation, Motivate, Whisper, Passion, cedarwood, Forgive, orange

—Creativity:

Oils: frankincense, sandalwood, Elevation, Motivate, Cheer, cypress, lemon

—Defeated:

Oils: Motivate, Passion, Peace, cypress, fir, Elevation, juniper berry, Balance

—Depression: *See also Depression*

Oils: Motivate, Cheer, lemon, frankincense, InTune, Console, lavender, bergamot, Elevation, Balance, Peace, Citrus Bliss

Primary Recommendations • Secondary Recommendations • Other Recommendations

232

—Emotional Trauma:

Oils: sandalwood, Forgive

—Expression (self-expression):

Oils: Balance, Elevation, Motivate, Passion

—Fear: *See also* **Fear**

Oils: Peace, Balance, ylang ylang, orange, sandalwood, Serenity, Motivate, Elevation, Passion

—Focus: *See Concentration*

—Grief/Sorrow: *See also* **Grief/Sorrow**

Oils: Cheer, Console, lemon, Elevation, Balance, Forgive, lavender, bergamot, orange, Citrus Bliss, grapefruit, wintergreen

—Guilt:

Oils: Peace, Elevation, Forgive, Deep Blue (on outer earlobes)

—Happiness/Joy:

Oils: Elevation, Cheer, Console, Citrus Bliss, Motivate, Passion, lemon, orange, spearmint, sandalwood, bergamot

—Loss:

Oils: Elevation, Forgive, tangerine, orange

—Mind (open):

Oils: frankincense, sandalwood, Balance

—Negative Emotions:

Oils: Elevation, Citrus Bliss, orange, grapefruit, Balance, fir, wintergreen, lavender

—Overburdened/Overwhelmed:

Oils: Peace, Balance, Citrus Bliss, orange

—Peace:

Oils: Serenity, lavender, Peace, In-Tune, ylang ylang, melissa, neroli

—Pity (self-pity):

Oils: Elevation, Forgive, Citrus Bliss, orange

—Positive (feeling):

Oils: Elevation, Motivate, Cheer, basil, peppermint, frankincense, cedarwood, juniper berry

—Rejection:

Oils: Motivate, Passion, Balance, lavender, geranium

—Release:

Oils: Forgive, Roman chamomile

—Stress: *See also* **Stress: Emotional Stress**

Oils: Elevation, Peace, clary sage, bergamot, Serenity

—Suicidal:

Oils: Elevation, AromaTouch, Citrus Bliss, Serenity

—Uplifting: *See also* **Uplifting**

Oils: Cheer, lemon, orange, Elevation, Brave, Console, Passion, Citrus Bliss, Forgive

—Worried:

Oils: Peace, bergamot, neroli, Serenity, Elevation, Balance, AromaTouch

: Inhale directly from bottle. Diffuse into the air. Apply oil to hands, tissue, or cotton wick, and inhale.

: Massage oils on back, chest, and/or legs. Gently massage 1–2 drops of oil into the outer lobes of the ear (avoid the ear canal). Add 1–2 drops of oil to a bath or shower gel or to bath salts, and use during a bath or shower.

: Add 1–2 drops to 1 cup (250 ml) distilled water or to ½ cup (125 ml) rice or almond milk before drinking. Add 1–2 drops to an empty capsule, and swallow.

: **Body System(s) Affected:** Emotional Balance and Nervous System.

: **Additional Research:**

Peppermint: Moss et al., 2008; **Ylang ylang:** Hongratanaworakit et al., 2004; Moss et al., 2008; Hongratanaworakit et al., 2006; **Lavender:** Huang et al., 2008; Lin et al., 2007; Bradley et al., 2007; Dimpfel et al., 2004; Dunn et al., 1995; Itai et al., 2000; Umezu, 2000; Field et al., 2005; Diego et al., 1998; Kim et al., 2005; Lee et al., 2006; Guillemain et al., 1989; **Melissa:** Ballard et al., 2002; **Orange:** Carvalho-Freitas et al., 2002; Lehrner et al., 2000; **Lemon:** Ceccarelli et al., 2004; Komiya et al., 2006; Komori et al., 1995; Kiecolt-Glaser et al., 2008; **Frankincense:** Moussaieff et al., 2008.

=Topical, =Aromatic, =Internal

Emphysema

Emphysema is a chronic pulmonary disease where airflow is restricted through the lungs due to destruction (typically caused by airborne toxins such as those in cigarette smoke) of the wall of the alveoli (small air sacs in the lungs where oxygen and carbon dioxide is exchanged with the blood). This destruction of the alveolar wall causes the alveoli to collapse when air is expelled from the lungs, trapping air inside.

> *Simple Solutions—Emphysema:* Add 1 drop eucalyptus to 1 tsp. (5 ml) fractionated coconut oil, and apply on chest and back.

Oils: ⊘☷eucalyptus, ⊘☷Breathe

⊘: Diffuse into the air.

☷: Dilute as recommended, and apply 1–2 drops to chest and back. Apply as a warm compress on chest.

⊕: **Body System(s) Affected:** Respiratory System and Cardiovascular System.

Endocrine System

See also Adrenal Glands, Ovaries, Pancreas, Pineal Gland, Pituitary Gland, Testes, Thymus, Thyroid

See Endocrine System Chart on previous page.

The endocrine system is the series of hormone-producing glands and organs that help regulate metabolism, reproduction, blood pressure, appetite, and many other body functions. The endocrine system is mainly controlled by the hypothalamus region of the brain that either produces hormones that stimulate the other endocrine glands directly, or that stimulates the pituitary gland located just below it to release the hormones needed to stimulate the other endocrine glands. These hormones are released into the bloodstream, where they travel to other areas of the body to either stimulate other endocrine glands or to stimulate tissues and organs of the body directly. Some essential oils may act as hormones or stimulate the endocrine system to produce hormones that have a regulating effect on the body.

Oils: O☷Zendocrine, ⊘☷rosemary, ⊘☷cinnamon

Other Products: OZendocrine Detoxification Complex to help support healthy endocrine cleansing and filtering.

—Hormonal Balance:

Oils: ☷⊘clary sage, ⊘clove, ⊘☷ylang ylang

Other Products: OPhytoestrogen Lifetime Complex

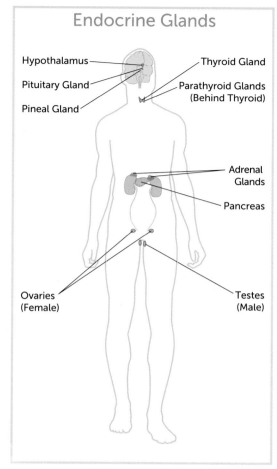

Endocrine Glands

Hypothalamus
Pituitary Gland
Pineal Gland

Thyroid Gland
Parathyroid Glands (Behind Thyroid)

Adrenal Glands
Pancreas

Ovaries (Female)
Testes (Male)

—Female:

Oils: ☷⊘ClaryCalm, ☷⊘Whisper

—Sexual Energy:

Oils: ⊘☷ylang ylang

O: Take capsules as directed on package. Place 1–2 drops of oil under the tongue, or add 3–5 drops of essential oil to an empty capsule; swallow capsule.

⊘: Diffuse into the air. Inhale directly from bottle. Apply oil to hands, tissue, or cotton wick, and inhale.

☷: Dilute as recommended, and apply 1–2 drops to the reflex points on the feet, lower back, thyroid, liver, kidneys, gland areas, the center of the body, or both sides of the spine and clavicle area. Add 1–2 drops to 1 Tbs. (15 ml) fractionated coconut oil, and use as massage oil.

⊕: **Body System(s) Affected:** Endocrine System.

Primary Recommendations • Secondary Recommendations • Other Recommendations

Endometriosis

Endometriosis is a chronic disorder in women where endometrium cells (cells from the lining of the uterus) grow outside of the uterus—typically around the ovaries, the ligaments that support the uterus, or the peritoneal (abdominal) cavity. These cells are often still responsive to the monthly hormone cycle that effects the changes in the uterus and can cause abnormal abdominal pain and irregularities in the menstrual cycle.

Oils: ○geranium, ○cypress, ○clary sage, ○On Guard, ○eucalyptus, ○Whisper

○: Dilute as recommended, and apply 1–2 drops on lower abdomen or on feet. Apply as a warm compress. Place 1–2 drops in warm bathwater, and bathe.

○: **Body System(s) Affected:** Reproductive System.

Endurance

> *Simple Solutions—Endurance:* Add 1 drop peppermint to a small bottle of water, and drink 15 minutes before exercising.

Oils: ○○peppermint○

Other Products: ○Mito2Max, ○Alpha CRS+, ○a2z Chewable, ○xEO Mega or vEO Mega, ○IQ Mega, ○Microplex VMz to provide nutrients and antioxidants that help support healthy cellular function and energy levels.

○: Diffuse into the air. Inhale directly from bottle. Apply oil to hands, tissue, or cotton wick, and inhale.

○: Take capsules as directed on package.

○: **Additional Research:**

Peppermint: (Meamarbashi et al., 2013).

Energy

> *Simple Solutions—Energy:* Inhale peppermint directly from the bottle for a quick energy boost.

Oils: ○○○peppermint○, ○○fir, ○○Elevation, ○○Balance, ○○Steady, ○○lemon, ○○litsea, ○○basil, ○○thyme, ○○rosemary, ○○orange, ○○lemongrass, ○○eucalyptus

Other Products: ○Mito2Max, ○Alpha CRS+, ○a2z Chewable, ○xEO Mega or vEO Mega, ○IQ Mega, ○Microplex VMz to provide nutrients and antioxidants that help support healthy cellular function and energy levels.

—Exhaustion:

Oils: First, work with one or more of the following nervous system oils to help calm and relax: ○lavender, ○ylang ylang, ○Roman chamomile, ○frankincense, ○clary sage. Secondly, use an energizing oil such as ○lemon, ○sandalwood, ○rosemary, ○○lime, ○basil, ○grapefruit.

—Fatigue:

Oils: ○○rosemary (nervous fatigue), ○○thyme (general fatigue)

—Mental Fatigue:

Oils: ○○Serenity, ○○Calmer, ○○lemongrass, ○○basil, ○petitgrain

Blend 1: Blend equal parts basil and lemongrass together. Apply to temples, back of neck, and feet. Diffuse into the air.

—Physical Fatigue:

Oils: ○○Serenity

—Physical:

Oils: ○lemon, ○cinnamon, ○bergamot

—Sexual:

Oils: ○ylang ylang

○: Diffuse into the air. Inhale directly from bottle. Apply oil to hands, tissue, or cotton wick, and inhale.

○: Dilute 1–2 drops in 1 Tbs. (15 ml) fractionated coconut oil, and massage into muscles. Place 1–2 drops in warm bathwater, and bathe. Dilute as recommended, and apply 1–2 drops on temples, back of neck, liver area, or feet.

○: Take capsules as directed on package.

○: **Body System(s) Affected:** Nervous System and Emotional Balance.

○: **Additional Research:**

Peppermint: (Meamarbashi et al., 2013).

Epilepsy

See **Seizure: Epilepsy**

Epstein-Barr

See **Mono;** *see also* **Antiviral: Epstein-Barr Virus**

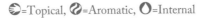
○=Topical, ○=Aromatic, ○=Internal

Estrogen

Estrogens are hormones produced by the ovaries that regulate the development of female characteristics and the menstrual cycle in females.

Oils: ⊘⊘ClaryCalm, ⊘⊘clary sage

Other Products: ⵔPhytoestrogen Lifetime Complex

⊖: Apply on the lower abdomen. Dilute 1–2 drops in 1 Tbs. (15 ml) fractionated coconut oil, and use as massage oil.

ⵔ: Take capsules as directed on package.

⊘: Diffuse into the air. Inhale directly from bottle. Apply oil to hands, tissue, or cotton wick, and inhale.

⊕: **Body System(s) Affected:** Reproductive System.

Exhaustion

See Energy: Exhaustion

Expectorant

See Congestion: Expectorant

Eyes

Eyes are the organs of the body responsible for detecting and adjusting to light and focusing images of the surrounding environment onto the optical nerve for transfer to the brain for processing.

Oils: ⊘lemongrass, ⊘sandalwood, ⊘cypress, ⊘lemon, ⊘fennel, ⊘eucalyptus, ⊘lavender, ⊘On Guard

Other Products: ⵔMicroplex VMz for nutrients that help support healthy eye cell function.

—Blocked Tear Ducts:

Tears from the eye normally drain through small tubes called tear ducts. The tear ducts carry tears from the surface of the eye into the nose where they are reabsorbed or evaporate. When these tear ducts are blocked, the eyes become watery and irritated. Blocked tear ducts are most common in babies and in older adults.

Oils: ⊘lavender

—Cataracts:

A cataract is a clouding of the normally transparent lens of the eye. This clouding results in blurry vision, seemingly faded colors, double vision, glare, and difficulty seeing at night. Over

time, the clouding can increase and lead to severe vision problems.

Oils: ⊘clove, ⊘lavender

Blend 1: Combine 8 drops lemongrass, 6 drops cypress, and 3 drops eucalyptus. Apply around the eye area twice a day. Do not get oil in the eyes.

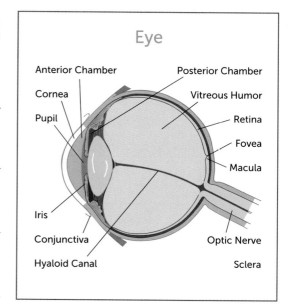

Eye

Anterior Chamber — Posterior Chamber
Cornea — Vitreous Humor
Pupil — Retina
— Fovea
— Macula
Iris
Conjunctiva — Optic Nerve
Hyaloid Canal — Sclera

—Dry/Itchy Eyes:

Oils: ⊘melaleuca (in humidifier)

—Eye Lid Drop/Drooping Eyelid:

A drooping eyelid is characterized by an excessive sagging of the upper eyelid. Drooping can be present at birth as a result of underdeveloped eyelid muscles, or it can occur with aging. Drooping eyelids can cause visual impairment if they droop enough to partially cover the eye.

Blend 2: Combine equal parts helichrysum and peppermint, and apply 1–2 drops on the eyelid. Do not get oil in the eyes.

—Improve Vision:

Oils: ⊘frankincense, ⊘lemongrass, ⊘juniper berry, ⊘On Guard, ⊘sandalwood, ⊘lavender

Blend 3: Combine 10 drops lemongrass, 5 drops cypress, and 3 drops eucalyptus with 2 Tbs. (25 ml) fractionated coconut oil. Apply around the eyes morning and night, or apply on reflex points on the feet or on the ears.

Primary Recommendations • Secondary Recommendations • Other Recommendations

—Iris Inflammation:

The iris is the colored part of the eye that regulates the amount of light entering the eye through the pupil. When the iris becomes inflamed, it results in a condition called iritis. Iritis is normally related to a disease or infection in another part of the body, but it can also be caused by injury to the eye. Symptoms of iritis include blurred vision, pain, tearing, light sensitivity, red eye, and a small pupil size.

Oils: ⊘eucalyptus

—Macular Degeneration:

Macular degeneration is an eye disease common in individuals 65 and older. It is marked by degeneration of a small, oval-shaped part of the retina called the macula. Because the macula is responsible for capturing the light from the central part of images coming into the eye, macular degeneration causes blurring or a blind spot in the central vision, making it difficult to drive, recognize faces, read, or do any kind of detail work.

Oils: ⊘clove

—Pink Eye:

Pink eye, also known as conjunctivitis, is an inflammation or infection of the membranes covering the whites of the eyes (conjunctiva) and the inner part of the eyelids. Swelling, redness, itching, discharge, and burning of the eyes are common symptoms of pink eye. Frequent causes include allergies, bacterial or viral infection, contact lenses, and eye drops.

Oils: ⊘⊘melaleuca, ⊘⊘lavender

—Retina (strengthen):

The retina is a layer of nerves lining the back of the eye. The retina is responsible for sensing light and then sending impulses (via the optic nerve) back to the brain so that visual images can be formed.

Oils: ⊘cypress, ⊘lemongrass, ⊘helichrysum, ⊘juniper berry, ⊘peppermint, ⊘lavender, ⊘sandalwood

—Swollen Eyes:

Oils: ⊘cypress, ⊘helichrysum, ⊘peppermint (allergies), ⊘lavender

◐: Caution: Never put essential oils directly in the eyes! Be careful when applying oils near the eyes. Be sure to have some fractionated coconut oil handy for additional dilution if irritation occurs. Never use water to wash off an oil that irritates. Dilute as recommended, and apply 1–2 drops

around eyes or to feet, thumbs, ankles, pelvis, base of neck, or reflex points on the feet.

⊘: Diffuse into the air.

◯: Take capsules as directed on package.

✛: **Body System(s) Affected:** Muscles, Nervous System, and Immune System.

Facial Oils
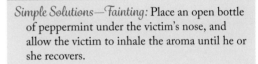

See Skin

Fainting

See also Shock

> *Simple Solutions—Fainting:* Place an open bottle of peppermint under the victim's nose, and allow the victim to inhale the aroma until he or she recovers.

Fainting is a temporary loss of consciousness caused by a momentary disruption of blood flow to the brain. Fainting can result from standing in one place too long, coughing very hard, fear, emotional trauma, heavy bleeding, or severe dehydration. Fainting can sometimes be a symptom of a more serious condition.

Oils: ⊘peppermint, ⊘rosemary, ⊘basil, ⊘lavender

⊘: Inhale directly from bottle.

✛: **Body System(s) Affected:** Nervous System.

Fatigue

See Energy: Fatigue

Fear

See also Anxiety, Calming

> *Simple Solutions—Fear:* Diffuse Peace in an aromatherapy diffuser.

> *Simple Solutions—Fear:* Add 3 drops lavender and 2 drops ylang ylang to 2 Tbs. (25 ml) of water in a small misting spray bottle. Allow children to spray into the air to help spray away fears.

Fear causes the blood vessels to tighten, restricting the amount of oxygen and nutrients that can reach the cells.

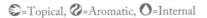

⊘=Topical, ⊘=Aromatic, ◯=Internal

Oils: 🌀🍃Peace, 🌀🍃Balance, 🌀🍃Steady, 🌀🍃ylang ylang🔲, 🍃orange🔲, 🌀🍃sandalwood, 🌀🍃clary sage, 🌀🍃geranium, 🌀🍃juniper berry, 🌀🍃myrrh, 🌀🍃bergamot, 🌀🍃fir, 🌀🍃cypress, 🌀🍃marjoram

🌀: Diffuse into the air. Inhale directly from bottle. Apply oil to hands, tissue, or cotton wick, and inhale.

🍃: Dilute as recommended, and apply 1–2 drops to temples, back of neck, or bottoms of feet.

🧍: **Body System(s) Affected:** Nervous System.

🔲: **Additional Research:**

Ylang ylang: (Hongratanaworakit et al., 2006); **Orange:** (Lehrner et al., 2000).

Feet

See Foot

Female-Specific Conditions

See also Endometriosis, Pregnancy/Motherhood

—Hemorrhaging: *See Blood: Hemorrhaging*

—Hot Flashes:

A hot flash is a sudden, intense feeling of heat in the face and upper body, often accompanied by an increased heart rate, sweating, dizziness, headache, weakness, or anxiety. Hot flashes are generally associated with the symptoms of menopause and premenopause.

> *Simple Solutions—Hot Flash:* Add 5 drops clary sage to 1 Tbs. (15 ml) jojoba oil, and add to bathwater as a bath oil.

Oils: 🍃🍃ClaryCalm, 🍃Balance, 🍃peppermint, 🍃clary sage

Other Products: ⭕Phytoestrogen Lifetime Complex, ⭕Daily Supplements Pack (contains Alpha CRS+, xEO Mega or vEO Mega, ⭕IQ Mega, and Microplex VMz)

Recipe 1: Both morning and evening, apply 1–2 drops each of Balance and peppermint to back of neck; then apply 1–2 drops clary sage to forearms in the morning and to ankles in the evening. The Daily Supplements Pack may also be taken to help regulate the hormonal system.

—Hormones (balancing):

Oils: 🍃🍃ClaryCalm, 🍃🍃ylang ylang, 🍃🍃clary sage

Other Products: ⭕Phytoestrogen Lifetime Complex

—Infertility:

Infertility is clinically defined as the inability to get pregnant after a year of trying. This could be due to any of several underlying causes.

Oils: 🍃clary sage, 🍃geranium, 🍃melissa, 🍃cypress, 🍃thyme, 🍃fennel, 🍃Roman chamomile, 🍃ylang ylang

—Menopause:

Menopause is the permanent ending of a female's menstruation and fertility. For most American women, Menopause occurs around age 51 and is often recognized by hot flashes, irregular periods, vaginal dryness, mood swings, difficulty sleeping, thinning hair, abdominal weight gain, and decreased fertility.

Oils: 🍃🍃ClaryCalm, 🍃cypress, 🍃lavender🔲, 🍃Roman chamomile, 🍃orange, 🍃clary sage, 🍃⭕fennel🔲, 🍃basil, 🍃geranium, 🍃rosemary, 🍃thyme

Other Products: ⭕Phytoestrogen Lifetime Complex, ⭕Bone Nutrient Lifetime Complex

–Premenopause:

Oils: 🍃🍃ClaryCalm, 🍃clary sage, 🍃lavender

Other Products: ⭕Phytoestrogen Lifetime Complex, ⭕Bone Nutrient Lifetime Complex

—Menstruation:

Menstruation, also known as a woman's "period," is the regular shedding of the uterus lining and vaginal discharge of blood when a woman is not pregnant. A woman's period lasts between 2 and 7 days and reoccurs on an average of every 28 days.

–Amenorrhea:

Amenorrhea is the absence of menstruation. The following oils may help induce menstrual flow (emmenagogic) and may need to be avoided during pregnancy for this reason. See Pregnancy/Motherhood for further safety data.

Oils: 🍃🍃ClaryCalm, 🍃basil, 🍃clary sage, 🍃peppermint, 🍃rosemary, 🍃juniper berry, 🍃marjoram, 🍃lavender, 🍃Roman chamomile

Other Products: ⭕Phytoestrogen Lifetime Complex

–Dysmenorrhea:

Dysmenorrhea is painful menstruation. Apply one or more of these oils to the abdomen. It may also help to use a hot compress.

Oils: ClaryCalm, clary sage, geranium, lavender, rose, cypress, peppermint, marjoram, Roman chamomile, basil, rosemary, fennel

Other Products: Phytoestrogen Lifetime Complex

–Irregular:

Oils: ClaryCalm, peppermint, rosemary, Roman chamomile, clary sage, fennel, lavender, spikenard, rose

Other Products: Phytoestrogen Lifetime Complex

–Menorrhagia:

Menorrhagia is abnormally heavy or extended menstrual flow. It may also refer to irregular bleeding at any time. This situation may be a sign of a more serious condition, so please see your doctor.

Oils: ClaryCalm, cypress, geranium, Roman chamomile, rose

Other Products: Phytoestrogen Lifetime Complex

–Scanty:

Oils: ClaryCalm, peppermint, lavender, melissa

Other Products: Phytoestrogen Lifetime Complex

—Ovaries:

Ovaries are the female reproductive organs in which eggs are produced and stored.

Oils: ClaryCalm, rosemary, geranium, DigestZen

Other Products: Phytoestrogen Lifetime Complex

–Ovarian Cyst:

Oils: basil

—PMS:

Premenstrual syndrome (PMS) is a group of symptoms such as irritability, anxiety, moodiness, bloating, breast tenderness, headaches, and cramping that occurs in the days or hours before menstruation begins and then disappear once menstruation begins. PMS is thought to be caused by the fluctuation in hormones during this time or by the way progesterone is broken down by the body. Caffeine intake from beverages or chocolate is also thought to enhance PMS symptoms.

> *Simple Solutions—PMS:* Combine 3 drops clary sage and 3 drops geranium with 1 tsp. (5 ml) almond oil. Add to warm bathwater for a soothing bath.

Oils: ClaryCalm, clary sage, geranium, fennel, lavender, bergamot, grapefruit, neroli

Other Products: Phytoestrogen Lifetime Complex, Bone Nutrient Lifetime Complex or Microplex VMz contain calcium, which has been found to help lessen PMS symptoms.

–Apathetic-Tired-Listless:

Oils: ClaryCalm, grapefruit, geranium, bergamot, fennel

Other Products: Phytoestrogen Lifetime Complex

–Irritable:

Oils: ClaryCalm, clary sage, bergamot, Roman chamomile

Other Products: Phytoestrogen Lifetime Complex

–Violent Aggressive:

Oils: ClaryCalm, geranium, bergamot

Other Products: Phytoestrogen Lifetime Complex

–Weeping-Depression:

Oils: ClaryCalm, clary sage, bergamot, geranium

Other Products: Phytoestrogen Lifetime Complex

—Postpartum Depression: *See Pregnancy/Motherhood: Postpartum Depression*

: Dilute as recommended, and apply to the abdomen, lower back, shoulders, or reflex points on the feet. Add 1–2 drops to 1 Tbs. (15 ml) fractionated coconut oil, and massage into abdomen, lower back, and shoulders. Apply as a warm compress

=Topical, =Aromatic, =Internal

to the abdomen. Add 1–2 drops to 2 tsp. (10 ml) olive oil, insert into vagina, and retain overnight with a tampon.

@: Place in hands and inhale. Diffuse into the air.

O: Take capsules as directed on package.

⊕: **Body System(s) Affected:** Reproductive System and Endocrine System.

⊕: **Additional Research:**

Lavender: Yamada et al., 2005; Fennel: Kim et al., 2012; Clary Sage: Han et al., 2006; Clary Sage, Lavender, and Marjoram: Ou et al., 2012; Rose: Bani et al., 2014; Thyme: Salmalian et al., 2014.

Fertility

See Female-Specific Conditions: Infertility, Male Specific Conditions: Infertility

Fever

See also Cooling Oils

Fever is an increase of the body's core temperature, typically in response to an infection or injury. A fever is the body's natural response to help enhance the immune system's ability to fight the infection.

> *Simple Solutions—Fever:* Blend 2 drops peppermint and 2 drops eucalyptus in a bowl of cool water. Moisten washcloth with water, and use to sponge the forehead, back of neck, and feet.

Oils: O⊜@peppermint, O⊜lemon, O⊜@lime, ⊜eucalyptus, Oclove, O⊜@patchouli, ⊜melaleuca, ⊜ginger, ⊜lavender, ⊜basil, ⊜fir, ⊜bergamot

—To Cool the System:

Oils: Oclove, O⊜@peppermint, ⊜eucalyptus, ⊜bergamot

—To Induce Sweating:

Oils: ⊜basil, ⊜fennel, ⊜melaleuca, ⊜peppermint, ⊜rosemary, ⊜lavender, ⊜cypress

O: Place 1–2 drops of oil under the tongue or place 1–2 drops of essential oil into capsule; then swallow capsule. Place 1–2 drops in 1 cup (250 ml) of rice milk or water, and sip slowly.

⊜: Dilute as recommended, and apply to back or to bottoms of the feet.

@: Diffuse into the air.

⊕: **Body System(s) Affected:** Immune System.

Fibrillation

See Cardiovascular System

Fibroids

Fibroids are noncancerous growths of muscle and connective tissue in the uterus. Fibroids can be painful and may affect fertility and pregnancy.

Oils: ⊜frankincense, ⊜helichrysum, ⊜oregano, ⊜Balance, ⊜lavender

⊜: Place 3 drops of oil in douche. Dilute as recommended, and apply to reflex points on the feet.

⊕: **Body System(s) Affected:** Reproductive System and Endocrine System.

Fibromyalgia

Fibromyalgia is long-term localized or generalized aches, pain, or tenderness in the muscles, ligaments, or other soft tissue that can interfere with normal movement, sleep, or other activities. There is no known cause of fibromyalgia, and many different factors may contribute to the development of this condition. Some have suggested eliminating refined sugar from the diet. Others have recommended reducing stress, stretching exercises, massage, or better sleep.

Oils: ⊜Deep Blue, ⊜wintergreen, ⊜helichrysum, ⊜lavender, ⊜rosemary, ⊜thyme

Other Products: OMito2Max, OAlpha CRS+, Oa2z Chewable, OxEO Mega or vEO Mega, OIQ Mega, OMicroplex VMz for nutrients needed for healthy muscle and nerve cell function.

⊜: Add 1–2 drops of oil to 1 Tbs. (15 ml) fractionated coconut oil, and massage on location. Apply as a warm compress over affected area.

O: Take capsules as directed on package.

⊕: **Body System(s) Affected:** Immune System and Muscles.

Finger (mashed)

Recipe 1: Apply 1 drop geranium (for bruising), 1 drop helichrysum (to stop the bleeding), 1 drop lavender, 1 drop lemongrass (for tissue repair), and 1 drop Deep Blue (for pain).

Flatulence

See Digestive System: Gas/Flatulence

Flu

See Influenza

Fluids

See Edema, Diuretic

Food Poisoning

See also Antibacterial, Antifungal, Antiviral, Digestive System, Parasites

Food poisoning refers to the effects on the digestive tract by pathogenic organisms—or the toxins they produce—that are ingested into the body in food. Symptoms of food poisoning can include stomach pain, cramps, diarrhea, nausea, and vomiting.

Oils: ⭕DigestZen🔲, ⭕⭕On Guard, ⭕rosemary

Other Products: ⭕DigestZen Softgels, ⭕⭕On Guard+ Softgels

⭕: Add 6 drops to 1 cup (250 ml) of water. Swish around in the mouth, and swallow. Place 1–2 drops in an empty capsule, and swallow.

🔆: **Body System(s) Affected:** Digestive System and Immune System.

🔲: **Additional Research:**

DigestZen: (Imai et al., 2001).

Foot

Oils: 🌀lemon, 🌀lavender, 🌀Roman chamomile

—**Athlete's Foot:** *See Antifungal: Athlete's Foot*

—**Blisters:**

Oils: 🌀lavender, 🌀geranium, 🌀melaleuca, 🌀Purify

—**Bunion:** *See also Bursitis*

A bunion is bursitis located at the base of the big toe. It is often caused by constrictive shoes that force the big toe to point inward and the base of the big toe to jut outward. This misplacement can irritate the bursa located at the base of the toe and cause it to become inflamed, which causes further irritation.

Oils: 🌀cypress

—**Calluses:**

A callus is a flat, thick growth of skin that develops on areas of the skin where there is constant friction or rubbing. Calluses typically form on the bottoms of the feet, but they can also form on the hands or other areas of the body exposed to constant friction.

Oils: 🌀oregano

—**Club Foot:**

Oils: 🌀ginger, 🌀rosemary, 🌀lavender, 🌀Roman chamomile

—**Corns:**

Corns are painful growths that develop on the small toes due to repetitive friction in that area (often from ill-fitting footwear). If untreated, corns can cause increased pressure on underlying tissue, causing tissue damage or ulcerations.

Oils: 🌀clove, 🌀peppermint, 🌀grapefruit, 🌀Citrus Bliss

🌀: Dilute as recommended, and apply to area. Combine 1–2 drops with fractionated coconut oil, and massage on location.

🔆: **Body System(s) Affected:** Muscles, Skeletal System, and Skin.

Forgetfulness

See Memory

Free Radicals

See Antioxidant

Frigidity

See Sexual Issues: Female Frigidity

Fungus

See Antifungal

Gallbladder

The gallbladder is a small sac that stores extra bile from the liver until it is needed to help with digestion in the small intestine. The gallbladder is located just below the liver.

Oils: 🌀geranium, 🌀rosemary, 🌀lavender, 🌀juniper berry

🌀=Topical, 🔆=Aromatic, ⭕=Internal

—Infection:

Oils: ◖helichrysum

—Stones:

> Gallstones are formed by cholesterol that has crystallized from the bile stored in the gallbladder. These stones can sometimes block the duct that comes from the gallbladder or the small opening from the common hepatic duct that allows bile to flow into the small intestine. Gallstones blocking these ducts can be painful and can lead to more serious complications, such as infections or jaundice.

> *Simple Solutions—Gallstones:* Apply 1 drop each of grapefruit and geranium over the gallbladder area. Hold a washcloth moistened with warm water over the area for 15 minutes.

Oils: ◖grapefruit, ◖geranium, ◖rosemary, ◖juniper berry, ◖wintergreen, ◖lime

◔: Dilute as recommended, and apply 1–2 drops over gallbladder area. Apply as a warm compress over the gallbladder area.

⊕: **Body System(s) Affected:** Endocrine System and Digestive System.

Gallstones

See Gallbladder: Stones

Gangrene

Gangrene is the localized decay of body tissue caused by a loss of blood to that area. Gas gangrene is caused by bacteria invading a deep wound that has lessened the blood supply or cut it off entirely. The bacteria create gases and pus in the infected area, causing severe pain and accelerating decay of the tissue.

Oils: ◖lavender, ◖On Guard, ◖thyme

◔: Dilute as recommended, and apply 1–3 drops on location.

⊕: **Body System(s) Affected:** Skin and Immune System.

Gas

See Digestive System: Gas/Flatulence

Gastritis

See Digestive System: Gastritis

Genitals

See Female-Specific Conditions, Male Specific Conditions/Issues

Germs

See Antibacterial, Antifungal, Antiviral

Gingivitis

See Oral Conditions: Gum Disease

Goiter

See Thyroid: Hyperthyroidism

Gout

Gout is a painful inflammation of a joint caused by a buildup of uric acid crystals deposited in the joint. Uric acid is formed during the natural breakdown of dead tissues in the body. An excess of uric acid in the bloodstream can lead to the formation of crystals in the joints or kidneys (kidney stones). Some good ways to prevent the formation of uric acid crystals include maintaining a healthy body weight (which leaves less body tissue to be broken down), exercising, and drinking plenty of water.

> *Simple Solutions—Gout:* Apply 1 drop Deep Blue on joint to help soothe pain.

Oils: ○◖lemon, ◖geranium, ◖Deep Blue, ◖wintergreen, ◖thyme

○: Place 1–2 drops in 1 cup (250 ml) of water, and drink. Place 1–2 drops of oil under the tongue or place 1–2 drops in an empty capsule, and swallow.

◔: Dilute as recommended, and apply on location. Add 1–2 drops to 1 Tbs. (15 ml) fractionated coconut oil, and massage on location.

⊕: **Body System(s) Affected:** Immune System.

Grave's Disease

See Thyroid: Hyperthyroidism

Grave's disease is an autoimmune disease caused by an abnormally shaped protein stimulating the thyroid to make and secrete more hormones. This can cause an enlargement of the thyroid (goiter), bulging eyes, increased heart rate, high blood pressure, and anxiety.

Oils: ⬤⬤lemongrass, ⬤⬤myrrh

Other Products: ⬤Microplex VMz for nutrients and minerals to help support thyroid function.

⬤: Dilute as recommended, and apply on thyroid area or on reflex points on the feet.

⬤: Diffuse into the air.

⬤: Take capsules as directed on package.

⬤: **Body System(s) Affected:** Endocrine System.

Grief/Sorrow

Simple Solutions—Grief: Diffuse citrus oils in an aromatherapy diffuser.

Oils: ⬤⬤Cheer, ⬤⬤Console, ⬤⬤lemon①, ⬤⬤Elevation, ⬤Balance, ⬤⬤Steady, ⬤⬤Forgive, ⬤⬤lavender, ⬤⬤bergamot①, ⬤⬤clary sage, ⬤⬤juniper berry, ⬤⬤eucalyptus, ⬤⬤helichrysum

⬤: Diffuse into the air. Inhale directly from bottle. Apply oil to hands, tissue, or cotton wick, and inhale. Wear 1–2 drops as perfume or cologne.

⬤: Dilute as recommended, and apply 1–2 drops to the forehead, shoulders, or feet. Add 1–2 drops to 1 Tbs. (15 ml) fractionated coconut oil, and massage over whole body.

⬤: **Body System(s) Affected:** Emotional Balance.

⬤: **Additional Research:**

Lemon: (Kiecolt-Glaser et al., 2008); Lemon: (Komiya et al., 2006); Lemon: (Komori et al., 1995); Lemon: (Komori et al., 1995); Bergamot: (Komori et al., 1995).

Gum Disease

See Oral Conditions: Gum Disease

Gums

See Oral Conditions: Gums

Habits

See Addictions

Hair

Other Products: ⬤Smoothing Conditioner, ⬤Protecting Shampoo, ⬤Root to Tip Serum, ⬤Healthy Hold Glaze.

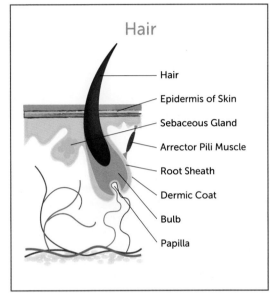

Hair

- Hair
- Epidermis of Skin
- Sebaceous Gland
- Arrector Pili Muscle
- Root Sheath
- Dermic Coat
- Bulb
- Papilla

—Beard:

Oils: ⬤rosemary, ⬤lemon, ⬤lavender, ⬤thyme, ⬤cypress

—Children:

Oils: ⬤lavender

—Damaged:

Other Products: ⬤Smoothing Conditioner, ⬤Protecting Shampoo, ⬤Root to Tip Serum

—Dandruff: *See also Antifungal*

Dandruff is a scalp condition characterized by the excessive shedding of dead skin cells. A small amount of flaking on the scalp is normal as old skin cells die off and fall away, but dandruff results when the amount of dead skin cells becomes excessive and visible. Dandruff can be caused by many possible factors: hormonal imbalance, poor hygiene, allergies, excessive use of hair sprays and gels, excessive use of curling irons, cold weather,

⬤=Topical, ⬤=Aromatic, ⬤=Internal

infrequent shampooing, etc. Many specialists believe that dandruff is caused by a tiny fungus called *Pityrosporum ovale*.

Simple Solutions—Dandruff: Combine 3 drops wintergreen with 1 tsp. (5 ml) jojoba oil, and apply to scalp in shower before washing hair.

Oils: lavender, wintergreen, cypress, rosemary, cedarwood, thyme, manuka

—Dry:

Oils: geranium, sandalwood, lavender, rosemary, wintergreen

Other Products: Smoothing Conditioner, Protecting Shampoo, Root to Tip Serum

—Estrogen Balance:

Estrogen is a steroid hormone that causes the development of female characteristics such as breasts and larger hips, helps with calcium uptake and balance, and plays many other important roles. Estrogen also helps hair to grow faster and to stay on the head longer. If estrogen levels fall, hair loss can quickly result.

Oils: clary sage

—Fragile Hair:

Oils: clary sage, lavender, thyme, sandalwood, wintergreen, Roman chamomile

Other Products: Smoothing Conditioner, Protecting Shampoo, Root to Tip Serum

—Greasy/Oily Hair:

Oils: basil, cypress, thyme, lemon, rosemary, petitgrain

Other Products: Smoothing Conditioner, Protecting Shampoo

—Growth (stimulate):

Oils: thyme, lavender, rosemary, ylang ylang, cedarwood, clary sage, geranium, ginger, lemon, grapefruit

—Itching:

Oils: peppermint, lavender

—Loss:

One common form of hair loss, especially in males, is androgenic alopecia (also known as male-pattern baldness in males). This condition is thought to be caused by a genetically predisposed sensitivity within the hair follicles to androgen hormones that causes them to shrink when exposed to this hormone. This shrinking of the hair follicles inhibits their ability to produce hair, leading to a receding hairline and partial baldness on the top and sides of the head in males and thinning hair in females. Another common form of baldness, especially in females, is alopecia areata, which is a condition in which hair loss occurs on all or part of the body. The most common form of alopecia areata involves the loss of round patches of hair on the scalp, leading this condition to be commonly referred to as "spot baldness."

Oils: rosemary, lavender, thyme, ylang ylang, cedarwood, wintergreen, lemon, clary sage, cypress, Roman chamomile

: Apply 1–2 drops of oil to hands, and massage into hair and scalp before bath or shower; then shampoo and rinse hair as normal. Add 1–2 drops of oil to 2 Tbs. (25 ml) of an unscented shampoo or shower gel, and use to shampoo hair. Use shampoo and conditioner as directed on bottles.

: **Body System(s) Affected:** Hair.

: **Additional Research:**

Thyme, Lavender, Rosemary, Cedarwood: Hay et al., 1998.

Halitosis

See **Oral Conditions: Halitosis**

Hands

Oils: geranium, lemon, lemongrass, sandalwood, rosemary, eucalyptus

—Dry:

Oils: geranium, sandalwood

—Neglected:

Oils: geranium, lemon

—Tingling In:

Oils: lemongrass

: Dilute as recommended, and apply 1–2 drops to hands. Dilute 1–2 drops in 1 Tbs. (15 ml) almond or olive oil, and use as massage oil to massage into hands.

: **Body System(s) Affected:** Skin and Muscles.

...ngovers

...ngover is a set of unpleasant physical effects that comes ...heavy alcohol consumption. Common symptoms of a ...over include nausea, headache, lack of energy, diarrhea, ...ncreased sensitivity to light and noise.

...mple Solutions—Hangover: Add 5 drops grapefruit, ...2 drops rosemary, and 1 drop juniper berry to 1 ...cup (250 g) Epsom salt. Dissolve ½ cup (125 g) of the salt in warm bathwater for a soothing bath.

lemon, grapefruit, lavender, rosemary, sandalwood

...Add 3–4 drops to warm bathwater, and bathe. Dilute as recommended, and apply 1–2 drops to back of neck or over liver. Add 1–2 drops to 1 Tbs. (15 ml) fractionated coconut oil, and massage onto back and neck.

- Inhale directly from bottle. Apply oil to hands, tissue, or cotton wick, and inhale. Drop 1–2 drops in bowl of hot water, and inhale vapors. Diffuse into the air.

- **Body System(s) Affected:** Digestive System.

Hashimoto's Disease

See also Thyroid: Hypothyroidism

Hashimoto's disease is an autoimmune disorder where the immune system attacks the thyroid, causing it to swell up and become irritated. Hashimoto's disease does not have a unique set of symptoms, but possible symptoms include abnormal fatigue, weight gain, muscle pain and stiffness, a hoarse voice, prolonged menstrual bleeding, constipation, a feeling of tightness in the throat, sensitivity to cold, dry skin, and depression.

Oils: lemongrass, myrrh

Other Products: Microplex VMz, Alpha CRS+, a2z Chewable to help provide nutrients essential for thyroid cell health.

- Dilute as recommended, and apply 1–2 drops over thyroid area or on reflex points on the feet.

- Diffuse into the air. Inhale oil applied to hands.

- Take capsules as directed on package.

- **Body System(s) Affected:** Immune System and Endocrine System.

Hay Fever

See Allergies: Hay Fever

Head Lice

See Insects/Bugs: Lice

Headaches

Simple Solutions—Headache: Apply 1 drop each of lavender, peppermint, and frankincense to the back of the neck and forehead.

Oils: PastTense, peppermint, rosemary, Deep Blue, Rescuer, cardamom, eucalyptus, frankincense, lavender, patchouli, basil, marjoram, neroli, clove

—Migraine Headache:

A migraine is a severe and painful type of headache. Symptoms of migraines include throbbing pain accompanied by nausea, vomiting, and heightened sensitivity to light. Women are much more likely than men to suffer from migraines. Migraines can be triggered by stress, anxiety, sleep or food deprivation, bright lights, loud noises, and hormonal changes.

Oils: PastTense, Rescuer, peppermint, basil, Deep Blue, wintergreen, spikenard, ylang ylang

—Tension Headache:

Tension headaches (also called "stress headaches") are the most common type of headache. Tension headaches are characterized by dull, constant pressure or pain (usually on both sides of the head). Tension headaches can last from 30 minutes to several days and tend to come back when a person is under stress.

Oils: PastTense, Rescuer, peppermint, Deep Blue

—Sugar Headache (caused by low blood sugar):

Oils: On Guard

- Dilute as recommended, and apply 1–2 drops to temples, back of neck, and forehead.

- Diffuse into the air. Inhale directly from bottle. Apply oil to hands, tissue, or cotton wick, and inhale.

- **Body System(s) Affected:** Nervous System.

- **Additional Research:**

 Peppermint: Göbel et al., 1994; **Lavender:** Sasannejad et al., 2012.

=Topical, =Aromatic, =Internal

Hearing

See **Ears**

Heart

See **Cardiovascular System: Heart**

Heartburn

See **Digestive System: Heartburn**

Heatstroke

Heatstroke is when the body's temperature rises dangerously high due to the body's inability to dissipate heat, typically because of high environmental temperatures and high levels of exertion. If not corrected, the body can overheat too much, causing organs and body systems to become damaged and possibly shut down—possibly leading to death. Symptoms of heatstroke include perspiration, dizziness, confusion, headaches, and nausea.

Simple Solutions—Heatstroke: Get to cooler location, and remove any excess clothing. Add 2 drops peppermint to cool water in a bowl, and use to sponge down body. Seek medical attention as soon as possible.

Oils: ○peppermint, ○lavender

○: Dilute as recommended, and apply 3–5 drops on neck and forehead. Cool the body as soon as possible in a cool bathtub, lake, river, or soaked linens.

⊕: **Body System(s) Affected:** Nervous System.

Hematoma

See also **Blood: Hemorrhaging.**

A hematoma is a collection of blood outside of the blood vessels. The most common form of a hematoma is a bruise. Hematomas can also form into hard, blood-filled sacs that look like welts and can move to different locations. These often dissolve on their own. Hematomas can also form in other organs as the result of injury or hemorrhaging.

Simple Solutions—Hematoma: Apply 1 drop helichrysum on location, and then hold a cloth soaked in cool water on top and hold in place for 15 minutes.

Oils: ○helichrysum

○: Dilute as recommended, and apply 1–2 drops on location.

⊕: **Body System(s) Affected:** Cardiovascular System.

Hemorrhaging

See **Blood: Hemorrhaging**

Hemorrhoids

Hemorrhoids are swollen, twisted veins that occur in the rectum or anus. They are caused by increased pressure within the veins, often due to pregnancy, frequent lifting, or constipation.

Simple Solutions—Hemorrhoids: Mix 1 drop cypress with 1 drop of either helichrysum or geranium, and apply on location.

Oils: ○cypress, ○geranium, ○clary sage, ○helichrysum, ○patchouli, ○copaiba, ○peppermint, ○sandalwood, ○juniper berry, ○frankincense, ○myrrh

○: Dilute as recommended, and apply 1–2 drops on location. Mix 1–2 drops with 1 tsp. (5 ml) fractionated coconut oil, and apply on location using a rectal syringe.

⊕: **Body System(s) Affected:** Cardiovascular System.

Hepatitis

See **Liver: Hepatitis**

Hernia

See also **Back: Herniated Discs**

A hernia is the protrusion of a tissue or organ through tissue or muscle outside of the body cavity in which it is normally contained. There are several different types of hernias, and the symptoms vary with each type.

—Hiatal:

A hiatal (hiatus) hernia is when a portion of the stomach protrudes through the diaphragm into the chest cavity above. This can cause pain, acid reflux, and heartburn. It can be caused by a birth defect or may be brought on by heavy lifting, stress, or being overweight.

Oils: ☍basil, ☍peppermint, ☍cypress, ☍ginger, ☍geranium, ☍lavender, ☍fennel, ☍rosemary

—Incisional:

An incisional hernia is caused by a protrusion through scar tissue from an abdominal wound or incision that hasn't healed correctly.

Oils: ☍basil, ☍helichrysum, ☍lemongrass, ☍geranium, ☍lavender, ☍ginger, ☍lemon, ☍melaleuca

—Inguinal:

An inguinal hernia is when the intestines protrude into the inguinal canal (a small opening that leads from the abdominal cavity into the groin area). This can sometimes be seen as a bulge in the groin area and is usually painless, but it may become painful if the blood supply to the herniated portion of the intestine is restricted (strangulated).

Oils: ☍lemongrass, ☍lavender

☍: Dilute as recommended, and apply on location, lower back, and reflex points on the feet.

✛: **Body System(s) Affected:** Muscles.

Herpes Simplex

See also **Antiviral**

Herpes simplex type 1 and type 2 viruses are the two viruses that cause genital and oral herpes infections. These viruses cause painful outbreaks of blisters and sores to occur in the affected area when the virus is active in the skin or mucus membranes, followed by periods of latency when the virus resides in the nerve cells around the infected area.

> *Simple Solutions—Cold Sores:* Combine 4 tsp. (5 g) beeswax pellets, 1 Tbs. (10 g) cocoa butter, and 3 Tbs. (45 ml) jojoba oil, and melt in the microwave (30 seconds at a time, stirring in between) or in a double boiler. Cool slightly, and add 5 drops melissa, 5 drops peppermint, and 5 drops helichrysum essential oil. Pour into small jars or lip balm containers, and allow to cool completely. Apply a small amount of balm on cold sores as needed.

Oils: ☍peppermint○, ☍melaleuca○, ☍helichrysum○, ☍clove○, ☍lavender, ☍eucalyptus○, ☍lemon, ☍cypress, ☍rose, ☍bergamot

☍: Dilute as recommended, and apply oil directly on the lesions at the first sign of outbreak.

✛: **Body System(s) Affected:** Immune System.

▭: **Additional Research:**

> Peppermint: Schuhmacher et al., 2003; **Melaleuca:** Schnitzler et al., 2001; **Helichrysum:** Nostro et al., 2003; **Clove:** Benencia et al., 2000; **Eucalyptus:** Schnitzler et al., 2001.

Hiccups/Hiccoughs

Hiccups, or hiccoughs, are the uncontrollable spasms of the diaphragm that cause a sudden intake of breath and the closure of the glottis (the opening that stops substances from entering the trachea while swallowing). Hiccups are thought to be caused either by a lack of carbon dioxide in the blood or by something irritating the diaphragm.

> *Simple Solutions—Hiccups:* Apply 1 drop sandalwood over the diaphragm (the bottom edge of the rib cage).

Oils: ⊘☍sandalwood

⊘: Diffuse into the air. Inhale directly from bottle. Apply oil to hands, tissue, or cotton wick, and inhale.

☍: Dilute as recommended, and apply 1–2 drops to the diaphragm area or reflex points on the feet.

✛: **Body System(s) Affected:** Respiratory System.

High Blood Pressure

See **Blood: Blood Pressure: High**

Hives

See also **Allergies, Antiviral**

Hives are itchy patches of inflamed spots on the skin surrounded by redness, typically caused by an allergic reaction or a viral infection.

> *Simple Solutions—Hives:* Mix 3 drops lavender and 2 drops melaleuca with 1 tsp. (5 ml) jojoba oil in a small roll-on bottle, and apply on location.

Oils: ☍melaleuca○, ☍peppermint, ☍lavender○

☍: Dilute as recommended, and apply 1–2 drops on location. Add 1–2 drops to 1 Tbs. (15 ml) fractionated coconut oil, and massage on location.

✛: **Body System(s) Affected:** Immune System and Skin.

: Additional Research:

Melaleuca: Koh et al., 2002; Brand et al., 2002; **Lavender:** Kim et al., 1999.

Hodgkin's Disease

See also **Cancer**

Hodgkin's disease (or Hodgkin's lymphoma) is a type of cancer that affects lymphocytes (white blood cells). It can cause enlarged lymph nodes, fever, sweating, fatigue, and weight loss.

Oils: clove

: Dilute as recommended, and apply 1–2 drops to the liver, kidney, and reflex points on the feet.

: **Body System(s) Affected:** Immune System.

Hormonal System/Imbalance

See **Endocrine System**

Hot Flashes

See **Female-Specific Conditions**

Housecleaning

—**Bathrooms/Kitchens:**

Oils: lemon, fir (for cleaning and disinfecting), litsea, pink pepper

Other Products: On Guard Cleaner Concentrate to help eliminate microorganisms from household surfaces.

: Place a few drops on your cleaning rag or dust cloth; or place 10 drops in a small spray bottle with distilled water, and mist on surfaces before cleaning.

—**Carpets:**

Oils: lemon, Purify

: Apply on carpet stains to help remove. To freshen carpet, add 50–70 drops of these (or another favorite oil) to ½ cup (100 g) baking soda. Sprinkle over carpets, wait 15 minutes, and then vacuum.

—**Dishes:**

Oils: lemon

Other Products: On Guard Cleaner Concentrate to help purify dishes.

: Add a couple of drops to dishwater for sparkling dishes and a great smelling kitchen. Can add to dishwasher as well.

—**Furniture Polish:**

Oils: lemon, fir, hinoki, Citrus Bliss, Purify

: Place a few drops on a clean rag, and use to polish furniture.

—**Gum/Grease:**

Oils: lemon, lime

: Place 1–2 drops on gum or grease to help dissolve.

—**Laundry:**

Oils: lemon, Purify

Other Products: On Guard Laundry Detergent to help naturally fight stains and brighten clothes.

: Add a few drops of oil to the water in the washer. Add a few drops on a washcloth with clothes in the dryer. Add a few drops to a small spray bottle of water, and mist on laundry in the dryer before drying. Any of these methods can increase the antibacterial benefits and help clothes to smell fresh and clean.

—**Mold/Fungus:** *See also* **Antifungal: Mold**

Oils: On Guard, Purify

: Diffuse into the air.

: Place a few drops on a cleaning rag, and wipe down the affected area.

—**Stains:**

Oils: lemon (has been used to remove black shoe polish from carpets)

: Apply on location.

Hyperactivity

See **Calming: Hyperactivity**

Hyperpnea

See **Respiratory System: Hyperpnea**

Hypertension

See **Blood: Blood Pressure: High**

Hypoglycemia

Hypoglycemia is a condition of low levels of sugar in the blood. It is most common in people with diabetes but can be caused by drugs or by a tumor in the pancreas that causes the pancreas to create too much insulin. Symptoms of hypoglycemia can include hunger, sweating, weakness, palpitations, shaking, dizziness, and confusion.

Oils: ⬤eucalyptus, ⬤On Guard, ⬤cinnamon, ⬤clove, ⬤thyme

Other Products: ⬤PB Assist+ to help maintain a healthy digestive system.

⬤: Dilute as recommended and apply 1–2 drops over pancreas and on reflex points on the feet.

⬤: Take capsules as directed on package.

⬤: **Body System(s) Affected:** Endocrine System.

Hysteria

*See **Calming***

Immune System

*See also **Allergies, Antibacterial, Antifungal, Antiviral, Cancer, Lymphatic System, Parasites***

The immune system is the body's defense against disease. The immune system protects the body by identifying and killing bacteria, viruses, parasites, other microorganisms, and tumor cells that would harm the body. The immune system is comprised of several different types of white blood cells (lymphocytes) that recognize, process, or destroy foreign objects, the bone marrow that creates several types of white blood cells, the thymus that creates white blood cells and teaches them to recognize foreign objects and distinguish them from the body's cells, lymphatic vessels that help transport lymph and white blood cells, and several other organs, such as the lymph nodes, tonsils, spleen, and appendix, that filter out foreign objects and serve as a place for white blood cells to gather, interact, and share information about infections.

Oils: ⬤⬤⬤On Guard, ⬤⬤⬤oregano⬤, ⬤⬤melaleuca, ⬤⬤rosemary, ⬤⬤clove, ⬤⬤frankincense, ⬤⬤geranium, ⬤⬤lemon, ⬤⬤thyme, ⬤⬤lavender, ⬤⬤lime

Other Products: ⬤On Guard+ Softgels, ⬤Mito2Max, ⬤Alpha CRS+, ⬤a2z Chewable, ⬤xEO Mega or vEO Mega, ⬤IQ Mega, ⬤Microplex VMz to

provide nutrients essential for healthy immune system function.

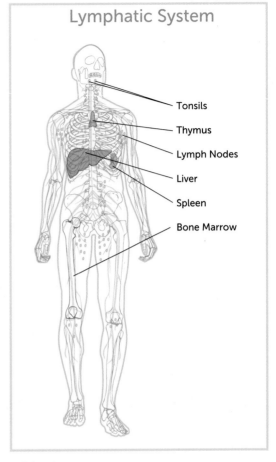

Lymphatic System

- Tonsils
- Thymus
- Lymph Nodes
- Liver
- Spleen
- Bone Marrow

—Stimulates:

Oils: ⬤⬤⬤oregano⬤, ⬤cinnamon, ⬤⬤frankincense, ⬤⬤melaleuca, ⬤On Guard, ⬤⬤lavender

⬤: Dilute as recommended, and apply 1–2 drops to bottoms of feet, along spine, or under arms (around lymph nodes). Add 1–2 drops to 1 Tbs. (15 ml) fractionated coconut oil, and massage onto back, arms, and feet.

⬤: Take capsules as recommended. Place 1–2 drops of oil under the tongue or place 2–3 drops in an empty capsule, and swallow.

⬤: Diffuse into the air.

⬤: **Body System(s) Affected:** Immune System.

⬤: **Additional Research:**

    Oregano: Walter et al., 2004

⬤=Topical, ⬤=Aromatic, ⬤=Internal

Impetigo

See Skin: Impetigo

Impotence

See Male Specific Conditions: Impotence

Incontinence

See Bladder: Bed Wetting and Incontinence

Indigestion

See Digestive System: Indigestion

Infection

See also Antibacterial, Antifungal, Antiviral

Oils: cinnamon, clary sage, On Guard, bergamot, myrrh (with oregano), Douglas fir (skin), basil, cypress, rosemary (with myrrh for oral infection), thyme (for urinary infection), lemongrass, lime, patchouli, lavender, oregano, juniper berry, fennel, peppermint

Other Products: On Guard+ Softgels. Microplex VMz for nutrients that help provide immune support.

—Infected Wounds:

Oils: frankincense, melaleuca, Douglas fir

Blend 1: Apply 1 drop thyme on location with hot compress daily. After infection and pus have been expelled, mix 3 drops lavender, 2 drops melaleuca, and 2 drops thyme combined with 1 tsp. (5 ml) fractionated coconut oil, and apply a little of this mixture on location twice daily.

: Dilute as recommended, and apply 1–2 drops on location. Mix 1–2 drops with 1 Tbs. (15 ml) fractionated coconut oil, and massage on location or on neck, arms, chest, or feet.

: Diffuse into the air. Add 1–2 drops to a bowl of hot water, and inhale the vapors.

: Take capsules as directed on package.

: **Body System(s) Affected:** Immune System.

Infertility

See Female-Specific Conditions: Infertility, Male Specific Conditions: Infertility

Inflammation

See also Antioxidant

Inflammation is the body's reaction to infection and injury. It is characterized by redness, swelling, warmth, and pain. Inflammation is an immune system response that allows the body to contain and fight infection or repair damaged tissue by dilating the blood vessels and allowing vascular permeability to increase blood supply to an injured or infected tissue. While a certain amount of inflammation can be beneficial in fighting disease and healing injuries, too much inflammation or chronic inflammation can actually be debilitating.

> *Simple Solutions—Inflammation from Injury:* Mix 3 drops frankincense and 2 drops lavender in a bowl of cold water. Dampen a washcloth with the water, and hold on location for 15–30 minutes.

Oils: frankincense, melaleuca, eucalyptus, oregano, Deep Blue, Rescuer, lavender, cardamom, patchouli, Roman chamomile, myrrh, rosemary, peppermint, wintergreen, clove, thyme, geranium, helichrysum, copaiba, Immortelle, juniper berry, cedarwood, Serenity, lemongrass, cypress

Other products: Alpha CRS+ and Microplex VMz or a2z Chewable for polyphenols and other antioxidants to help relieve oxidative stress associated with inflammation. xEO Mega or vEO Mega or IQ Mega for omega-3 fatty acids that help balance the inflammatory response.

: Dilute as recommended, and apply 1–2 drops on location and on the back of neck by the base of the skull. Add 3–4 drops to 1 Tbs. (15 ml) fractionated coconut oil, and massage on location.

: Place 1–2 drops of oil under the tongue, or place 2–3 drops of oil in an empty capsule, and swallow. Place 1–2 drops in 1 cup (250 ml) of rice or almond milk, and drink. Take supplements as directed on package.

: Diffuse into the air. Add 1–2 drops to a bowl of hot water or humidifier, and inhale the vapors to help relieve inflammation within the respiratory system.

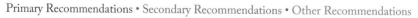

Primary Recommendations • Secondary Recommendations • Other Recommendations

⊕: Body System(s) Affected: Immune System.

⊡: Additional Research:

Frankincense: Zhou et al., 2004; Blain et al., 2009; Gayathri et al., 2007; Fan et al., 2005; Moussaieff et al., 2008; **Melaleuca:** Caldefie-Chézet et al., 2004; Brand et al., 2002; Brand et al., 2002; Brand et al., 2001; Hart et al., 2000; Golab et al., 2007; Koh et al., 2002; Pearce et al., 2005; **Eucalyptus:** Grassmann et al., 2000; Santos et al., 2000; Lu et al., 2004; Silva et al., 2003; Vigo et al., 2004; **Lavender:** Hajhashemi et al., 2003; Peana et al., 2002; **Cardamom:** al-Zuhair et al., 1996; **Roman Chamomile:** Safayhi et al., 1994; **Myrrh:** Tipton et al., 2003; Tipton et al., 2006; **Rosemary:** Cheung et al., 2007; González-Trujano et al., 2007; Takaki et al., 2008; **Peppermint:** Adam et al., 2006; Juergens et al., 1998; **Wintergreen:** Trautmann et al., 1991; **Clove:** Reddy et al., 1994; Halder et al., 2011; **Thyme:** Vigo et al., 2004; **Geranium:** Maruyama et al., 2005; **Helichrysum:** Appendino et al., 2007; **Cedarwood:** Tumen et al., 2013; **Dill:** Naseri et al., 2012.

Influenza

See also Antiviral

Influenza, commonly referred to as "the flu," is a highly contagious viral infection of the respiratory system. Influenza is marked by a sudden onset of high fever, dry cough, sore throat, muscle aches and pains, headache, fatigue, loss of appetite, nausea, and nasal congestion.

> *Simple Solutions—Influenza:* Diffuse Breathe in a misting aromatherapy diffuser.

Oils: ⊘⊘Breathe, ⊘⊘melaleuca⊡, ⊘⊘Opeppermint, ⊘⊘rosemary, ⊘⊘eucalyptus, ⊘⊘Douglas fir, ⊘⊘On Guard, ⊘⊙fir (aches/pains), ⊘⊙lavender, ⊘⊘oregano, ⊘⊘thyme, ⊘orange, ⊘Ocopaiba, ⊘⊘clove, O⊘ginger

Other Products: OOn Guard+ Softgels. ⊙On Guard Foaming Hand Wash to help prevent the spread of influenza viruses. OMicroplex VMz for nutrients to help support immune function.

⊘: Diffuse into the air.

⊙: Dilute as recommended, and apply to thymus area, chest, back, sinuses, or reflex points on the feet. Add 1–2 drops to hot bathwater, and bathe. Dilute 1–2 drops in 1 Tbs. (15 ml) fractionated coconut oil, and massage on chest, back, and feet.

O: Place 1–2 drops of ginger or peppermint oil in an empty capsule, and swallow to help reduce feelings of nausea. Take supplements as directed on package.

⊕: Body System(s) Affected: Immune System and Respiratory System.

⊡: Additional Research:

Melaleuca: Li et al., 2013.

Injuries

See Skeletal System, Bruises, Cuts, Inflammation, Joints, Muscles/Connective Tissue, Pain, Skin: Scarring, Tissue: Scarring, Wounds

Insects/Bugs

See also Bites/Stings

> *Simple Solutions—Bugs:* Avoid bug bites and stings by repelling the bugs. Diffuse TerraShield, or apply TerraShield to exposed skin.

—Bees, Wasps, and Hornet Stings:

Oils: ⊙Roman chamomile, ⊙basil, ⊙Purify, ⊙Stronger, ⊙lavender, ⊙lemongrass, ⊙lemon, ⊙peppermint, ⊙thyme.

Recipe 1: Remove the stinger, and apply a cold compress of Roman chamomile to the area for several hours or as long as possible.

⊙: Dilute as recommended, and apply 1–2 drops on location after making certain that the stinger is removed.

—Gnats and Midges:

Oils: ⊙lavender, ⊙⊘TerraShield

Recipe 2: Mix 3 drops thyme in 1 tsp. (5 ml) cider vinegar or lemon juice. Apply to bites to stop irritation.

⊙: Dilute as recommended, and apply 1–2 drops to bite area.

⊘: Diffuse into the air. Place 1–2 drops on small ribbons, strings, or cloth, and hang around area to help repel mosquitoes.

—Itching:

Oils: ⊙lavender

⊙: Dilute as recommended, and apply 1–2 drops to affected area.

—Lice:

Oils: ⊙eucalyptus⊡, ⊙⊘TerraShield, ⊙rosemary, ⊙melaleuca⊡, ⊙geranium, ⊙lemon, ⊙lavender

⊙: Dilute as recommended, and rub 1–2 drops into the scalp three times a day, and apply to feet.

—Mosquitoes:

Oils: ⊙⊘TerraShield, ⊙⊘patchouli⊡, ⊙lavender, ⊙Stronger, ⊙helichrysum

⊙: Dilute as recommended, and apply 1–2 drops to feet and exposed skin. Add 3–5 drops to 1 Tbs. (15 ml) fractionated coconut oil, and apply to exposed skin. Add 2–3 drops to 2–4 Tbs. (25–50 ml) distilled water in a small spray bottle; shake well, and mist onto the skin or into small openings where bugs may come through.

⊘: Diffuse into the air. Place 1–2 drops on small ribbons, strings, or cloth, and hang around area to help repel mosquitoes.

—Repellent:

Oils: ⊜⊘TerraShield, ⊜⊘patchouli, ⊜⊘basil, ⊜⊘lavender⊡, ⊜⊘lemongrass, ⊜⊘cedarwood⊡, ⊜⊘eucalyptus, ⊜⊘arborvitae, ⊜⊘thyme, ⊜⊘Purify

Blend 1: Combine 5 drops lavender, 5 drops lemongrass, 3 drops peppermint, and 1 drop thyme. Place neat on feet. Add to 1 cup (250 ml) of water, and spray on using a fine-mist spray bottle. Or place drops of this blend on ribbons or strings and tie near windows or around picnic or camping area.

Blend 2: Combine equal parts clove, lemon, and orange, and apply 2–3 drops on skin.

Blend 3: Place 5 drops lemon and 5 drops Purify in a small spray bottle with distilled water. Shake well, and mist on your skin to help protect against insects, flies, and mosquitoes.

⊙: Dilute as recommended, and apply 1–2 drops to feet and exposed skin. Add 3–5 drops to 1 Tbs. (15 ml) fractionated coconut oil, and apply to exposed skin. Add 20–30 drops to 2–4 Tbs. (25–50 ml) distilled water in a small spray bottle; shake well, and mist onto the skin or into small openings where bugs may come through.

⊘: Diffuse into the air. Place 1–2 drops on small ribbons, strings, or cloth, and hang around area to help repel insects.

—Spiders:

Oils: ⊜basil, ⊜Purify (with melaleuca), ⊜lavender, ⊜lemongrass, ⊜lemon, ⊜peppermint, ⊜thyme

⊙: Dilute as recommended, and apply 1–2 drops to affected area. Apply oil as a cold compress.

—Termites:

Oils: ⊜⊘patchouli⊡, ⊜⊘vetiver⊡ (repels), ⊜⊘clove⊡ (kills)

⊙: Apply oils around foundation and to soil around wood structures to help repel termites.

⊘: Diffuse into the air.

—Ticks:

Oils: ⊜⊘TerraShield, ⊜lavender⊡, ⊜⊘Stronger,

Removing Ticks:

Do not apply mineral oil, Vaseline, or anything else to remove the tick as this may cause it to inject the spirochetes into the wound.

Be sure to remove the entire tick. Get as close to the mouth as possible, and firmly tug on the tick until it releases its grip. Don't twist. If available, use a magnifying glass to make sure that you have removed the entire tick.

Save the tick in a jar, and label it with the date, where you were bitten on your body, and the location or address where you were bitten for proper identification by your doctor, especially if you develop any symptoms.

Do not handle the tick.

Wash hands immediately.

Check the site of the bite occasionally to see if any rash develops. If it does, seek medical advice promptly.

⊙: After getting the tick out, apply 1 drop lavender every 5 minutes for 30 minutes.

⊕: **Body System(s) Affected:** Skin.

⬚: **Additional Research:**

Melaleuca: Williamson et al., 2007; Canyon et al., 2007; Patchouli: Trongtokit et al., 2005; Lavender: van Tol et al., 2007; Mkolo et al., 2007; Eucalyptus: Choi et al., 2010; Greive et al., 2017; Patchouli: Zhu et al., 2003; Vetiver: Zhu et al., 2001; Clove: Zhu et al., 2001; Cedarwood: Singh et al., 1984; Cassia: Chang et al., 2006; Geranium: Tabanca et al., 2013; Grapefruit: Flor-Weiler et al., 2011.

Insomnia

Insomnia is difficulty falling or staying asleep. It can be triggered by stress, medications, drug or alcohol use, anxiety, or depression.

Simple Solutions—Insomnia: Add 5 drops lavender and 3 drops Roman chamomile to 2 Tbs. (25 ml) water in a small spray bottle. Spray on kids' pillows and sheets at bedtime.

Oils: ⊘⊜Serenity, ⊘⊜Calmer, ⊘⊜lavender⊡, ⊘⊜orange⊡, ⊘⊜Roman chamomile, ⊘⊜spikenard, ⊘⊜cypress, ⊘⊜ylang ylang, ⊘⊜Citrus Bliss, ⊘⊜marjoram, ⊘⊜petitgrain, ⊘⊜lemon, ⊘⊜rosemary, ⊘⊜sandalwood, ⊘⊜clary sage, ⊘⊜bergamot

Blend 1: Combine 6 drops Citrus Bliss with 6 drops lavender. Apply blend to big toes, bottoms of the feet, 2 drops around the navel, and 3 drops on the back of the neck.

Recipe 1: Combine 2 drops Roman chamomile, 6 drops geranium, 3 drops lemon, and 4 drops sandalwood. Add 6 drops of this blend to your bath at bedtime, and combine 5 drops with 2 tsp. (10 ml) fractionated coconut oil for a massage after the bath.

—For Children:

—1–5 years:

Oils: ⊜⊘Calmer, ⊘lavender, ⊘Roman chamomile

—5+ years:

Oils: ⊜⊘Calmer, ⊜⊘clary sage, ⊜⊘geranium, ⊜⊘ylang ylang

⊘: Diffuse into the air. Dissolve 3 drops essential oil in 1 tsp. (5 ml) pure grain alcohol (such as vodka) or perfumer's alcohol, and combine with distilled water in a 2 oz. spray bottle; shake well, and spray into the air before sleep. Place 1–2 drops on bottom of pillow or stuffed animal.

⊜: Dilute as recommended, and apply 1–2 drops on feet and back of neck. Combine 1–2 drops essential oil with 1 Tbs. (15 ml) fractionated coconut oil, and massage onto back, legs, feet, and arms.

⊕: **Body System(s) Affected:** Nervous System.

⊕: **Additional Research:**

Lavender: Lee et al., 2006; Chien et al., 2012; Kim et al., 2016; **Orange:** Carvalho-Freitas et al., 2002.

Intestinal Problems

See Digestive System

Invigorating

Oils: ⊜⊘wintergreen, ⊜⊘eucalyptus, ⊜⊘peppermint

⊜: Dilute as recommended, and apply 1–2 drops to back of neck or temples.

⊘: Diffuse into the air. Inhale directly from bottle. Apply oil to hands, tissue, or cotton wick, and inhale.

⊕: **Body System(s) Affected:** Emotional Balance.

Irritability

See Calming

Irritable Bowel Syndrome

See Digestive System

Itching

Itching is a tingling or irritation of the skin that produces a desire to scratch. Itching can be brought on by many factors including stress, bug bites, sunburns, allergic reactions, infections, and dry skin.

> *Simple Solutions—Itching:* Combine 10 drops lavender with 1 tsp. (5 ml) jojoba oil in a small roll-on bottle, and apply on location.

Oils: ⊜lavender, ⊜Serenity, ⊜peppermint, ⊜blue tansy

⊜: Dilute as recommended, and apply 1–2 drops on location and on ears. Add 2–3 drops to 1 Tbs. (15 ml) fractionated coconut oil, and apply a small amount on location.

⊕: **Body System(s) Affected:** Skin.

Jaundice

Jaundice is a condition characterized by a yellow appearance of the skin and the whites of the eyes. Jaundice is a result of excessive levels in the blood of a chemical called bilirubin. Bilirubin is a pigment that is made when hemoglobin from old or dead red blood cells is broken down. Jaundice occurs when the liver is unable to pass bilirubin from the body as fast as it is being produced. Jaundice is often a symptom of other diseases or conditions.

Oils: ⊜⊘geranium, ⊜⊘lemon, ⊜⊘rosemary

⊜: Dilute as recommended, and apply 1–2 drops to liver area, abdomen, and reflex points on the feet.

⊘: Diffuse into the air.

⊕: **Body System(s) Affected:** Cardiovascular System.

Jet Lag

See also Insomnia

Jet lag is the disruption of normal sleep patterns experienced while the body's internal clock adjusts to rapid changes in daylight and nighttime hours when flying to different areas of the world. Jet lag can cause tiredness, fatigue, and insomnia during normal sleeping hours. It is recommended to drink lots of fluids and to avoid alcohol or caffeine while flying to help prevent jet lag. Avoiding naps and forcing yourself to stay awake until

⊜=Topical, ⊘=Aromatic, ◯=Internal

your normal bedtime the first day can also help the body recover more quickly.

Oils: ⬤Balance, ⬤⬤Steady, ⬤peppermint, ⬤eucalyptus, ⬤geranium, ⬤lavender, ⬤grapefruit, ⬤lemongrass

⬤: Use invigorating oils such as peppermint and eucalyptus in the morning and calming oils such as lavender and geranium at night. Dilute as recommended, and apply 1–2 drops to temples, thymus, lower back, and bottoms of feet. Add 2–3 drops to 1 Tbs. (15 ml) fractionated coconut oil, and massage onto back, legs, shoulders, and feet. Add 1–2 drops to warm bathwater, and bathe.

⬤: **Body System(s) Affected:** Emotional Balance.

Joints

See also Arthritis, Inflammation, Muscles/Connective Tissue, Skeletal System

A joint is an area where 2 bones come together. Joints can offer limited or no movement between the bones (such as in the skull) or can offer a wide range of motion (such as in the shoulders, hands, and knees).

> *Simple Solutions—Joint Soreness:* Combine 3 drops eucalyptus, 3 drops peppermint, and 3 drops rosemary with 1 tsp. (5 ml) fractionated coconut oil in a small roll-on bottle. Apply on location, and then apply an ice pack on top.

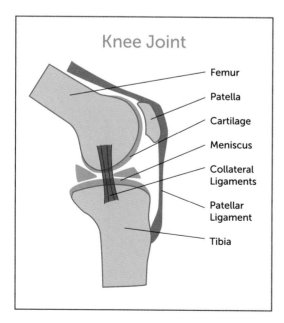

Knee Joint

- Femur
- Patella
- Cartilage
- Meniscus
- Collateral Ligaments
- Patellar Ligament
- Tibia

Oils: ⬤Deep Blue, ⬤Rescuer, ⬤wintergreen, ⬤Roman chamomile (inflammation)

Other Products: ⬤Deep Blue Rub and ⬤TriEase Softgels to help comfort joint stiffness and soreness.

—Rotator Cuff (sore):

The rotator cuff is the group of muscles and tendons that connect and hold the upper arm in the shoulder joint. The rotator cuff can become sore due to repetitive stressful shoulder motions or injury.

Oils: ⬤wintergreen, ⬤Deep Blue, ⬤Rescuer, ⬤lemongrass, ⬤peppermint, ⬤fir

Other Products: ⬤Deep Blue Rub and ⬤TriEase Softgels to help comfort joint stiffness and soreness.

—Shoulder (frozen): *See also Inflammation*

A frozen shoulder refers to a condition where the range of motion of the shoulder is severely limited and painful. This can be caused by inflammation, stiffness, abnormal tissue growth within the joint capsule (connective tissue that helps cushion, lubricate, and protect the joint) around the shoulder, arthritis, or inflammation of the bursa (small fluid-filled sacs that cushions muscle, ligament, and tendon tissue from the bones as they move across them). These conditions can be extremely painful and can take a long time to heal.

Oils: ⬤Deep Blue, ⬤fir, ⬤lemongrass, ⬤basil, ⬤wintergreen, ⬤Rescuer, ⬤oregano, ⬤peppermint

Other Products: ⬤Deep Blue Rub and ⬤TriEase Softgels to help comfort joint stiffness and soreness.

Regimen 1: Begin by applying 1–2 drops of fir to the shoulder reflex point on the foot on the same side as the frozen shoulder to help with any inflammation. Check for any improvement in pain and/or range of motion. Repeat these steps using lemongrass (for torn or pulled ligaments), basil (for muscle spasms), and wintergreen (for bone problems). After determining which of these oils gets the best results for improving pain and/or range of motion, apply 1–2 drops of the oil (or oils) to the shoulder. Then apply 1–2 drops of peppermint (to help soothe the nerves) and 1–2 drops oregano (to help enhance muscle flexibility). Finally, apply fir to the opposite shoulder to create balance as it compensates for the sore one. Drink lots of water.

—Tennis Elbow:

Tennis elbow (epicondylitis) is an injury to the tendons that connect the humerus bone near the elbow to the muscles that pull the hand backwards (lateral) and forward (medial) at the wrist. This type of injury is often associated with the repetitive forehand and backhand motions of playing tennis but can be caused by other activities that stress these tendons as well.

Oils: 🜄Deep Blue, 🜄Rescuer, 🜄eucalyptus, 🜄peppermint, 🜄helichrysum, 🜄wintergreen, 🜄rosemary, 🜄lemongrass

Other Products: 🜄Deep Blue Rub and ⦾TriEase Softgels to help comfort joint stiffness and soreness.

Blend 1: Combine 1 drop each of lemongrass, helichrysum, marjoram, and peppermint. Apply on location; then apply an ice pack.

🜄: Dilute as recommended, and apply 1–2 drops on location or on reflex points on the feet. Combine 5–10 drops with 1 Tbs. (15 ml) fractionated coconut oil, and massage on location.

🜁: **Body System(s) Affected:** Skeletal System.

Kidneys

The kidneys are paired organs located just below the rib cage on either side of the spine that function to filter waste and extra water from the blood. The kidneys convert the waste and extra water into urine that is then excreted through urination. The kidneys also play an important role in hormone production.

> *Simple Solutions—Kidney Stones:* Drink a glass of water with 1 tsp. (5 ml) lemon juice daily to help prevent kidney stones.

Oils: 🜄lemongrass, ⦾thyme🜁, ⦾Zendocrine, ⦾bergamot🜁, 🜄juniper berry, 🜄grapefruit, 🜄geranium, 🜄clary sage

Other Products: ⦾xEO Mega or vEO Mega or ⦾IQ Mega to provide omega-3 fatty acids that help support kidney function. ⦾Zendocrine Detoxification Complex to help support healthy kidney functioning.

🜄: Dilute as recommended, and apply to kidneys and reflex points on the feet. Apply as a hot compress.

⦾: Take capsules as directed on package. Add 1–2 drops of essential oil to an empty capsule; swallow capsule.

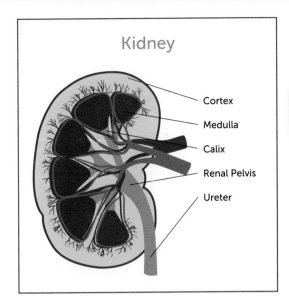

Kidney

- Cortex
- Medulla
- Calix
- Renal Pelvis
- Ureter

—Diuretic: *See Diuretic*

—Infection:

Kidney infections occur when bacteria enters the urinary tract. They are marked by fever, abdominal pain, chills, painful urination, dull kidney pain, nausea, vomiting, and a general feeling of discomfort.

Oils: 🜄rosemary

🜄: Dilute as recommended, and apply to kidneys and reflex points on the feet.

⦾: Drink 1 gallon (4 L) of distilled water and 8 cups (2 L) cranberry juice in 1 day.

—Inflammation (nephritis):

⦾: Drink 1 gallon (4 L) of distilled water and 8 cups (2 L) cranberry juice in 1 day.

—Kidney Stones:

A kidney stone is a solid piece of material that forms as chemicals in the urine crystallize and adhere together in the kidney. Small stones may pass through urination without causing pain. Larger stones with sharp edges and corners, however, can cause an extreme amount of pain as they are passed out of the body through the urinary tract.

Oils: ⦾lemon, 🜄eucalyptus, 🜄juniper berry

🜄: Apply as a hot compress over kidneys. Dilute as recommended, and apply 1–2 drops on location.

⦾: Add 1–2 drops oil to 1 cup (250 ml) of water, and drink. To help pass a stone, drink ½ cup (125 ml)

🜄=Topical, 🜁=Aromatic, ⦾=Internal

distilled water with juice from ½ lemon every 30 minutes for 6 hours; then take 2 Tbs. (25 ml) light extra-virgin olive oil with the juice from 1 full lemon, and repeat daily until stone passes. Drinking plenty of water can help prevent the formation of kidney stones.

⊕: **Body System(s) Affected:** Digestive System and Endocrine System.

▭: **Additional Research:**

Thyme: Youdim et al., 1999; **Bergamot:** Trovato et al., 2010.

Knee Cartilage Injury

See Muscles/Connective Tissue: Cartilage Injury

Labor

See Pregnancy/Motherhood: Labor

Lactation

See Pregnancy/Motherhood: Lactation

Lactose Intolerance

Lactose intolerance is the inability of the body to fully digest lactose, a sugar found in milk and in other dairy products. Symptoms of lactose intolerance include abdominal pain and bloating, diarrhea, nausea, and gas.

Oils: O⬤lemongrass

◑: Add 1–2 drops to 1 tsp. (5 ml) honey, and swallow; or add 1–2 drops to ½ cup (125 ml) rice or almond milk, and drink. Place 1–2 drops in an empty capsule, and swallow.

◔: Dilute as recommended, and apply 1–2 drops on abdomen or reflex points on the feet.

⊕: **Body System(s) Affected:** Digestive System.

Laryngitis

See also Allergies, Antiviral

Laryngitis is an inflammation and swelling of the voice box (called the larynx) that causes the voice to sound hoarse or raspy. Laryngitis is most commonly caused by viruses, allergies, or overuse of the voice and will generally go away by itself within two weeks.

Simple Solutions—Laryngitis: Apply 1 drop sandalwood to throat. Add 1 drop lemon to 1 tsp. (5 ml) honey, dissolve in a small cup of warm water, and sip.

Oils: ⬤⬤sandalwood, ⬤frankincense, ⬤thyme, ⬤lavender

⟳: Diffuse into the air.

◔: Dilute as recommended, and apply to neck and reflex points on the feet.

⊕: **Body System(s) Affected:** Immune System.

Laundry

See Housecleaning: Laundry

Leukemia

See Cancer: Leukemia

Libido

See Sexual Issues: Libido

Lice

See Insects/Bugs: Lice

Ligaments

See Muscles/Connective Tissue: Ligaments

Lipoma

See Tumor: Lipoma

Lips

Simple Solutions—Chapped Lips: Combine 4 tsp. (5 g) beeswax pellets, 1 Tbs. (10 g) cocoa butter, and 3 Tbs. (45 ml) jojoba oil, and melt in the microwave (30 seconds at a time, stirring in between) or in a double boiler. Cool slightly, and add 15 drops myrrh. Pour into small jars or lip balm containers, and allow to cool completely. Apply a small amount of lip balm as desired.

Oils: ⬤lavender, ⬤melaleuca, ⬤lemon

Other Products: ☙Lip Balm

—Dry lips:

Blend 1: Combine 2–5 drops geranium with 2–5 drops
lavender. Apply 1–2 drops on lips.

☙: Dilute as recommended, and apply 1 drop on lips.
Combine 1–2 drops essential oil with 1 Tbs. (15
ml) fractionated coconut oil, and apply a small
amount to lips.

☺: **Body System(s) Affected:** Skin.

Liver

The liver is the largest internal organ of the body. It is
located in the upper abdomen and helps with digestion,
produces cholesterol used to make several hormones
and cellular membranes, removes waste products and
old cells from the blood, and metabolizes harmful
substances and toxins into harmless chemicals. The
liver also has amazing regenerative abilities. Left with
as little as 25% of its original mass, the liver can regrow
what was lost and return to normal size.

Oils: ☙⊘geranium, ☙helichrysum, ☙ODigest-
Zen, Ocilantro⊕, Orosemary⊕, Oginger⊕,
☙cypress⊕, ☙⊘Ograpefruit, OZendocrine,
☙Omyrrh, ☙⊘Serenity, ☙⊘Roman chamomile

Other Products: OxEO Mega or vEO Mega, OIQ
Mega, OAlpha CRS+, OMicroplex VMz, Oa2z
Chewable for omega-3 fatty acids and other nutri-
ents that help support healthy liver cell functions.
OZendocrine Detoxification Complex to help
support healthy liver functioning.

—Cirrhosis:

Cirrhosis is scarring of the liver that occurs as the
liver tries to repair damage done to itself. When
extensive liver damage occurs, the massive scar
tissue buildup makes it impossible for the liver to
function. The most common causes of cirrhosis
are fatty liver (resulting from obesity or diabetes)
and alcohol abuse; but any damage done to the
liver can cause cirrhosis.

Oils: ☙⊘frankincense, ☙⊘myrrh, ☙⊘geranium,
☙⊘rosemary⊕, ☙⊘juniper berry, ☙⊘rose,
☙⊘Roman chamomile

—Cleansing:

Oils: ☙⊘clove, ☙⊘geranium, ☙⊘helichrysum,
☙⊘myrrh

—Hepatitis: *See also **Antiviral**.*

Hepatitis is any swelling or inflammation of
the liver. This can interfere with normal liver
functioning and can possibly lead to cirrhosis or
cancer over time. The most common cause of
hepatitis is from one of the five different forms
of hepatitis viruses, but it can also be caused by
alcohol consumption, other viruses, or medications. Possible symptoms of hepatitis include
diarrhea, jaundice, stomach pain, loss of appetite,
dark-colored urine, pale bowel movements,
nausea, and vomiting.

Oils: ☙⊘myrrh, ☙⊘melaleuca, ☙⊘frankincense⊕,
☙cypress⊕, ☙⊘rosemary, ☙⊘oregano,
☙⊘thyme, ☙⊘basil, ☙⊘cinnamon, ☙⊘eucalyp-
tus, ☙⊘peppermint

—Viral:

Oils: O☙myrrh, ☙⊘rosemary, ☙⊘basil

Other Products: OPB Assist+ or OPB Assist
Jr to help maintain friendly intestinal
flora that help prevent toxins from pathogenic bacteria and viruses.

—Jaundice: *See **Jaundice***

—Stimulant:

Oils: ☙⊘helichrysum

☙: Dilute as recommended, and apply 1–2 drops over
liver area and on reflex points on the feet. Apply
1–2 drops on spine and liver area for viral infections. Apply as a warm compress over the liver area.

⊘: Diffuse into the air. Inhale directly from bottle.
Apply oil to hands, tissue, or cotton wick, and inhale.

O: Take capsules as directed on package. Add 1–2 drops
essential oil to an empty capsule; swallow capsule.

☺: **Body System(s) Affected:** Digestive System and
Endocrine System.

⊕: **Additional Research:**

Frankincense: Hussein et al., 2000; **Cypress:** Ali et al., 2010;
Cilantro: Pandey et al., 2011; Moustafa et al., 2012; **Rosemary:**
Ra Kovi et al., 2014; **Ginger:** Liu et al., 2013.

Loss of Smell

*See **Nose: Olfactory Loss***

Lou Gehrig's Disease

Lou Gehrig's disease (also known as amyotrophic lateral sclerosis) is a progressive and fatal neurological disease that affects nerve cells in the brain and spinal cord. As the disease progresses, motor neurons die and the brain loses its ability to control muscle movement. Later stages of the disease can lead to complete paralysis. Eventually, control of the muscles needed to breathe, to speak, and to eat is lost.

Oils: cypress, Balance, frankincense, sandalwood, Serenity, geranium, rosemary, thyme

Other Products: OxEO Mega or vEO Mega or OIQ Mega for omega fatty acids essential for nerve cell function.

: Dilute as recommended, and apply 1–2 drops on brain stem, neck, spine, and reflex points on the feet. Add 1–2 drops to 1 Tbs. (15 ml) fractionated coconut oil, and apply on back, neck, and feet.

: Diffuse into the air. Inhale directly from bottle. Apply oil to hands, tissue, or cotton wick, and inhale.

: Take capsules as directed on package.

: **Body System(s) Affected:** Nervous System.

Lumbago

See Back: Lumbago/Lower Back Pain

Lungs

See Respiratory System: Lungs

Lupus

Lupus is an autoimmune disease that occurs when the immune system begins attacking its own tissues and organs. Lupus can cause pain, damage, and inflammation in the joints, blood vessels, skin, and organs. Common symptoms include joint pain or swelling, fever, muscle pain, and red rashes (often on the face). Lupus is more common in women than in men.

Oils: clove, Elevation, On Guard, Balance, melissa

: Dilute as recommended, and apply 1–2 drops on adrenal glands, under the arms, on neck, or on bottoms of the feet.

: Diffuse into the air. Inhale directly from bottle. Apply oil to hands, tissue, or cotton wick, and inhale.

: **Body System(s) Affected:** Immune System.

Lyme Disease

*See also **Antibacterial, Insects/Bugs: Ticks***

Lyme disease is a bacterial infection that comes from the bite of an infected tick. The first symptom is usually a red rash, which may look like a bullseye. As the infection spreads to other parts of the body, flu-like symptoms will occur, such as fever, chills, headache, body aches, stiff neck, and fatigue. If untreated, serious neurological and joint problems may develop after months or even years after the initial infection. Prevention of tick bites and quick removal of ticks reduce the chances of developing Lyme disease.

Oils: oregano, cinnamon, clove, TerraShield (prevent), lavender (prevent)

: Dilute as recommended, and apply 1–2 drops over location or on bottoms of the feet.

: Diffuse into the air. Inhale directly from bottle. Apply oil to hands, tissue, or cotton wick, and inhale.

: **Body System(s) Affected:** Immune System.

: **Additional Research:**

Oregano, Cinnamon, Clove: Feng et al., 2017.

Lymphatic System

*See also **Immune System***

The lymphatic system is made up of the tissues and organs (bone marrow, thymus, spleen, lymph nodes, etc.) that produce and store the cells used to fight infection and disease. The lymphatic system transports immune cells through a fluid called lymph.

Oils: cypress, sandalwood, DigestZen

Blend 1: Combine 5 drops Roman chamomile, 5 drops lavender, and 5 drops orange with 2 Tbs. (25 ml) fractionated coconut oil, and massage onto the skin over lymph nodes.

Other Products: OAlpha CRS+, Oa2z Chewable, OxEO Mega or vEO Mega or OIQ Mega, and OMicroplex VMz for nutrients that help support healthy immune function.

—**Cleansing:**

Oils: lemon, lime

—Decongestant For:

Oils: 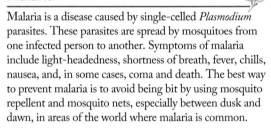cypress, grapefruit, Citrus Bliss, lemongrass, helichrysum, orange, rosemary, thyme

—Drainage Of:

Oils: helichrysum, lemongrass

—Eliminates Waste Through:

Oils: lavender

—Increase Function of:

Oils: lemon

🌀: Diffuse into the air. Inhale directly from bottle. Apply oil to hands, tissue, or cotton wick, and inhale.

💧: Dilute as recommended, and apply 1–2 drops on neck, arms, thyroid area, and reflex points on the feet. Add 1–2 drops to warm bathwater, and bathe.

⃝: Take capsules as directed on package.

Malaria

Malaria is a disease caused by single-celled *Plasmodium* parasites. These parasites are spread by mosquitoes from one infected person to another. Symptoms of malaria include light-headedness, shortness of breath, fever, chills, nausea, and, in some cases, coma and death. The best way to prevent malaria is to avoid being bit by using mosquito repellent and mosquito nets, especially between dusk and dawn, in areas of the world where malaria is common.

Simple Solutions—Malaria: To keep mosquitoes at bay, add 2–3 drops TerraShield to 2–4 Tbs. (25–50 ml) distilled water in a small spray bottle; shake well, and mist onto exposed skin or into small openings where bugs may come through.

Simple Solutions—Malaria: Mix 1 drop lemon with 1 tsp. (5 ml) honey and 1 cup (250 ml) warm water, and drink slowly.

Oils: TerraShield, eucalyptus, lemongrass, lavender, lemon

💧: Dilute as recommended, and apply 1–2 drops to feet and exposed skin. Add 3–5 drops to 1 Tbs. (15 ml) fractionated coconut oil, and apply to exposed skin. Add 2–3 drops to 2–4 Tbs. (25–50 ml) distilled water in a small spray bottle; shake well, and mist onto the skin or into small openings where bugs may come through.

🌀: Diffuse into the air. Place 1–2 drops on small ribbons, strings, or cloth, and hang around area to help repel mosquitoes.

⃝: Mix 1–2 drops lemon with 1 tsp. (5 ml) honey and 1 cup (250 ml) distilled water, and drink.

☤: **Body System(s) Affected:** Immune System.

⃤: **Additional Research:**

Eucalyptus: Trigg, 1996.

Male-Specific Conditions/Issues

Simple Solutions—Jock Itch: Combine 15 drops melaleuca with 2 Tbs. (15 g) cornstarch. Sprinkle a small amount on location once or twice a day as needed.

—Genital Area

  –Infection:

    Oils: melaleuca, oregano, eucalyptus, lavender

  –Inflammation:

    Oils: lavender, Roman chamomile

  –Swelling:

    Oils: cypress, lavender, rosemary, eucalyptus

—Impotence:

Impotence, also known as erectile dysfunction, is the frequent inability to have or sustain an erection. This may be caused by circulation problems, nerve problems, low levels of testosterone, medications, or psychological stresses.

Oils: clary sage, cassia, clove, ginger, dill, sandalwood

—Infertility:

Infertility is clinically defined as the inability to achieve pregnancy after a year of trying.

Oils: basil, clary sage, thyme, geranium, cinnamon

—Jock Itch: *See also Antifungal: Ringworm*

Jock itch is a type of fungal infection that infects the skin of the genital area, causing itching or painful red patches of skin. It occurs more often during warm weather.

Oils: melaleuca, lavender, cypress

💧=Topical, 🌀=Aromatic, ⃝=Internal

Recipe 1: Place 2 drops of any of the above oils in 1 tsp. (5 ml) fractionated coconut oil, and apply to area morning and night. Alternately, place 2 drops oil in a small bowl of water, and wash the area with the water and then dry well each morning and night.

: Dilute as recommended, and apply 1–2 drops on location or on reflex points on the feet. Dilute 1–2 drops in 1 Tbs. (15 ml) fractionated coconut oil, and massage on location. Add 1–2 drops essential oil to warm water, and bathe.

: Place 1–2 drops in an empty capsule, and swallow.

: Diffuse into the air. Inhale directly from bottle. Apply oil to hands, tissue, or cotton wick, and inhale.

: **Body System(s) Affected:** Reproductive System.

: **Additional Research:**

Cassia: Goswami et al., 2013; **Dill:** Monsefi et al., 2011; **Geranium:** Slima et al., 2013; **Cinnamon:** Yüce et al., 2014; **Cassia:** Goswami et al., 2014.

Massage

*For oils that can be used of an aromatic massage for a specific purpose, see also **Anxiety, Arthritis, Asthma, Back, Calming, Cardiovascular System, Cooling Oils, Edema, Energy, Fever, Foot, Hair, Hands, Headaches, Inflammation, Invigorating, Joints, Lymphatic System, Muscles/Connective Tissue, Nervous System, Pain, Pregnancy/Motherhood, Respiratory System, Skeletal System, Skin, Sleep, Stress, Tissue, Uplifting, Warming Oils***

Massage is the manipulation of the soft tissues in the body through holding, moving, compressing, or stroking. Massage can be done to help aid circulation, relax muscles, relieve pain, reduce swelling, speed healing after strains and sprains, restore function to the body, and release tension and stress.

> *Simple Solutions—Massage:* Add 10 drops of your favorite essential oil or blend to 1 Tbs. (15 ml) fractionated coconut oil or another carrier oil such as almond, olive, jojoba, sesame seed, or flaxseed to create your own personal massage oil.

Oils: AromaTouch—a blend specifically created to aid in therapeutic massage to relax and soothe muscles, to increase circulation, and to stimulate tissues. See other conditions for specific oils that can be used to create a massage oil for that condition.

Other Products: Deep Blue Rub and TriEase Softgels to help soothe tired, achy, and sore muscles and improve circulation within the tissue.

Blend 1: Combine 5 drops Roman chamomile, 5 drops lavender, and 5 drops orange with 2 Tbs. (25 ml) fractionated coconut oil, and use as massage oil for a relaxing massage.

: Add 1–10 drops of essential oil to 1 Tbs. (15 ml) fractionated coconut oil or another carrier oil such as almond, olive, jojoba, sesame seed, or flaxseed to create a massage oil. *See also the section on the Aroma Massage Technique in the Science and Application of Essential Oils section of this book.*

: **Body System(s) Affected:** Muscles and Skin.

Measles

*See **Childhood Diseases: Measles***

Melanoma

*See **Cancer: Skin/Melanoma***

Memory

*See also **Alzheimer's Disease***

Memory is the mental capacity to retain and recall facts, events, past experiences, and impressions. Memory retention can be enhanced by memory exercises, adequate sleep, and associations with previous knowledge. Aroma also plays a role in memory. At least one study has indicated that individuals exposed to an aroma while learning had an easier time remembering what they had learned when exposed to the same aroma, while those who were exposed to a differing aroma had a more difficult time remembering what they had learned.

> *Simple Solutions—Memory:* Place 5 drops of rosemary on a natural stone or unglazed clay pendant, and wear while studying and again while taking a test to help recall facts.

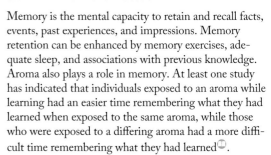

Oils: rosemary, peppermint, Thinker, frankincense, basil, Citrus Bliss, clove, lemon, juniper berry, cedarwood, ginger, grapefruit, lime, bergamot, rose, dill, lavender, lemongrass, petitgrain

Other Products: 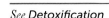OxEO Mega or vEO Mega, OIQ Mega, OMicroplex VMz for omega-3 fatty acids and other nutrients essential to brain cell health.

—Improve:

Oils: ⊘⊜clove, ⊜⊘Thinker, ⊘clary sage

—Stimulate:

Oils: ⊘rosemary, ⊜⊘Thinker

⊘ Diffuse into the air. Inhale directly from bottle. Apply oil to hands, tissue, or cotton wick, and inhale. Wear as a perfume or cologne.

⊜ Dilute as recommended, and apply 1–2 drops on temples or back of neck.

O Take capsules as directed on package.

⊕: **Body System(s) Affected:** Nervous System.

⊕ **Additional Research:**

Smith et al., 1992; **Rosemary:** Moss et al., 2003; **Peppermint:** Moss et al., 2008; **Basil:** Sarahroodi et al., 2012; **Clove:** Halder et al., 2011; **Rose:** Esfandiary et al., 2014; **Dill:** Thukham-Mee et al., 2012.

Menopause

See Female-Specific Conditions: Menopause

Menstruation

See Female-Specific Conditions: Menstruation

Mental

See Alertness, Brain, Energy, Memory, Stress

Metabolism

Metabolism refers to the processes involved in converting ingested nutrients into substances that can be used within the cells of the body for energy or to create needed cellular structures. This process is carried out by various chemical reactions facilitated by enzymes within the body.

—Balance:

Oils: ⊘clove, ⊘⊜Balance, ⊜⊘Steady, ⊘⊜oregano

⊘ Diffuse into the air. Inhale oil applied to tissue or cotton wick.

⊜ Dilute as recommended, and apply 1–2 drops on neck or on bottoms of the feet.

⊕: **Body System(s) Affected:** Digestive System and Endocrine System.

Metals

See Detoxification

Mice (Repel)

Oils: ⊜⊘Purify

⊜ Apply 1–2 drops in small openings or crevices where mice are likely to appear. Add 1–5 drops to small cotton balls, and place in openings where mice may come in.

⊘ Diffuse into the air.

Migraines

See Headaches: Migraine Headache

Mildew

See also Antifungal

Mildew is a whitish fungus that forms a flat growth on plants and organic material. Mildew attacks clothing, leather, paper, ceilings, walls, floors, shower walls, windowsills, and other places with high moisture levels. Mildew can produce a strong musty odor, especially in places with poor air circulation.

> *Simple Solutions—Mildew:* Add 25 drops Purify to ¼ cup (50 ml) water in a small spray bottle, and spray on surface to help neutralize mildew.

Oils: ⊜Purify

⊜: Place a few drops in a small spray bottle with distilled water, and spray into air or on surface to help neutralize mildew.

Mind

See Alertness, Brain, Energy: Fatigue: Mental Fatigue, Memory

Minerals (Deficiency)

Minerals are naturally occurring, inorganic substances with a chemical composition and structure. Some minerals are essential to the human body. A person is considered to have a mineral deficiency when the concentration level of any mineral needed to maintain optimal health is abnormally low in the body.

⊜=Topical, ⊘=Aromatic, O=Internal

Other Products: ⬤Microplex VMz contains a balanced blend of minerals essential for optimal cellular health, including calcium, magnesium, zinc, selenium, copper, manganese, chromium, and molybdenum; ⬤TerraGreens for a whole food source of essential nutrients.

⬤: Take capsules as directed on package.

❤: **Body System(s) Affected:** Digestive System.

Miscarriage

See Pregnancy/Motherhood: Miscarriage

Moles

See Skin: Moles

Mono (Mononucleosis)

See also Antiviral

Mononucleosis is a viral disease caused by the Epstein-Barr virus that usually spreads through contact with infected saliva, tears, and mucus. Most adults have been exposed to this virus sometime in their lives, but many display no symptoms or only very mild flu-like symptoms. Mononucleosis symptoms are most often seen in adolescents and young adults. Symptoms of this disease include fatigue, weakness, severe sore throat, fever, swollen lymph nodes, swollen tonsils, headache, loss of appetite, and a soft or swollen spleen. Once individuals are exposed to the Epstein-Barr virus, they carry the virus for the rest of their lives. The virus sporadically becomes active, but the symptoms do not appear again. Whenever the virus is active, however, it can be spread to others—even if the person carrying it shows no symptoms.

> *Simple Solutions—Mono:* Combine 3 drops oregano, 3 drops On Guard, and 3 drops thyme. Rub 3 drops of this blend on the feet.

Oils: ⬤⬤Breathe, ⬤⬤On Guard

Other Products: ⬤On Guard+ Softgels

⬤: Dilute as recommended, and apply 1–3 drops on throat and feet.

⬤: Diffuse into the air. Inhale oil directly from bottle, or inhale oil that is applied to the hands.

❤: **Body System(s) Affected:** Immune System.

Mood Swings

A mood swing is a rapid change of mood caused by fatigue or by a sudden shift in the body's hormonal balance.

> *Simple Solutions—Mood Swing:* Diffuse Balance to help balance emotions.

Oils: ⬤clary sage, ⬤Serenity, ⬤⬤Calmer, ⬤lavender, ⬤Balance, ⬤⬤Steady, ⬤rosemary, ⬤Elevation, ⬤geranium, ⬤rose, ⬤ylang ylang, ⬤sandalwood, ⬤lemon, ⬤peppermint, ⬤bergamot, ⬤fennel

⬤: Diffuse into the air. Inhale oil directly or applied to the hands.

❤: **Body System(s) Affected:** Emotional Balance.

Morning Sickness

See Pregnancy/Motherhood: Morning Sickness

Mosquitoes

See Insects/Bugs: Mosquitoes

Motion Sickness

See Nausea: Motion Sickness

MRSA

See Antibacterial

Mucus

See Congestion

Multiple Sclerosis

See also Brain: Myelin Sheath

Multiple sclerosis (MS) is an autoimmune disease in which the immune system attacks and gradually destroys the myelin sheath (which covers and insulates the nerves) and the underlying nerve fibers of the central nervous system. This destruction of the myelin sheath interferes with communication between the brain and the rest of the body. Symptoms of MS include partial or complete loss of vision, tingling, burning, pain in parts of the body, tremors, loss of coordination, unsteady gait, dizziness, and memory problems.

Oils: 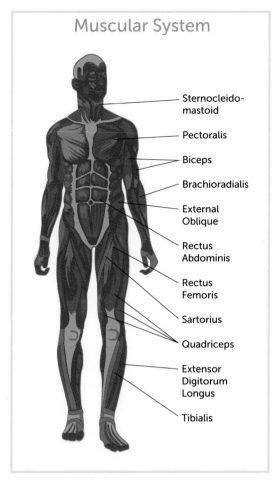frankincense, sandalwood, peppermint, clove, cypress, juniper berry, Serenity, oregano, thyme, birch, rosemary, wintergreen

Other Products: OxEO Mega or vEO Mega or OIQ Mega for omega-3 fatty acids that help support nerve and brain function.

: Dilute as recommended, and apply 1–2 drops to spine, back of neck, and feet. Dilute 1–3 drops in 1 Tbs. (15 ml) fractionated coconut oil, and massage on back and neck.

: Take capsules as directed on package.

: Diffuse into the air. Inhale directly from bottle. Apply oil to hands, tissue, or cotton wick, and inhale.

: **Body System(s) Affected:** Nervous System and Immune System.

: **Additional Research:**

Multiple Sclerosis: (Alberti et al., 2017).

Mumps

See Childhood Diseases: Mumps

Muscles

See also Cardiovascular System: Heart Tissue

Muscle is the tissue in the body that has the ability to contract, making movement possible. The three main types of muscle in the body are smooth muscle (such as that in the stomach, intestines, and blood vessels), cardiac muscle (found in the heart), and skeletal muscle (attached to the bones). Skeletal muscles are connected to the bones with tough fibrous tissue called tendons and allow for coordinated, controlled movement of the body, such as walking, pointing, or eye movement. Smooth muscles and cardiac muscles move automatically without conscious control to perform their functions.

Oils: marjoram, Deep Blue, Rescuer, peppermint, AromaTouch, copaiba, birch, cypress, wintergreen, lemongrass, lavender

Other Products: Deep Blue Rub and OTriEase Softgels to help relieve sore muscles, OMito-2Max, OAlpha CRS+, Oa2z Chewable, OxEO Mega or vEO Mega, OIQ Mega, OMicroplex VMz for coenzyme Q10 and other nutrients to support muscle cell energy and function.

Muscular System

Sternocleido-mastoid

Pectoralis

Biceps

Brachioradialis

External Oblique

Rectus Abdominis

Rectus Femoris

Sartorius

Quadriceps

Extensor Digitorum Longus

Tibialis

—Aches and Pains: *See also Pain*

Muscle pain usually results from overuse, tension, stress, strain, or injury. However, muscle pain can also be caused by a disease or infection affecting the whole body, such as the flu, fibromyalgia, or a connective tissue disorder.

Simple Solutions—Muscle Aches/Pains: Blend 10 drops Deep Blue in 1 Tbs. (15 ml) fractionated coconut oil. Gently massage oil into aching muscles.

Oils: marjoram, Deep Blue, Rescuer, copaiba, birch, clove, AromaTouch, oregano, peppermint, wintergreen, fir (with inflammation), vetiver, Roman chamomile, helichrysum, ginger, lavender, rosemary, thyme

Other Products: Deep Blue Rub and OTriEase Softgels to help relieve sore muscles.

=Topical, =Aromatic, O=Internal

263

—Bruised: *See Bruises*

—Cardiac Muscle: *See also* **Cardiovascular System: Heart**

Cardiac muscle is the type of muscle found in the walls of the heart.

Oils: 🌿🍃marjoram, 🌿🍃lavender, 🌿🍃peppermint, 🌿🍃rosemary, 🍃cinnamon

—Cartilage Injury:

Cartilage is a type of connective tissue in the body. It is firmer than other tissues and is used to provide structure and support without being as hard or as rigid as bone. Types of cartilage include hyaline cartilage, elastic cartilage, and fibrocartilage. Hyaline cartilage lines the bones and joints, helping them move smoothly. Elastic cartilage is found in the ear and larynx and is used to keep other tubular structures, such as the nose and trachea, open. Fibrocartilage is the strongest and most rigid cartilage. It is found in the intervertebral discs and other high-stress areas and serves to connect tendons and ligaments to bones. The hyaline cartilage surrounding bones and joints can become torn or injured if the joint is bent or twisted in a traumatic way. This can cause pain, swelling, tenderness, popping, or clicking within the joint and can limit movement.

Oils: 🍃birch, 🍃wintergreen, 🍃marjoram, 🍃Rescuer, 🍃lemongrass, 🍃fir, 🍃peppermint

—Cramps/Charley Horses:

A muscle cramp or charley horse is the sudden, involuntary contraction of a muscle. Muscle cramps can occur in any muscle in the body, but they usually occur in the thigh, calf, or arch of the foot. Cramps can be caused by excessive strain to the muscle, injury, overuse, dehydration, or lack of blood flow to the muscle. Muscle cramps can happen during or after a physical activity and while lying in bed.

Simple Solutions—Charley Horse: Blend 5 drops lemongrass and 5 drops peppermint in 1 Tbs. (15 ml) fractionated coconut oil. Gently massage oil into cramping muscles.

Oils: 🍃lemongrass with 🍃peppermint, 🍃marjoram, 🍃Deep Blue, 🍃Rescuer, 🍃rosemary, 🍃basil, 🍃thyme, 🍃vetiver, 🍃Roman chamomile, 🍃cypress, 🍃grapefruit, 🍃clary sage, 🍃lavender

—Development:

When muscles are stretched or used during exercise, they produce a substance that activates stem cells already present in the tissue. Once these cells are activated, they begin to divide—creating new muscle fiber and thereby increasing the size and strength of the muscles.

Oils: 🍃birch, 🍃wintergreen, 🍃Deep Blue

—Fatigue:

Muscle fatigue is the muscle's temporary reduction in strength, power, and endurance. This happens when there is an increase in lactic acid and blood flow to the muscle, a depletion of glycogen, or a deprivation of oxygen to the tissue.

Oils: 🍃marjoram, 🍃fir, 🍃cypress, 🍃peppermint, 🍃eucalyptus, 🍃grapefruit, 🍃rosemary, 🍃thyme

Other Products: 🍃Deep Blue Rub and ⭕TriEase Softgels

—Inflammation: *See Inflammation*

—Ligaments:

A ligament is a sheet or band of tough connective tissue and fibers that connects bones together or helps bind and support a joint.

Simple Solutions—Ligament Injury: Add 10 drops lemongrass to 1 tsp. (5 ml) fractionated coconut oil in a small roll-on bottle. Apply on location, and then apply an ice pack on top.

Oils: 🍃lemongrass

—Over Exercised:

When a person overexercises, his or her muscles do not get sufficient rest or time to heal. This continued muscle strain can cause muscle sprains, strain, and even tears to soft tissue. It may also cause stiffness and soreness to the neck, upper or lower back, shoulder, arm, or joint.

Oils: 🍃fir, 🍃eucalyptus, 🍃copaiba⃝, 🍃Rescuer, 🍃lavender, 🍃thyme, 🍃ginger

Other Products: 🍃Deep Blue Rub and ⭕TriEase Softgels to help provide comfort to tired and sore muscles.

Recipe 1: Add 3 drops marjoram and 2 drops lemon to warm bathwater, and soak.

Blend 1: Combine 2 drops eucalyptus, 2 drops peppermint, and 2 drops ginger with 1 Tbs. (15 ml) fractionated coconut oil, and massage into muscles.

—Rheumatism (Muscular): *See Fibromyalgia*

—Smooth Muscle:

Oils: marjoram, rosemary, peppermint, fennel, cypress, juniper berry, clary sage, melissa, lavender, sandalwood, bergamot

—Spasms:

A muscle spasm is a sudden, involuntary contraction or twitching of a muscle. This may or may not cause pain.

Oils: basil, marjoram, Deep Blue, Rescuer, Roman chamomile, peppermint, cypress, clary sage, lavender

—Sprains:

A sprain is an injury to a ligament caused by excessive stretching. The ligament can have little tears in it or it can be completely torn apart to be considered a sprain. The most common areas to receive a sprain are the ankle, knee, and wrist. After a person receives a sprain, the area will swell rapidly and be quite painful. If the ligament is torn apart, surgery may be required.

Oils: marjoram, lemongrass, fir, Rescuer, helichrysum, rosemary, thyme, copaiba, vetiver, eucalyptus, clove, ginger, lavender

—Strain:

A strain is a tear of the muscle tissue due to excessive strain or overstretching. Strains can cause inflammation, pain, and discoloration of the skin around the injured area.

Oils: lemongrass, Deep Blue, Rescuer, ginger (circulation), helichrysum (pain)

—Stiffness:

Oils: Deep Blue

Other Products: Deep Blue Rub and TriEase Softgels

—Tendinitis:

Tendinitis is the inflammation of a tendon due to injury, repetitive exercise or strain, or diseases such as arthritis, gout, and gonorrhea. This can cause swelling and pain in the affected tendon.

Simple Solutions—Tendinitis: Apply 1 drop marjoram on location, and cover with a cool pack for 15 minutes.

Oils: marjoram, lavender

—Tension (especially in shoulders and neck):

Muscle tension is a condition in which the muscle remains in a semi-contracted state for an extended period of time. This is usually due to physical or emotional stress.

Oils: marjoram, Deep Blue, Rescuer, peppermint, helichrysum, juniper berry, lavender, Roman chamomile, spikenard

Other Products: Deep Blue Rub and TriEase Softgels

—Tone:

Apply these oils before exercise to help tone muscles.

Oils: birch, cypress, wintergreen, marjoram, basil, peppermint, orange, thyme, rosemary, juniper berry, grapefruit, lavender

: Dilute as recommended, and apply 1–2 drops on location. Add 2–4 drops to 1 Tbs. (15 ml) fractionated coconut oil, and massage into desired muscles or joints. Add 1–2 drops to warm bathwater, and bathe. Apply as hot or cold (for strains or sprains) compress.

: Take capsules as directed on package. Place 1–2 drops of oil under the tongue or add 1–2 drops essential oil to empty capsule, and swallow.

: Diffuse into the air.

: Body System(s) Affected: Muscles.

: Additional Research:

Peppermint: Göbel et al., 1994; Rosemary: Aqel, 1991.

Muscular Dystrophy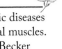

Muscular dystrophy is any of several genetic diseases that cause gradual weakening of the skeletal muscles. The most common forms, Duchenne and Becker muscular dystrophies, are caused by a gene defect that inhibits or alters the production of dystrophin, a protein necessary for proper muscle cell structure.

Oils: marjoram, lemongrass, basil, rosemary, AromaTouch, Deep Blue, geranium, lavender, lemon, orange, ginger

Other Products: Deep Blue Rub and TriEase Softgels to help relieve and relax tense and aching muscles.

: Dilute as recommended, and apply 1–2 drops on location. Add 2–4 drops to 1 Tbs. (15 ml) fractionated coconut oil, and massage into desired

=Topical, =Aromatic, =Internal

muscles. Add 1–2 drops to warm bathwater and bathe. Apply as cold compress.

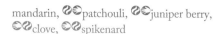: **Body System(s) Affected:** Nervous System and Muscles.

Myelin Sheath

See Brain: Myelin Sheath

Nails

Oils: lemon, frankincense, myrrh, Citrus Bliss, melaleuca (infection), eucalyptus, lavender, grapefruit, rosemary, cypress, oregano, thyme

Blend 1: Combine 2 drops frankincense, 2 drops lemon, and 2 drops myrrh with 2 drops wheat germ oil. Apply 2–3 times per week.

Other Products: Microplex VMz for nutrients essential to healthy nail growth.

: Dilute as recommended, and apply 1–2 drops to nails. Add 1–2 drops to 1 tsp. (5 ml) fractionated coconut oil, and apply to nails.

: Take capsules as directed on package.

: **Body System(s) Affected:** Skin.

: **Additional Research:**

Melaleuca: Buck et al., 1994.

Nasal

See Nose

Nausea

Nausea is a sick feeling in the stomach producing an urge to vomit.

Simple Solutions—Motion Sickness: Inhale the aroma of peppermint.

Simple Solutions—Nausea: Add 2 drops ginger to a bowl of hot water, and inhale the warm vapor coming from the water.

Oils: ginger, peppermint, lavender, cardamom, DigestZen, green

mandarin, patchouli, juniper berry, clove, spikenard

Other Products: DigestZen Softgels

—Morning Sickness: *See Pregnancy/Motherhood: Morning Sickness*

—Motion Sickness:

Motion sickness is a feeling of illness that occurs as a result of repeated movement, such as that experienced in a car, on a boat, or on a plane. These motions interfere with the body's sense of balance and equilibrium. The most common symptoms of motion sickness include dizziness, fatigue, and nausea.

Oils: peppermint, DigestZen, ginger

—Vomiting:

Oils: ginger, peppermint, patchouli, fennel, rose, Roman chamomile

: Place 1–2 drops essential oil in an empty capsule, and swallow. Take supplements as directed.

: Diffuse into the air. Inhale directly from bottle. Apply oil to hands, tissue, or cotton wick, and inhale.

: Dilute as recommended, and apply 1–2 drops to the feet, temples and wrists. Dilute 1–2 drops essential oil in 1 Tbs. (15 ml) fractionated coconut oil, and massage on stomach. Apply oil as a warm compress.

: **Body System(s) Affected:** Digestive System.

: **Additional Research:**

Ginger: Vutyavanich et al., 2001; Nanthakomon et al., 2006; Bone et al., 1990; Peppermint: Tayarani-Najaran et al., 2013.

Neck

Oils: lemon, geranium, clary sage, orange, basil, helichrysum

: Dilute 1–5 drops oil in 1 Tbs. (15 ml) fractionated coconut oil, and massage on neck.

: **Body System(s) Affected:** Skeletal System and Muscles.

See also **Back, Brain**

> *Simple Solutions—Neuralgia:* Blend 5 drops marjoram and 5 drops eucalyptus with 1 tsp. (5 ml) carrier oil in a small roll-on bottle, and apply along nerve.

The nervous system is a network of nerve cells that regulates the body's reaction to external and internal stimuli. The nervous system sends nerve impulses to organs and muscles throughout the body. The body relies on these impulses to function. The nervous system is comprised of the central nervous system (the brain and spinal cord) and the peripheral nervous system (all other nerves). The peripheral nervous system is comprised of the somatic nervous system (nerves that connect to the skeletal muscles and sensory nerve receptors in the skin) and the autonomic nervous system (nerves that connect to the cardiac and smooth muscles and other organs, tissues, and systems that don't require conscious effort to control). The autonomic system is divided further into two main parts: the sympathetic and parasympathetic nervous systems. The sympathetic nervous system functions to accelerate heart rate, increase blood pressure, slow digestion, and constrict blood vessels. It activates the "fight or flight" response in order to deal with threatening or stressful situations. The parasympathetic nervous system functions to slow heart rate, store energy, stimulate digestive activity, and relax specific muscles. It allows the body to return to a normal and calm state after experiencing pain or stress.

Oils: peppermint (soothes and strengthens damaged nerves), basil (stimulates), lavender, lemon, grapefruit, frankincense, turmeric, bergamot, cedarwood (nervous tension), lemongrass (for nerve damage), marjoram (soothing), geranium (regenerates), Serenity, Roman chamomile, juniper berry, vetiver, cinnamon, neroli, ginger, orange, sandalwood

Other Products: Mito2Max to help support healthy nerve function. xEO Mega or vEO Mega or IQ Mega for essential omega fatty acids that help support nerve cell health. Microplex VMz, a2z Chewable for nutrients and minerals necessary for proper nerve cell function. Alpha CRS+ for nutrients that help support nerve cell health and energy.

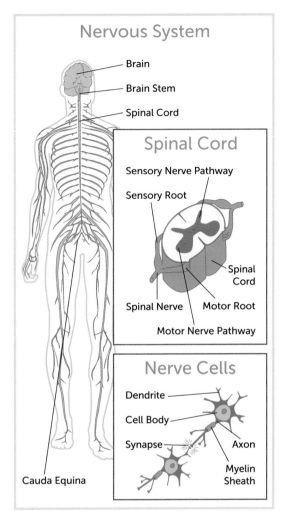

Nervous System

- Brain
- Brain Stem
- Spinal Cord

Cauda Equina

Spinal Cord

- Sensory Nerve Pathway
- Sensory Root
- Spinal Cord
- Spinal Nerve
- Motor Root
- Motor Nerve Pathway

Nerve Cells

- Dendrite
- Cell Body
- Synapse
- Axon
- Myelin Sheath

—Bell's Palsy:

Bell's palsy is a weakness or paralysis of muscles on one side of the face. Bell's palsy tends to set in quickly, normally in a single day. Symptoms include numbness of one side of the face, loss of ability to taste, drooling, pain in or behind the ear, facial droop, headache, and change in the amount of saliva or tears produced. In most cases Bell's palsy symptoms will begin to improve within a few weeks. But in some few cases the symptoms continue for life.

Oils: peppermint, rosemary, thyme

—Carpal Tunnel Syndrome: *See Carpal Tunnel Syndrome*

=Topical, =Aromatic, =Internal

—Huntington's Disease:

Huntington's disease (HD) is a progressive neurodegenerative disorder passed genetically from one generation to the next. As the disease develops, it causes nerve cells in the brain to waste away, resulting in a loss of control over body movement, emotions, and mental reasoning. Early symptoms include unsteady walking and decreased coordination. Later symptoms include sudden involuntary jerking body movements, slurred speech, decreased mental capacity, and psychological and emotional problems. Those carrying the HD gene have a 50% chance of passing it on to each of their children.

Oils: ⊜⊘peppermint, O⊜⊘turmeric⊡, ⊜⊘basil

Other Products: Oils: OMito2Max to help support healthy nerve function. OxEO Mega or vEO Mega

—Lou Gehrig's Disease (ALS): *See Lou Gehrig's Disease*

—Multiple Sclerosis (MS): *See Multiple Sclerosis*

—Neuralgia:

Neuralgia is intense pain felt along the path of a nerve. Neuralgia results from damage or irritation to a nerve. Causes can include certain drugs, diabetes, infections, inflammation, trauma, and chemical irritation.

Oils: ⊜marjoram, ⊜eucalyptus⊡, ⊜Roman chamomile, ⊜lavender, ⊜juniper berry, ⊜helichrysum, ⊜cedarwood

—Neuritis:

Neuritis is the inflammation of a nerve or of a group of nerves. Neuritis causes pain, poor reflexes, and muscle atrophy.

Oils: ⊜eucalyptus⊡, ⊜Roman chamomile, ⊜lavender, ⊜juniper berry, ⊜clove, ⊜cedarwood

—Neurotonic:

Oils: ⊜melaleuca, ⊜thyme

—Paralysis:

Paralysis is the loss of one's ability to move and control one or more specific sets of muscles. Paralysis generally occurs as a result of damage to the nervous system, especially damage to the spinal cord. Primary causes include injury, stroke, multiple sclerosis, amyotrophic lateral sclerosis (Lou Gehrig's disease), botulism, spina bifida, and Guillain-Barré syndrome.

Oils: ⊜⊘peppermint, ⊜⊘lemongrass, ⊜⊘geranium, ⊜⊘Balance, ⊜⊘Purify, ⊜⊘cypress, ⊜⊘juniper berry, ⊜⊘ginger, ⊜⊘helichrysum

—Parasympathetic Nervous System:

The parasympathetic nervous system functions to slow heart rate, store energy, stimulate digestive activity, and relax specific muscles. It allows the body to return to a normal and calm state after experiencing pain or stress.

Oils: ⊘⊜lavender⊡ (stimulates), ⊘⊜lemongrass (regulates), ⊘⊜marjoram (tones), ⊘⊜Serenity, ⊘⊜Balance

—Parkinson's Disease: *See Parkinson's Disease*

—Sympathetic Nervous System:

The sympathetic nervous system functions to accelerate heart rate, increase blood pressure, slow digestion, and constrict blood vessels in most tissues and organs, while dilating arterioles in the skeletal muscles where increased blood flow is needed. It activates the "fight or flight" response in order to deal with threatening or stressful situations.

Oils: ⊘⊜grapefruit⊡ (stimulates), ⊘⊜eucalyptus, ⊘⊜peppermint, ⊘⊜ginger

—Virus of Nerves: *See also Antiviral*

Oils: ⊜frankincense, ⊜clove

⊜: Dilute as recommended, and apply 1–3 drops on location, spine, back of neck, and reflex points on the feet. Add 2–4 drops to 1 Tbs. (15 ml) fractionated coconut oil, and massage on location. Add 1–2 drops to warm bathwater, and bathe.

⊘: Diffuse into the air. Inhale directly from bottle. Apply oil to hands, tissue, or cotton wick, and inhale.

O: Take 1–2 drops of oil in a capsule, or with a beverage. Take capsules as directed on package.

⊕: **Body System(s) Affected:** Nervous System.

⊡: **Additional Research:**

Peppermint: Koo et al., 2001; **Lavender:** Tanida et al., 2006; Shen et al., 2005; **Lemon:** Aloisi et al., 2002; Fukumoto et al., 2006; Koo et al., 2002; **Grapefruit:** Shen et al., 2005; Haze et al., 2002; **Frankincense:** Moussaieff et al., 2008; **Turmeric:** Preeti et al., 2008; Chen et al., 2018; **Eucalyptus:** Santos et al., 2000.

Nervousness

Nervousness is a state of high anxiety, distress, agitation, or psychological uneasiness.

Oils: orange, spikenard, neroli

: Diffuse into the air. Inhale directly from bottle. Apply oil to hands, tissue, or cotton wick, and inhale.

: Dilute as recommended, and apply 1–2 drops to temples.

: **Body System(s) Affected:** Emotional Balance.

Nose

Oils: melaleuca, rosemary

—Bleeding:

A nosebleed (medically called *epistaxis*) is the loss of blood through the nose. Nosebleeds are fairly common and can be caused by many factors. The most common causes of nosebleed are dry air that causes the nasal membrane to dry out and crack, allergies, nose trauma/injury, and colds and other viruses.

Oils: helichrysum, cypress, lemon, frankincense, lavender

—Nasal Nasopharynx:

The nasopharynx is the upper part of the throat (pharynx) situated behind the nose. The nasopharynx is responsible for carrying air from the nasal chamber into the trachea.

Oils: eucalyptus

—Nasal Polyp:

A nasal polyp is an abnormal tissue growth inside the nose. Since nasal polyps are not cancerous, very small polyps generally do not cause any problems. But larger polyps can obstruct the nasal passage and make it difficult to breath or smell and can cause frequent sinus infections. Possible symptoms of polyps include runny nose, decreased sense of smell, decreased sense of taste, snoring, facial pain or headache, itching around the eyes, and persistent congestion.

Oils: frankincense, oregano, Breathe, peppermint, Purify, basil

—Olfactory Loss:

Olfactory loss (or anosmia) is the loss of one's ability to smell. The most common causes for olfactory loss are sinonasal disease, head injury, and infection of the upper respiratory tract.

Oils: peppermint, basil

—Rhinitis: *See also* **Allergies, Antiviral, Colds**

Rhinitis is an inflammation of the nasal mucous membrane (the moist lining inside the nasal cavity where mucus is produced that acts as an air filtration system by trapping incoming dirt particles and moving them away for disposal). Rhinitis can cause runny nose, nasal congestion, sneezing, ear problems, and phlegm in the throat. Rhinitis is commonly caused by viral infections and allergies and can be acute (short-term) or chronic (long-term).

Oils: eucalyptus, peppermint, lemon, lavender, basil

Other Products: TriEase Softgels

: Dilute as recommended, and apply 1–2 drops on nose (use extreme caution to avoid getting oil in the eye). Dilute as recommended, and apply 1 drop to a cotton swab, and swab the inside of the nose.

: Diffuse into the air, and inhale the vapors through the nose. Inhale directly from bottle. Apply oil to hands, tissue, or cotton wick, and inhale.

: **Body System(s) Affected:** Respiratory System.

: **Additional Research:**

Lemon: Ferrara et al., 2012.

Nursing

*See **Pregnancy/Motherhood: Lactation***

Obesity

*See **Weight: Obesity***

Odors

*See **Deodorant, Deodorizing***

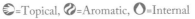

=Topical, =Aromatic, =Internal

See also **Antibacterial, Antifungal: Thrush.**

—Abscess:

A tooth abscess is a collection of pus at the root of an infected tooth. The main symptom of a tooth abscess is a painful, persistent, throbbing toothache. The infected tooth may be sensitive to heat, cold, and pressure caused by chewing. Later symptoms may include swelling in the face, swollen lymph nodes in the neck or jaw, and a fever. Abscesses may eventually rupture, leaving a foul-tasting fluid in the mouth. If left untreated, an abscess can spread to other areas of the head and neck.

Oils: 🜁clove, 🜁On Guard, 🜁Purify, 🜁helichrysum, 🜁melaleuca, 🜁frankincense, 🜁Roman chamomile, 🜁wintergreen

Other Products: 🜁On Guard Natural Whitening Toothpaste, 🜁On Guard Mouthwash

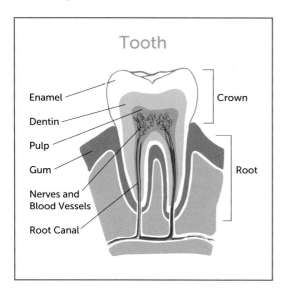

Tooth

Enamel

Dentin

Pulp

Gum

Nerves and Blood Vessels

Root Canal

Crown

Root

Blend 1: Blend 1 drop each of clove, wintergreen, myrrh, and helichrysum to help with infection.

—Cavities:

A cavity is a decayed area or hole in a tooth caused by bacteria in the mouth. A cavity that is allowed to progress without treatment can result in pain, infection, and loss of the tooth. Good oral hygiene and eating less sugar can help to reduce the risk of cavities.

Simple Solutions—Cavity: Apply 1 drop clove on location to help soothe pain.

Oils: 🜁On Guard, 🜁melaleuca, 🜁peppermint, 🜁eucalyptus, 🜁cinnamon

Other Products: 🜁On Guard Natural Whitening Toothpaste, 🜁On Guard Mouthwash

—Gums:

The gums (also called "gingiva") are the soft pink tissue surrounding the teeth. The gums form a seal around the teeth and are snugly attached to the bone underneath to withstand the friction of food passing over them in chewing.

Oils: 🜁myrrh, 🜁lavender, 🜁melaleuca, 🜁helichrysum, 🜁Roman chamomile

Other Products: 🜁On Guard Natural Whitening Toothpaste, 🜁On Guard Mouthwash

—Gum Disease:

Gum disease is an infection of the tissue and bones surrounding the teeth and is caused by a buildup of plaque. Gum disease consists of two parts: first gingivitis and then periodontal disease. Gingivitis is an inflammation of the gums because of bacteria associated with plaque buildup. When infected with gingivitis, the gums become red and swollen and often bleed during teeth brushing. Periodontal disease occurs when gingivitis is left untreated and becomes progressively worse. The inflamed gums begin pulling away from the teeth and leave empty pockets where food particles can easily collect and become infected. As the disease progresses, the gums pull farther away from the teeth and the bacteria eats away at the tissue and bone. As this occurs, the teeth lose their anchoring and can fall out.

Simple Solutions—Gingivitis/Gum Disease: Add 2 drops myrrh to ¼ tsp. (2 g) baking soda. Apply on gum lines, and leave for 60 seconds. Rinse mouth with water, and spit out.

Oils: 🜁melaleuca, 🜁On Guard, 🜁myrrh, 🜁helichrysum, 🜁rose

Other Products: 🜁On Guard Natural Whitening Toothpaste, 🜁On Guard Mouthwash

—Halitosis (Bad Breath):

Halitosis is the technical term for "bad breath." Common causes of halitosis include smoking, drinking, poor oral hygiene, gum disease, dry mouth, tooth decay, and certain foods.

> *Simple Solutions—Halitosis:* Add 10–15 drops peppermint or spearmint to 1 tsp. (5 ml) water in a small spray bottle. Shake, and spray 1–2 sprays in mouth as needed.

Oils: peppermint◐, On Guard, patchouli, lavender

Other Products: On Guard Natural Whitening Toothpaste, On Guard Mouthwash

—Mouth Ulcers:

Mouth ulcers are open, often painful, sores that occur in the mouth. Common mouth ulcers include canker sores and cold sores. Stress, anxiety, fatigue, injury, illness, hormonal changes, and food allergies can often trigger mouth ulcers.

Oils: basil, myrrh, orange

Other Products: On Guard Natural Whitening Toothpaste, On Guard Mouthwash

—Teeth Grinding:

Teeth grinding (also called bruxism) is the habit of clenching the teeth and rubbing them against one another. Teeth grinding often occurs unconsciously while a person is asleep. If teeth grinding is frequent, it can lead to tooth damage, jaw pain, and headaches.

Oils: Serenity

—Teething Pain:

Around ages 4–7 months, a baby will get his or her first teeth. Some infants teethe without discomfort; but for other infants, teething can be a painful process. Common symptoms of teething include irritability or fussiness, drooling, chin rash, biting, difficulty sleeping, and low-grade fever.

Oils: lavender

—Toothache:

A toothache is a pain around a tooth. Toothaches can result from many factors, including infection, injury, decay, jaw problems, cavities, damaged fillings, and gum disease. Common symptoms of a toothache include sharp or throbbing pain, swelling around the tooth, fever, headache, and foul-tasting drainage from the infected tooth.

Oils: clove, melaleuca, Purify, Roman chamomile

Other Products: On Guard Natural Whitening Toothpaste, On Guard Mouthwash

—Toothpaste:

Oils: On Guard

Other Products: On Guard Natural Whitening Toothpaste

Recipe 1: Mix 1–2 drops On Guard with ½ tsp. (3 g) baking soda to form a paste, and use as toothpaste to brush onto the teeth.

: Dilute as recommended, and apply 1–2 drops on location or along jawbone. Apply the oils with a hot compress on the face. Use On Guard Natural Whitening Toothpaste as directed. Dilute as recommended, and apply 1–2 drops to a small cotton ball or cotton swab; swab on location. Mix 1–2 drops with ½ cup (125 ml) of water, and use as mouth-rinse. Add 1–2 drops to toothpaste. Place 5–6 drops with 2 Tbs. (25 ml) distilled water in a small spray bottle, and mist into the mouth.

: Diffuse into the air.

: **Body System(s) Affected:** Skeletal System and Skin.

: **Additional Research:**

Melaleuca: Takarada et al., 2004; Shapiro et al., 1994; Filoche et al., 2005; Santamaria et al., 2014; **Peppermint:** Shayegh et al., 2008; Rasooli et al., 2008; **Eucalyptus:** Takarada et al., 2004; Charles et al., 2000; **Cinnamon:** Filoche et al., 2005.

Osteomyelitis

See Skeletal System: Osteomyelitis

Osteoporosis

See Skeletal System: Osteoporosis

Ovaries

Ovaries are the female reproductive organs in which eggs are produced and stored.

Oils: rosemary (regulates), geranium, Whisper, DigestZen

—Ovarian Cyst:

An ovarian cyst is a fluid-filled sac within the ovary. While ovarian cysts are common, and most cause no problems, they may cause feelings of aching or pressure and can cause pain, bleeding, and other problems if they become too large or become twisted or rupture.

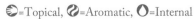

=Topical, =Aromatic, =Internal

Oils: ♨♨basil

♨: Dilute as recommended, and apply 1–2 drops on abdomen and reflex points on the feet. Add 1–2 drops to 1 Tbs. (15 ml) fractionated coconut oil, and massage into abdomen and lower back. Apply as a warm compress to the abdomen. Add 1–2 drops to 2 tsp. (10 ml) olive oil, insert into vagina, and retain overnight with a tampon.

♨: Diffuse into the air. Inhale directly from bottle. Apply oil to hands, tissue, or cotton wick, and inhale.

♨: **Body System(s) Affected:** Reproductive Systems.

Overeating

See Eating Disorders: Overeating

Overweight

See Weight

Oxygenating

The term "oxygenate" means to supply, to treat, or to infuse with oxygen. All of the cells in the body require oxygen to create the energy necessary to live and function correctly. The brain consumes 20% of the oxygen we inhale.

Oils: ♨♨sandalwood, ♨♨frankincense, ♨♨oregano, ♨♨fennel

♨: Diffuse into the air. Inhale directly from bottle. Apply oil to hands, tissue, or cotton wick, and inhale.

♨: Dilute as recommended, and apply 1–2 drops to forehead, chest, and sinuses.

Pain

> *Simple Solutions—Pain:* Add 25 drops Deep Blue to 1 Tbs. (15 ml) fractionated coconut oil to make a soothing massage oil for sore muscles.

> *Simple Solutions—Pain:* Combine 15 drops lavender with 1 tsp. (5 ml) jojoba oil in a small roll-on bottle, and apply on small cuts or scrapes to help soothe pain.

Oils: ♨♨lavender⊕, ♨eucalyptus⊕, ♨Deep Blue, ♨Rescuer, ♨lemon⊕, ♨rosemary⊕, ♨clove⊕, ♨cypress, ♨fir, ♨helichrysum, ♨geranium,

♨frankincense, ♨lemongrass, ♨marjoram, ♨melaleuca, ♨peppermint, ♨rosemary, ♨wintergreen, ♨blue tansy

Other Products: ♨Deep Blue Rub and ⊙TriEase Softgels to help soothe muscles and joints. ⊙Alpha CRS+, ⊙a2z Chewable to help relieve oxidation associated with inflammation that contributes to pain.

—Bone:

Bone pain is a gnawing, throbbing sensation in the bones and has many possible causes, including fractures, cancer, infection, injury, leukemia, and osteoporosis.

Oils: ♨Deep Blue, ♨Rescuer, ♨wintergreen, ♨lavender, ♨cypress, ♨juniper berry, ♨fir, ♨cedarwood, ♨helichrysum, ♨peppermint, ♨sandalwood

—Chronic:

Chronic pain is generally defined as pain that lasts three months or longer.

Oils: ♨Deep Blue, ♨Rescuer, ♨wintergreen, ♨cypress, ♨fir, ♨juniper berry, ♨helichrysum, ♨cedarwood, ♨ginger ⊕, ♨peppermint, ♨sandalwood

—General:

Oils: ♨Deep Blue, ♨Rescuer, ♨wintergreen, ♨lavender, ♨cypress, ♨marjoram, ♨fir, ♨helichrysum, ♨peppermint, ♨sandalwood

—Inflammation: *See also Inflammation*

Oils: ♨rosemary⊕, ♨eucalyptus⊕, ♨lavender⊕, ♨Deep Blue, ♨Rescuer

Other Products: ♨Deep Blue Rub and ⊙TriEase Softgels

—Joints:

Oils: ♨Deep Blue, ♨Rescuer, ♨wintergreen, ♨Roman chamomile

Other Products: ♨Deep Blue Rub and ⊙TriEase Softgels

—Muscle:

Oils: ♨Deep Blue, ♨Rescuer, ♨fir, ♨clove, ♨lavender, ♨lemongrass (ligaments), ♨cypress, ♨marjoram, ♨helichrysum, ♨peppermint, ♨sandalwood, ♨wintergreen

Other Products: ♨Deep Blue Rub and ⊙TriEase Softgels

—Tissue:

Oils: ♨Deep Blue, ♨Rescuer, ♨helichrysum

Primary Recommendations • Secondary Recommendations • Other Recommendations

Other Products: 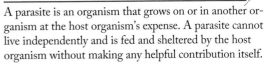Deep Blue Rub and TriEase Softgels

 : Dilute as recommended, and apply 1–2 drops on location. Combine with carrier oil, and massage into affected muscles and joints. Apply as a warm compress over affected areas.

 : Take capsules as directed on package.

 : Diffuse into the air. Inhale oil that is applied to a tissue or cotton wick.

 : **Body System(s) Affected:** Nervous and Skeletal Systems, Muscles, and Skin.

 : **Additional Research:**

Lavender: Ghelardini et al., 1999; Hajhashemi et al., 2003; Kane et al., 2004; Kim et al., 2005; **Eucalyptus:** Göbel et al., 1994; Liapi et al., 2007; Santos et al., 2000; **Lemon:** Aloisi et al., 2002; Ceccarelli et al., 2004; **Rosemary:** Kim et al., 2005; Göbel et al., 1994; Liapi et al., 2007; González-Trujano et al., 2007; Takaki et al., 2008; **Clove:** Ghelardini et al., 2001; **Rosemary:** Santos et al., 2000; González-Trujano et al., 2007; Takaki et al., 2008; **Coriander:** Taherian et al., 2012; **Ginger:** Yip et al., 2008.

Painting

Add one 15 ml bottle of your favorite essential oil (or oil blend) to any 5-gallon bucket of paint. Stir vigorously, mixing well, and then either spray paint or paint by hand. This should eliminate the paint fumes and after-smell.

Palpitations

See Cardiovascular System: Palpitations

Pancreas

The pancreas is a gland organ located behind the stomach. The pancreas is responsible for producing insulin and other hormones and for producing "pancreatic juices" that aid in digestion.

Oils: cypress, rosemary, Breathe, lemon, On Guard

—Pancreatitis:

Pancreatitis is the term used to describe pancreas inflammation. Pancreatitis occurs when the pancreatic juices that are designed to aid in digestion in the small intestine become active while still inside the pancreas. When this occurs, the pancreas literally begins to digest itself. Acute pancreatitis lasts for only a short time and then resolves itself. Chronic pancreatitis does not resolve itself but instead gradually destroys the pancreas.

Oils: lemon, marjoram

—Stimulant For:

Oils: helichrysum

—Support:

Oils: cinnamon, geranium, fennel

 : Dilute as recommended, and apply 1–2 drops over pancreas area or on reflex points on the feet.

 : Diffuse into the air. Inhale directly from bottle. Apply oil to hands, tissue, or cotton wick, and inhale.

 : **Body System(s) Affected:** Endocrine System and Digestive System.

Panic

See Anxiety

Paralysis

See Nervous System: Paralysis

Parasites

A parasite is an organism that grows on or in another organism at the host organism's expense. A parasite cannot live independently and is fed and sheltered by the host organism without making any helpful contribution itself.

Oils: oregano , thyme, fennel, Roman chamomile, DigestZen, lavender , melaleuca , clove

Other Products: DigestZen Softgels

—Intestinal:

Intestinal parasites are parasites that infect the intestinal tract. These parasites enter the intestinal tract through the mouth by unwashed or uncooked food, contaminated water, and unclean hands. Symptoms of intestinal parasites include diarrhea, abdominal pain, weight loss, fatigue, gas or bloating, nausea or vomiting, stomach pain, passing a worm in a stool, stools containing blood and mucus, and rash or itching around the rectum or vulva.

Oils: lemon, oregano , Roman chamomile

—Worms:

Parasitic worms are worm-like organisms that live inside another living organism and feed off their host organism at the host organism's expense,

 =Topical, =Aromatic, =Internal

causing weakness and disease. Parasitic worms can live inside of animals as well as humans.

Oils: 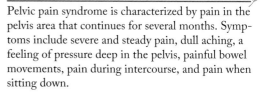DigestZen, lavender, rosemary, thyme, peppermint, Roman chamomile, bergamot, melaleuca

Blend 1: Combine 6 drops Roman chamomile, 6 drops eucalyptus, 6 drops lavender, and 6 drops lemon with 2 Tbs. (25 ml) fractionated coconut oil. Apply 10–15 drops over abdomen with a hot compress, and apply 1–2 drops on intestine and colon reflex points on the feet.

: Place 2–4 drops essential oil in empty capsule, and swallow. Add 1–2 drops to ½ cup (125 ml) rice or almond milk; drink.

: Apply as warm compress over abdomen. Add 2–3 drops to 1 Tbs. (15 ml) fractionated coconut oil, and apply as rectal retention enema for 15 minutes or more. Dilute as recommended, and apply to abdomen and reflex points on the feet.

: Body System(s) Affected: Immune System and Skin.

: Additional Research:

Oregano: Force et al., 2000; **Lavender:** Moon et al., 2006; **Melaleuca:** Gómez-Rincón et al., 2014.

Parasympathetic Nervous System

See **Nervous System: Parasympathetic Nervous System**

Parkinson's Disease

Parkinson's disease is a progressive neurodegenerative disease marked by impairment of muscle movement and speech. Symptoms of Parkinson's disease include slowed motion, muscle stiffness, difficulty maintaining balance, impaired speech, loss of automatic movements (such as blinking, smiling, and swinging the arms while walking), and hand tremors.

Oils: cinnamon, marjoram, lavender, clary sage, frankincense, Balance, sandalwood, Serenity, vetiver, cypress (circulation), bergamot, geranium, helichrysum, juniper berry, lemon, orange, peppermint, rosemary, thyme

Other Products: Mito2Max to help support healthy nerve function. Alpha CRS+, a2z Chewable contain Coenzyme Q10, which has been studied

for its potential benefits in alleviating Parkinson's disease. xEO Mega or vEO Mega for essential omega fatty acids that help support healthy nerve cell function.

: Add 5–10 drops essential oil to 1 Tbs. (15 ml) fractionated coconut oil and massage on affected muscles, back, legs, and neck. Dilute as recommended and apply 1–2 drops to base of neck or reflex points on the feet. Add 3–5 drops to warm bathwater, and bathe.

: Take capsules as directed on package.

: Diffuse into the air. Inhale directly from bottle. Apply oil to hands, tissue, or cotton wick, and inhale.

: Body System(s) Affected: Nervous System and Muscles.

: Additional Research:

Cinnamon: Shaltiel-Karyo et al., 2012; **Eugenol found in cassia, cinnamon, and clove :** Kabuto et al., 2007; **Coenzyme Q10:** Hargreaves et al., 2008; Kooncumchoo et al., 2006; Winkler-Stuck, 2004.

Pelvic Pain Syndrome

Pelvic pain syndrome is characterized by pain in the pelvis area that continues for several months. Symptoms include severe and steady pain, dull aching, a feeling of pressure deep in the pelvis, painful bowel movements, pain during intercourse, and pain when sitting down.

> *Simple Solutions—Pelvic Pain Syndrome:* Add 3 drops ginger and 2 drops geranium to 1 tsp. (5 ml) jojoba oil. Place oil mixture in warm bathwater as a soothing bath oil.

Oils: ginger, geranium, clove, bergamot, thyme, rose

: Place 2–3 drops in warm bathwater, and soak for 10 minutes. Add 5–10 drops to 1 Tbs. (15 ml) fractionated coconut oil, and massage on pelvis and upper legs.

Periodontal Disease

See **Oral Conditions: Gum Disease**

Pests

See **Insects/Bugs, Mice**

Phlebitis

See **Cardiovascular System: Phlebitis**

Pimples

See **Acne**

Pink Eye

See **Eyes: Pink Eye**

Pineal Gland

The pineal gland is a tiny endocrine gland located close to the center of the brain. It is responsible for producing the hormone melatonin that regulates the sleep/wake cycle. The pineal gland also serves to regulate blood pressure, sexual development, growth, body temperature, and motor function.

Oils: frankincense, sandalwood, vetiver, ginger, cedarwood

🌀: Diffuse into the air. Inhale oil directly from bottle. Apply oil to hands, tissue, or cotton wick, and inhale.

⊕: **Body System(s) Affected:** Endocrine System.

Pituitary Gland

The pituitary gland is a small endocrine gland located at the base of the brain that secretes hormones directly into the bloodstream. It is composed of three different lobes, each responsible for producing a different set of hormones. The anterior lobe secretes the human growth hormone (stimulates overall body growth), adreno-corticotropic hormone (controls hormone secretion by the adrenal cortex), thyrotropic hormone (stimulates activity of the thyroid gland), and the gonadotropic hormones (control growth and reproductive activity of the ovaries and testes). The intermediate lobe stimulates melanocytes (control pigmentation such as skin color) The posterior lobe secretes antidiuretic hormone (causes water retention by the kidneys) and oxytocin (stimulates the mammary glands to release milk and causes uterine contractions). The pituitary gland is often referred to as the "master" endocrine gland because it controls the functioning of the other endocrine glands.

Oils: frankincense, sandalwood, vetiver, ginger

—**Balances:**

Oils: ylang ylang, geranium

—**Increases Oxygen:**

Oils: frankincense, sandalwood

🌀: Diffuse into the air. Inhale oil directly from bottle. Apply oil to hands, tissue, or cotton wick, and inhale.

🜄: Dilute as recommended, and apply 1–2 drops to forehead, back of neck, and reflex points on big toes.

⊕: **Body System(s) Affected:** Endocrine System.

Plague

See also **Antibacterial**

Plague is a potentially deadly bacterial disease that is caused by the *Yersinia pestis* bacteria, which is transmitted to humans and animals through close contact or through bites from fleas that have previously bitten infected animals. Symptoms include fever, headaches, and extremely swollen and hot lymph nodes. If left untreated, plague can quickly invade the lungs—causing severe pneumonia, high fever, bloody coughing, and death.

Oils: clove, On Guard, frankincense, oregano

🜄: Dilute as recommended, and apply to neck, chest, and reflex points on the feet.

🌀: Diffuse into the air.

⊕: **Body System(s) Affected:** Immune System.

Plague

See **Antibacterial, Oral Conditions**

Pleurisy

See **Antibacterial, Respiratory System: Pleurisy**

PMS

See **Female-Specific Conditions: PMS**

Pneumonia

See also **Respiratory System, Antibacterial, Antifungal, Antiviral**

Pneumonia is an illness characterized by lung inflammation in which the lungs are infected by a bacteria, fungus, or virus. The result is a cough, chest pain, difficulty breathing, fever, shaking chills, headache, muscle pain, and fatigue. Pneumonia is a special concern for young

🜄=Topical, 🌀=Aromatic, ◯=Internal

children and individuals over the age of 65. Pneumonia ranges in seriousness from mild to life threatening.

> *Simple Solutions—Pneumonia:* Diffuse Breathe in a misting aromatherapy diffuser for 15 minutes every hour throughout the day.

Oils: 🌀🌿Breathe, 🌀🌿On Guard, 🌀🌿thyme⬭, 🌿cinnamon⬭, 🌀🌿oregano⬭, 🌀🌿eucalyptus, 🌀🌿melaleuca, 🌀🌿lavender, 🌿lemon, 🅾🌿tangerine⬭, 🌀🌿frankincense, 🌀🌿myrrh

Other Products: 🅾On Guard+ Softgels

🌀: Diffuse into the air. Place 4 drops in ½ cup (125 ml) hot water, and inhale steam deeply.

🅾: Take capsules as directed on package.

🌿: Dilute as recommended, and apply to chest, back, and reflex points on the feet. Apply as warm compress to the chest. Place 2–3 drops in 1 tsp. (5 ml) fractionated coconut oil; place oil in rectum, and retain overnight.

🔆: **Body System(s) Affected:** Immune System and Respiratory System.

⬭: **Additional Research:**

Thyme: Inouye et al., 2001; Fabio et al., 2007; **Cinnamon:** Inouye et al., 2001; Fabio et al., 2007; **Oregano:** Preuss et al., 2005; **Tangerine:** Zhou et al., 2012.

Poison Ivy/Oak

Poison oak and poison ivy are plants with an oily sap called urushiol that causes an itchy rash when it comes into contact with the skin. Infection by poison oak or poison ivy is recognized by redness and itching of the skin, a rash, red bumps, and later oozing blisters. A rash caused by poison oak or by poison ivy usually lasts from 5 to 12 days.

> *Simple Solutions—Poison Oak/Ivy:* Wash skin with soap and water as soon as possible after contact. If rash and itching develop, add 10 drops lavender and 10 drops Roman chamomile to ½ cup (125 ml) calamine lotion. Apply a small amount on affected areas up to twice per day as needed.

Oils: 🌿rose, 🌿lavender, 🌿Elevation, 🌿Roman chamomile

🌿: Dilute as recommended, and apply 1–2 drops on location. Add 2–3 drops to 1 tsp. (5 ml) fractionated coconut oil, and apply on location.

🔆: **Body System(s) Affected:** Skin.

Pollution

See **Purification**

Polyps

See **Colon: Polyps, Nose: Nasal Polyp**

Pregnancy/Motherhood

Pregnancy is the period of time (generally 9 months) in which a woman carries a developing fetus in her uterus.

Oils: 🌀🌿geranium, 🌀🌿ylang ylang, 🌀🌿lavender⬭, 🌀🌿grapefruit, 🌀🌿Roman chamomile

Other Products: 🅾Alpha CRS+, 🅾a2z Chewable, 🅾xEO Mega or vEO Mega, 🅾Microplex VMz for nutrients essential to support cellular health and body function.

—Anxiety/Tension: *See* **Calming**

—Baby (Newborn):

Oils: 🌿frankincense (1 drop on crown), 🌿myrrh (1 drop on umbilical cord and navel), 🌿Balance (1 drop on feet and spine)

🌿: Apply as indicated above.

—Breasts:

In the first trimester of pregnancy, a woman's breasts become sore and tender as the body begins to prepare itself for breast-feeding. During pregnancy the breasts enlarge, the nipples grow larger and become darker, and the breasts may begin to leak colostrum—the first milk the body makes in preparation for the developing baby.

Oils: 🌿lavender (soothes), 🌿geranium (soothes), 🌿Roman chamomile (sore nipples), 🌿fennel (tones)

🌿: Add 3–5 drops to 1 Tbs. (15 ml) fractionated coconut oil, and massage on location.

—Delivery:

Delivery is the act or process of giving birth.

Oils: 🌀🌿lavender (stimulates circulation, calming, antiseptic), 🌿clary sage, 🌿Balance

🌿: Dilute as recommended, and apply 1–2 drops on hips, bottoms of feet, or abdomen. Add 3–5 drops to 1 Tbs. (15 ml) fractionated coconut oil, and massage on hips, bottoms of feet, or abdomen.

🜄: Diffuse into the air. Inhale directly from bottle. Apply oil to hands, tissue, or cotton wick, and inhale.

–Avoid Episiotomy:

Oils: 🜄geranium

🜄: Add 5–10 drops to ½ tsp. (2.5 ml) olive oil, and massage perineum.

–Diffuse:

Oils: 🜄Serenity, 🜄Elevation

🜄: Diffuse into the air.

–Uterus:

Oils: 🜄clary sage

🜄: Apply 1–3 drops around the ankles to help tone uterus.

–Transition:

Oils: 🜄basil

🜄: Dilute as recommended, and apply 1–2 drops to temples or abdomen.

—Early Labor:

Preterm labor is labor that begins before the 37th week of pregnancy. Babies born before the 37th week are considered premature. Signs of preterm labor include contractions every 10 minutes or more often, cramps, low backache, pelvic pressure, and change in vaginal discharge (fluid or blood).

Oils: 🜄lavender

🜄: Gently apply 1–3 drops on stomach or on heart area to help stop.

—Energy:

Blend 1: Combine 2 drops Roman chamomile, 2 drops geranium, and 2 drops lavender in 2 tsp. (10 ml) fractionated coconut oil, and massage into the skin.

—Hemorrhaging:

Postpartum hemorrhaging is excessive bleeding following childbirth. It is commonly defined as losing 500 ml of blood after vaginal birth and 1000 ml of blood after a cesarean birth. Postpartum hemorrhaging generally occurs within 24 hours following the birth and can be life threatening if not stopped.

Oils: 🜄helichrysum

🜄: Apply 1–3 drops on lower back to help prevent hemorrhaging.

—High Blood Pressure:

High blood pressure can potentially be dangerous in pregnancy. High blood pressure can cause a decreased flow of blood to the placenta, slowing down the baby's growth; premature placenta separation from the uterus, taking away the baby's oxygen and nutrients and causing heavy bleeding in the mother; premature birth; and the risk of future disease. Pregnancy can in some cases actually cause a woman's blood pressure to increase.

Oils: 🜄🜄ylang ylang⬜, 🜄🜄eucalyptus⬜, 🜄🜄lavender, 🜄🜄clove, 🜄🜄clary sage, 🜄🜄lemon. **Note:** Avoid rosemary, thyme, and possibly peppermint.

Bath 1: Place 3 drops ylang ylang in bathwater, and bathe in the evening twice a week.

Blend 2: Combine 5 drops geranium, 8 drops lemongrass, and 3 drops lavender in 2 Tbs. (25 ml) fractionated coconut oil. Rub over heart and on reflex points on left foot and hand.

🜄: Dilute as recommended, and apply on location, on reflex points on feet and hands, and over heart.

🜄: Diffuse into the air. Apply oils to hands, and inhale oils from hands cupped over the nose. Inhale oil applied to a tissue or cotton wick.

—Labor (during):

Oils: 🜄clary sage (may combine with fennel), 🜄lavender⬜

🜄: Apply 3 drops around ankles or on abdomen.

—Labor (post):

Oils: 🜄lavender, 🜄geranium

🜄: Dilute as recommended, and apply 1–3 drops on abdomen, ankles, or bottoms of feet.

—Lactation (Milk Production):

Lactation is the production and secretion of milk from the mammary glands of females for the nourishment of their young offspring. Lactation is commonly referred to as "breast-feeding."

Simple Solutions—Nursing: Blend 3 drops lavender, 2 drops geranium, and 1 drop Roman chamomile with 1 Tbs. (15 ml) almond oil. Apply a small amount on breasts to help soothe. Wash off before feeding the baby.

Oils: 🜄clary sage (start production), 🜄fennel or 🜄basil (increase production), 🜄peppermint (decrease production), 🜄Whisper (contains jasmine⬜ that may help decrease production)

🜄=Topical, 🜄=Aromatic, 🌕=Internal

: Dilute as recommended, and apply 1–2 drops on breasts. Apply peppermint with cold compress to help reduce production. *Caution: Fennel should not be used for more than 10 days, as it will excessively increase flow through the urinary tract.*

—Mastitis: *See also **Antibacterial**.*

Mastitis is a breast infection occurring in women who are breast-feeding. Mastitis causes the breast to become red, swollen, and very painful. Symptoms of mastitis include breast tenderness, fever, general lack of well-being, skin redness, and a breast that feels warm to the touch. Mastitis generally occurs in just one breast, not in both.

Oils: lavender, Citrus Bliss (combine with lavender), patchouli

: Dilute as recommended, and apply 1–2 drops on breasts.

—Miscarriage (after):

A miscarriage is a pregnancy that ends on its own within the first 20 weeks. Signs of a miscarriage include vaginal bleeding, fluid or tissue being ejected from the vagina, and pain and cramping in the abdomen or lower back. Miscarriages occur before the baby is developed enough to survive. About half of all pregnancies end in miscarriage, but most happen too early for the mother to be aware that it has occurred. Women who miscarry after about 8 weeks of pregnancy should consult their doctor as soon as possible afterwards to prevent any future complications.

Oils: frankincense, grapefruit, geranium, lavender, Roman chamomile

: Dilute 5–6 drops in 1 Tbs. (15 ml) fractionated coconut oil, and massage on back, legs, and arms. Add 3–4 drops to warm bathwater, and bathe.

—Morning Sickness:

Morning sickness is the nauseated feeling accompanying the first trimester of pregnancy for many women. Morning sickness can often include vomiting. For most women, morning sickness begins around the sixth week of pregnancy and ends around the twelfth week. Although it is called "morning" sickness, the symptoms can occur at any time during the day.

Simple Solutions—Morning Sickness: Add 2 drops ginger to a bowl of hot water, and inhale the warm vapor coming from the water.

Oils: ginger, peppermint, lemon

: Dilute as recommended, and apply 1–3 drops on ears, down jaw bone, and on reflex points on the feet.

: Place 1–3 drops in empty capsule; swallow capsule.

: Diffuse into the air. Inhale directly from bottle. Apply oil to hands, tissue, or cotton wick, and inhale. Apply 1 drop on pillow to inhale at night.

—Placenta:

The placenta is the organ responsible for sustaining life in an unborn baby. The placenta attaches to the uterus wall and connects to the mother's blood supply to provide nutrients and oxygen for the fetus. The placenta plays other essential roles as well: It removes waste created by the fetus, triggers labor and delivery, and protects the fetus against infection.

Oils: basil (to help retain)

: Dilute as recommended, and apply 1–2 drops on lower abdomen and reflex points on the feet.

—Postpartum Depression:

Postpartum depression is depression sometimes experienced by mothers shortly after giving birth. New mothers may experience symptoms such as irritableness, sadness, uncontrollable emotions, fatigue, anxiety, difficulty sleeping, thoughts of suicide, hopelessness, and guilt. Postpartum depression is typically thought to result from a hormonal imbalance caused by the pregnancy and childbirth.

Oils: Elevation, lemon, lavender, frankincense, clary sage, geranium, grapefruit, bergamot, Balance, myrrh, orange

: Diffuse into the air. Inhale directly from bottle. Apply oil to hands, tissue, or cotton wick, and inhale.

: Dilute as recommended, and apply 1–2 drops to temple or forehead. Add 5–10 drops to 1 Tbs. (15 ml) fractionated coconut oil, and use as massage oil. Add 1–3 drops to warm bathwater, and bathe.

—Preeclampsia: *See also **Pregnancy/Motherhood: High Blood Pressure***

Preeclampsia, also known as toxemia, is pregnancy-induced high blood pressure. Symptoms include protein in the urine, elevated blood pressure levels, sudden weight gain, blurred vision, abdominal pains in the upper-right side, and swelling in the hands and face. Women suffering from preeclampsia are often put on bed rest for the remainder of the pregnancy to ensure the safety of the mother and baby.

Oils: 🔄🔄cypress

🔄: Dilute 1:1 in fractionated coconut oil, and apply 1–2 drops on bottoms of feet and on abdomen.

🔄: Diffuse into the air. Inhale directly from bottle. Apply oil to hands, tissue, or cotton wick, and inhale.

—Self Love:

Oils: 🔄Elevation

🔄: Diffuse into the air. Wear as perfume.

—Stretch Marks: *See Skin: Stretch Marks*

🔄: **Body System(s) Affected:** Reproductive System and Endocrine System.

⬜: **Additional Research:**

Lavender: Olapour et al., 2013; **Ylang ylang:** Hongratanaworakit et al., 2006; Hongratanaworakit et al., 2004; **Eucalyptus:** Lahlou et al., 2002; **Jasmine:** Shrivastav et al., 1988; **Ginger:** Vutyavanich et al., 2001; **Lemon:** Yavari kia et al., 2014; **Patchouli:** Li et al., 2014; Komiya et al., 2006; Komori et al., 1995; Komori et al., 1995; **Lavender:** Lee et al., 2006; Moussaieff et al., 2008; Yazdkhasti et al., 2016

Prostate

The prostate gland is a small organ just beneath that bladder that is part of the male reproductive system. Its primary function is to create and store fluid that helps nourish and protect the sperm.

Oils: 🔄helichrysum, 🔄frankincense, 🔄juniper berry

—Benign Prostatic Hyperplasia:

The size of the prostate begins at about the same size as a walnut but increases in size as a male ages. If the prostate grows too large, it can block passage of urine from the bladder through the urethra. This blockage can lead to increased risk for developing urinary tract stones, infections, or damaged kidneys.

Oils: 🔄fennel

—Prostate Cancer: *See Cancer: Prostate*

—Prostatitis:

Prostatitis is an inflamed prostate, typically due to infection. This can cause pain in the lower back and groin area, painful urination, and the need to urinate frequently.

Oils: 🔄thyme, 🔄cypress, 🔄lavender

🔄: Dilute as recommended, and apply to the posterior, scrotum, ankles, lower back, or bottoms of feet.

🔘: Add 5 drops to 1 Tbs. (15 ml) fractionated coconut oil, insert into rectum, and retain throughout the night.

🔄: **Body System(s) Affected:** Reproductive System.

Psoriasis

Psoriasis is a skin condition characterized by patches of red, scaly skin that may itch or burn. The most commonly affected areas are the elbows, knees, scalp, back, face, palms, and feet. But other areas can be affected as well. Psoriasis doesn't have a known cure or cause, but it is thought an auto-immune disorder may play a role. Psoriasis tends to be less severe in the warmer months.

> *Simple Solutions—Psoriasis:* Combine 2 drops Roman chamomile with 2 drops lavender, and apply on location.

Oils: 🔄helichrysum, 🔄thyme, 🔄lavender, 🔄melaleuca, 🔄Roman chamomile, 🔄cedarwood, 🔄bergamot

🔄: Dilute as recommended, and apply 1–2 drops on location.

🔄: **Body System(s) Affected:** Skin.

Pulmonary

See Respiratory System: Lungs

Purification

Oils: 🔄Purify, 🔄lemon, 🔄lemongrass, 🔄eucalyptus, 🔄melaleuca, 🔄cedarwood, 🔄orange, 🔄fennel

—Air:

Oils: 🔄lemon, 🔄peppermint, 🔄Purify

—Cigarette Smoke:

Oils: 🔄Purify

—Dishes:

Oils: 🔄lemon

—Water:

Oils: 🔘🔄lemon, 🔄Purify, 🔘🔄peppermint

🔄: Diffuse into the air. Add 10–15 drops to 2 Tbs. (25 ml) distilled water in a small spray bottle; shake well, and mist into the air.

🔄=Topical, 🔄=Aromatic, 🔘=Internal

: Add 1–2 drops to dishwater for sparkling dishes and a great smelling kitchen. Add 1–2 drops to warm bathwater, and bathe. Add 1–2 drops to bowl of water, and use to clean the outside of fruit and vegetables.

: Add 1 drop oil to 1½–2 cups (375–500 ml) of drinking water to help purify.

Pus

See **Infection**

Radiation

Radiation is energy emitted from a source and sent through space or matter. Different forms of radiation can include light, heat, sound, radio, micro-waves, gamma rays, or X-rays, among others. While many forms of radiation are around us every day and are perfectly safe (such as light, sound, and heat), frequent or prolonged exposure to high-energy forms of radiation can be detrimental to the body, possibly causing DNA mutation, damaged cellular structures, burns, cancer, or other damage.

Oils: peppermint, sandalwood

—**Gamma Radiation:**

Oils: peppermint

—**Radiation Therapy:**

Radiation treatments can produce tremendous toxicity within the liver. Cut down on the use of oils with high phenol content to prevent increasing liver toxicity. Oils with high phenol content include wintergreen, birch, clove, basil, fennel, oregano, thyme, melaleuca, and cinnamon.

—**Ultraviolet Radiation:**

Oils: sandalwood, frankincense, melaleuca, thyme, clove

—**Weeping Wounds From:**

Oils: melaleuca, thyme, oregano

: Place 1–2 drops under the tongue or place 2–3 drops in an empty capsule, and swallow.

: Dilute as recommended, and apply 1–2 drops on location.

: **Additional Research:**

Peppermint: Samarth et al., 2004; Samarth et al., 2009; Samarth et al., 2006; Samarth et al., 2003; Samarth et al., 2007; **Sandalwood:** Arasada et al., 2008; Dwivedi et al., 2006; **Melaleuca:** Caldefie-Chézet et al., 2004; **Thyme:** Wei et al., 2007; **Clove:** Wei et al., 2007.

Rashes

See **Skin: Rashes**

Raynaud's Disease

See also **Arteries, Cardiovascular System: Circulation**

Raynaud's disease is a condition that causes the arteries supplying blood to the skin to suddenly narrow and inhibit blood circulation. As a result, specific areas of the body feel numb and cool. The most commonly affected areas are the toes, fingers, nose, and ears. During an attack, the skin turns white and then blue. As circulation returns and warms the affected areas, a prickling, throbbing, stinging, or swelling sensation often accompanies it. These attacks are often triggered by cold temperatures and by stress.

Oils: cypress, rosemary, geranium, helichrysum, fennel, clove, lavender

: Dilute as recommended, and apply 1–2 drops on the affected area, to carotid arteries, and on reflex points on the feet.

: Diffuse into the air. Inhale oil directly from bottle, or inhale oil that is applied to hands, tissue, or cotton wick.

: **Body System(s) Affected:** Cardiovascular System.

Relaxation

Relaxation is a state of rest and tranquility, free from tension and anxiety.

> *Simple Solutions—Relaxing:* Combine 3 drops lavender and 3 drops Roman chamomile with 1 cup (250 g) Epsom salt. Add ½ cup (125 g) of salt to warm bathwater for a relaxing bath.

Oils: lavender, ylang ylang, lemon, AromaTouch, neroli, star anise, Roman chamomile, geranium, frankincense, fir, sandalwood, clary sage

: Diffuse into the air. Inhale directly from bottle. Apply oil to hands, tissue, or cotton wick, and inhale.

: Add 5–10 drops to 1 Tbs. (15 ml) fractionated coconut oil (or another carrier oil), and use as massage oil. Place 1–2 drops in warm bathwater, and bathe.

: **Body System(s) Affected:** Emotional Balance.

⏱: **Additional Research:**

Lavender: Pemberton et al., 2008; Field et al., 2005; Diego et al., 1998; Buchbauer et al., 1991; **Ylang ylang:** Hongratanaworakit et al., 2006; **Lemon:** Komiya et al., 2006.

Respiratory System

The respiratory system's primary purposes are to supply the blood with oxygen that is then delivered to all parts of the body and to remove waste carbon dioxide from the blood and eliminate it from the body. The respiratory system consists of the mouth, nose, and pharynx (through which air is first taken in), larynx (voice box), trachea (airway leading from the larynx to the lungs), bronchi (which branch off from the trachea and into the lungs), bronchioles (smaller tubes that branch off from the bronchi), alveoli (tiny sacs filled with capillaries that allow inhaled oxygen to be transferred into the blood and carbon dioxide to be expelled from the blood into the air in the lungs), pleura (which covers the outside of the lungs and the inside of the chest wall), and diaphragm (a large muscle at the bottom of the chest cavity that moves to pull air into the lungs (inhale) and to push air out of the lungs (exhale)).

Oils: ⊘⊜Breathe, ⊘⊜eucalyptus⊖, ⊘⊜peppermint⊖, ⊘⊜Douglas fir, ⊘⊜cinnamon⊖, ⊘⊜manuka, ⊘⊜On Guard, ⊘⊜cardamom⊖, ⊘⊜melaleuca, ⊘⊜fir, ⊘⊜clary sage, ⊘⊜fennel, ⊘⊜helichrysum, ⊘⊜marjoram, ⊘⊜oregano, ⊘⊜bergamot⊖, ⊘⊜clove, ⊘⊜frankincense, ⊘⊜lemon, ⊘⊜rosemary, ⊘⊜lime

Blend 1: Combine 5 drops eucalyptus, 8 drops frankincense, and 6 drops lemon. Apply to bottoms of feet; or add to 2 Tbs. (25 ml) fractionated coconut oil, and apply as a hot compress on chest.

Recipe 1: Combine 10 drops eucalyptus and 10 drops myrrh with 1 Tbs. (15 ml) fractionated coconut oil. Insert rectally for overnight retention enema.

Other Products: ⊖Breathe Respiratory Drops, ⊜⊘Breathe Vapor Stick, ⊖TriEase Softgels

—Asthma: *See Asthma*

—Breathing:

Oils: ⊘⊜Breathe, ⊘⊜cinnamon, ⊘⊜frankincense, ⊘⊜rosemary, ⊘⊜Douglas fir, ⊘⊜thyme, ⊘⊜marjoram, ⊘⊜juniper berry, ⊘⊜ginger

Other Products: ⊜⊘Breathe Vapor Stick, ⊖Breathe Respiratory Drops

—Bronchitis: *See Bronchitis*

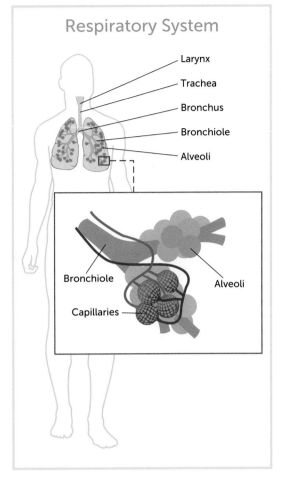

Respiratory System

Larynx
Trachea
Bronchus
Bronchiole
Alveoli

Bronchiole
Capillaries
Alveoli

—Congestion: *See Congestion*

—Cough: *See Cough*

—Cystic Fibrosis:

Cystic fibrosis is an inherited genetic condition that causes glands the lungs and other organs to secrete less hydrated, more sticky secretions. The stickiness of these secretions cause blockages and inflammation, damaging the lungs and other organs over time.

Simple Solutions—Cystic Fibrosis: Diffuse bergamot in an aromatherapy diffuser.

Oils: ⊘⊜bergamot⊖

—Hyperpnea:

Hyperpnea is rapid or heavy breathing that occurs normally as a result of strenuous physical exertion and abnormally in conjunction with fever and disorders.

Oils: ⊘☉ylang ylang

—Lungs:

The lungs are paired organs located on either side of the heart. The lungs function to exchange oxygen and carbon dioxide (breathing). Oxygen passes into the blood by inhaling, and exhaling expels carbon dioxide. The lungs keep the body supplied with the oxygen necessary to keep cells alive. The lung on the right side of the body contains three lobes (sections) and is slightly larger than the lung on the left side of the body, which has two lobes.

Oils: ⊘☉Breathe, ⊘☉eucalyptus, ⊘☉sandalwood, ⊘☉frankincense, ⊘☉Elevation, ⊘☉On Guard (for infections)

Other Products: ○Zendocrine Detoxification Complex to help support healthy lung functioning.

—Oxygen:

Oils: ⊘frankincense, ⊘sandalwood, ⊘cedarwood

—Pleurisy:

Pleurisy is an inflammation of the moist membrane (pleura) that surrounds the lungs and lines the rib cage. Pleurisy is characterized by a dry cough, chest pain, and difficulty breathing. Viral infection is the most common cause of pleurisy; but lung infections, chest injuries, and drug reactions are also possible causes. Pleurisy usually lasts between a few days and a couple weeks.

Oils: ⊘☉cypress, ⊘☉thyme

—Pneumonia: *See Pneumonia*

⊘: Diffuse into the air. Inhale directly from bottle. Apply oil to hands, tissue, or cotton wick, and inhale.

☉: Dilute as recommended, and apply to chest, sinuses, neck, or reflex points on the feet. Add 2–3 drops to water, and gargle. Apply to chest as warm compress. Add 20 drops to 1 Tbs. (15 ml) fractionated coconut oil, and insert rectally for overnight retention enema.

○: Take supplements as directed on package.

✛: **Body System(s) Affected:** Respiratory System.

▥: **Additional Research:**

Eucalyptus: Vigo et al., 2004; Lu et al., 2004; Juergens et al., 1998; **Peppermint:** Juergens et al., 1998; **Cinnamon:** Singh et al., 1995; Inouye et al., 2001; **Cardamom:** Kumari et al., 2013; **Bergamot:** Borgatti et al., 2011.

Restlessness

See Calming

Rheumatic Fever

See also Antibacterial

Rheumatic fever is the inflammation of the heart and joints in response to a strep throat or scarlet fever infection. This inflammation can cause permanent damage to the heart. Symptoms of rheumatic fever include painful and swollen joints, chest pain, fever, fatigue, the sensation of a pounding heartbeat, shortness of breath, rash, sudden jerky body movements, and unusual displays of emotion. Rheumatic fever is most common in children between ages 5 and 15.

Oils: ☉ginger (for pain)

☉: Dilute as recommended, and apply 1–2 drops on location.

✛: **Body System(s) Affected:** Immune System and Cardiovascular Systems.

Rheumatism

See Arthritis: Rheumatoid Arthritis

Rhinitis

See Nose: Rhinitis

Ringworm

See Antifungal: Ringworm

Rocky Mountain Spotted Fever

See also Antibacterial, Insects/Bugs: Ticks

Rocky Mountain spotted fever is a bacterial disease that spreads through the bite of an infected tick. Symptoms include high fever, severe headache, and a red, non-itchy rash that first appears on the wrists and ankles, then spreads from there.

Oils: ○☉⊘On Guard, ☉⊘cinnamon, ☉Purify, ☉⊘TerraShield (prevent), ☉⊘lavender (prevent)

☉: Dilute as recommended, and apply 1–2 drops over location or on bottoms of the feet.

⊘: Diffuse into the air. Inhale directly from bottle. Apply oil to hands, tissue, or cotton wick, and inhale.

Primary Recommendations • Secondary Recommendations • Other Recommendations

◐: Place 1–2 drops of oil under the tongue, or place oils in empty capsules and swallow.

◆: **Body System(s) Affected:** Immune System.

Sadness

See Grief/Sorrow

Salmonella

See Antibacterial, Food Poisoning

Scabies

See Skin: Scabies

Scarring

See Skin: Scarring, Tissue: Scarring

Schmidt's Syndrome

See Adrenal Glands: Schmidt's Syndrome

Sciatica

Sciatica is pain resulting from the irritation of the sciatic nerve. The sciatic nerve is the longest nerve in the body. It runs from the spinal cord through the buttock and hip area and down the back of each leg. When the sciatic nerve is pinched or irritated due to something such as a herniated disk, the pain experienced along the sciatic nerve is called "sciatica." Symptoms of sciatica include pain in the area, numbness and weakness along the sciatic nerve, tingling sensations, or a loss of bladder or bowel control.

> *Simple Solutions—Sciatica:* Mix 5 drops peppermint with 1 tsp. (5 ml) fractionated coconut oil in a small roll-on bottle. Apply on lower back every 3 hours as needed.

Oils: ◐peppermint, ◐Roman chamomile, ◐helichrysum, ◐thyme, ◐Deep Blue (for pain), ◐Balance, ◐fir, ◐sandalwood, ◐lavender, ◐wintergreen

◐: Dilute as recommended, and apply 1–2 drops on lower back, buttocks, or legs. Add 5–10 drops to 1 Tbs. (15 ml) fractionated coconut oil, and massage on spine, back, legs, and bottoms of feet.

◆: **Body System(s) Affected:** Nervous System.

Scrapes

See Wounds

Scurvy

Scurvy is a disease caused by a deficiency of ascorbic acid (vitamin C). Some results of scurvy are general weakness, anemia, gum disease (gingivitis), skin hemorrhages, spots on the skin (usually the thighs and legs), and bleeding from the mucous membranes.

Oils: ◐ginger

Other Products: ◐Microplex VMz contains vitamin C necessary for preventing scurvy.

◐: Dilute as recommended, and apply 1–2 drops over kidneys, liver, and reflex points on the feet.

◐: Take capsules as directed on package.

◆: **Body System(s) Affected:** Skin and Digestive System.

Sedative

See Calming: Sedative

Seizure

A seizure is an uncontrolled, abnormal electrical discharge in the brain which may produce a physical convulsion, minor physical signs, thought disturbances, or a combination of symptoms. The symptoms depend on what parts of the brain are involved.

Oils: ◐clary sage, ◐lavender◐, ◐rose◐, ◐◐peppermint◐, ◐Balance, ◐clove◐, ◐Serenity, ◐Elevation

Other Products: ◐Mito2Max to help support healthy nerve function. ◐xEO Mega or vEO Mega, ◐Microplex VMz contain omega fatty acids, minerals, and other nutrients that support healthy brain function.

—Convulsions:

A convulsion is the repeated, rapid contracting and relaxing of muscles resulting in the uncontrollable shaking of the body. Convulsions usually last about 30 seconds to 2 minutes and are often associated with seizures.

Oils: ◐lavender◐, ◐clary sage, ◐Balance

◐=Topical, ◐=Aromatic, ◐=Internal

—Epilepsy:

Epilepsy is a neurological condition where the person has recurring, unpredictable seizures. Epilepsy has many possible causes; although in many cases the cause is unknown. Possible causes may include illness, injury to the brain, or abnormal brain development.

Oils: ◐clary sage

—Grand Mal Seizure:

The grand mal seizure, also known as the tonic-clonic seizure, is the most common seizure. The tonic phase lasts about 10–20 seconds. During this stage, the person loses consciousness, and the muscles contract—causing the person to fall down. During the clonic phase, the person experiences violent convulsions. This phase usually lasts less than two minutes.

Oils: ◐Balance (on feet), ◐◑Serenity (around navel), ◐Elevation (over heart)

Other Products: ○Microplex VMz contains zinc and copper—an imbalance of zinc and copper has been theorized to play a role in grand mal seizures.

◐: Dilute as recommended, and apply 1–2 drops to back of neck, navel, heart, or reflex points on the feet.

○: Take capsules as directed on package.

◑: Diffuse into the air.

✛: **Body System(s) Affected:** Nervous System.

○: **Additional Research:**

Lavender: Brum et al., 2001; **Rose:** Hosseini et al., 2011; **Rose:** Ramezani et al., 2008; **Peppermint:** Koutroumanidou et al., 2013; **Clove:** Hosseini et al., 2012; **Dill:** Arash et al., 2013.

Sexual Issues

Simple Solutions—Low Libido: Blend 5 drops ylang ylang and 1 drop cinnamon with 1 Tbs. (15 ml) fractionated coconut oil to make a romantic massage oil.

—Arousing Desire: *See Aphrodisiac*

—Frigidity:

Female frigidity is a female's lack of sexual drive or her inability to enjoy sexual activities. This disorder has many possible physical and psychological causes, including stress, fatigue, guilt, fear, worry, alcoholism, or drug abuse.

Oils: ◐◑clary sage, ◐◑ylang ylang, ◐◑Whisper, ◐◑rose

—Impotence:

Impotence in men, also known as erectile dysfunction, is the frequent inability to have or sustain an erection. This may be caused by circulation problems, nerve problems, low levels of testosterone, medications, or psychological stresses.

Oils: ◑○clary sage, ◑○clove, ◑○rose, ◑○ginger, ◑○sandalwood

—Libido (low):

Libido is a term used by Sigmund Freud to describe human sexual desire. Causes for a lack of sexual desire can be both physical and psychological. Some possible causes include anemia, alcoholism, drug abuse, stress, anxiety, past sexual abuse, and relationship problems.

Oils: ◐◑ylang ylang, ◐◑Elevation

Other Products: ○Mito2Max

—Men:

Oils: ◐◑cinnamon, ◐◑ginger, ◐◑myrrh

—Women:

Oils: ◐◑clary sage, ◑geranium

◑: Diffuse into the air. Dissolve 2–3 drops in 2 tsp. (10 ml) pure grain or perfumer's alcohol, combine with distilled water in a 1–2 oz. spray bottle, and spray into the air or on clothes or bed linens.

◐: Dilute as recommended, and wear on temples, neck, or wrists as perfume or cologne. Combine 3–5 drops of your desired essential oil with 1 Tbs. (15 ml) fractionated coconut oil to use as a massage oil. Combine 1–2 drops with ¼ cup (50 g) Therapeutic Bath Salts, and dissolve in warm bathwater for a romantic bath.

○: Take capsules as directed. Place 1–2 drops oil in an empty capsule, and swallow.

✛: **Body System(s) Affected:** Reproductive System.

Sexually Transmitted Diseases (STD)

See AIDS/HIV, Herpes Simplex

Shingles

See also **Antiviral, Childhood Diseases: Chicken-pox, Nervous System: Neuralgia**

Shingles is a viral infection caused by the same virus that causes chickenpox. After a person has had chickenpox, the virus lies dormant in the nervous system. Years later, that virus can be reactivated by stress, immune deficiency, or disease and cause shingles. Symptoms of shingles start with tingling, pain, neuralgia, or itching of an area of skin and become visually obvious as red blisters form in that same area along the nerve path, forming a red band on the skin. Blisters most commonly appear wrapping from the middle of the back to the middle of the chest but can form on the neck, face, and scalp as well. Another name for shingles is herpes zoster.

> *Simple Solutions—Shingles:* Blend 3 drops lavender, 3 drops melaleuca, and 3 drops thyme with 1 tsp. (5 ml) fractionated coconut oil. Apply on feet and on location.

Oils: ⊘melaleuca, ⊘eucalyptus, ⊘lavender, ⊘lemon, ⊘geranium, ⊘bergamot

⊘: Dilute as recommended, and apply 1–2 drops on location. Add 5–10 drops essential oil to 1 Tbs. (15 ml) fractionated coconut oil, and massage on location and on bottoms of feet.

♁: **Body System(s) Affected:** Skin, Nervous System, and Immune System.

Shock

See also **Cardiovascular System: Circulation, Cardiovascular System: Heart**

Shock is a life-threatening condition where the body suffers from severely low blood pressure. This can be caused by low blood volume due to bleeding or dehydration, inadequate pumping of the heart, or dilation of the blood vessels due to head injury, medications, or poisons from bacterial infections. Shock can cause pale or bluish skin that feels cold or clammy to the touch, confusion, rapid breathing, and a rapid heartbeat. Without the needed oxygen being sent to the body's tissues and cells, the organs can shut down and, in severe cases, can lead to death. Shock often accompanies severe injuries or other traumatic situations. A person suffering from shock should be made to lie down with the feet elevated above the head, be kept warm, and have the head turned to the side in case of vomiting. Check breathing often, and ensure that any visible bleeding is stopped. Get emergency medical help as soon as possible.

> *Simple Solutions—Shock:* Follow the instructions outlined above, and hold an open bottle of peppermint under the victim's nose.

Oils: ⊘⊘peppermint, ⊘Roman chamomile, ⊘helichrysum (may help stop bleeding), ⊘melaleuca, ⊘Elevation, ⊘⊘ylang ylang, ⊘Balance, ⊘⊘myrrh, ⊘⊘melissa, ⊘⊘basil, ⊘rosemary

⊘: Dilute as recommended, and apply 1–2 drops on back of neck, feet, over heart, or on front of neck.

⊘: Diffuse into the air. Inhale directly from bottle. Apply oil to hands, tissue, or cotton wick, and inhale.

♁: **Body System(s) Affected:** Cardiovascular System and Nervous System.

Shoulder

See **Joints: Shoulder**

Sinuses

Sinuses are several hollow cavities within the skull that allow the skull to be more lightweight without compromising strength. These cavities are connected to the nasal cavity through small channels. When the mucous membrane lining these channels becomes swollen or inflamed due to colds or allergies, these channels can become blocked—making it difficult for the sinuses to drain correctly. This can lead to infection and inflammation of the mucous membrane within the sinuses (sinusitis). There are sinus cavities behind the cheek bone and forehead and near the eyes and nasal cavity.

> *Simple Solutions—Sinusitis:* Add 2 drops eucalyptus to a bowl of hot water, and inhale the vapor.

Oils: ⊘⊘helichrysum, ⊘⊘eucalyptus, ⊘⊘Breathe, ⊘⊘peppermint, ⊘⊘On Guard, ⊘cedarwood

—Sinusitis:

Oils: ⊘⊘eucalyptus, ⊘⊘rosemary, ⊘⊘Breathe, ⊘DigestZen, ⊘⊘peppermint, ⊘⊘melaleuca, ⊘⊘fir, ⊘⊘ginger

Recipe 1: For chronic sinusitis, apply 1–2 drops DigestZen around navel 4 times daily; apply 2 drops peppermint under tongue 2 times daily.

⊘=Topical, ⊘=Aromatic, ○=Internal

⊘: Diffuse into the air. Inhale directly from bottle. Apply oil to hands, tissue, or cotton wick, and inhale. Place 1–2 drops in a bowl of hot water, and inhale vapors.

⊜: Dilute as recommended, and apply 1–2 drops along the sides of the nose or forehead (often clears out sinuses immediately).

⊕: **Body System(s) Affected:** Respiratory System.

Skeletal System

In an adult individual, the skeletal system comprises 206 bones. These bones provide structure to the body and allow for movement, as well as provide protection for vital organs and tissues. Bones contain bone marrow where blood cells are created. Bones also act as storage reservoirs for calcium and other minerals that the body needs.

Oils: ⊘wintergreen, ⊘fir, ⊘cypress, ⊘juniper berry, ⊘⊜cedarwood, ⊘lavender, ⊘lemongrass, ⊘marjoram, ⊘peppermint, ⊘sandalwood

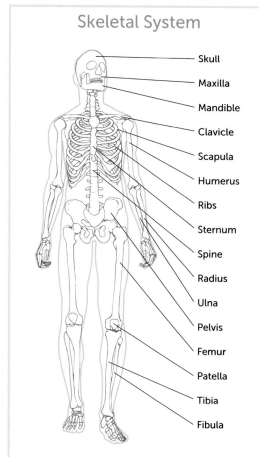

Skeletal System

- Skull
- Maxilla
- Mandible
- Clavicle
- Scapula
- Humerus
- Ribs
- Sternum
- Spine
- Radius
- Ulna
- Pelvis
- Femur
- Patella
- Tibia
- Fibula

Other Products: ⊙Microplex VMz contains nutrients essential for bone development, such as calcium, magnesium, zinc, and vitamin D.

—Bone Spurs:

A bone spur (osteophyte) is a bony projection formed on a normal bone. Bone spurs form as the body tries to repair itself by building extra bone in response to continued pressure, stress, or rubbing. Bone spurs can cause pain if they rub against soft tissues or other bones.

Oils: ⊘wintergreen, ⊘cypress, ⊘marjoram

—Broken:

> *Simple Solutions—Broken Bone :* Combine 1 drop each of lemongrass, clove, eucalyptus, and melaleuca. Apply gently over bone once daily until healed.

Oils: ⊘Deep Blue (for pain), ⊘⊙frankincense

Recipe 1: Apply wintergreen and cypress oils at night before bed. Apply helichrysum, oregano, and Balance in the morning.

Blend 1: Combine equal parts lemongrass, clove, eucalyptus, and melaleuca. Apply on location.

Other Products: ⊙Microplex VMz contains essential bone nutrients calcium, magnesium, zinc, and vitamin D.

—Bruised

Oils: ⊘Deep Blue, ⊘helichrysum

—Cartilage:

Cartilage is a type of connective tissue in the body that provides structure and support for other tissues without being hard and rigid like bone. Unlike other connective tissues, cartilage does not have blood vessels. Cartilage is found in many areas of the body, including the joints, ears, nose, bronchial tubes, and intervertebral discs.

Oils: ⊘sandalwood (helps regenerate), ⊘fir (inflammation)

—Development:

Other Products: ⊙Microplex VMz contains essential bone nutrients necessary for development, such as calcium, magnesium, zinc, and vitamin D.

—Osteomyelitis: *See also **Antibacterial, Antifungal***

Osteomyelitis is a bone infection that is usually caused by bacteria. The infection often starts in another area of the body and then spreads to the bone. Symptoms include fever, pain, swelling, nausea, drainage of pus, and uneasiness. Diabetes, hemodialysis, recent trauma, and IV drug abuse are risk factors for osteomyelitis.

Simple Solutions—Osteomyelitis: Combine 3 drops lemongrass, 2 drops clove, 2 drops eucalyptus, and 2 drops melaleuca with 1 tsp. (5 ml) fractionated coconut oil. Apply once or twice a day on location as needed.

Recipe 1: Apply equal parts lemongrass, clove, eucalyptus, and melaleuca, either blended together or applied individually on location.

—Osteoporosis:

Osteoporosis is a disease characterized by a loss of bone density, making the bones extremely fragile and susceptible to fractures and breaking. Osteoporosis develops when bone resorption exceeds bone formation. Osteoporosis is significantly more common in women than in men, especially after menopause; but the disease does occur in both genders.

Oils: ⊜clove, ⊜geranium, ⊜peppermint, ⊜wintergreen, ⊜fir, ⊜Deep Blue, ⊜thyme, ⊜rosemary⊡, ⊜lemon, ⊜cypress

Other Products: OBone Nutrient Lifetime Complex, OPhytoestrogen Lifetime Complex

—Pain:

Oils: ⊜Deep Blue, ⊜Rescuer, ⊜wintergreen, ⊜juniper berry, ⊜fir

—Rotator Cuff: *See Joints: Rotator Cuff*

⊜: Dilute as recommended, and apply on location or on reflex points on feet.

O: Take capsules as directed. Place 1–2 drops of oil in an empty capsule; swallow.

⊕: **Body System(s) Affected:** Skeletal System.

▭: **Additional Research:**

Rosemary and Eucalyptus: Mühlbauer et al., 2003.

Skin

See also Acne, Antibacterial, Antifungal, Boils, Burns, Foot, Cancer: Skin/Melanoma

The skin is the organ the covers the body, offering the first layer of protection to the internal organs and tissues from exposure to the environment and fungal,

bacterial, and other types of infection. It helps regulate body heat and helps prevent evaporation of water from the body. The skin also carries nerve endings that allow the body to sense touch, heat, and pain. The skin is comprised of three layers. The upper layer is the epidermis, the middle layer is the dermis, and the deeper layer is the hypodermis (or subcutis layer).

Oils: ⊜peppermint, ⊜melaleuca, ⊜HD Clear, ⊜Immortelle, ⊜sandalwood, ⊜frankincense, ⊜lavender, ⊜magnolia, ⊜neroli, ⊘⊜manuka, ⊜Oyarrow Pom, ⊜myrrh, ⊜geranium, ⊜rosemary, ⊜spikenard, ⊜Balance, ⊜ylang ylang, ⊜marjoram, ⊜cypress, ⊜juniper berry, ⊜green mandarin, ⊜cedarwood, OZendocrine, ⊜turmeric, ⊜vetiver, ⊜arborvitae, ⊜helichrysum, ⊜lemon, ⊜orange, ⊜lime, ⊜patchouli

Other Products: ⊜Anti-Aging Moisturizer, ⊜Baby Lotion, ⊜Baby Hair and Body Wash, ⊜Detoxifying Mud Mask, ⊜Diaper Rash Cream, ⊜Exfoliating Body Scrub, ⊜Anti-Aging Eye Cream, ⊜Facial Cleanser, ⊜Hydrating Body Mist with Beautiful, ⊜Hydrating Cream, ⊜Hydrating Serum, ⊜Invigorating Scrub, ⊜Refreshing Body Wash, ⊜Replenishing Body Butter, ⊜Bightening Gel, ⊜Pore Reducing Toner, ⊜Reveal Facial System, and ⊜Skin Serum for vibrant, youthful-looking skin. ⊜HD Clear Foaming Face Wash and ⊜HD Clear Facial Lotion to help improve tone and texture of the skin. ⊜On Guard Foaming Hand Wash to help protect against harmful microorganisms on the skin. ⊜Citrus Bliss and ⊜Serenity Bath Bar, or ⊜Hand and Body Lotion to help cleanse and moisturize the skin. ⊜Correct-X to help cleanse and support the skin's natural healing process. OxEO Mega or vEO Mega, OIQ Mega, OAlpha CRS+, Oa2z Chewable, OMicroplex VMz contain omega fatty acids and other nutrients essential for healthy skin cell function. OZendocrine Detoxification Complex to help support healthy cleansing and filtering of the skin.

⊜: Dilute as recommended, and apply 1–2 drops on location. Add 5–10 drops to 2 Tbs. (25 ml) fractionated coconut oil, and use as massage oil. Add 1 drop essential oil to 1 tsp. (5 ml) unscented lotion, and apply on the skin. Add 1–2 drops to 1 Tbs. (15 ml) bath or shower gel, and apply to skin. Apply foaming hand wash to skin instead of soap, or use bath bars when washing hands or bathing.

⊜=Topical, ⊘=Aromatic, O=Internal

Skin

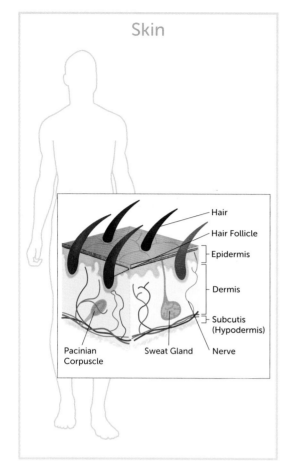

Hair
Hair Follicle
Epidermis
Dermis
Subcutis (Hypodermis)
Pacinian Corpuscle
Sweat Gland
Nerve

◐: Take capsules as directed on package. Add 3–5 drops of oil to an empty capsule; swallow capsule.

—Acne: *See Acne*

—Boils: *See Boils*

—Burns: *See Burns*

—Calluses:

A callus is a flat, thick growth of skin that develops on areas of the skin where there is constant friction or rubbing. Calluses typically form on the bottoms of the feet but can also form on the hands or other areas of the body exposed to constant friction.

Simple Solutions—Callus: Combine 5 drops oregano oil with 1 Tbs. (15 ml) jojoba oil. Apply a small amount daily over calluses.

Oils: ⬬oregano, ⬬HD Clear, ⬬Roman chamomile

⬬: Dilute as recommended, and apply 1–2 drops on area.

—Chapped/Cracked:

Chapped or cracked skin is the result of the depletion of natural oils (sebum) in the skin, leading to dehydration of the skin beneath it. Some common causes for chapped skin include exposure to the cold or wind, repeated contact with soap or chemicals that break down oils, or a lack of essential fatty acids in the body.

Oils: ⬬myrrh, ⬬HD Clear, ⬬Immortelle, ⬬◐Yarrow Pom

Other Products: ⬬Baby Lotion, ⬬Diaper Rash Cream, ⬬Hand and Body Lotion, ⬬Hydrating Body Mist with Beautiful, ⬬Hydrating Cream and ⬬Hydrating Serum to help moisturize and protect. ⬬Correct-X to help cleanse and support the skin's natural healing process. ◐xEO Mega or vEO Mega or ◐IQ Mega to help supply essential omega fatty acids necessary for healthy skin. ⬬Citrus Bliss and ⬬Serenity Bath Bar contain natural oils that help moisturize and soften the skin.

⬬: Dilute as recommended, and apply 1–2 drops on location. Add 5–10 drops to 1 Tbs. (15 ml) fractionated coconut oil, and massage on location.

◐: Take capsules as directed on package.

—Corns: *See Foot: Corns*

—Dehydrated:

Oils: ⬬geranium, ⬬lavender, ⬬Immortelle

Other Products: ⬬Baby Lotion, ⬬Baby Hair and Body Wash, ⬬Hand and Body Lotion, ⬬Hydrating Body Mist with Beautiful, ⬬Hydrating Cream and ⬬Hydrating Serum to help moisturize and protect. ⬬Citrus Bliss and ⬬Serenity Bath Bar contain natural oils that help moisturize and soften.

⬬: Dilute as recommended, and apply 1–2 drops on location. Add 5–10 drops to 2 Tbs. (25 ml) fractionated coconut oil, and use as massage oil. Add 1 drop essential oil to 1 tsp. (5 ml) unscented lotion, and apply on the skin. Add 1–2 drops to 1 Tbs. (15 ml) bath or shower gel, and apply to skin.

—Dermatitis/Eczema:

Dermatitis is any inflammation of the upper layers of the skin that results in redness, itching, pain, or possibly blistering. It can be caused by contact with an allergen or irritating substance, fungal infection, dehydration, or possibly another medical condition.

Oils: ⊜HD Clear, ⊜helichrysum, ⊜juniper berry, ⊜thyme, ⊜geranium, ⊜arborvitae, ⊜melaleuca, ⊜lavender, ⊜magnolia, ⊜patchouli, ⊜bergamot, ⊜rosemary

⊜: Add 5–10 drops to 1 Tbs. (15 ml) fractionated coconut oil, and apply on location. Dilute as recommended, and apply 1–2 drops on location.

—**Diaper Rash:** *See Children and Infants: Diaper Rash*

—**Dry:**

Oils: ⊜geranium, ⊜lavender, ⊜Roman chamomile, ⊜Immortelle, ⊜sandalwood, ⊜lemon

Other Products: ⊜Anti-Aging Moisturizer, ⊜Hydrating Body Mist with Beautiful, ⊜Hydrating Cream, and ⊜Hydrating Serum to help relieve dryness and reduce the visible signs of aging. ⊜Baby Lotion, ⊜Baby Hair and Body Wash, and ⊜Hand and Body Lotion to help moisturize and protect. ⊜Reveal Facial System to help promote healthy skin matrix building and moisture retention.

⊜: Add 5–10 drops to 1 Tbs. (15 ml) fractionated coconut oil, and use as massage oil. Add 2–3 drops essential oil to 1 tsp. (5 ml) Hand and Body Lotion, and apply on the skin.

—**Energizing:**

Oils: ⊜bergamot, ⊜lemon

Other Products: ⊜Invigorating Scrub to polish and exfoliate the skin. ⊜Citrus Bliss Invigorating Bath Bar contains natural oatmeal kernels that help exfoliate.

⊜: Dilute as recommended, and apply 1–2 drops on location. Add 5–10 drops to 2 Tbs. (25 ml) fractionated coconut oil, and use as massage oil. Add 1 drop essential oil to 1 tsp. (5 ml) Hand and Body Lotion, and apply on the skin. Add 1–2 drops to 1 Tbs. (15 ml) bath or shower gel, and apply to skin. Massage Invigorating Scrub over wet skin for up to one minute before rinsing with warm water.

—**Facial Oils:** *See also **Dehydrated, Dry, Energizing, Oily/Greasy,** and **Revitalizing** in this section for other oils that can be used for specific skin types/conditions.*

Oils: ⊜myrrh, ⊜sandalwood, ⊜vetiver

⊜: Add 5–10 drops to 1 Tbs. (15 ml) fractionated coconut oil, and apply to face. Add 1–2 drops essential oil to 1 tsp. (5 ml) unscented lotion, and apply on the skin.

—**Fungal Infections:** *See Antifungal: Athlete's Foot, Antifungal: Ringworm*

—**Impetigo:**

Impetigo is a bacterial skin infection that causes sores and blisters full of a yellowish fluid. These sores can be itchy and painful and can easily be spread to other areas of the skin or to another person.

Oils: ⊜geranium, ⊜lavender, ⊜HD Clear, ⊜myrrh

⊜: Boil ½ cup (125 ml) of water, and let cool. Add 5–10 drops essential oil. Wash sores with this water, and then cover sores for an hour. Apply oils as a hot compress on location.

—**Itching:**

An itch is a tingling and unpleasant sensation that evokes the desire to scratch. Itching can be caused by various skin disorders or diseases, parasites such as scabies and lice, allergic reactions to chemicals or drugs, dry skin, insect bites, etc. Scratching the itching area too hard or too often can damage the skin.

Oils: ⊜peppermint, ⊜lavender, ⊜magnolia, ⊜manuka, ⊜Serenity

Other Products: ⊜Citrus Bliss Invigorating Bath Bar contains natural oatmeal kernels that can help exfoliate skin and soothe itching.

⊜: Dilute as recommended, and apply 1–2 drops on location and on ears. Wash body with Bath Bar.

—**Melanoma:** *See Cancer: Skin/Melanoma*

—**Moles:**

Moles are small growths on the skin of pigment-producing skin cells that usually appear brown or black in color. Moles typically appear within a person's first 20 years of life and usually stay with a person throughout his or her life. While moles are not dangerous, melanoma (a type of skin cancer that develops in pigment cells) can resemble a mole at first. Moles that

⊜=Topical, ⊘=Aromatic, ⬤=Internal

vary in color or that appear to change fairly quickly in size or shape could be cancerous and should be examined.

> *Simple Solutions—Moles:* Apply 1 drop frankincense on location. Seek medical attention if appearance or color of moles changes.

Oils: ⬦frankincense, ⬦sandalwood, ⬦geranium, ⬦lavender

⬦: Dilute as recommended, and apply 1 drop on location.

—Oily/Greasy:

Oils: ⬦lemon, ⬦HD Clear, ⬦cypress, ⬦frankincense, ⬦geranium, ⬦lavender, ⬦marjoram, ⬦orange, ⬦rosemary

Other Products: ⬦HD Clear Foaming Face Wash and ⬦HD Clear Facial Lotion to help balance skin sebum levels. ⬦Facial Cleanser to cleanse the skin and leave it feeling smooth and fresh.

⬦: Add 5–10 drops to 1 Tbs. (15 ml) fractionated coconut oil, and use as massage oil. Use Facial Cleanser as directed on package.

—Psoriasis: *See Psoriasis*

—Rashes:

A rash is an area of irritated skin, redness, or red bumps on the body. Rashes may be localized or may cover large patches of the body. A rash may be caused by a chemical or allergen irritating the skin or may occur as a symptom of another medical condition or infection.

> *Simple Solutions—Rashes:* Combine 2 drops lavender and 2 drops Roman chamomile with 1 tsp. (5 ml) jojoba oil in a small roll-on container. Apply on affected areas once or twice a day to help soothe.

Oils: ⬦melaleuca, ⬦spikenard, ⬦OYarrow Pom, ⬦lavender, ⬦magnolia, ⬦Roman chamomile, ⬦hinoki, ⬦turmeric, ⬦spikenard

⬦: Dilute as recommended, and apply 1–2 drops on location. Add 1–5 drops to 1 Tbs. (15 ml) fractionated coconut oil, and apply on location.

—Revitalizing:

Oils: ⬦cypress, ⬦lemon, ⬦Immortelle, ⬦HD Clear, ⬦fennel, ⬦lime, ⬦green mandarin

Other Products: ⬦Hydrating Body Mist with Beautiful. ⬦Invigorating Scrub to polish and exfoliate the skin. ⬦Reveal Facial System to help promote healthy skin matrix building and moisture retention. ⬦Citrus Bliss Invigorating Bath Bar contains natural oatmeal kernels that help exfoliate.

⬦: Add 5–10 drops to 1 Tbs. (15 ml) fractionated coconut oil, and use as massage oil. Add 2–3 drops essential oil to 1 tsp. (5 ml) unscented lotion, and apply on the skin. Massage Invigorating Scrub over wet skin for up to one minute before rinsing with warm water.

—Ringworm: *See Antifungal: Ringworm*

—Scabies:

Scabies is an infestation of the skin by mites (*Sarcoptes scabei*) that burrow into the upper layers of the skin, causing small, extremely itchy bumps.

> *Simple Solutions—Scabies:* Blend 10 drops On Guard with 1 Tbs. (15 ml) fractionated coconut oil. Apply a small amount on location once or twice a day as needed.

Oils: ⬦On Guard, ⬦HD Clear, ⬦melaleuca, ⬦peppermint, ⬦lavender, ⬦bergamot

⬦: Add 5–10 drops to 1 Tbs. (15 ml) fractionated coconut oil, and apply a small amount on location morning and night. Dilute as recommended, and apply 1–2 drops on location.

—Scarring:

Scars are fibrous connective tissue that is used to quickly repair a wound or injury in place of the regular skin or tissue.

> *Simple Solutions—Scars:* Add 2 drops frankincense and 2 drops helichrysum to 1 tsp. (5 ml) almond oil in a small roll-on container. Apply a small amount on scars daily as needed..

Oils: ⬦lavender (burns), ⬦rose (helps prevent), ⬦frankincense (helps prevent), ⬦OYarrow Pom, ⬦helichrysum (reduces), ⬦geranium, ⬦myrrh, ⬦neroli

Other Products: ⬦Correct-X to help cleanse and support the skin's natural healing process.

Blend 1: Combine 5 drops helichrysum and 5 drops lavender with 1 Tbs. (15 ml) sunflower oil or with liquid lecithin (an emulsifier extracted from eggs or soy), and apply on location.

Primary Recommendations • Secondary Recommendations • Other Recommendations

Blend 2: Combine 1 drop lavender, 1 drop lemongrass, and 1 drop geranium; apply on location to help prevent scar formation.

⬡: Dilute as recommended, and apply 1–2 drops on location.

—Sensitive:

Oils: ⬡lavender, ⬡neroli, ⬡magnolia, ⬡geranium

⬡: Dilute as recommended, and apply 1–2 drops on location.

—Skin Ulcers:

A skin ulcer is an open sore where the epidermis and possibly part or all of the dermis is missing, exposing the deeper layers of the skin. This can be caused by burns, pressure, friction, irritation, or infections damaging the upper layers of the skin.

Oils: ⬡lavender, ⬡myrrh, ⬡HD Clear, ⬡helichrysum, ⬡Purify

⬡: Dilute as recommended, and apply 1–2 drops on location.

—Stretch Marks:

Stretch marks are thin purple or red areas of the skin that appear as the skin is rapidly stretched over a short period of time, stretching and tearing the dermis layer (middle layer) of the skin. Many women notice the appearance of stretch marks in the last few months of pregnancy, but stretch marks can also appear on men or women during any period of rapid weight gain. These marks most often appear on the breasts, stomach, buttocks, thighs, and hips. Stretch marks tend to fade over time, but it is difficult to eliminate them completely.

> *Simple Solutions—Stretch Marks:* Add 2 drops lavender and 3 drops myrrh to 1 tsp. (5 ml) hazelnut oil in a small roll-on bottle. Apply on location once per day.

Oils: ⬡lavender, ⬡myrrh, ⬡neroli

⬡: Add 5–10 drops to 1 Tbs. (15 ml) fractionated coconut oil or hazelnut oil, and apply on location.

—Sunburn: *See Burns: Sunburn*

—Tones:

Oils: ⬡lemon, ⬡green mandarin

⬡: Add 4–5 drops to 1 Tbs. (15 ml) fractionated coconut oil, and use as massage oil (avoid direct sunlight for 24 hours after application).

—Vitiligo:

Vitiligo is white patches of the skin caused by the death or dysfunction of pigment-producing cells in the area. While the exact cause is unknown, vitiligo may be caused by an immune or genetic disorder or may have a relationship to thyroid problems.

Oils: ⬡sandalwood, ⬡vetiver, ⬡frankincense, ⬡myrrh, ⬡Purify

⬡: Dilute as recommended, and apply 1–2 drops behind ears and on back of neck or on reflex points on the feet; then cup hands together, and inhale the aroma from the hands.

—Wrinkles:

A wrinkle is a fold or crease in the skin that develops as part of the normal aging process. Wrinkles are thought to be caused by a breakdown of collagen (a protein that gives structure to cells and tissue) in the skin, causing the skin to become more fragile and loose.

> *Simple Solutions—Wrinkles:* Blend 3 drops myrrh, 2 drops dill, and 1 drop cilantro with 1 tsp. (5 ml) jojoba oil in a small roll-on bottle. Apply on location once per day.

Oils: ⬡Immortelle, ⬡lavender, ⬡myrrh⊖, ⬡fennel, ⬡dill⊖, ⬡geranium, ⬡frankincense, ⬡spikenard, ⬡rose, ⬡rosemary, ⬡clary sage, ⬡cypress, ⬡helichrysum, ⬡lemon, ⬡orange, ⬡oregano, ⬡sandalwood, ⬡thyme, ⬡neroli, ⬡ylang ylang

Other Products: ⬡Anti-Aging Moisturizer and ⬡Veráge Moisturizer to help relieve dryness and reduce the visible signs of aging. ⬡Tightening Serum and ⬡Youthful Pore Reducing Toner to help tighten the skin to eliminate fine lines and wrinkles. ⬡Hydrating Body Mist with Beautiful, ⬡Hydrating Cream, and ⬡Veráge Immortelle Hydrating Serum to help promote fuller, smoother looking skin. ⬡Reveal Facial System and ⬡Veráge Cleanser to help promote healthy skin matrix building and moisture retention.

Blend 1: Combine 1 drop frankincense, 1 drop lavender, and 1 drop lemon. Rub on morning and night around the eyes (be careful not to get in eyes).

Blend 2: Combine 1 drop sandalwood, 1 drop helichrysum, 1 drop geranium, 1 drop lavender, and 1 drop frankincense. Add to 2 tsp. (10 ml) unscented lotion, and apply to skin.

⬡=Topical, ⬡=Aromatic, ⬡=Internal

: Dilute as recommended, and apply 1–2 drops to skin. Add 5–10 drops to 1 Tbs. (15 ml) fractionated coconut oil or other carrier oil such as jojoba, apricot, hazelnut, or sweet almond, and apply on areas of concern. Add 3–5 drops to ½ cup (125 g) Therapeutic Bath Salts, and dissolve in warm bathwater before bathing.

: **Body System(s) Affected:** Skin.

: **Additional Research:**

Myrrh: Auffray, 2007; **Dill:** Cenizo et al., 2006; **Cilantro:** Park et al., 2012.

Sleep

See also **Insomnia**

Sleep is a regular period in which the body suspends conscious motor and sensory activity. Sleep is thought to play a role in restoring and healing the body and processing the memories of the day.

Oils: lavender, Serenity, Calmer, spikenard, Roman chamomile, marjoram

Recipe 1: Combine 5 drops geranium and 5 drops lavender with ¼ cup (50 g) Therapeutic Bath Salts; dissolve in warm bathwater, and bathe in the evening to help promote a good night's sleep.

: Dilute as recommended, and apply 1–2 drops essential oil to spine, bottoms of feet, or back of neck. Add 1–2 drops to warm bathwater, and bathe before sleeping. Add 5–10 drops to 1 Tbs. (15 ml) fractionated coconut oil, and massage on back, arms, legs, and feet.

: Diffuse into the air. Add 1–2 drops to bottom of pillow before sleeping. Add 2–5 drops to 2 Tbs. (25 ml) distilled water in a small spray bottle, and mist into the air or on linens before sleeping.

: **Body System(s) Affected:** Nervous System, Endocrine System, and Emotional Balance.

: **Additional Research:**

Lavender and Roman Chamomile: Cho et al., 2013; **Lavender:** Kim et al., 2016.

Slimming and Toning Oils

See **Weight: Slimming/Toning**

Smell (loss of)

See **Nose: Olfactory Loss**

Smoking

See **Addictions: Smoking, Purification: Cigarette Smoke**

Snake Bite

See **Bites/Stings: Snakes**

Sores

See **Wounds, Antibacterial, Antifungal, Antiviral**

Sore Throat

See **Throat: Sore, Antibacterial, Antiviral, Infection**

Spasms

See **Muscles/Connective Tissue, Digestive System**

Spina Bifida

Spina bifida is a birth defect in which the vertebrae of the lower spine do not form correctly, leaving a gap or opening between them. In the most severe cases, this can cause the meninges (the tissue surrounding the spinal cord), or even the spinal cord itself, to protrude through the gap. If the spinal cord protrudes through the gap, it can prevent the nerves from developing normally, causing numbness, paralysis, back pain, and loss of bladder and bowel control and function. This latter type often also develops with a defect in which the back part of the brain develops in the upper neck rather than within the skull, often causing a mental handicap.

Oils: eucalyptus, lavender, Roman chamomile, lemon, orange, rosemary

Other Products: Alpha CRS+ contains 400 mg of folic acid, which has been found to significantly reduce the chance of spina bifida developing in infants if taken as a daily supplement by their mothers before conception (Centers for Disease Control and Prevention, 2004).

: Take capsules as directed on package

: Dilute as recommended, and apply 1–2 drops to bottoms of feet, along spine, on forehead, and on back of neck.

: Diffuse into the air.

⊕: Body System(s) Affected: Skeletal and Nervous Systems.

Spine

See Back

Spleen

See also Lymphatic System

The spleen is a fist-sized spongy tissue that is part of the lymphatic system. Its purpose is to filter bacteria, viruses, fungi, and other unwanted substances out of the blood and to create lymphocytes (white blood cells that create antibodies).

Oils: ◐marjoram

◐: Dilute as recommended and apply 1–2 drops over spleen or on reflex points on the feet. Apply as a warm compress over upper abdomen.

⊕: Body System(s) Affected: Cardiovascular System and Immune System.

Sprains

See Muscles/Connective Tissue: Sprains

Spurs

See Skeletal System: Bone Spurs

Stains

See Housecleaning: Stains

Staph Infection

See Antibacterial: Staph Infection

Sterility

See Female-Specific Conditions: Infertility, Male Specific Conditions: Infertility

Stimulating

Oils: ◑◐peppermint, ◑◐Elevation, ◑◐eucalyptus○, ◑◐orange, ◑◐ginger, ◑◐grapefruit, ◑◐rose, ◑◐rosemary○, ◑◐basil

◐: Diffuse into the air. Inhale directly from bottle. Apply oil to hands, tissue, or cotton wick, and inhale.

◐: Dilute as recommended, and apply 1–2 drops to forehead, neck, or bottoms of feet. Add 1–2 drops to an unscented bath gel, and add to warm bathwater while filling; bathe. Add 5–10 drops to 1 Tbs. (15 ml) fractionated coconut oil, and use as massage oil.

⊕: Body System(s) Affected: Emotional Balance.

◻: **Additional Research:**

Eucalyptus: Nasel et al., 1994; Rosemary: Nasel et al., 1994.

Stings

See Bites/Stings

Stomach

See Digestive System: Stomach

Strep Throat

See Throat: Strep

Stress

> *Simple Solutions—Stress:* Diffuse lavender or grapefruit oil in an aromatherapy diffuser.

> *Simple Solutions—Stress:* Add 10 drops lavender to 1 cup (250 g) Epsom salt. Dissolve ½ cup (125 g) of the salt in warm bathwater for a relaxing bath.

Stress is the body's response to difficult, pressured, or worrisome circumstances. Stress can cause both physical and emotional tension. Symptoms of stress include headaches, muscle soreness, fatigue, insomnia, nervousness, anxiety, and irritability.

Oils: ◑◐lavender○, ◑◐InTune, ◑◐Thinker, ◑◐lemon○, ◑◐ylang ylang○, ◑◐bergamot, ◑◐petitgrain, ◑◐neroli, ◑◐Elevation, ◑◐Serenity, ◑◐Calmer, ◑◐grapefruit, ◐Rescuer, ◐AromaTouch, ◑◐Roman chamomile, ◑◐geranium, ◑◐spikenard, ◑◐Balance, ◑◐frankincense, ◑◐marjoram

◐=Topical, ◐=Aromatic, ○=Internal

—Chemical:

Oils: ⊘⊜lavender, ⊘⊜rosemary, ⊘⊜grapefruit, ⊘⊜geranium, ⊘⊜clary sage, ⊘⊜lemon

—Emotional Stress:

Oils: ⊘⊜Elevation, ⊘⊜clary sage, ⊘⊜Peace, ⊘⊜bergamot, ⊘⊜Console, ⊘⊜petitgrain, ⊘⊜geranium, ⊜⊘Roman chamomile, ⊘⊜sandalwood

—Environmental Stress:

Oils: ⊘⊜bergamot, ⊘⊜cypress, ⊘⊜geranium, ⊜cedarwood

—Mental Stress:

Oils: ⊘⊜lavender⊕, ⊜⊘InTune, ⊜⊘Thinker, ⊘⊜grapefruit, ⊘⊜bergamot, ⊘⊜petitgrain, ⊘⊜sandalwood, ⊘⊜geranium

—Performance Stress:

Oils: ⊘⊜grapefruit, ⊘⊜bergamot, ⊘⊜ginger, ⊘⊜rosemary

—Physical Stress:

Oils: ⊘⊜Serenity, ⊘⊜lavender, ⊘⊜bergamot, ⊘⊜geranium, ⊘⊜marjoram, ⊜Rescuer, ⊜⊘Roman chamomile, ⊘⊜rosemary, ⊘⊜thyme

—Stress Due to Tiredness or Insomnia:

Blend 1: Add 15 drops clary sage, 10 drops lemon, and 5 drops lavender to 2 Tbs. (25 ml) fractionated coconut oil. Massage on skin.

⊘: Diffuse into the air. Inhale directly from bottle. Apply oil to hands, tissue, or cotton wick, and inhale. Wear as perfume or cologne.

⊜: Add 5–10 drops to 1 Tbs. (15 ml) fractionated coconut oil, and massage on skin. Add 1–2 drops to ¼ cup (50 g) Therapeutic Bath Salts, and dissolve in warm bathwater before bathing. Dilute as recommended, and apply 1–2 drops on neck, back, or bottoms of feet.

⊕: **Body System(s) Affected:** Emotional Balance and Nervous System.

⊡: **Additional Research:**

Lavender: Pemberton et al., 2008; Motomura et al., 2001; Lemon: Komiya et al., 2006; Ylang ylang: Hongratanaworakit et al., 2006.

Stretch Marks

See Skin: Stretch Marks

Stroke

See also Brain, Blood: Clots, Cardiovascular System

A stroke occurs when the blood supply to the brain is interrupted. Within a few minutes, brain cells begin to die. The affected area of the brain is unable to function, and one or more limbs on one side of the body become weak and unable to move. Strokes can cause serious disabilities, including paralysis and speech problems.

Oils: ⊘⊜cypress, ⊘⊜helichrysum, ⊘fennel⊕, ⊘cedarwood⊕, ⊘basil⊕

—Muscular Paralysis:

Oils: ⊜lavender

Blend 1: Combine 1 drop basil, 1 drop lavender, and 1 drop rosemary, and apply to spinal column and paralyzed area.

⊘: Inhale oil directly or applied to hands, tissue, or cotton wick. Diffuse into the air.

⊜: Dilute as directed, and apply 1–2 drops to the back of the neck and the forehead.

⊕: **Body System(s) Affected:** Cardiovascular System and Nervous System.

⊡: **Additional Research:**

Fennel: Tognolini et al., 2007; Cedarwood: Asakura et al., 2000; Basil: Bora et al., 2011.

Sudorific

A sudorific is a substance that induces sweating.

Oils: ⊜thyme, ⊜rosemary, ⊜lavender, ⊜Roman chamomile, ⊜juniper berry

⊜: Add 5–10 drops to 1 Tbs. (15 ml) fractionated coconut oil, and apply to skin.

⊕: **Body System(s) Affected:** Endocrine System.

Suicidal Feelings

See Depression

Sunburn

See Burns: Sunburn

Sunscreen

Oils: ⊜helichrysum, ⊜arborvitae⊕, ⊜sandalwood

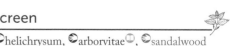

Primary Recommendations • Secondary Recommendations • Other Recommendations

⬙: Add 5–10 drops to 1 Tbs. (15 ml) fractionated coconut oil, and apply to the skin.

✚: Body System(s) Affected: Skin.

⬚: Additional Research:

Arborvitae: Baba et al., 1998.

Swelling

See Edema, Inflammation

Sympathetic Nervous System

See Nervous System: Sympathetic Nervous System

Tachycardia

See Cardiovascular System: Tachycardia

Taste (Impaired)

See also Nose: Olfactory Loss

Taste is the sensation of sweet, sour, salty, or bitter by taste buds on the tongue when a substance enters the mouth. This sensation, combined with the smell of the food, helps create the unique flavors we experience in food.

Oils: ⬙helichrysum, ⬙peppermint

⬙: Dilute as recommended, and apply 1 drop on the tongue or reflex points on the feet.

Teeth

See Oral Conditions

Temperature

See Cooling Oils, Warming Oils

Tendinitis

See Muscles/Connective Tissue: Tendinitis

Tennis Elbow

See Joints: Tennis Elbow

Tension

Oils: ⬙⬙Serenity, ⬙⬙Calmer, ⬙⬙lavender, ⬙Aroma-Touch, ⬙Rescuer, ⬙⬙cedarwood, ⬙⬙ylang ylang, ⬙⬙Roman chamomile, ⬙⬙frankincense, ⬙⬙basil (nervous), ⬙⬙bergamot (nervous), ⬙⬙grapefruit

⬙: Inhale oil applied to hands. Diffuse into the air.

⬙: Add 3–5 drops to ½ cup (125 g) Therapeutic Bath Salts, and dissolve in warm bathwater before bathing. Add 5–10 drops to 1 Tbs. (15 ml) fractionated coconut oil, and use as massage oil.

✚: Body System(s) Affected: Emotional Balance.

Testes

Testes are the male reproductive organs. The testes are responsible for producing and storing sperm and male hormones such as testosterone. Hormones produced in the testes are responsible for the development of male characteristics: facial hair, wide shoulders, low voice, and reproductive organs.

Oils: ⬙⬙rosemary

—**Regulation:**

Oils: ⬙⬙clary sage, ⬙⬙sandalwood, ⬙⬙geranium

⬙: Dilute as recommended, and apply 1–2 drops on location or on reflex points on the feet.

⬙: Diffuse into the air. Inhale directly from bottle. Apply oil to hands, tissue, or cotton wick, and inhale.

✚: Body System(s) Affected: Reproductive System.

Throat

See also Respiratory System, Neck

Oils: ⬙cypress, ⬙oregano

—**Congestion:**

Oils: ⬙⬙peppermint, ⬙⬙myrrh

—**Cough:** *See Respiratory System*

—**Dry:**

Oils: O⬙lemon, O⬙grapefruit

—**Infection In:**

Oils: ⬙⬙Olemon, O⬙⬙On Guard, ⬙⬙Opeppermint, ⬙⬙oregano, ⬙⬙clary sage

Other Products: OOn Guard+ Softgels

—**Laryngitis:** *See Laryngitis*

⬙=Topical, ⬙=Aromatic, O=Internal

—Sore:

Oils: 🌿🌿melaleuca, 🌿🌿🌿🌿On Guard, 🌿🌿oregano, 🌿🌿sandalwood, 🌿🌿lime, 🌿🌿bergamot, 🌿🌿geranium, 🌿🌿ginger, 🌿🌿myrrh

> *Simple Solutions—Sore Throat:* Add 4 drops On Guard and 1 tsp. (5 g) salt to ¼ cup (50 ml) warm water, and stir until salt is dissolved. Gargle with the solution for 30 seconds, then spit out. Repeat up to 2 times a day until sore throat is gone.

> *Simple Solutions—Sore Throat:* Add 3 drops eucalyptus and 2 drops lemon to 1 tsp. (5 ml) honey, and dissolve in 2 Tbs. (25 ml) of water. Place in a small spray bottle. Shake well, and mist 3–4 sprays into throat as needed to help soothe.

Other Products: ⭕On Guard Protecting Throat Drops to soothe irritated and sore throats.

—Strep:

Strep throat is a throat infection caused by streptococci bacteria. This infection causes the throat and tonsils to become inflamed and swollen, resulting in a severe sore throat. Symptoms of strep throat include a sudden severe sore throat, pain when swallowing, high fever, swollen tonsils and lymph nodes, white spots on the back of the throat, skin rash, and sometimes vomiting. Strep throat should be closely monitored so that it doesn't develop into a more serious condition such as rheumatic fever or kidney inflammation.

Oils: ⭕🌿🌿On Guard🌐, 🌿🌿melaleuca, 🌿🌿ginger, 🌿🌿geranium, 🌿🌿oregano

—Tonsillitis:

Tonsillitis is inflammation of the tonsils, typically due to infection. Tonsillitis causes the tonsils to become swollen and painful. Symptoms of tonsillitis include sore throat, red and swollen tonsils, painful swallowing, loss of voice, fever, chills, headache, and white patches on the tonsils.

Oils: 🌿🌿melaleuca, 🌿🌿On Guard, 🌿ginger, 🌿🌿lavender, 🌿🌿lemon, 🌿🌿bergamot, 🌿🌿clove, 🌿thyme, 🌿🌿Roman chamomile

⭕: Add 1 drop to 1 cup (250 ml) water (1 liter for On Guard), and drink. Place 1 drop oil under the tongue. Take supplement as directed.

🌿: Dilute as recommended, and apply 1–2 drops on throat or reflex points on the feet. Add 1–2 drops to ½ cup (125 ml) water, and gargle.

🌀: Diffuse into the air. Inhale directly from bottle. Apply oil to hands, tissue, or cotton wick, and inhale.

➕: **Body System(s) Affected:** Respiratory System and Immune System.

⊕: **Additional Research:**

On Guard: Fabio et al., 2007; Cermelli et al., 2008.

Thrush

See Antifungal: Candida, Antifungal: Thrush, Children and Infants: Thrush

Thymus

See also Immune System, Lymphatic System

The thymus is an organ responsible for the development of T cells needed for immune system functioning. The thymus is located just behind the sternum in the upper part of the chest.

Oils: 🌿On Guard

🌿: Dilute as recommended, and apply over thymus or on bottoms of feet.

➕: **Body System(s) Affected:** Immune System.

Thyroid

See also Endocrine System

The thyroid is a gland located in the front of the neck that plays a key role in regulating metabolism. The thyroid produces and secretes the hormones needed to regulate blood pressure, heart rate, body temperature, and energy production.

—Dysfunction:

Oils: 🌿🌿clove

—Hyperthyroidism: *See also Grave's Disease*

Hyperthyroidism is when the thyroid gland produces too much of its hormones, typically due to the thyroid becoming enlarged. This can result in a noticeably enlarged thyroid gland (goiter), sudden weight loss, sweating, a rapid or irregular heartbeat, shortness of breath, muscle weakness, nervousness, and irritability.

Oils: 🌿🌿myrrh, 🌿🌿lemongrass

Blend 1: Combine 1 drop myrrh and 1 drop lemongrass, and apply on base of throat and on reflex points on the feet.

—Hypothyroidism: *See also **Hashimoto's Disease***

Hypothyroidism is the result of an underactive thyroid. Consequently, the thyroid gland doesn't produce enough of necessary hormones. Symptoms include fatigue, a puffy face, a hoarse voice, unexplained weight gain, higher blood cholesterol levels, muscle weakness and aches, depression, heavy menstrual periods, memory problems, and low tolerance for the cold.

Oils: ⚬⚬peppermint, ⚬⚬clove, ⚬⚬lemongrass

Blend 2: Combine 1 drop lemongrass with 1 drop of either peppermint or clove, and apply on base of throat and on reflex points on the feet.

—Supports:

Oils: ⚬myrrh

⚬: Dilute as recommended, and apply 1–2 drops on base of throat, hands, or reflex points on the feet.

⚬: Diffuse into the air. Inhale oils applied to hands.

⚬: **Body System(s) Affected:** Endocrine System.

Tinnitus

*See **Ears: Tinnitus***

Tired

*See **Energy***

Tissue

Tissue refers to any group of similar cells that work together to perform a specific function in an organ or in the body. Some types of tissue include muscle tissue, connective tissue, nervous tissue, or epithelial tissue (tissue that lines or covers a surface, such as the skin or the lining of the blood vessels).

Oils: ⚬lemongrass, ⚬helichrysum, ⚬basil, ⚬marjoram, ⚬sandalwood, ⚬Roman chamomile, ⚬lavender

Other Products: ⚬Deep Blue Rub and ⚬TriEase Softgels to help soothe muscle and connective tissues.

—Cleanses Toxins From:

Oils: ⚬fennel

—Connective Tissue: *See **Muscles/Connective Tissue***

—Deep Tissue Pain: *See **Pain: Tissue***

—Repair:

Oils: ⚬lemongrass, ⚬helichrysum, ⚬orange

—Regenerate:

Oils: ⚬lemongrass, ⚬helichrysum, ⚬geranium, ⚬patchouli

—Scarring:

Scar tissue is the dense and fibrous tissue that forms over a healed cut or wound. The scar tissue serves as a protective barrier but is still inferior to the healthy, normal tissue. In an area of scar tissue, sweat glands are nonfunctional, hair does not grow, and the skin is not as protected against ultraviolet radiation. Scars fade and become less noticeable over time but cannot be completely removed.

Oils: ⚬lavender (burns), ⚬rose (helps prevent), ⚬frankincense (helps prevent), ⚬helichrysum (reduces), ⚬geranium, ⚬myrrh

Blend 1: Combine 5 drops helichrysum and 5 drops lavender with 1 Tbs. (15 ml) sunflower oil or with liquid lecithin (an emulsifier extracted from eggs or soy), and apply on location.

Blend 2: Combine 1 drop lavender, 1 drop lemongrass, and 1 drop geranium, and apply on location to help prevent scar formation.

⚬: Dilute as recommended, and apply 1–2 drops on location or on reflex points on the feet. Apply as warm compress. Add 5–10 drops to 1 Tbs. (15 ml) fractionated coconut oil, and massage on location.

Tonic

A tonic is a substance given to invigorate or strengthen an organ, tissue, or system or to stimulate physical, emotional, or mental energy and strength.

—General:

Oils: ⚬⚬lemongrass, ⚬⚬cinnamon, ⚬⚬sandalwood, ⚬⚬clary sage, ⚬⚬grapefruit, ⚬⚬ginger, ⚬⚬geranium, ⚬⚬marjoram, ⚬⚬myrrh, ⚬⚬orange, ⚬⚬Roman chamomile, ⚬⚬ylang ylang

—Heart:

Oils: ⚬⚬thyme, ⚬⚬lavender

—Nerve:

Oils: ⚬⚬clary sage, ⚬⚬melaleuca, ⚬⚬thyme

—Skin:

Oils: ⚬lemon

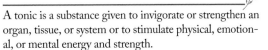
⚬=Topical, ⚬=Aromatic, ⚬=Internal

—Uterine:

Oils: ⊙∅thyme

⊙: Add 5–10 drops to 1 Tbs. (15 ml) fractionated coconut oil, and massage on location. Dilute as recommended, and apply 1–2 drops to area or to reflex points on the feet. Add 1–2 drops to warm bathwater before bathing.

⊘: Diffuse into the air. Inhale directly from bottle. Apply oil to hands, tissue, or cotton wick, and inhale.

Tonsillitis

See Throat: Tonsillitis

Toothache

See Oral Conditions: Toothache

Toxemia

See also Antibacterial, Pregnancy/Motherhood: Preeclampsia

Toxemia is the general term for toxic substances in the bloodstream. This is typically caused by a bacterial infection in which bacteria release toxins into the blood.

Oils: ⊙∅cypress

⊙: Dilute as recommended, and apply 1–2 drops on neck, over heart, or on bottoms of feet. Add 5–10 drops to 1 Tbs. (15 ml) fractionated coconut oil, and massage on neck, back, chest, and legs.

⊘: Diffuse into the air.

✛: **Body System(s) Affected:** Immune System and Cardiovascular System.

Toxins

See Detoxification

Travel Sickness

See Nausea: Motion Sickness

Tuberculosis (T.B.)

See also Antibacterial, Respiratory System

Tuberculosis is a bacterial disease spread through the air (via coughing, spitting, sneezing, etc.). Tuberculosis most commonly infects the lungs, but it can infect oth-

er bodily systems as well. Symptoms of tuberculosis include a chronic cough (often with blood), fever, chills, weakness and fatigue, weight loss, and night sweats. Tuberculosis is contagious and sometimes deadly.

Oils: ⊙∅eucalyptus, ⊙∅cypress, ⊙∅Breathe, ⊙∅thyme, ⊙∅cedarwood, ⊙∅On Guard, ∅lemon, ⊙∅melissa, ⊙∅vetiver⊙, ⊙∅peppermint, ⊙∅sandalwood

Other Products: ⊙Breathe Respiratory Drops, ⊙∅Breathe Vapor Stick

—Airborne Bacteria:

Oils: ∅On Guard, ∅lemongrass⊙, ∅geranium⊙, ∅Purify, ∅Breathe

—Pulmonary:

Oils: ⊙∅oregano, ⊙∅cypress, ⊙∅eucalyptus, ⊙∅frankincense

⊘: Diffuse into the air. Inhale directly from bottle. Apply oil to hands, tissue, or cotton wick, and inhale. Add 2–3 drops to bowl of hot water, and inhale vapors.

⊙: Dilute as recommended, and apply 1–2 drops on chest, back, or reflex points on the feet. Add 1–2 drops to 1 tsp. (5 ml) fractionated coconut oil, and apply as rectal implant. Add 5–10 drops to 1 Tbs. (15 ml) fractionated coconut oil, and massage on chest, back, and feet.

✛: **Body System(s) Affected:** Respiratory System and Immune System.

▢: **Additional Research:**

Vetiver: Saikia et al., 2012; **Lemongrass:** Doran et al., 2009; **Geranium:** Doran et al., 2009.

Tumor

See also Cancer

A tumor is an abnormal growth of cells in a lump or mass. Some tumors are malignant (cancerous) and some are benign (noncancerous). Benign tumors in most parts of the body do not create health problems. *For information on cancerous (malignant) tumors, see Cancer.*

Oils: ⊙∅frankincense, ⊙DDR Prime, ⊙∅clove, ⊙∅sandalwood

—Lipoma:

Lipoma is a benign tumor of the fatty tissues that most commonly forms just below the surface of the skin; but it can also form in any other area of the body where fatty tissue is present.

Oils: ⬢frankincense, ⬢clove, **O**DDR Prime, ⬢grapefruit, ⬢ginger

⬢: Dilute as recommended, and apply 1–2 drops on location.

O: Take 3–5 drops in an empty capsule, or with food and beverage. Take up to twice per day as needed.

⬢: Diffuse into the air. Inhale directly from bottle. Apply oil to hands, tissue, or cotton wick, and inhale.

Typhoid

See also **Antibacterial**

Typhoid fever is a bacterial infection caused by the bacteria *Salmonella typhi*. Typhoid is spread through food and water infected with the feces of typhoid carriers. Possible symptoms of typhoid include abdominal pain, severe diarrhea, bloody stools, chills, severe fatigue, weakness, chills, delirium, hallucinations, confusion, agitation, and fluctuating mood.

Oils: ⬢⬢cinnamon, ⬢⬢peppermint, ⬢⬢Purify, ⬢⬢lemon, ⬢⬢Breathe

⬢: Dilute as recommended, and apply over intestines or on reflex points on the feet.

⬢: Diffuse into the air.

⬢: **Body System(s) Affected:** Immune System and Digestive System.

Ulcers

See also **Digestive System**

An ulcer is an open sore either on the skin or on an internal mucous membrane (such as that lining the stomach).

> *Simple Solutions—Ulcers:* Mix 1 drop lemon in 1 tsp. (5 ml) honey. Dissolve in 1 cup (250 ml) of warm water, and drink.

Oils: O⬢frankincense, O⬢myrrh, O⬢marjoram⬚, O⬢lemon⬚, O⬢dill⬚, O⬢oregano, O⬢rose, O⬢thyme, O⬢clove, O⬢bergamot

—Duodenal:

A duodenal ulcer is an ulcer in the upper part of the small intestine.

Oils: O⬢frankincense, O⬢myrrh, O⬢lemon, O⬢oregano, O⬢rose, O⬢thyme, O⬢clove, O⬢bergamot

—Gastric: *See also* **Digestive System: Gastritis.**

A gastric ulcer is an ulcer in the stomach.

Oils: O⬢geranium, O⬢peppermint, O⬢marjoram⬚, O⬢lemon⬚, O⬢dill⬚, O⬢frankincense, O⬢orange, O⬢bergamot

—Leg:

An ulcer on the leg may be due to a lack of circulation in the lower extremities or possibly due to a bacterial, fungal, or viral infection. *See also* **Cardiovascular System: Circulation, Antibacterial, Antifungal, Antiviral.**

Oils: ⬢Purify, ⬢lavender, ⬢Roman chamomile, ⬢geranium

—Mouth: *See* **Canker Sores**

—Peptic:

A peptic ulcer is an ulcer that forms in an area of the digestive system where acid is present, such as in the stomach (gastric), esophagus, or upper part of the small intestine (duodenal). *See also* **Duodenal, Gastric** in this section.

Recipe 1: Flavor 4 cups (1 L) of water with 1 drop cinnamon, and sip all day.

—Varicose Ulcer:

A varicose ulcer is an ulcer on the lower leg where varicose (swollen) veins are located.

Oils: ⬢melaleuca, ⬢geranium, ⬢lavender, ⬢eucalyptus, ⬢thyme

O: Add 1 drop oil to rice or almond milk, and drink. Place oil in an empty capsule and swallow. Add 1 drop or less as flavoring to food after cooking.

⬢: Dilute as recommended, and apply 1–2 drops over area. Apply as warm compress.

⬢: **Body System(s) Affected:** Skin and Digestive System.

⬚: **Additional Research:**

Marjoram: Al-Howiriny et al., 2009; **Lemon:** Rozza et al., 2011; **Dill:** Hosseinzadeh et al., 2002.

Unwind

See **Calming**

⬢=Topical, ⬢=Aromatic, **O**=Internal

Uplifting

Oils: ⚫️🔵Cheer, ⚫️lemon🔘, ⚫️orange, ⚫️🔵petitgrain, ⚫️Elevation, ⚫️🔵Brave, ⚫️🔵Console, ⚫️🔵Passion, ⚫️Citrus Bliss, ⚫️🔵Forgive, ⚫️bergamot, ⚫️grapefruit, ⚫️yarrow, ⚫️Whisper, ⚫️myrrh, ⚫️wintergreen, ⚫️lavender

⚫️: Diffuse into the air. Inhale directly from bottle. Apply oil to hands, tissue, or cotton wick; inhale. Wear as perfume or cologne.

🔵: **Body System(s) Affected:** Emotional Balance.

🔘: **Additional Research:**

Lemon: Kiecolt-Glaser et al., 2008; Komori et al., 1995.

Ureter

See Urinary Tract

Urinary Tract

The urinary tract is the collection of organs and tubes responsible for producing and excreting urine. The urinary tract is comprised of the kidneys, bladder, ureters, and urethra.

Oils: 🔵⚫️sandalwood, 🔵⚫️thyme, 🔵⚫️melaleuca, 🔵⚫️bergamot, 🔵⚫️lavender, 🔵⚫️rosemary

—General Stimulant:

Oils: 🔵⚫️eucalyptus, 🔵⚫️bergamot

—Infection: *See also Bladder: Cystitis/Infection*

Oils: 🔵Purify, 🔵⚫️lemongrass, 🔵cedarwood, 🔵⚫️geranium, 🔵bergamot, 🔵⚫️juniper berry

Blend 1: Combine 1 drop On Guard with 1 drop oregano; apply as a hot compress over abdomen and pubic area.

Other Products: ⭕️On Guard+ Softgels

—Stones In: *See also Kidneys: Kidney Stones*

Stones are solid masses that form as minerals and other chemicals crystallize and adhere together. They can form in the bladder or kidneys. While small stones generally cause no problems, larger stones may block the ureters or urethra, causing intense pain and possibly injury.

Oils: 🔵fennel, 🔵geranium

—Support:

Oils: 🔵⚫️geranium, 🔵⚫️cypress, 🔵⚫️melaleuca

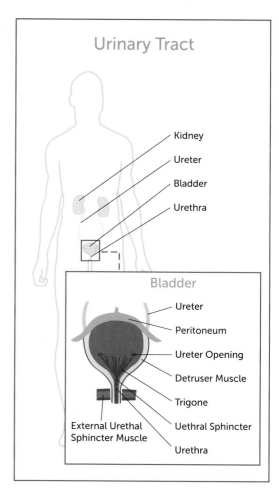

Urinary Tract

- Kidney
- Ureter
- Bladder
- Urethra

Bladder

- Ureter
- Peritoneum
- Ureter Opening
- Detruser Muscle
- Trigone
- Uethral Sphincter
- External Urethal Sphincter Muscle
- Urethra

🔵: Dilute as recommended, and apply 1–2 drops over lower abdomen, lower back, or pubic area. Add 5–10 drops to 1 Tbs. (15 ml) fractionated coconut oil, and massage on abdomen, lower, back, or pubic area. Apply as a warm compress.

⭕️: Take supplement as directed.

⚫️: Diffuse into the air.

🔵: **Body System(s) Affected:** Endocrine System and Digestive System.

Uterus

See also Endometriosis, Female-Specific Conditions

The uterus is the female reproductive organ in which a fetus is formed and develops until birth.

Oils: 🔵frankincense, 🔵lemon, 🔵myrrh, 🔵cedarwood, 🔵geranium

—Regeneration of Tissue:

Oils: ⬭frankincense

—Uterotonic:

An uterotonic is a medication used to stimulate contractions of the uterus. Uterotonics should be avoided or used with extreme caution during pregnancy as they may be abortive. Uterotonics are used to start or speed up labor, to reduce hemorrhaging, and to cause contractions after a miscarriage.

Oils: ⬭thyme

—Uterine Cancer: *See Cancer: Uterine*

⬭: Dilute as recommended, and apply 1–2 drops on lower abdomen or on reflex points on the feet and ankles. Add 2–5 drops essential oil to 1 tsp. (5 ml) fractionated coconut oil, and insert into vagina for overnight retention (a tampon may be used if necessary to help retain the oil). Apply as a warm compress.

⊕: **Body System(s) Affected:** Reproductive System.

Vaginal

—Candida: *See also Antifungal: Candida*

Candida refers to a genus of yeast that are normally found in the digestive tract and on the skin of humans. These yeast are typically symbiotically beneficial to humans. However, several species of *Candida*, such as *Candida albicans*, can cause infections, such as vaginal candidiasis, that cause localized itching, soreness, and redness.

Oils: ⬭melaleuca⊕, ⬭⬭oregano⊕, ⬭clove⊕, ⬭On Guard, ⬭bergamot, ⬭peppermint⊕, ⬭thyme⊕, ⬭lavender⊕, ⬭eucalyptus, ⬭rosemary, ⬭⬭DigestZen

—Infection: *See also Candida (above), Antibacterial, Antifungal, Antiviral*

Vaginal infections occur when there is a disruption in the normal balance of vaginal organisms, such as the sudden presence of yeast, bacteria, or viruses. Common signs of vaginal infection include redness, swelling, itching, pain, odor, change in discharge color or amount, a burning sensation when urinating, and pain or bleeding during intercourse. The most common vaginal infections are yeast infection, trichomoniasis, and bacterial vaginosis.

Oils: ⬭rosemary, ⬭cinnamon (dilute heavily), ⬭melaleuca, ⬭oregano, ⬭thyme, ⬭myrrh, ⬭clary sage, ⬭cypress, ⬭juniper berry, ⬭eucalyptus, ⬭lavender

—Vaginitis:

Vaginitis is vaginal inflammation, typically due to infection, characterized by redness, swelling, itching, irritation, discharge, and pain of the vaginal area.

Oils: ⬭rosemary, ⬭cinnamon (dilute heavily), ⬭eucalyptus, ⬭melaleuca, ⬭lavender

Recipe 1: Valerie Worwood suggests combining 1 drop lavender, 1 drop melaleuca, 1 tsp. (5 ml) vinegar, ½ tsp. (2.5 ml) lemon juice, and 2½ cups (625 ml) of warm water for a douche that can be used 3 days a week.

⬭: Dilute oils as recommended, and apply 1–2 drops on location. Add 2–3 drops to 1 tsp. (5 ml) fractionated coconut oil, insert using vaginal syringe, and retain using tampon overnight. Add 2–3 drops to 1 tsp. (5 ml) fractionated coconut oil, soak tampon in mixture, insert, and leave in all day or overnight. Add 1–2 drops to warm water, and use in a douche. Add 1–2 drops to warm bathwater, and bathe.

◯: Place 1–2 drops under the tongue, or place 2–3 drops in an empty capsule, and swallow.

⊕: **Body System(s) Affected:** Reproductive System.

Varicose Ulcers

See Ulcers: Varicose Ulcer

Varicose Veins

Varicose veins are twisted, enlarged, blue and purple veins most often found on the legs and ankles. They have several possible causes, including weakened valves causing blood to pool around the vein. In some cases, varicose veins are merely a cosmetic problem because of their appearance, but in other cases they can be quite painful. *See also Hemorrhoids for varicose veins of the anus or rectum.*

> *Simple Solutions—Varicose Veins:* Add 3 drops cypress and 1 drop lemongrass to 1 Tbs. (15 ml) fractionated coconut oil. Gently massage a small amount on location daily.

Oils: ⬭cypress, ⬭lemongrass, ⬭lemon, ⬭peppermint, ⬭helichrysum, ⬭Citrus Bliss, ⬭geranium, ⬭lavender, ⬭rosemary, ⬭juniper berry, ⬭orange

⬭: Dilute as recommended, and apply oils gently from ankles up the legs. *Consistent application of oils for an extended period of time is the key.* Add 3–5 drops to 1

⬭=Topical, ⊘=Aromatic, ◯=Internal

Tbs. (15 ml) fractionated coconut oil, and massage above the veins towards the heart. Wearing support hose and elevating the feet can also help keep blood from pooling in the legs.

🌀: **Body System(s) Affected:** Cardiovascular System and Skin.

🛈: **Additional Research:**

Melaleuca: Bagg et al., 2006; Banes-Marshall et al., 2001; Cox et al., 2000; D'Auria et al., 2001; Hammer et al., 2004; Mondello et al., 2006; Vazquez et al., 2000; Oregano: Manohar et al., 2001; Clove: Chaieb et al., 2007; Peppermint: Mimica-Dukić et al., 2003; Thyme: Pina-Vaz et al., 2004; Lavender: D'Auria et al., 2005.

Vascular System

See **Cardiovascular System;**
see also **Arteries, Capillaries, Veins**

Vasodilator

See **Arteries: Arterial Vasodilator**

Veins

A vein is a blood vessel that carries blood from the capillaries back to the heart. Veins may also have one-way valves on the inside that help keep blood from flowing backwards and pooling in the lower extremities due to gravity.

Oils: 🌢lemongrass, 🌢cypress, 🌢lemon, 🌢helichrysum

—Blood Clot in Vein:

Blend 1: Apply 1 drop cypress and 1 drop helichrysum on location of clot to help dissolve.

🌀: Dilute as recommended, and apply 1–2 drops on location. Add 5–10 drops to 1 Tbs. (15 ml) fractionated coconut oil, and massage on location.

🌀: **Body System(s) Affected:** Cardiovascular System.

Vertigo

See also **Ears, Nausea: Motion Sickness**

Vertigo refers to the sensation that the environment and objects around an individual are moving or spinning, usually causing a loss of balance or feelings of nausea. Vertigo may be caused by ear infections, ear disorders, or motion sickness.

Oils: 🌢🌀ginger, 🌢helichrysum, 🌢geranium, 🌢basil, 🌢lavender

Recipe 1: Apply 1–2 drops each of helichrysum, geranium, and lavender to the tops of each ear (massaging slightly); then apply the oils behind each ear, pulling your hands down behind the jaw bone to just below the jaw. Finish by applying 1–2 drops of basil behind and down each ear. This can be performed multiple times a day until symptoms decrease.

🌀: Dilute as recommended, and apply 1–2 drops around ears and on reflex points on the feet.

🌀: Inhale oil directly from bottle. Apply oil to hands, tissue, or cotton wick, and inhale.

🌀: **Body System(s) Affected:** Nervous, Respiratory, and Digestive Systems.

Viral Disease/Viruses

See **Antiviral**

Vitiligo

See **Skin: Vitiligo**

Voice (Hoarse)

See also **Laryngitis**

A hoarse voice is typically caused by laryngitis (inflammation of the larynx due to infection), but it can also be caused by other problems such as an ulcer, sore, polyp, or tumor on or near the vocal cords.

Oils: 🅞bergamot

Recipe 1: Add 1 drop melaleuca, 1 drop rosemary, 1 drop clove, and 1 drop lemon to 1 tsp. (5 ml) honey. Swish around in the mouth for a couple of minutes to liquefy with saliva; then swallow.

🌀: Add 1 drop to 1 tsp. (5 ml) honey, and swallow.

🌀: **Body System(s) Affected:** Respiratory System.

Vomiting

See **Nausea: Vomiting**

Warming Oils

Oils: 🌢cinnamon, 🌢oregano, 🌢yuzu, 🌢thyme, 🌢marjoram, 🌢rosemary, 🌢juniper berry

🌀: Add 5–10 drops to 1 tsp. (5 ml) fractionated coconut oil, and massage briskly into skin.

🌀: **Body System(s) Affected:** Skin.

Warts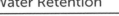

A wart is a small, firm, hard growth on the skin, usually located on the hands and feet, that is typically caused by a virus.

> *Simple Solutions—Wart:* Combine 5 drops cypress, 10 drops lemon, and 2 Tbs. (25 ml) apple cider vinegar. Apply on location twice daily; bandage. Keep a bandage on until wart is gone.

Oils: ◐frankincense, ◐On Guard, ◐melaleuca, ◐oregano (layer with On Guard), ◐clove, ◐cypress, ◐arborvitae, ◐cinnamon, ◐lemon, ◐lavender

Recipe 1: Combine 5 drops cypress, 10 drops lemon, and 2 Tbs. (25 ml) apple cider vinegar. Apply on location twice daily; bandage. Keep a bandage on until wart is gone.

—Genital:

A genital wart is a small, painful wart or cluster of warts located in the genital area or in the mouth or throat. This type of wart is typically spread by contact with the skin through sexual activity.

Oils: ◐frankincense, ◐On Guard, ◐melaleuca, ◐oregano, ◐thyme

—Plantar:

Plantar warts are painful warts that grow on the bottoms of the feet. They are usually flattened and embedded into the skin due to the pressure caused by walking on them.

Oils: ◐oregano

◐: Dilute as recommended, or dilute 1–2 drops of oil in a few drops fractionated coconut oil; then apply 1–2 drops on location daily.

◐: **Body System(s) Affected:** Skin and Immune System.

Water Purification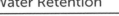

Oils: ◐◐lemon, ◐◐Purify, ◐peppermint, ◐orange

◐: Add 1 drop of oil to 1½–2 cups (375–500 ml) of drinking water to help purify.

◐: Add 1–2 drops to dishwater for sparkling dishes and a great smelling kitchen. Add 1–2 drops to warm bathwater, and bathe. Add 1–2 drops to a bowl of water, and use the water to clean the outsides of fruits and vegetables.

Water Retention

*See **Edema, Diuretic***

Weakness

*See **Energy***

Weight

Proper exercise and nutrition are the most critical factors for maintaining a healthy weight. Other factors that may influence weight include an individual's metabolism, level of stress, hormonal imbalances, low or high thyroid function, or the level of insulin being produced by the body.

> *Simple Solutions—Overeating:* Diffuse Slim & Sassy to help reduce cravings during the day.

—Obesity:

Obesity is the condition of being overweight to the extent that it affects health and lifestyle. By definition, obesity is considered as a body mass index (BMI) of 30 kg/m² or greater.

Oils: ◐◐grapefruit◐ ◐◐Slim & Sassy, ◐◐oregano◐, ◐◐thyme◐, ◐Yarrow Pom, ◐◐orange◐, ◐rosemary, ◐◐juniper berry, ◐fennel

Other Products: ◐Slim & Sassy TrimShakes, ◐Slim & Sassy Contrōl Instant Drink Mix, ◐Slim & Sassy Contrōl Bars, ◐Mito2Max for enhanced cellular energy. ◐TerraGreens for a whole food source of essential nutrients and antioxidants. ◐Alpha CRS+ contains polyphenols resveratrol and epigallocatechin-3-gallate (EGCG), which have been studied for their abilities to help prevent obesity.

—Slimming/Toning:

Oils: ◐◐grapefruit◐, ◐◐Slim & Sassy, ◐Yarrow Pom, ◐◐orange, ◐lemongrass, ◐rosemary, ◐thyme, ◐lavender

Other Products: ◐Slim & Sassy TrimShakes.

—Weight Loss:

Oils: ◐◐Slim & Sassy, ◐Elevation, ◐Yarrow Pom, ◐◐patchouli

Other Products: ◐Slim & Sassy TrimShakes, ◐Slim & Sassy Contrōl Instant Drink Mix, ◐Slim & Sassy Contrōl Bars. ◐TerraGreens for a whole food source of essential nutrients.

◐=Topical, ◐=Aromatic, ◐=Internal

Recipe 1: Add 5 drops lemon and 5 drops grapefruit to 1 gallon (4 L) of water, and drink throughout the day.

⊘: Diffuse oil into the air. Inhale oil directly from bottle; or inhale oil that is applied to hands, tissue, or cotton wick.

○: Add 8 drops of Slim & Sassy to 2 cups (½ L) of water, and drink throughout the day between meals. Add 1 drop of oil to 1½–2 cups (375–500 ml) of water, and drink. Drink Trim or V Shake 1–2 times per day as a meal alternative. Take capsules as directed on package.

⊕: **Body System(s) Affected:** Digestive System.

⊙: **Additional Research:**

Grapefruit: Shen et al., 2005; Haze et al., 2010; **Carvacrol found in oregano and thyme essential oils :** Cho et al., 2012; **D-Limonene found in lime, lemon, bergamot, dill, grapefruit, lavender, lemongrass, Roman chamomile, tangerine, and wild orange essential oils :** Jing et al., 2013; **Lime:** Asnaashari et al., 2010; **Cinnamon:** Boque et al., 2013.

Whiplash

Whiplash is the over-stretching or tearing of the muscles, ligaments, and/or tendons in the neck and head. This is typically caused by a sudden collision or force pushing the body in one direction, while the head's tendency to remain in the same place causes the head to quickly rock in the opposite direction the body is going.

> *Simple Solutions—Whiplash:* Blend 3 drops lemongrass and 2 drops marjoram with 1 Tbs. (15 ml) fractionated coconut oil. Gently massage a small amount into the neck and shoulders daily.

Oils: ⊘Deep Blue, ⊘Rescuer, ⊘lemongrass (ligaments), ⊘marjoram (muscles), ⊘birch, ⊘basil, ⊘juniper berry, ⊘helichrysum, ⊘vetiver, ⊘clove, ⊘peppermint, ⊘Roman chamomile

⊘: Dilute as recommended, and apply 1–2 drops on back of neck. Add 5–10 drops to 1 Tbs. (15 ml) fractionated coconut oil, and massage on back of neck, on shoulders, and on upper back.

⊕: **Body System(s) Affected:** Skeletal System and Muscles.

Whooping Cough

See Childhood Diseases: Whooping Cough

Withdrawal

See Addictions: Withdrawal

Women

See Female-Specific Conditions

Workaholic

See Addictions: Work

Worms

See Antifungal: Ringworm, Parasites: Worms

Wounds

See also Antibacterial, Blood: Bleeding

A wound is a general term for an injury that involves tissue (typically the skin or underlying skeletal muscles) being torn, cut, punctured, scraped, or crushed.

> *Simple Solutions—Wounds:* Apply 1 drop helichrysum on area to help stop bleeding. Add 1 drop each lavender, melaleuca, and basil to a bowl of warm water. Use water to wash wound.

Oils: ⊘clove, ⊘melaleuca, ⊘helichrysum, ⊘lavender, ⊘lemongrass, ⊘Purify, ⊘⊘Stronger, ⊘basil⊙, ⊘yarrow, ⊘cypress, ⊘eucalyptus, ⊘frankincense, ⊘Roman chamomile, ⊘⊘copaiba, ⊘peppermint (after wound has closed), ⊘myrrh, ⊘rose, ⊘⊘blue tansy, ⊘sandalwood, ⊘thyme, ⊘juniper berry, ⊘bergamot

Recipe 1: Place 1–3 drops of helichrysum on fresh wound to help stop bleeding. Add 1 drop clove⊙ to help reduce pain. Once bleeding has stopped, apply a drop of lavender (to help start healing), a drop of melaleuca (to help fight infection), and a drop of lemongrass (for possible ligament damage). Bandage the wound. When changing the bandage, apply 1 drop basil or sandalwood to help promote further healing. Add 1 drop Purify or On Guard to help prevent infection.

Other Products: ⊘Correct-X to help cleanse and support the skin's natural healing process.

Blend 1: Add 1 drop lavender to 1 drop Purify and apply to wound.

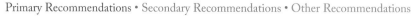

—Children/Infants:

Oils: ⬤Roman chamomile, ⬤⬤Stronger,

Recipe 2: Add 1–3 drops each of helichrysum and lavender to 1 tsp. (5 ml) fractionated coconut oil, and apply a small amount to wound.

—Bleeding:

Oils: ⬤helichrysum, ⬤rose, ⬤lavender, ⬤lemon

Blend 2: Combine 1 drop Roman chamomile, 1 drop geranium, and 1 drop lemon, and apply with a warm compress 2–3 times a day for 3–4 days, then reduce to once a day until healed.

—Disinfect:

Oils: ⬤melaleuca, ⬤⬤Stronger, ⬤thyme, ⬤lavender

—Healing:

Oils: ⬤basil⬤, ⬤helichrysum, ⬤⬤Stronger, ⬤melaleuca, ⬤lavender, ⬤myrrh, ⬤sandalwood

—Inflammation: *See Inflammation*

—Scarring: *See Skin: Scarring, Tissue: Scarring*

—Surgical:

Oils: ⬤peppermint, ⬤melaleuca

Blend 2: Add 3 drops helichrysum, 3 drops frankincense, and 4 drops lavender to 2 tsp. (10 ml) fractionated coconut oil. Apply a few drops when changing bandages.

—Weeping:

Oils: ⬤myrrh, ⬤patchouli

⬤: Dilute as recommended, and apply 1–2 drops on location.

⬤: **Body System(s) Affected:** Skin and Immune System.

⬤: **Additional Research:**

Basil: Orafidiya et al., 2003; Clove: Ghelardini et al., 2001; Cinnamon: Ghosh et al., 2013.

Wrinkles

See Skin: Wrinkles

Yeast

See Antifungal: Candida

Yoga

Oils: ⬤⬤Align, ⬤⬤Anchor, ⬤⬤Arise, ⬤sandalwood, ⬤cedarwood, ⬤⬤litsea

⬤: Diffuse into the air.

⬤: **Body System(s) Affected:** Emotional Balance.

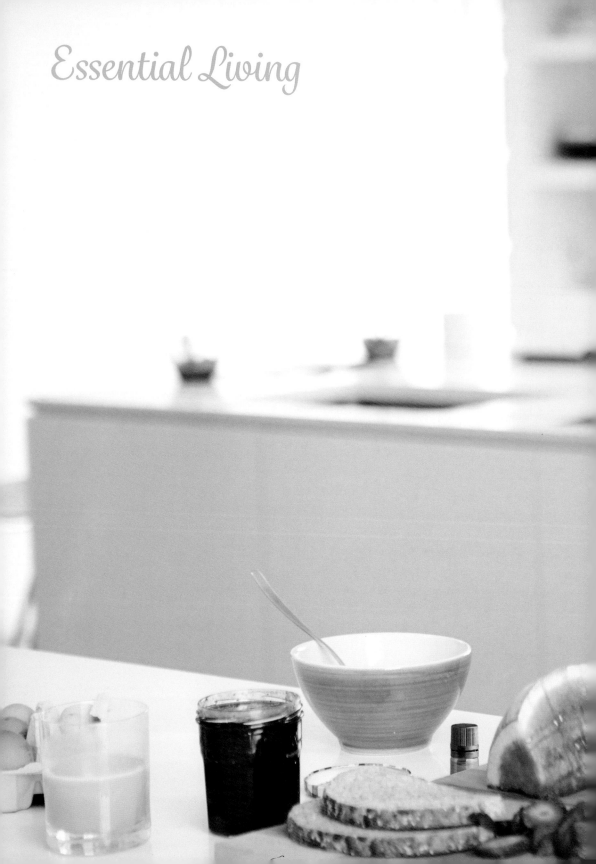

Essential Living

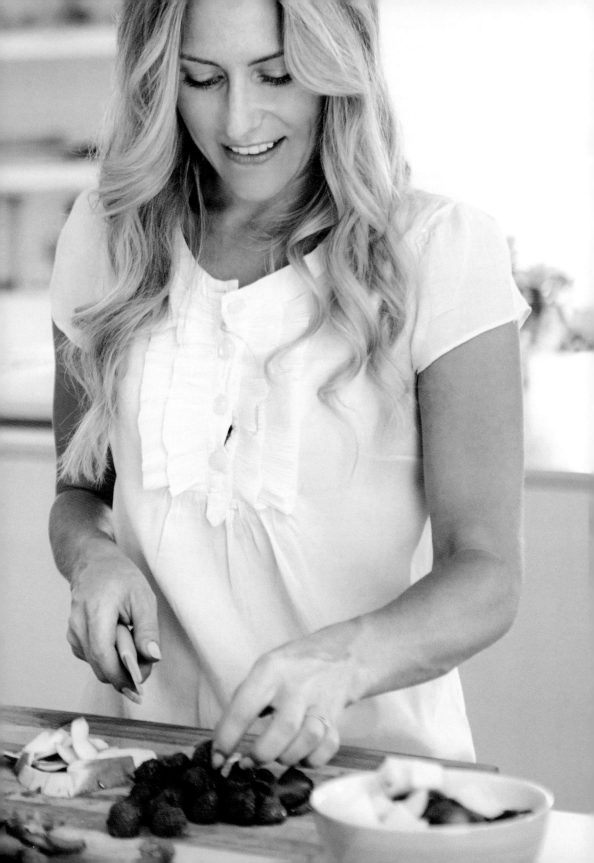

Using essential oils in the bath or shower instead of products with artificial perfumes and fragrances allows one to simultaneously enjoy the topical and aromatic benefits of an essential oil or blend.

Bath and Shower Tips

Bathwater: Add 3–6 drops of oil to the bathwater while the tub is filling. Because the individual oils will separate as the water calms down, the skin will quickly draw the oils from the top of the water. Some people have commented that they were unable to endure more than 6 drops of oil. Such individuals may benefit from adding the oils to a bath and shower gel base first. Soak in the tub for 15 minutes.

Bath and Shower Gel: Add 3–6 drops of oil to 1 Tbs. (15 ml) of a natural bath and shower gel base; add to the water while the tub is filling. Adding the oils to a bath and shower gel base first allows one to obtain the greatest benefit from the oils, as they are more evenly dispersed throughout the water and not allowed to immediately separate.

Washcloth: When showering, add 3–6 drops of oil to a bath and shower gel base before applying to a washcloth and using to wash the body.

Body Sprays: Fill a small spray bottle with distilled water, and add 10–15 drops of your favorite essential oil or blend. Shake well, and spray onto the entire body just after taking a bath or shower.

Footbath: Add enough hot water to a basin to cover the ankles. Add 1–3 drops of your desired essential oil. Soak feet for 5–10 minutes, inhaling the aroma of the oils.

Hand Bath: Pour enough hot water in a basin to cover hands up to the wrists. Add 1–3 drops of your desired essential oil. Soak hands for 5–10 minutes while bending, pulling, and massaging the fingers and hands to stimulate. Try combining essential oils with 1 Tbs. (15 ml) honey in a hand bath or regular bath to help moisturize the skin.

Shower: With the water turned on, drop peppermint, rosemary, or Breathe on the shower floor as you enter to help invigorate and open the nasal passages. Use soothing oils at night to help promote a feeling of calmness and relaxation. Alternately, fill a tub/shower combo with about an inch or two of water; then place oils in the water before turning on the shower. This will allow the oils to more easily be drawn into the feet during the shower and also allow the aroma to be inhaled.

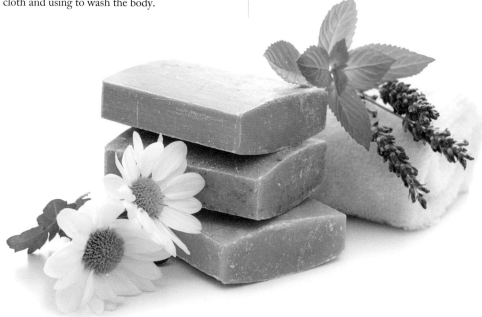

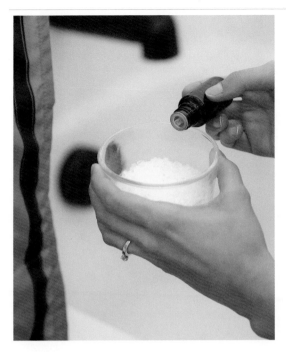

Bath Salts Base

1 c. (250 g) Epsom salt (or sea salt)

15 drops EO *(see blend ideas below)*

Combine essential oils with salt in a container. Dissolve ¼–½ cup (50–125 g) of this bath salt mixture in warm bathwater before bathing.

Bath Oils Base

2 T. (25 ml) fractionated coconut oil
(or jojoba or sweet almond oil)

15 drops EO *(see blend ideas below)*

Blend vegetable oil with essential oils in a small container. Add 1 tsp. (5 ml) of this bath oil to warm bathwater before bathing.

Relaxing Bliss

 + + +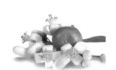

5 drops lavender   5 drops petitgrain   3 drops fennel   2 drops orange

Soothe Your Troubles

 + 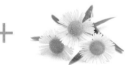 + +

4 drops lavender   4 drops R. chamomile   4 drops cedarwood   3 drops lemongrass

Refreshed and Ready to Go

 + + +

5 drops peppermint   4 drops lavender   3 drops grapefruit   3 drops lemongrass

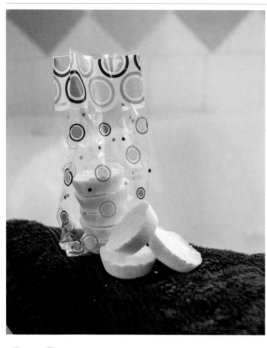

Fizzing Bath Bomb Base

⅔ c. (125 g) baking soda   ½ c. (75 g) cornstarch

⅓ c. (75 g) Epsom salt   2 t. (10 ml) water

2 t. (10 g) coconut oil   Spray bottle with water

15 drops EO *(see blend ideas below)*

Combine the dry ingredients in one bowl and the wet ingredients in another. Add the wet ingredients to the dry ingredients slowly while stirring with a whisk. Knead the mixture until it has the texture of mildly wet sand and clumps together when pressed. If it is too dry, moisten it slightly with a mist from the spray bottle, one spritz at a time, just until it holds together. Form into balls, or mold in small soap or candy molds or a mini muffin tin (lined with paper muffin cups). Allow to dry for 1–2 hours, then remove from molds or tins, and allow to dry overnight.

To use, place a bath bomb in warm bathwater, and enjoy!

Sweet Dreams

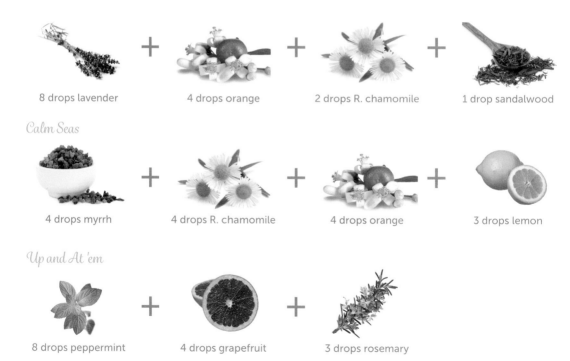

8 drops lavender   +   4 drops orange   +   2 drops R. chamomile   +   1 drop sandalwood

Calm Seas

4 drops myrrh   +   4 drops R. chamomile   +   4 drops orange   +   3 drops lemon

Up and At 'em

8 drops peppermint   +   4 drops grapefruit   +   3 drops rosemary

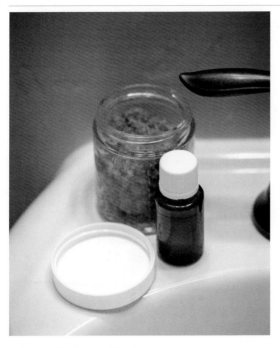

Simple Sugar Scrub Base

¼ c. (50 g) raw sugar   ¼ c. (50 ml) sweet almond oil

8 drops vitamin E oil (optional natural preservative)

15 drops EO *(see blend ideas below)*

Mix all ingredients together in a glass bowl. Store in airtight containers. To use, place a small amount of the scrub in the palm, and scrub over moistened skin. Rinse off in a shower or tub. (Note: The oils in this scrub can make the floor of the bathtub or shower slippery, so use caution when rinsing off.)

Try using different coarsenesses of sugar to create progressively smoother scubs (e.g., a course raw sugar "buffing" scrub followed by a fine white sugar "polishing" scrub.

Lemon Rosemary Scrub

 +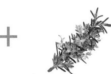

10 drops lemon   5 drops rosemary

Skin-Toning Scrub

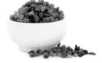 +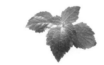

9 drops myrrh   4 drops patchouli   2 drops geranium

Invigorating Scrub

 + 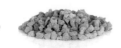 +

5 drops ginger   5 drops frankincense   5 drops grapefruit

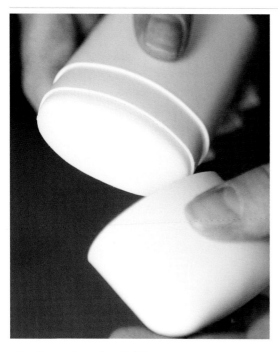

Deodorant Base

3 T. (35 g) coconut oil	1 T. (5 g) beeswax pellets
¼ c. (30 g) cornstarch	¼ c. (50 g) baking soda
6 drops vitamin E oil	Deodorant container

15 drops EO *(see blend ideas below)*

Melt beeswax and coconut oil in a double boiler or in the microwave (stirring every 30 seconds until just melted). Stir in cornstarch, baking soda, and vitamin E oil. Allow to cool slightly; then add essential oils. Pour into an empty deodorant container. Allow to cool and harden completely. Apply deodorant as needed.

Purifying Lavender Melaleuca

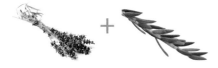

8 drops lavender   7 drops melaleuca

Flower Power

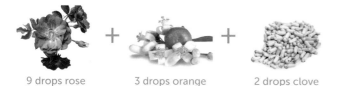

9 drops rose   3 drops orange   2 drops clove

Spicy Fresh

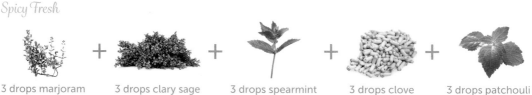

3 drops marjoram   3 drops clary sage   3 drops spearmint   3 drops clove   3 drops patchouli

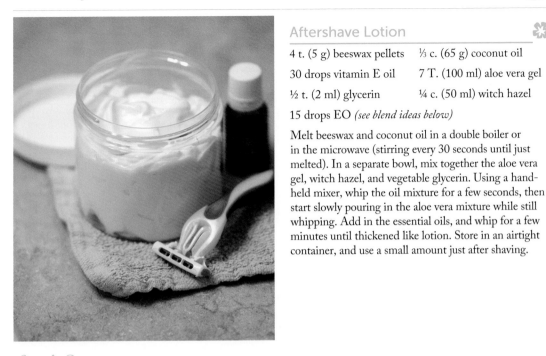

Aftershave Lotion

4 t. (5 g) beeswax pellets	⅓ c. (65 g) coconut oil
30 drops vitamin E oil	7 T. (100 ml) aloe vera gel
½ t. (2 ml) glycerin	¼ c. (50 ml) witch hazel

15 drops EO *(see blend ideas below)*

Melt beeswax and coconut oil in a double boiler or in the microwave (stirring every 30 seconds until just melted). In a separate bowl, mix together the aloe vera gel, witch hazel, and vegetable glycerin. Using a hand-held mixer, whip the oil mixture for a few seconds, then start slowly pouring in the aloe vera mixture while still whipping. Add in the essential oils, and whip for a few minutes until thickened like lotion. Store in an airtight container, and use a small amount just after shaving.

Ease the Burn

 +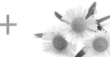

9 drops lavender   6 drops R. chamomile

Skin-Toning

 + 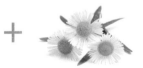 +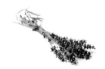

6 drops myrrh   6 drops R. chamomile   3 drops lavender

Sensitive Skin

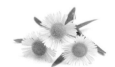 + + +

8 drops R. chamomile   3 drops lavender   1 drop peppermint   1 drop lemon

Natural Perfumes

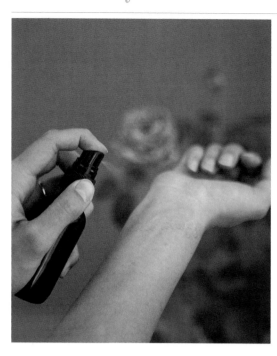

Simple Perfume Base

1 t. (5 ml) pure grain or perfumer's alcohol
OR 1 t. (5 ml) jojoba oil

15 drops EO *(see blend ideas below)*

Mix essential oils with a pure grain alcohol (like vodka or Everclear) or perfumer's alcohol, and pour into a small spray bottle. Alternately, mix with jojoba oil in a small roll-on bottle for an alcohol-free perfume. Apply a small amount on wrists, neck, or other desired points.

Solid Perfume Base

1 t. (2 g) beeswax pellets   1 T. (15 ml) jojoba oil

15 drops EO *(see blend ideas below)*

Combine beeswax and jojoba oil, and melt in the microwave (stirring every 30 seconds until just melted) or in a double boiler. Let cool slightly, and add essential oils and vitamin E oil. Pour into a small jar or lockets. Apply a small amount on the wrists, neck, or other points on the skin as desired.

Romance

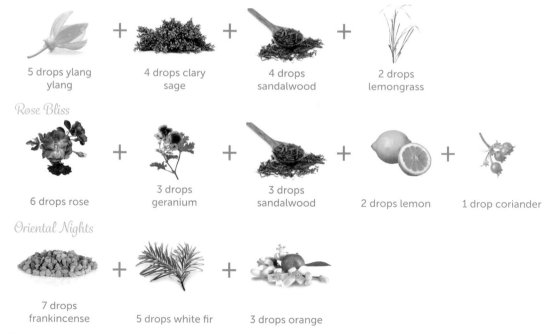

| 5 drops ylang ylang | + | 4 drops clary sage | + | 4 drops sandalwood | + | 2 drops lemongrass |

Rose Bliss

6 drops rose + 3 drops geranium + 3 drops sandalwood + 2 drops lemon + 1 drop coriander

Oriental Nights

7 drops frankincense + 5 drops white fir + 3 drops orange

Tip: Combine your alcohol-based perfume with 2 tsp. (10 ml) water for a lighter eau de toilette, or ¼ cup (50 ml) water for a room or body spray.

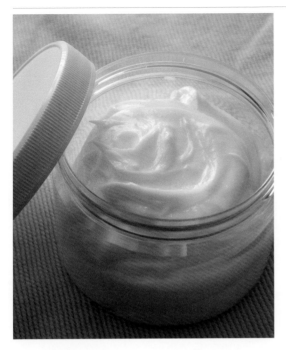

Simple Lotion Base

¼ c. (20 g) beeswax pellets

½ c. (100 g) coconut oil

½ c. (125 ml) aloe vera gel

15 drops EO *(see blend ideas below)*

Combine beeswax and coconut oil, and melt in the microwave (stirring every 30 seconds until just melted) or in a double boiler. Allow mixture to cool to room temperature (about an hour). Using a handheld mixer, whip the mixture, and slowly add in the aloe vera gel and essential oils. Whip together until well incorporated and fluffy. Store in an airtight jar or lotion dispenser in a cool location. Apply a small amount on the skin as desired. This lotion is great when feeling warm on a hot summer day!

Cool Mint

 +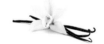

12 drops peppermint   3 drops vanilla extract

Skin-Soothing

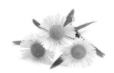 + 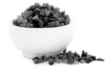 +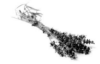

6 drops R. chamomile   6 drops myrrh   3 drops lavender

Lavender Fields

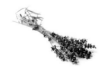 +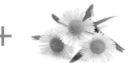

10 drops lavender   5 drops R. chamomile

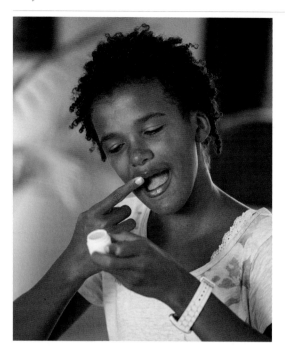

Lip Balm Base

4 t. (5 g) beeswax pellets

1 T. (15 g) cocoa butter

3 T. (45 ml) jojoba oil

15 drops EO *(see blend ideas below)*

Combine beeswax and cocoa butter, and melt in the microwave (stirring every 30 seconds until just melted) or in a double boiler. Mix in jojoba oil until incorporated. Let cool slightly, and add essential oils. Pour into small jars or lip balm dispensers. Allow to cool and solidify completely. Apply a small amount on the lips as desired.

Minty Fresh

 +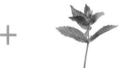

10 drops peppermint   5 drops spearmint

Creamsicle

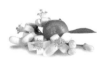 + +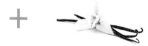

10 drops orange   3 drops grapefruit   2 drops vanilla extract

Lemon Thyme

 +

12 drops lemon   3 drops thyme

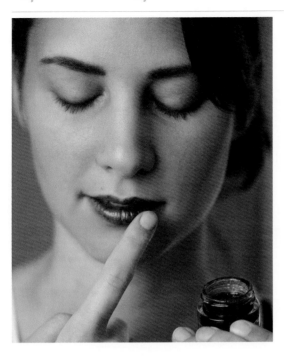

Berry Mint Lip Stain

3 blackberries

3 raspberries

1 small strawberry (no stem)

½ t. (3 ml) sweet almond oil

1 drop peppermint essential oil OR 1 drop of a blend from the previous page

Heat the berries in the microwave or over a double boiler until soft. Mash the berries with a fork until well blended. Allow to cool slightly, and mix in the sweet almond oil and essential oil. Strain the mixture through a coffee filter or cheesecloth to remove pulp and seeds. Place in a small salve or lip gloss jar, and store in the refrigerator. To use, dip your finger into the stain and apply to the lips. Wash finger immediately after application to avoid staining the finger.

Brown Sugar Mint Lip Scrub

3 T. (40 g) brown sugar

1 T. (15 g) coconut oil

2 drops peppermint essential oil OR 2 drops of a blend from the previous page

Mix together all of the ingredients. Store in a small glass jar. To use, place a small amount on the lips, and rub lips together for a couple minutes to help exfoliate. Rinse lips with water.

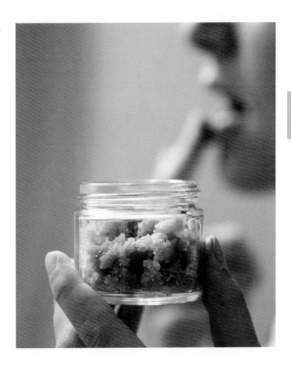

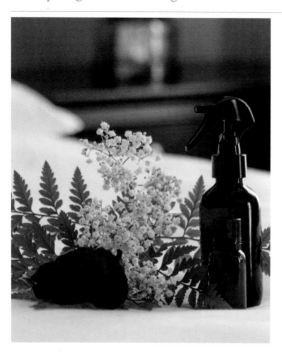

"Time to Sleep" Linen Spray

1 t. (5 ml) pure grain or perfumer's alcohol

¼ c. (50 ml) water

Small misting spray bottle

15 drops Serenity or another soothing essential oil *(see below)*

Mix essential oils withw a pure grain alcohol (like vodka or Everclear) or perfumer's alcohol in a small spray bottle. Add water. To use this spray, shake well, then mist a few spritzes on pillows, sheets, or other linens before bed time.

Soothing Essential Oils:

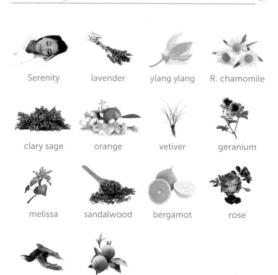

Serenity · lavender · ylang ylang · R. chamomile

clary sage · orange · vetiver · geranium

melissa · sandalwood · bergamot · rose

spikenard · petitgrain

More Sleeping/Relaxation Tips:

Diffusion: Diffuse soothing essential oils or blends to help you feel calm and relaxed before going to sleep.

Pillow: Place 1–2 drops of a soothing essential oil or blend on a pillow or stuffed animal before you sleep to help calm your mind and body.

Relaxing Bath: Mix 1–3 drops of a soothing essential oil with bath salts or directly in warm bathwater for a relaxing bath.

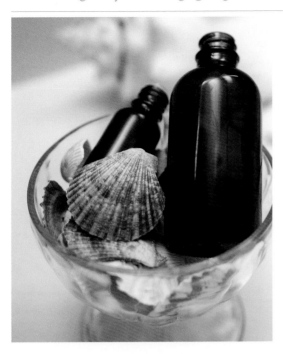

Invigorating Shower

3 drops Elevation or another invigorating essential oil *(see below)*

Place 3 drops of the essential oil or blend on the floor of a shower just before entering for an invigorating morning shower.

Invigorating Essential Oils:

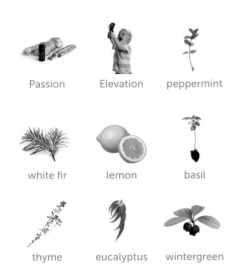

Passion Elevation peppermint

white fir lemon basil

thyme eucalyptus wintergreen

More Energizing/Invigorating Tips:

Diffusion: Diffuse an invigorating oil in the morning. Some individuals like to use a timer to start their diffuser a few minutes before their alarm clock goes off to help the body begin to wake up naturally.

Morning Beverage: Add a few drops of peppermint, lemon, or orange to water, a fresh fruit/vegetable smoothie, or another healthy beverage.

Kitchen

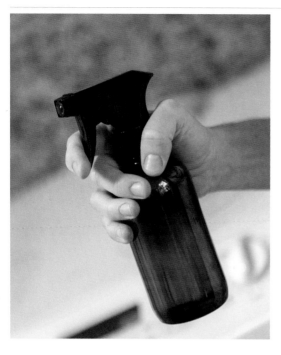

Disinfecting Spray

½ c. (125 ml) white vinegar

½ c. (125 ml) water

Small spray bottle

15 drops On Guard or another disinfecting essential oil *(see below)*

Combine all ingredients in a small spray bottle. Shake well, and spray on counters, cutting boards, microwave, refrigerator, garbage cans, or other desired surfaces; use a rag to wipe off.

Other Kitchen Cleaning Tips:

Counter Cleaning: Add 1–2 drops of lemon, On Guard, or another disinfecting oil to a damp rag. Use to wipe down counters, tables, or stoves.

Trash Can Deodorizer: Add 3–5 drops of a deodorizing essential oil or blend *(see bottom right)* to 1 Tbs. (15 g) baking powder. Sprinkle into trash can.

Dishes: Add a few drops of lemon to dishwater for sparkling dishes and a great-smelling kitchen. You can add the essential oil to a dishwasher as well.

Disinfecting Essential Oils:

 On Guard   lemon   Purify   melaleuca

 lime   cinnamon   thyme   peppermint

Deodorizing Essential Oils:

  Purify   peppermint   clary sage   melaleuca

  lavender   geranium   eucalyptus

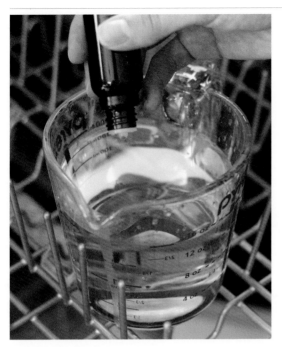

Dishwasher Cleaner

2 c. (½ L) white vinegar

10 drops lemon essential oil

Remove the lower rack from your dishwasher. Using a rag soaked in warm, soapy water, wipe down the bottom of the dishwasher to remove any loose food or dirt. Replace the bottom rack. Place the vinegar and lemon oil in a dishwasher-safe bowl or cup. Place this on the top rack of the dishwasher. Run your dishwasher on the hottest setting without any other dishes for a full cycle. Open and enjoy a clean, great-smelling dishwasher!

Streak-Free Glass & Mirror Spray

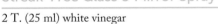

2 T. (25 ml) white vinegar

2 T. (25 ml) rubbing alcohol

1½ t. (5 g) cornstarch

¾ c. (175 ml) water

5 drops lemon and 5 drops lime essential oil

Small spray bottle

Combine vinegar, alcohol, cornstarch, and essential oils in the spray bottle. Screw on the spray top, and shake to combine. Unscrew the top, and add water. Screw on the spray top, and shake again to combine. To use, shake, then spray on glass or mirror. Wipe glass or mirror with a rag.

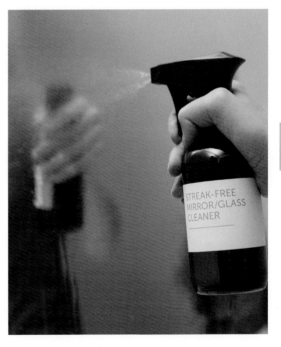

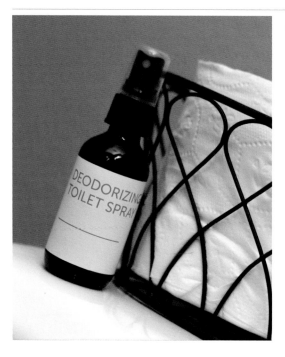

Toilet Spray

1 t. (5 ml) vegetable glycerin

1 t. (5 ml) rubbing alcohol

¼ c. (50 ml) water

Small spray bottle

15 drops EO *(see blend ideas below)*

Blend glycerin, alcohol, and essential oils in spray bottle, and shake to combine. Add water, and shake again to combine. To use, shake the bottle, then spray a few times in the toilet before you do your business.

Sweet Citrus

 + 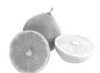 +

5 drops lemongrass   5 drops bergamot   5 drops grapefruit

Ocean Breeze

 + +

7 drops cedarwood   5 drops lemon   3 drops rosemary

Herbal Bliss

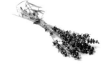 + + +

4 drops lavender   4 drops peppermint   4 drops rosemary   2 drops melaleuca

Other Bathroom Cleaning Tips:

Mildew Spray: Mix 5 drops lemon and 5 drops white fir with ¼ cup (50 ml) water in a small spray bottle. Spray on areas with mildew.

Deodorizing Spray: Place 5–8 drops of a deodorizing essential oil (try 5 drops grapefruit and 1 drop peppermint) in a 1 oz. spray bottle, and fill the remainder of the bottle with water. Shake well, and spray into the air.

Mold: Diffuse On Guard into the air to help eliminate mold.

Laundry Tips:

Gum/Grease: Use lemon or Citrus Bliss to help take gum or grease out of clothes (test in a small, in-conspicuous area first to ensure that the oil won't affect delicate dyes or fabrics).

Washing: Add a few drops of Purify to the wash water to help kill bacteria and germs in clothes.

Drying: Put Purify, Elevation, lemongrass, or another favorite oil or blend on a wet rag, and then place the rag in the dryer with clothing. Or mist oils from a spray bottle directly into the dryer to keep clothes smelling great—without artificial perfumes or fragrances.

Furniture Tips:

Polish: For a simple furniture polish, put a few drops of lemon, Purify, or white fir oil on a dust cloth, and use to wipe down wood.

Clothes/Closets:

Clothing Deodorizer: Place a tissue or cotton ball with several drops of Purify, lavender, lemongrass, mela-leuca, peppermint, Citrus Bliss, or another favorite oil in a perforated wood, glass, or stone container. Place container in a closet, shoe cupboard, or drawer to keep clothes naturally smelling great.

Painting Tips:

Paint Fumes: To effectively remove paint fumes and after smell, add one 15 ml bottle of oil to any 5-gallon bucket of paint. Purify and citrus single oils have been favorites, but Citrus Bliss and Elevation would work just as well. Either a paint sprayer or brush and roller can be used to apply the paint after mixing the oils into the paint by stirring vigorously. Oils may eventually rise to the top if using a water-based paint. Occasional stirring may be necessary to keep the oils mixed.

Carpet Care Tips:

Carpet Cleaner/Deodorizer: Mix 1 cup (200 g) baking soda and 20–50 drops melaleuca, lemon, Purify, or another favorite oil in a glass jar. Close jar, shake together, and let stand overnight. Sprinkle lightly over carpets, let sit for 15 minutes, and then vacuum.

Grease/Gum Remover: Try lemon or lime oil on stubborn greasy stains, or use to help dissolve gum stuck to the carpet (be certain to test oil in a small, inconspicuous area of the carpet first to ensure it won't affect any delicate dyes in the carpet).

Bug/Pest Repellent Tips:

Bug-Repelling Oils: TerraShield, lavender, lemongrass, patchouli, basil, Purify.

Mice-Repelling Oil: Purify.

Personal Bug Repellent: Apply repelling oils directly on the skin (dilute with fractionated coconut oil if you are covering a large area).

Bug Spray: Add 10–15 drops of repelling oil to 2 Tbs. (25 ml) water in a small misting spray bottle. Shake well, and mist over exposed skin and clothing.

Diffusion: Diffuse repelling oils in a room.

Pest Repellent: Place repelling oils on a string, ribbon, or cotton ball, and hang near air vents or windows, or place in cracks and other areas where bugs or pests come through.

Wipes

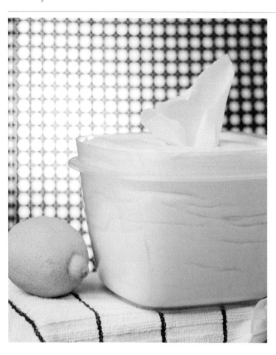

Wipe Base

2 T. (25 ml) Castile soap (or other unscented soap)

2 T. (25 ml) jojoba oil

2 c. (½ L) water

8 drops vitamin E oil

1 roll paper towels (heavy-duty work best) OR dry bamboo wipes

2 round plastic storage containers

15 drops EO *(see blend ideas below)*

Cut the roll of paper towels in half with a serrated knife, remove the cardboard tube from the center, and place each half in one of the round plastic storage containers. Combine the soap, jojoba oil, water, vitamin E oil, and essential oils together. Pour half of the liquid over each of the paper towel halves, and allow liquid to soak into the paper towels. To use, pull wipes from the center of the roll. Seal the storage container afterwards to keep wipes moist. Use within 1–2 weeks.

Baby Wipes

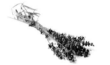 +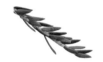

10 drops lavender · 5 drops melaleuca

Facial Cleansing Wipes

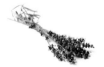 + +

5 drops lavender · 5 drops lemon · 5 drops melaleuca

Disinfecting Wipes

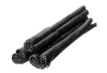 + 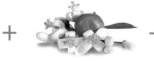 + +

4 drops cinnamon · 4 drops orange · 4 drops lemon · 3 drops rosemary

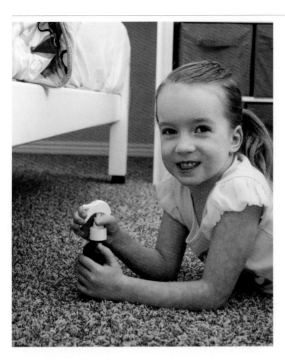

Kid's Room Spray Base

½ c. (125 ml) water

Small spray bottle

15 drops EO *(see blend ideas below)*

Combine water and essential oils in a small spray bottle (the kind with a trigger spray is easiest for kids to use). Give to older children to spray into the air as needed or desired.

Kid's Diffuser Blends

Diffuser

15 drops EO *(see blend ideas below)*

Diffuse one of the blends below in a water misting home or car diffuser.

Sweet Dreams

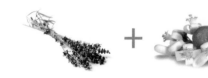 + 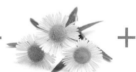 + 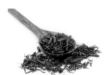 +

8 drops lavender   4 drops orange   2 drops R. chamomile   1 drop sandalwood

Laser Focus

 + +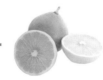

7 drops white fir   5 drops rosemary   3 drops bergamot

Calm Car Trip

 +

10 drops ginger   5 drops peppermint

The aroma of essential oils can be a major contributor to helping create the right atmosphere at home. Studies have shown that certain aromas can help a space feel warm and inviting, while other aromas, like orange, can help relax and reduce anxiety. Here are a few ideas to get you started, but try experimenting with other oils to see what kind of mood they contribute to.

CALMING SCENT

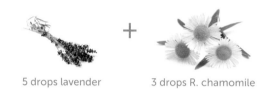

5 drops lavender   3 drops R. chamomile

FLOWERS APLENTY

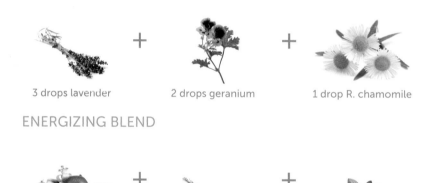

3 drops lavender   2 drops geranium   1 drop R. chamomile

ENERGIZING BLEND

3 drops orange   1 drop rosemary   4 drops peppermint

REFRESHING BLEND

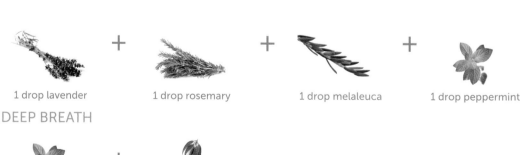

1 drop lavender   1 drop rosemary   1 drop melaleuca   1 drop peppermint

DEEP BREATH

3 drops peppermint   3 drops eucalyptus

RELAXING BREATH

 +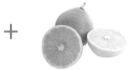

3 drops lavender   3 drops bergamot

CITRUS SPICE

 + 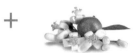 + +

3 drops lemon   4 drops orange   2 drops grapefruit   1 drop clove

STRESS LESS

 + + 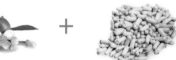 +

2 drops lemon   2 drops orange   2 drops clove   2 drops cedarwood

SPRINGTIME BLISS

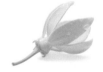 + +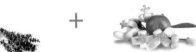

1 drop ylang ylang   2 drops lavender   5 drops orange

HOLIDAY GLOW

 + 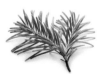 +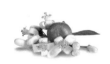

3 drops cinnamon   7 drops white fir   5 drops orange

WINTER WONDERLAND

 + +

1 drop frankincense   2 drops orange   1 drop peppermint

Clove	Use as an analgesic (for topical pain relief) and a drawing salve (to pull toxins/infection from the body). Good for acne, constipation, headaches, nausea, and toothaches.
Frankincense	Enhances effect of any other oil. It facilitates clarity of mind, accelerates all skin recovery issues, and reduces anxiety and mental and physical fatigue. Reduces hyperactivity, impatience, irritability, and restlessness. Helps with focus and concentration.
Lavender	Use for agitation, bruises, burns (can mix with melaleuca), leg cramps, herpes, heart irregularities, hives, insect bites, neuropathy, pain (inside and out), bee stings, sprains, sunburn (combine with frankincense), and sunstroke. Relieves insomnia, depression, and PMS and is a natural antihistamine (asthma or allergies).
Lemon	Use for arthritis, colds, constipation, coughs, cuts, sluggishness, sore throats, sunburn, and wounds. It lifts the spirits and reduces stress and fatigue. Internally it counteracts acidity, calms an upset stomach, and encourages elimination.
Lemongrass	Use for sore and cramping muscles and charley horses (with peppermint; drink lots of water). Apply to bottoms of feet in winter to warm them.
Melaleuca	Use for bug bites, colds, coughs, cuts, body odor, eczema, fungus, infections (ear, nose, or throat), microbes (internally), psoriasis, rough hands, slivers (combine with clove to draw them out), sore throats, and wounds.
Oregano	Use as heavy-duty antibiotic (internally with olive oil or coconut oil in capsules or topically on bottoms of feet—follow up with lavender and peppermint). Also for fungal infections and for reducing pain and inflammation of arthritis, backache, bursitis, carpal tunnel syndrome, rheumatism, and sciatica. Always dilute.
Peppermint	Use as an analgesic (for topical pain relief, bumps, and bruises). Can also be used for circulation, fever, headache, indigestion, motion sickness, nausea, nerve problems, or vomiting.

Purify	Use for airborne pathogens, cuts, germs (on any surface), insect bites, itches (all types and varieties), and wounds. Also boosts the immune system.
DigestZen	Use for all digestion issues such as bloating, congestion, constipation, diarrhea, food poisoning (internal), heartburn, indigestion, motion sickness, nausea, and stomachache. Also works well on diaper rash.
AromaTouch	Use for relaxation and stress relief. It is soothing and anti-inflammatory and enhances massage.
On Guard	Use to disinfect all surfaces. It eliminates mold and viruses and helps to boost the immune system (bottoms of feet or internally; use daily).
TerraShield	Deters all flying insects and ticks from human bodies and pets.
Breathe	Use for allergies, anxiety, asthma, bronchitis, congestion, colds, coughs, flu, and respiratory distress.
Deep Blue	Use for pain relief. Works well in cases of arthritis, bruises, carpal tunnel, headaches, inflammation, joint pain, migraines, muscle pain, sprains, and rheumatism. Follow with peppermint to enhance effects.

Essential oils are great for adding flavor or spice to your favorite meal. Essential oils can impart the natural, fresh taste of fresh herbs and spices but are more concentrated and can easily be used year-round when fresh herbs are not available. Essential oils are also a great substitute for dried or powdered spices, since dried spices have lost many of the liquid essential oils that impart much of the flavor and aroma found in the natural plant. Additionally, while many commercially available flavoring extracts use artificial flavors or are diluted in alcohol or propylene glycol, essential oils provide a concentrated, pure flavor that is extracted naturally from the plant.

Many great essential oil cookbooks are available that can help you get started using essential oils in cooking. But it is fairly easy (and a lot of fun) to substitute essential oils into your own favorite recipes in place of spices, flavoring extracts, and fresh or dried herbs.

Essential Oils Commonly Used in Cooking

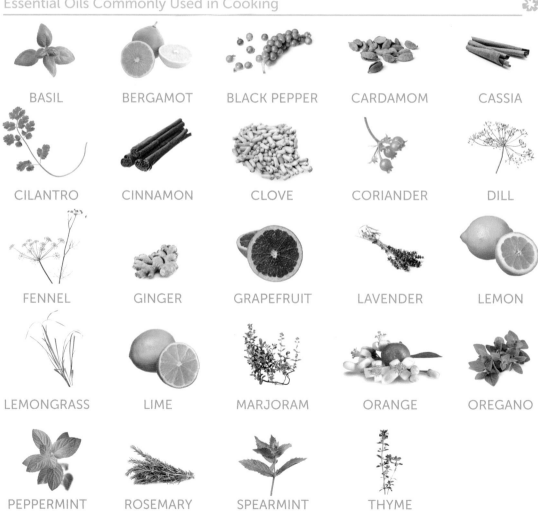

BASIL	BERGAMOT	BLACK PEPPER	CARDAMOM	CASSIA
CILANTRO	CINNAMON	CLOVE	CORIANDER	DILL
FENNEL	GINGER	GRAPEFRUIT	LAVENDER	LEMON
LEMONGRASS	LIME	MARJORAM	ORANGE	OREGANO
PEPPERMINT	ROSEMARY	SPEARMINT	THYME	

1. Know what part of the plant the oil came from. Citrus oils are pressed from the peel, so they can substitute for the zest but not the juice.

2. Getting the exact amount of oil drops can be tricky due to the different viscosity levels of the oils. If using the regular bottle with the orifice reducer, place your drops on a spoon; then stir into your mixture to ensure you have the right amount.

3. Putting your cooking oils in dropper bottles allows you to easily control the number of drops used and provides sufficient space to dip a toothpick into the oil when needed.

4. A little goes a long way. Start with only a drop of oil, taste, and repeat until you are satisfied with the flavor. Some oils are really strong, and a toothpick dipped in the oil, then stirred into your mixture, may be sufficient.

5. Use glass or stainless steel mixing bowls. Try to avoid plastic cookware, as the oils can damage certain types of plastic.

6. Always keep your oils away from heat, light, and humid conditions to maintain a long shelf life. Refrigerator storage is fine.

7. Make sure to recap your bottles so the oils don't evaporate out.

8. Because oils are altered by heat and may evaporate, it is always best to add the oils at the end of cooking if possible.

9. Give a subtle hint of herbs to your savory baked goods by creating a spray in a 4 oz. glass trigger spray bottle. Add a few drops of essential oil and 2 Tbs. (25 ml) of olive oil to the spray bottle, and then fill the bottle the rest of the way with distilled water. Use this mixture to spray items like empanadas, tortilla chips, baked french fries, egg rolls, etc.

10. If you are cooking with kids, make sure to keep the oils out of their reach.

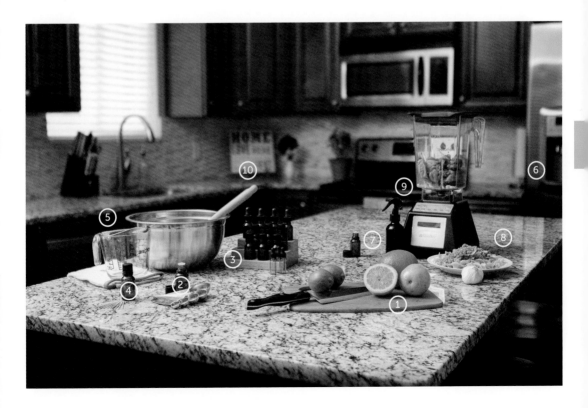

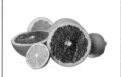

Typically, 1 drop of a citrus oil can substitute for 1 tsp. (2 g) of citrus zest. If the recipe calls for the zest from 1 citrus fruit, you can use 3–10 drops of the citrus essential oil instead.

For minty oils such as peppermint and spearmint, try substituting 1 drop of essential oil for 1 tsp. (500 mg) dried mint leaves or 1 Tbs. (3 g) fresh mint leaves.

Cinnamon and cassia are pretty similar, and typically what we know as ground cinnamon is really ground cassia; however, the strength of their flavor is quite a bit different. You will want to start by substituting 1 drop of cinnamon for 1–2 Tbs. (8–15 g) ground cinnamon and 1 drop of cassia for 1 tsp. (2 g) ground cinnamon or cassia.

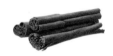

For herbaceous oils like basil, marjoram, oregano, rosemary, cilantro, dill, etc., start with a toothpick dipped in the oil and stirred into the mixture, and then add more to taste as needed.

Floral herbs like lavender can be used in cooking; but because floral flavors are uncommon, you want just a hint of this flavor. Start with a toothpick, and add more if needed.

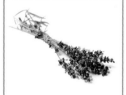

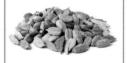

For other flavors, a good rule of thumb is to substitute 1 drop of oil for 1–2 tsp. (500 mg–1 g) of dried spice or herb and 1 drop of oil for 1–2 Tbs. (3–5 g) of fresh herb. If you think the oil is strong or if the recipe calls for less than the above quantities, start with a toothpick dip instead. Taste, and add more if needed.

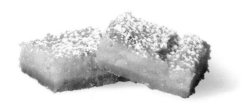

Luscious Lemon Bars

2 c. (240 g) flour	1 t. (4 g) baking powder
½ c. (100 g) sugar	Dash of salt
1 c. (225 g) butter	½ c. (125 ml) water
¼ t. (2 g) salt	½ c. (125 ml) lemon juice
4 eggs	3 drops lemon EO
6 T. (45 g) flour	1 T. (8 g) powdered sugar
1½ c. (300 g) sugar	Lemon zest (optional)

Preheat oven to 350° F. Mix together flour, sugar, and salt. Cut in the butter until the dough reaches a fine crumb consistency. Press the dough into the bottom of a 9" × 13" pan. Bake for 20 minutes till golden. While crust is baking, beat eggs in a large mixing bowl. In a separate dish, stir together flour, sugar, baking powder, and salt. Add flour mixture to eggs, and stir till smooth. Gradually stir in lemon juice, water, and lemon oil. Pour mixture over baked crust, and return to the oven. Bake 30 minutes or until set. Allow to cool completely, and sift powdered sugar over the top. Garnish with zest if desired. *Substitute orange oil and orange juice to make orange bars.

Rosemary Roasted Red Potatoes

16–24 red potatoes, washed and dried
½–¾ c. (125–175 ml) all-natural ranch dressing
1 drop ea. rosemary and oregano essential oils
2 T. (20 g) garlic powder
1–2 t. (2–5 g) smoked paprika
Sea salt and black pepper to taste

Preheat oven to 450° F. Dice potatoes into 1" pieces, and place in 9" × 13" pan. Blend essential oils with ranch dressing, and toss with potatoes to coat. Sprinkle potato mixture with garlic, paprika, salt, and pepper. Cover with aluminum foil, and bake for 25–40 minutes. Remove foil, stir potatoes, and bake uncovered for 15–20 minutes, stirring once more, until golden.

Basil Pesto Chicken

2 t. (10 ml) olive oil	2 garlic cloves, minced
¼ c. (50 ml) olive oil	2 c. (60 g) spinach leaves
¼ c. (35 g) pine nuts	2 T. (25 ml) lemon juice
2 drops lemon EO	1 drop basil EO
⅓ c. (25 g) parmesan cheese	
Salt and pepper to taste	
2–3 chicken breasts, cooked and sliced	

Sauté garlic cloves in 2 tsp. (10 ml) olive oil for 2 minutes. Blend together spinach, pine nuts, sautéed garlic, ¼ cup (50 ml) olive oil, lemon juice, and essential oils in a blender, pulsing and scraping the sides as needed. Add parmesan cheese, salt, and pepper, and blend in. Serve over chicken and your choice of cooked pasta.

Strawberry Citrus Breakfast Ice Cream*

¼ ripe avocado
1 c. (150 g) frozen strawberries
2 T. (25 ml) plain yogurt
1 T. (15 ml) honey or agave
1 drop ea. orange and lime essential oils

Place all ingredients minus oils into a food processor, and purée on high. Remove from food processor, and stir in oils. Serve immediately. *Prepare the night before and freeze in ice-pop molds for a quick, on-the-go breakfast.

Creamy, Creamless, Raw Tomato Soup*

6 ripe tomatoes, seeded and chopped
½ c. (125 ml) water
1 t. minced garlic (1 clove)
½ t. (1 g) onion powder
1 t. (5 g) sea salt
1 ripe avocado, chopped
2 T. (25 ml) extra virgin olive oil
2 drops basil essential oil

Place tomatoes, water, garlic, onion powder, and salt in blender, and blend until smooth. Add the avocado and olive oil, and blend again until smooth. Pour soup into a ceramic or wooden bowl, and add basil oil, stirring to combine. Serve immediately. For a chilled soup, refrigerate for 2 hours. For warm soup, heat over stove.

Appendix and References

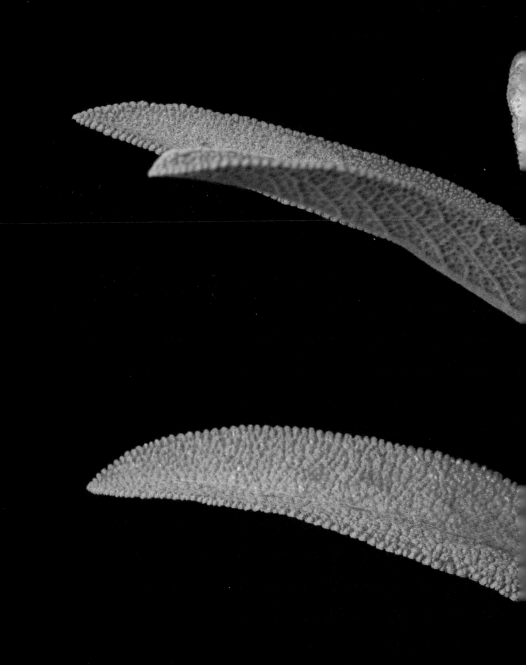

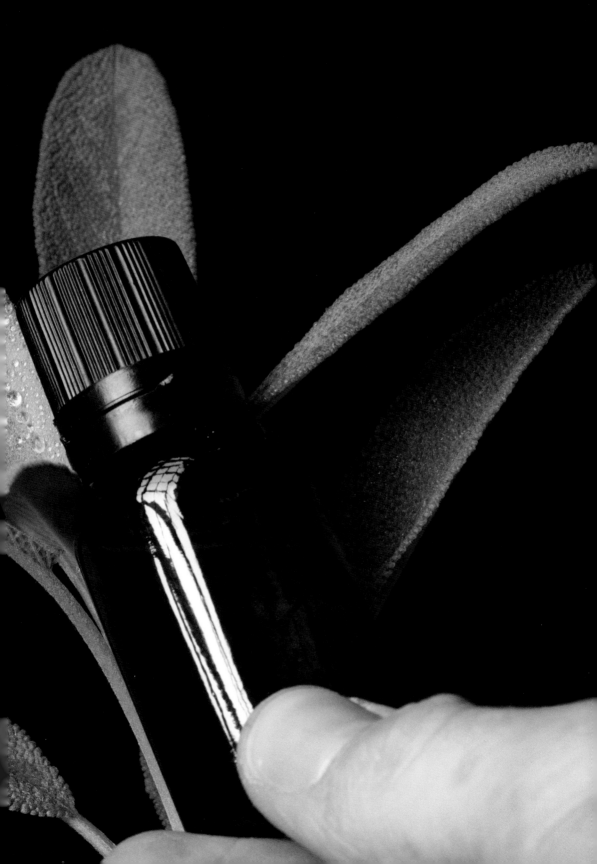

Appendix A: Body Systems Chart

The following chart lists the oils and products discussed within this book and indicates which body systems they primarily affect. While this chart does not include every system that could possibly be affected by each formulation, it attempts to list the primary systems that are most often affected. It is provided to give the beginning aromatherapy student a starting point for personal use and analysis.

Product Name	Cardiovascular System	Digestive System	Emotional Balance	Hormonal System	Immune System	Muscles and Skeletal System	Nervous System	Respiratory System	Skin and Hair
A2z Chewable	•	•		•	•	•	•	•	•
Alpha CRS+	•				•	•	•	•	•
Arborvitae			•					•	•
AromaTouch			•	•	•	•	•		
Balance			•			•	•		•
Basil	•					•			
Bergamot		•	•						•
Birch						•			
Black Pepper		•					•		
Blue Tansy							•		
Bone Nutrient Lifetime Complex			•			•	•		•
Brave			•				•		
Breathe								•	
Calmer			•				•		
Cardamom		•						•	
Cassia					•				
Cedarwood							•	•	
Cheer			•						
Cilantro		•	•						
Cinnamon Bark					•				
Citrus Bliss			•		•		•		
ClaryCalm			•	•					•
Clary Sage				•					
Clove	•	•			•			•	
Console			•						
Copaiba	•	•	•		•	•			•
Coriander		•		•					
Cypress	•					•			
DDR Prime	•				•	•		•	
Deep Blue						•	•		
DigestZen		•							
Dill	•	•							
Douglas Fir						•		•	

Product Name	Cardiovascular System	Digestive System	Emotional Balance	Hormonal System	Immune System	Muscles and Skeletal System	Nervous System	Respiratory System	Skin and Hair
Elevation			•	•					
Eucalyptus								•	•
Fennel		•		•					
Forgive			•						
Frankincense			•		•		•		•
Geranium			•						•
Ginger		•					•		
Grapefruit	•								
Green Mandarin		•	•		•				•
GX Assist		•			•				
HD Clear					•				•
Helichrysum	•					•			
Hinoki			•		•			•	•
InTune			•	•	•		•		
IQ Mega	•	•			•		•		•
Jasmine			•	•					
Juniper Berry		•	•				•		•
Lavender	•		•				•		•
Lemon		•			•			•	
Lemon Myrtle					•	•		•	
Lemongrass					•	•			
Lime		•			•			•	
Litsea		•			•			•	
Magnolia				•	•				•
Manuka						•		•	•
Marjoram	•					•			
Melaleuca					•	•		•	•
Melissa			•						•
Microplex MVp	•	•	•	•	•	•	•	•	•
Mito2Max	•			•		•	•		
Motivate			•						
Myrrh				•	•		•		•
Neroli		•	•						•
On Guard					•				•
Orange		•	•		•				•
Oregano					•	•		•	
Passion			•						
PastTense						•	•		
Patchouli									•

Appendix A: Body Systems Chart *(continued)*

Product Name	Cardiovascular System	Digestive System	Emotional Balance	Hormonal System	Immune System	Muscles and Skeletal System	Nervous System	Respiratory System	Skin and Hair
Peace			●						
Peppermint		●				●	●	●	●
Petitgrain			●		●				
Phytoestrogen Lifetime Complex			●	●		●			●
Pink Pepper					●			●	●
Purify		●	●		●				●
Rescuer						●	●		
Roman Chamomile			●				●		●
Rose			●						●
Rosemary					●		●	●	
Sandalwood			●			●	●		●
Serenity							●		
Siberian Fir						●		●	
Slim & Sassy		●	●						
Slim & Sassy TrimShake and V Shake		●		●		●			
Spearmint		●	●						
Spikenard			●						●
Star Anise	●	●		●				●	
Steady			●				●		
Stronger					●				●
TerraShield									●
Terrazyme		●							
Thinker			●				●		
Thyme					●	●			
Turmeric		●			●				●
Vetiver			●	●			●		●
Whisper			●	●			●		
White Fir								●	
Wintergreen						●			
xEO Mega	●	●			●				●
Yarrow				●	●				●
Yarrow Pom	●		●	●	●		●		●
Ylang Ylang	●		●	●					
Yoga Blends			●	●			●		
Yuzu		●			●				●
Zendocrine		●		●	●			●	●

Appendix B: Single Essential Oils Property Chart

The following chart presents some of the properties of each of the single oils. An attempt has been made to indicate the effectiveness of the oils for each property, where supporting information existed. However, this information should not be considered conclusive. It is provided to give the beginning aromatherapy student a starting point for personal use and analysis. Also, keep in mind the applicable safety data when applying an oil for its property. For example, cinnamon bark is one of the best known antiseptics, but it is also extremely irritating to the skin. It may work well to sanitize the bathroom with, but it should be used with extreme caution on the skin.

Properties of Essential Oils

Antibacterial: an agent that prevents the growth of (or destroys) bacteria.

Anticatarrhal: an agent that helps remove excess catarrh from the body. Expectorants help promote the removal of mucus from the respiratory system.

Antidepressant: an agent that helps alleviate depression.

Antifungal: an agent that prevents and combats fungal infection.

Anti-infectious: an agent that prevents and combats the spread of germs.

Anti-inflammatory: an agent that alleviates inflammation.

Antimicrobial: an agent that resists or destroys pathogenic microorganisms.

Antiparasitic: an agent that prevents and destroys parasites.

Antirheumatic: an agent that helps prevent and relieve rheumatism.

Antiseptic: an agent that destroys and prevents the development of microbes.

Antispasmodic: an agent that prevents and eases spasms or convulsions.

Antiviral: a substance that inhibits the growth of a virus.

Analgesic: a substance that relieves pain.

Immune-stimulant: an agent that stimulates the natural defense mechanism of the body.

Single Oil Name	Antibacterial	Anticatarrhal	Antidepressant	Antifungal	Anti-infectious	Anti-inflammatory	Antimicrobial	Antiparasitic	Antirheumatic	Antiseptic	Antispasmodic	Antiviral	Analgesic	Immune-stimulant
Arborvitae	++			+++	+		++	++		++				
Basil	++	+	+		+	+++				+	+	+		
Bergamot					+	+++		+		+	+		+	
Birch					+			+	+++	+				
Black Pepper	+						+			+	+	+	++	
Blue Tansy	+			++		+	++			+			+	
Cardamom	++				+	++	+			+	+			
Cassia	+		+	+	+	+	++	+		++++	+	+		
Cedarwood					+	+				++				
Cilantro	+				+									
Cinnamon	+		+	+	+	+	++	+		++++	+	+		
Clary Sage	+		+		+					+	+			
Clove	+++	+		++	+			++	+	+		+++		
Copaiba	++					++++				++			++	
Coriander	++		++		++			+			+		+	
Cypress	+				+			+	+	+	+			
Dill	+			+		+					++			
Douglas Fir		+++			+		+			+				
Eucalyptus	++	++			+	+						+++	++	+

Single Oil Name	Antibacterial	Anticatarrhal	Antidepressant	Antifungal	Anti-infectious	Anti-inflammatory	Antimicrobial	Antiparasitic	Antirheumatic	Antiseptic	Antispasmodic	Antiviral	Analgesic	Immune-stimulant
Fennel	+	++				+	+	+		+	+			
Frankincense		++	++		+++	+				+				+++
Geranium	+++		++	++	+	+			+					
Ginger		++								++			++	
Grapefruit	++									++				
Green Mandarin						++	+			+	+			
Helichrysum	++	+++		+		++	++			+	+++			
Hinoki	++			+	+	++				+		+		
Jasmine		+	++				++			+	+	+		
Juniper Berry										++	+	+		
Lavender			++		+	++	+	+	+	+	++		++	
Lemon	++				+		++	+		+++	+			++
Lemon Myrtle	++			+++		+	++						+	
Lemongrass	+		+	+		++	+			+			++	
Lime	++									++		+		
Litsea	++			+			+			+		+		
Magnolia	+					+	+						++	
Manuka	+++	+		++	+		+			+++		+	+	
Marjoram	+	+		+	+					++	++	+	++	
Melissa	+		++				+				++	++		
Melaleuca	+++			++++	+	+		+		+		+++		++
Myrrh		+		+	+	+++	++	+		+		+++		
Neroli	+		++		+			+		++	++	+		
Orange	++		++	+		+				++				
Oregano	+++	+		+++	+++			+++	++	+	+	++	++	++
Patchouli	+		+	+	+	+	+			+		+		
Peppermint	+	+		+	+	++	+			+	+	+	++	
Petitgrain	++				+	+	+			++				
Pink Pepper	++			+		+						+		
Roman Chamomile	+		+		+	+++				+	+		++	
Rose					+									
Rosemary	+++	+		+++	+	+++							+++	
Sandalwood	+	+++	++	+						++	+			
Siberian Fir		+								++		+		
Spearmint	++			+		+				+	+			+
Spikenard	+		++	+		+		+						+
Star Anise				++						+	+			
Thyme	+	+		+++			++	+	++	+		+		++
Turmeric						++	+						+	
Vetiver					+					+	+			+
White Fir		+								++			+	
Wintergreen						+++			+	+	+		+	
Yarrow						+				++				
Ylang Ylang			+		+					+	+			
Yuzu	+													+

Research References

Aalinkeel R et al. (2008 Aug 25). "The dietary bioflavonoid, quercetin, selectively induces apoptosis of prostate cancer cells by down-regulating the expression of heat shock protein 90," Prostate.

Abbasi M N, Abbasi M S, Bekhradi R (2013). "Suppressive effects of rosa damascena essential oil on naloxone-precipitated morphine withdrawal signs in male mice," Iran J Pharm Res. 12(3):357-61.

Abdel-Aal el, S. M., Akhtar, H., Zaheer, K., & Ali, R. (2013 Apr). Dietary sources of lutein and zeaxanthin carotenoids and their role in eye health. Nutrients, 5(4), 1169-1185.

Abdel-Sattar E, Zaitoun AA, Farag MA, El Gayed SH, Harraz FM (2009 Feb 25). "Chemical composition, insecticidal and insect repellent activity of Schinus molle L. leaf and fruit essential oils against Trogoderma granarium and Tribolium castaneum," Nat Prod Res. Epub ahead of print: 1-10.

Abdullah, D., Ping, Q. N., & Liu, G. J. (1996 Jan). Enhancing effect of essential oils on the penetration of 5-fluorouracil through rat skin. Yao Xue Xue Bao, 31(3), 214-221.

Abebe, W. (2002). Herbal medication: potential for adverse interactions with analgesic drugs. Journal of Clinical Pharmacy and Therapeutics, 27(6), 391-401.

Abedon, B (2008). "Essentra - a patented extract that reduces stress and enhances sleep," (http://www.nutragenesisnutrition.com/images/stories/pdf/ess_stress_wp.pdf):1-4.

Abenavoli L, Capasso R, Milic N, Capasso F (2010 Jun 7). "Milk thistle in liver diseases: past, present, future," Phytother Res. Epub ahead of print.

Adam B, Liebregts T, Best J, Bechmann L, Lackner C, Neumann J, Koehler S, Holtmann G (2006 Feb). "A combination of peppermint oil and caraway oil attenuates the post-inflammatory visceral hyperalgesia in a rat model," Scand J Gastroenterol. 41(2):155-60.

Adib-Hajbaghery M, Mousavi SN (2017 Dec). "The effects of chamomile extract on sleep quality among elderly people: A clinical trial," Complement Ther Med. 35:109-114.

Agero A.L.C., Verallo-Rowell V.M (2004 Sep). "A randomized double-blind controlled trial comparing extra virgin coconut oil with mineral oil as a moisturizer for mild to moderate xerosis," Dermatitis. 15(3):109-116.

Agrawal, P., Rai, V., & Singh, R. B. (1996 Sep). Randomized placebo-controlled, single blind trial of holy basil leaves in patients with noninsulin-dependent diabetes mellitus. Int J Clin Pharmacol Ther, 34(9), 406-409.

Ahmad A, Khan A, Kah L.A., Manzoor N (2012 Oct). "In vitro synergy of eugenol and methyleugenol with fluconazole against clinical Candida isolates," J. Med. Microbiol. 59(10):1178-1184.

Ahmad S, Beg Z.H. (2013 Jun). "Hypolipidemic and antioxidant activities of thymoquinone and limonene in atherogenic suspension fed rats," Food Chem. 138(2-3):1116-1124.

Ahmed H.H., Abd-Rabou A.A., Hassan A.Z., "Phytochemical Analysis and Anticancer Investigation of Bswellia serrata Bioactive Constituents In Vitro," Asian Pac. J. Cancer Prev. 16(16):7179-7188.

Akha, O., Rabiei, K., Kashi, Z., Bahar, A., Zaeif-Khorasani, E., Kosaryan, M., . . . Emadian, O. (2014). The effect of fennel (Foeniculum vulgare) gel 3% in decreasing hair thickness in idiopathic mild to moderate hirsutism, A randomized placebo controlled clinical trial. Caspian J Intern Med, 5(1), 26-29.

Akhondzadeh S, Naghavi HR, Vazirian M, Shayeganpour A, Rashidi H, Khani M (2001 Oct). "Passionflower in the treatment of generalized anxiety: a pilot double-blind randomized controlled trial with oxazepam," J Clin Pharm Ther. 26(5):363-7.

Akhtar, S., Ismail, T., & Riaz, M. (2013). Flaxseed - a miraculous defense against some critical maladies. Pak J Pharm Sci, 26(1), 199-208.

Al-Ali, K. H., El-Beshbishy, H. A., El-Badry, A. A., & Alkhalaf, M. (2013 Dec). Cytotoxic activity of methanolic extract of Mentha longifolia and Ocimum basilicum against human breast cancer. Pak J Biol Sci, 16(23), 1744-1750.

Alam, P., Ansari, M.J., Anwer, M.K., Raish, M. Kamal, Y.K., & Shakeel, F. (2017 May). "Wound healing effects of nanoemulsion containing clove essential oil," Artif Cells Nanomed Biotechnol. 45(3):591-597.

Al-Anati L, Essid E, Reinehr R, Petzinger E (2009 Apr). "Silibinin protects OTA-mediated TNF-alpha release from perfused rat livers and isolated rat Kupffer cells," Mol Nutr Food Res. 53(4):460-6.

al-Bagieh N.H., Idowu A, Salako N.O. (1994). "Effect of aqueous extract of miswak on the in vitro growth of Candida albicans," Microbios. 80(323):107-113.

Alberti, T.B., Barbosa, W. L.R., Vieira, J.L.F., Raposo, N.R.B., & Dutra, R.C. (2017). "(-)-β-Caryophyllene, a CB2 Receptor-Selective Phytocannabinoid, Suppresses Motor Paralysis and Neuroinflammation in a Murine Model of Multiple Sclerosis," Int J Mol Sci. 18(4):691.

Alberts, B., Bray, D., Hopkin, K., Johnson, A., Lewis, J., Raff, M., . . . Walter, P. (2013). Essential cell biology. New York, NY: Garland Science.

Albertsson, P. A., Kohnke, R., Emek, S. C., Mei, J., Rehfeld, J. F., Akerlund, H. E., & Erlanson-Albertsson, C. (2007 Feb 1). Chloroplast membranes retard fat digestion and induce satiety: effect of biological membranes on pancreatic lipase/co-lipase. Biochem J, 401(3), 727-733.

Alexandrovich I, Rakovitskaya O, Kolmo E, Sidorova T, Shushunov S (2003 Jul-Aug). "The effect of fennel (Foeniculum Vulgare) seed oil emulsion in infantile colic: a randomized, placebo-controlled study," Altern Ther Health Med. 9(4):58-61.

Alfthan G, Tapani K, Nissinen K, et al. (2004). "The effect of low doses of betaine on plasma homocysteine in healthy volunteers," Br J Nutr. 92:665-669.

al-Hader AA, Hasan ZA, Aqel MB (1994 Jul 22). "Hyperglycemic and insulin release inhibitory effects of Rosmarinus officinalis," J Ethnopharmacol. 43(3):217-21.

Al-Harrasi A. et al (2014 Sep). "Analgesic effects of crude extracts and fractions of Omani frankincense obtained from traditional medicinal plant Boswellia sacra on animal models," Asian Pac J Trop Med. 7S1:S485-49

Al-Howiriny, T., Alsheikh, A., Alqasoumi, S., Al-Yahya, M., ElTahir, K., & Rafatullah, S. (2009 Aug). Protective Effect of Origanum majorana L. 'Marjoram' on various models of gastric mucosal injury in rats. Am J Chin Med, 37(3), 531-545.

Ali, S. A., Rizk, M. Z., Ibrahim, N. A., Abdallah, M. S., Sharara, H. M., & Moustafa, M. M. (2010 Dec). Protective role of Juniperus phoenicea and Cupressus sempervirens against CCl(4). World J Gastrointest Pharmacol Ther, 1(6), 123-131.

Allman-Farinelli, M. A., Gomes, K., Favaloro, E. J., & Petocz, P. (2005 Jul 29). A diet rich in high-oleic-acid sunflower oil favorably alters low-density lipoprotein cholesterol, triglycerides, and factor VII coagulant activity. J Am Diet Assoc, 105(7), 1071-1079.

Almas K., Al-Zeid Z (2004 Feb 6). "The immediate antimicrobial effect of a toothbrush and miswak on cariogenic bacteria: a clinical study," J. Contemp. Dent. Pract. 5(1):105-114.

Almela L, Sánchez-Muñoz B, Fernández-López JA, Roca MJ, Rabe V (2006 Jul). "Liquid chromatograpic-mass spectrometric analysis of phenolics and free radical scavenging activity of rosemary extract from different raw material," J Chromatogr A. 1120(1-2):221-9.

Aloisi AM, Ceccarelli I, Masi F, Scaramuzzino A (2002 Oct 17). "Effects of the essential oil from citrus lemon in male and female rats exposed to a persistent painful stimulation," Behav Brain Res. 136(1):127-35.

Alqareer A, Alyahya A, Andersson L (2006 Nov). "The effect of clove and benzocaine versus placebo as topical anesthetics," J Dent. 34(10):747-50.

Al-Saidi S, Rameshkumar K.B., Hisham A, Sivakumar N, Al-Kind (2012 Mar). "Composition and antibacterial activity of the essential oils of four commercial grades of Omani frankincense from the oleo-gum resin of Boswellia sacra FLUECK," Chem. Biodivers. 9(3):615-624.

Al-Snafi, A.E. (2015). "The Pharmacological importance of Bellis perennis - A review," Int J Phytotherapy. 5(2):63-69.

al-Zuhair H, el-Sayeh B, Ameen HA, al-Shoora H (1996 Jul-Aug). "Pharmacological studies of cardamom oil in animals," Pharmacol Res. 34(1-2):79-82.

Amano S, Akutsu N, Ogura Y, Nishiyama T (2004 Nov). "Increase of laminin 5 synthesis in human keratinocytes by acute wound fluid, inflammatory cytokines and growth factors, and lysophospholipids," Br J Dermatol. 151(5):961-70.

Amantea D, Fratto V, Maida S, Rotiroti D, Ragusa S, Nappi G, Bagetta G, Corasaniti MT (2009). "Prevention of Glutamate Accumulation and Upregulation of Phospho-Akt may Account for Neuroprotection Afforded by Bergamot Essential Oil against Brain Injury Induced by Focal Cerebral Ischemia in Rat," Int Rev Neurobiol. 85:389-405.

Ambrosone CB, McCann SE, Freudenheim JL, Marshall JR, Zhang Y, Shields PG (2004 May). "Breast cancer risk in premenopausal women is inversely associated with consumption of broccoli, a source of isothiocyanates, but is not modified by GST genotype," J Nutr. 134(5):1134-8.

American Cancer Society (2008). "Cancer Facts and Figures." Downloaded at http://www.cancer.org/downloads/STT/2008CAFFfinalsecured.pdf.

Amine, E., Baba, N., Belhadj, M., Deurenberg-Yap, M., Djazayery, A., Forrester, T., ... & Yoshiike, N. (2002). Diet, nutrition and the prevention of chronic diseases: Report of a Joint WHO/FAO Expert Consultation. World Health Organization.

Ammar, A.H., Bouajila, J., Lebrihi, A., Mathieu, F., Romdhane, M., Za-grouba, F. (2012). "Chemical composition and in vitro antimicrobial and antioxidant activities of Citrus aurantium l. flowers essential oil (Neroli oil)," Pak J Biol Sci. 15(21):1034-40.

Ammon HP (2002). "Boswellic acids (components of frankincense) as the active principle in treatment of chronic inflammatory diseases," Wien Med Wochenschr. 152(15-16):373-8.

Amoian B, Moghadamnia A.A., Barzi S, Sheykholeslami S, Rangiani A (2010 Aug). "Salvadora Persica extract chewing gum and gingival health: Improve-ment of gingival and probebleeding index," Complement. Ther. Clin. Pract. 16(3):121-123.

An, R., Chiu, C. Y., Zhang, Z., & Burd, N. A. (2014). Nutrient intake among US adults with disabilities. Journal of Human Nutrition and Dietetics.

Anderson, J. W., Weiter, K. M., Christian, A. L., Ritchey, M. B., & Bays, H. E. (2014 Jan 1). Raisins compared with other snack effects on glycemia and blood pressure: a randomized, controlled trial. Postgrad Med, 126(1), 37-43.

Anderson KJ, Teuber SS, Gobeille A, Cremin P, Waterhouse AL, Steinberg FM (2001 Nov). "Walnut polyphenolics inhibit in vitro human plasma and LDL oxidation," J Nutr. 131(11):2837-42.

Ando Y (1994 Aug). "[Breeding control and immobilizing effects of wood microingredients on house dust mites]," Nihon Koshu Eisei Zasshi. 41(8):741-50.

Andradea, E. H. A., Alves, C. N., Guimarães, E. F., Carreira, L. M. M., & Maia, J. G. S. (2011 Sep). Variability in essential oil composition of Piper dilatatum L.C. Rich. Biochemical Systematics and Ecology, 39, 669-675.

Andrews R.E., Parks L.W., Spence K.D. (1980) Some Effects of Douglas Fir Terpenes on Certain Microorganisms. Applied and Environmental Microbiology. 40: 301-304.

Andrian E., Grenier D., Rouabhia M. (2006) Porphyromonas gingivalis-Ep-ithelial Cell Interactions in Periodontitis. Journal of Dental Research. 85: 392-403.

Antimutagenic effects of extracts from sage (Salvia officinalis) in mammalian system in vivo. (2006 Jul 19). "Relaxant effects of Rosa damascena on guinea pig tracheal chains and its possible mechanism(s)," J Ethnopharmacol. 106(3):377-82.

Apay S.E., Arslan S, Akpinar R.B., Celebioglu A (2012 Dec). "Effect of aromatherapy massage on dysmenorrhea in Turkish students," Pain Manag. Nurs. Off. J. Am. Soc. Pain Manag. Nurses. 13(4): 236-240.

Appendino G, Ottino M, Marquez N, Bianchi F, Giana A, Ballero M, Sterner O, Fiebich BL, Munoz E (2007 Apr). "Arzanol, an anti-inflammatory and anti-HIV-1 phloroglucinol alpha-Pyrone from Helichrysum italicum ssp. microphyllum," J Nat Prod. 70(4):608-12.

Aqel MB (1991 May-Jun). "Relaxant effect of the volatile oil of Rosmarinus officinalis on tracheal smooth muscle," J Ethnopharmacol. 33(1-2):57-62.

Arasada BL, Bommareddy A, Zhang X, Bremmon K, Dwivedi C. (2008 Jan-Feb). "Effects of alpha-santalol on proapoptotic caspases and p53 expression in UVB irradiated mouse skin," Anticancer Res. 28(1A):129-32.

Arash, A., Mohammad, M. Z., Jamal, M. S., Mohammad, T. A., & Azam, A. (2013 Oct). Effects of the Aqueous Extract of Anethum graveolens Leaves on Seizure Induced by Pentylenetetrazole in Mice. Malays J Med Sci, 20(5), 23-30.

Archana R, Namasivayam A (1999 Jan). "Antistressor effect of Withania somnifera," J Ethnopharmacol. 64(1):91-3.

Arima, Y., Nakai, Y., Hayakawa, R., & Nishino, T. (2003 Jan). Antibacterial effect of beta-thujaplicin on staphylococci isolated from atopic dermatitis: relationship between changes in the number of viable bacterial cells and clinical improvement in an eczematous lesion of atopic dermatitis. J Antimi-crob Chemother, 51(1), 113-122.

Arunakul M, Thaweboon B, Thaweboon S, Asvanund Y, Charoenchaikorn K (2011 Dec). "Efficacy of xylitol and fluoride mouthrinses on salivary Mutans streptococci," Asian Pac. J. Trop. Biomed. 1(6):488-490.

Arzi A, Sela L, Green A, Givaty G, Dagan Y, Sobel N (2010 Jan). "The influence of odorants on respiratory patterns in sleep," Chem. Senses. 35(1):31-40.

Asakura, K., Matsuo, Y., Oshima, T., Kihara, T., Minagawa, K., Araki, Y., . . . Ninomiya, M. (2000 Apr). omega-agatoxin IVA-sensitive Ca(2+) channel blocker, alpha-eudesmol, protects against brain injury after focal ischemia in rats. Eur J Pharmacol, 394(1), 57-65.

Asao T, Kuwano H, Ide M, Hirayama I, Nakamura JI, Fujita KI, Horiuti R (2003 Apr). "Spasmolytic effect of peppermint oil in barium during double-contrast barium enema compared with Buscopan," Clin Radiol. 58(4):301-5.

Asensio, C. M., Nepote, V., & Grosso, N. R. (2011 Sep). Chemical stability of extra-virgin olive oil added with oregano essential oil. J Food Sci, 76(7), S445-450.

Asnaashari, S., Delazar, A., Habibi, B., Vasfi, R., Nahar, L., Hamedeyazdan, S., & Sarker, S. D. (2010 Dec). Essential oil from Citrus aurantifolia

prevents ketotifen-induced weight-gain in mice. Phytother Res, 24(12), 1893-1897.

Astani A, Reichling J, Schnitzler P (2011). "Screening for antiviral activities of isolated compounds from essential oils," Evid.-Based Complement. Altern. Med. ECAM. 2011:253643.

Atsumi T, Tonosaki K (2007 Feb). "Smelling lavender and rosemary increases free radical scavenging activity and decreases cortisol level in saliva," Psychi-atry Res. 150(1):89-96.

Auffray, B. (2007 Feb). Protection against singlet oxygen, the main actor of se-bum squalene peroxidation during sun exposure, using Commiphora myrrha essential oil. Int J Cosmet Sci, 29(1), 23-29.

Australia Rural Industries Research and Development Corporation. (n.d.). Essential Oils and Plant Extracts. Retrieved Sept. 29, 2014 from http://www.rirdc.gov.au/research-programs/plant-industries/essential-oils-and-plant-extracts.

Awale, S., Tohda, C., Tezuka, Y., Miyazaki, M., & Kadota, S. (2011). Protec-tive Effects of Rosa damascena and Its Active Constituent on Abeta(25-35)-Induced Neuritic Atrophy. Evid Based Complement Alternat Med, 2011, 1-8.

Azanchi, T., Shafaroodi, H., and Asgarpanah, J. (2014). "Anticonvulsant activity of Citrus aurantium blossom essential oil (neroli): involvment of the GABAergic system," Nat Prod Commun. 9(11):1615-8.

Baba, T., Nakano, H., Tamai, K., Sawamura, D., Hanada, K., Hashimoto, I., & Arima, Y. (1998 Jan). Inhibitory effect of beta-thujaplicin on ultraviolet B-induced apoptosis in mouse keratinocytes. J Invest Dermatol, 110(1), 24-28.

Babu, K. G., Singh, B., Joshi, V. P., & Singh, V. (2002). Essential oil com-position of Damask rose (Rosa damascena Mill.) distilled under different pressures and temperatures. Flavour and Fragrance Journal, 17(2), 136-140.

Badia P, Wesensten N, Lammers W, Culpepper J, Harsh J (1990 Jul). "Responsiveness to olfactory stimuli presented in sleep," Physiol Behav. 48(1):87-90.

Bae GS et al (2012 Oct). "Protective effects of alpha-pinene in mice with ceru-lein-induced acute pancreatitis," Life Sciences. 91(17-18):866-871.

Bagchi D, Hassoun EA, Bagchi M, Stohs SJ (1993 Aug). "Protective effects of antioxidants against endrin-induced hepatic lipid peroxidation, DNA damage, and excretion of urinary lipid metabolites," Free Radic Biol Med. 15(2):217-22.

Bagchi D, Sen CK, Ray SD, Das DK, Bagchi M, Preuss HG, Vinson JA (2003 Feb-Mar). "Molecular mechanisms of cardioprotection by a novel grape seed proanthocyanidin extract," Mutat Res. 523-24:87-97.

Bagg J, Jackson MS, Petrina Sweeney M, Ramage G, Davies AN (2006 May). "Susceptibility to Melaleuca alternifolia (tea tree) oil of yeasts isolated from the mouths of patients with advanced cancer," Oral Oncol. 42(5):487-92.

Bagheri-Nesami M, Espahbodi F, Nikkhah A, Shorofi S.A., Charati J.Y. (2014 Feb). "The effects of lavender aromatherapy on pain following needle insertion into a fistula in hemodialysis patients," Complement. Ther. Clin. Pract. 20(1):1-4.

Bahramikia, S., & Yazdanparast, R. (2009 Aug). Efficacy of different fractions of Anethum graveolens leaves on serum lipoproteins and serum and liver oxidative status in experimentally induced hypercholesterolaemic rat models. Am J Chin Med, 37(4), 685-699.

Bakirel T, Bakirel U, Keleş OU, Ulgen SG, Yardibi H (2008 Feb 28). "In vivo assessment of antidiabetic and antioxidant activities of rosemary (Rosmarinus officinalis) in alloxan-diabetic rabbits," J Ethnopharmacol. 116(1):64-73.

Balazs L, Okolicany J, Ferrebee M, Tolley B, Tigyi G (2001 Feb). "Topical application of the phospholipid growth factor lysophosphatidic acid pro-motes wound healing in vivo," Am J Physiol Regul Integr Comp Physiol. 280(2):R466-72.

Balestrieri, E., Pizzimenti, F., Ferlazzo, A., Giofre, S. V., Iannazzo, D., Piperno, A., . . . Macchi, B. (2011 Mar). Antiviral activity of seed extract from Citrus bergamia towards human retroviruses. Bioorg Med Chem, 19(6), 2084-2089.

Balick, MJ, Cox PA. (1996). Plants, People and Culture: The Science of Ethnobotany. Scientific American Library, New York.

Ballard CG, O'Brien JT, Reichelt K, Perry EK (2002 Jul). "Aromatherapy as a safe and effective treatment for the management of agitation in severe de-mentia: the results of a double-blind, placebo-controlled trial with Melissa," J Clin Psychiatry. 63(7):553-8.

Baldissera MD, Da Silva AS, Oliveira CB, Zimmermann CE, Vaucher RA, Santos RC, Rech VC, Tonin AA, Giongo JL, Mattos CB, Koester L, Santurio JM, Monteiro SG (2013 Apr). "Trypanocidal activity of the essential oils in their conventional and nanoemulsion forms: in vitro tests," Exp Parasitol. 134(3):356-61.

Ballabeni V, Tognolini M, Bertoni S, Bruni R, Guerrini A, Rueda GM, Ba-rocelli E (2007 Jan). "Antiplatelet and antithrombotic activities of essential oil from wild Ocotea quixos (Lam.) Kosterm. (Lauraceae) calices from Amazonian Ecuador," Pharmacol Res. 55(1):23-30.

Ballabeni V, Tognolini M, Giorgio C, Bertoni S, Bruni R, Barocelli E (2009 Oct 13). "Ocotea quixos Lam. essential oil: In vitro and in vivo investigation on its anti-inflammatory properties," Fitoterapia. Epub ahead of print.

Banerjee S, Ecavade A, Rao AR (1993 Feb). "Modulatory influence of sandalwood oil on mouse hepatic glutathione S-transferase activity and acid soluble sulphydryl level," Cancer Lett. 68(2-3):105-9.

Banes-Marshall L, Cawley P, Phillips CA (2001). "In vitro activity of Melaleuca alternifolia (tea tree) oil against bacterial and Candida spp. isolates from clinical specimens," Br J Biomed Sci. 58(3):139-45.

Bani, S., Hasanpour, S., Mousavi, Z., Mostafa Garehbaghi, P., & Gojazadeh, M. (2014 Jan). The Effect of Rosa Damascena Extract on Primary Dysmenorrhea: A Double-blind Cross-over Clinical Trial. Iran Red Crescent Med J, 16(1), 1-6.

Banno N, Akihisa T, Yasukawa K, Tokuda H, Tabata K, Nakamura Y, Nishimura R, Kimura Y, Suzuki T (2006 Sep 19). "Anti-inflammatory activities of the triterpene acids from the resin of Boswellia carteri," J Ethnopharmacol. 107(2):249-53.

Bao L, Yao XS, Tsi D, Yau CC, Chia CS, Nagai H, Kurihara H (2008 Jan 23). "Protective effects of bilberry (Vaccinium myrtillus L.) extract on KbrO3-induced kidney damage in mice," J Agric Food Chem. 56(2):420-5.

Baqui, A. A., Kelley, J. I., Jabra-Rizk, M. A., Depaola, L. G., Falkler, W. A., & Meiller, T. F. (2001 Jul). In vitro effect of oral antiseptics on human immunodeficiency virus-1 and herpes simplex virus type 1. J Clin Periodontol, 28(7), 610-616.

Barak AJ, Beckenlauer HC, Badkhsh S, Tuma DJ (1997). "The effect of betaine in reversing alcoholic steatosis", Alcohol Clin Exp Res. 21(6):1100-1102.

Barceloux D.G. (2009 Jun). "Cinnamon (Cinnamomum Species)," Disease-a-Month. 55(6):327-335.

Barchiesi, F., Silvestri, C., Arzeni, D., Ganzetti, G., Castelletti, S., Simonetti, O., Cirioni, O., Kamysz, W., Kamysz, E., Spreghini, E., Abruzzetti, A., Riva, A., Offidani, A.M., Giacometti, A., and Scalise, G. "In vitro susceptibility of dermatophytes to conventional and alternative antifungal agents," Med. Mycol. 2009;47(3):321–326.

Barker S, Grayhem, Koon J, Perkins J, Whalen A, Raudenbush (2003 Dec). "Improved performance on clerical tasks associated with administration of peppermint odor," Percept. Mot. Skills. 97(3):1007-1010.

Barocelli E et al (2004 Nov). "Antinociceptive and gastroprotective effects of inhaled and orally administered Lavandula hybrida Reverchon 'Grosso' essential oil," Life Sci. 76(2):213-23.

Barthelman M., Chen W., Gensler H.L., Huang C., Dong Z., Bowden G.T. (1998) Inhibitory Effects of Perillyl Alcohol on UVB-induced Murine Skin Cancer and AP-1 Transactivation. Cancer Research. 58: 711-716.

Basholli-Salihu, M., Schuster, R., Hajardi, A., Mulla, D., Viernstein, H., Mustafa, B., & Mueller, M. (2017 Dec.). "Phytochemical composition, anti-inflammatory activity and cytotoxic effects of essential oils from three Pinus spp," Pharm Biol. 55(1):1553-1560.

Bassett IB, Pannowitz DL, Barnetson RS (1990 Oct 15). "A comparative study of tea-tree oil versus benzoylperoxide in the treatment of acne," Med J Aust. 153(8):455-8.

Bastiaens M, Hoefnagel J, Westendorp R, Vermeer BJ, Bouwes Bavinck JN (2004 Jun). "Solar lentigines are strongly related to sun exposure in contrast to ephelides," Pigment Cell Res. 17(3).

Bastos J.F.A., Moreira I.J.A., Ribeiro T.P., Medeiros I.A., Antoniolli A.R., De Sousa D.P., Santos M.R.V. (2009) Hypotensive and Vasorelaxant Effects of Citronellol, a Monoterpene Alcohol, in Rats. Basic & Clinical Pharmacology & Toxicology. 106: 331-337.

Basu A, Lucas EA (2007 Aug). "Mechanisms and effects of green tea on cardiovascular health," Nutr Rev. 65(8 Pt 1):361-75.

Batista LC, Cid YP, De Almeida AP, Prudêncio ER, Riger CJ, De Souza MA, Coumendouros K, Chaves DS (2016 Feb). "In vitro efficacy of essential oils and extracts of Schinus molle L. against Ctenocephalides felis felis," Parasitology. 143(5):627-38.

Bayala B. et al (2014 Mar). "Chemical Composition, Antioxidant, Anti-Inflammatory and Anti-Proliferative Activities of Essential Oils of Plants from Burkina Faso," PLoS ONE. 9(3):92122.

Baylac S (2003). "Inhibition of 5-lipoxygenase by essential oils and other natural fragrant extracts," Int. J. Aromather. 13(2-3):138-142.

Behnam S, Farzaneh M, Ahmadzadeh M, Tehrani AS (2006). "Composition and antifungal activity of essential oils of Mentha piperita and Lavendula angustifolia on post-harvest phytopathogens," Commun Agric Appl Biol Sci. 71(3 Pt B):1321-6.

Belardinelli R, Mucaj A, Lacalaprice F, Solenghi M, Principi F, Tiano L, Littarru GP (2005). "Coenzyme Q10 improves contractility of dysfunctional myocardium in chronic heart failure," Biofactors. 25(1-4):137-45.

Belhamel K, Abderrahim A, Ludwig R (2008). "Chemical composition and antibacterial activity of the essential oil of Schinus molle L. grown in Algeria," Int. J. Essent. Oil Ther. 2(4):175-177.

Benencia F, Courrèges MC (2000 Nov). "In vitro and in vivo activity of eugenol on human herpes virus," Phytother Res. 14(7):495-500.

Benencia, F., & Courreges, M. C. (1999 May). Antiviral activity of sandalwood oil against herpes simplex viruses-1 and -2. Phytomedicine, 6(2), 119-123.

Ben Othman, S., Katsuno, N., Kanamaru, Y., & Yabe, T. (2015). Water-soluble extracts from defatted sesame seed flour show antioxidant activity in vitro. Food Chemistry, 175(0), 306-314

Bemben, Michael G, Massey Benjamin H, Bemben, Debra A, Boileau Richard A, Misner James E (1995 Feb). "Age-related patterns in body composition for men aged 20-79 yr," Med Sci Sports Exerc, 27(2):264-9.

Bendaoud H, Romdhane M, Souchard J.P., Cazaux S, Bouajila J (2010 Aug). "Chemical composition and anticancer and antioxidant activities of Schinus molle L. and Schinus terebinthifolius Raddi berries essential oils," J. Food Sci. 75(6):C466-472.

Benedek B. et al (2008 Jan). "Yarrow (Achillea millefolium L. s.l.): pharmaceutical quality of commercial samples," Pharm. 63(1):23-26.

Benzi VS, Murrayb AP, Ferrero AA (2009 Sep). "Insecticidal and insect-repellent activities of essential oils from Verbenaceae and Anacardiaceae against Rhizopertha dominica," Nat Prod Commun. 4(9):1287-90.

Berić T, Nikolić B, Stanojević J, Vuković-Gacić B, Knezević-Vukcević J (2008 Feb). "Protective effect of basil (Ocimum basilicum L.) against oxidative DNA damage and mutagenesis," Food Chem Toxicol. 46(2):724-32.

Bezanilla F. (2006) The action potential: From voltage-gated conductances to molecular structures. Biological Research. 39: 425-435.

Bhalla Y, Gupta V.K., Jaitak V (2013 Dec). "Anticancer activity of essential oils: a review: Anticancer activity of essential oils," Journal of the Science of Food and Agriculture. 93(15):3643-3

Bhatia S.P., McGinty D, Letizia C.S., Api A.M. (2008 Nov). "Fragrance material review on cedrol," Food and Chemical Toxicology. 46(11):S100-S102.

Bhattacharya SK, Goel RK (1987 Mar). "Anti-stress activity of sitoindosides VII and VIII, new acylsterylglucosides from Withania somnifera," Phytother Res. 1(1):32-7.

Bhattacharya SK, Kumar A, Ghosal S (1995). "Effects of glycowithanolides from Withania somnifera on animal model of Alzheimer's disease and perturbed central cholinergic markers of cognition in rats," Phytother. Res. 9:110-3.

Bhuinya T, Singh P, Mukherjee S et al (2010). "Litsea cubeba—Medicinal values—Brief summary," J. Trop. Med. Plants. 11(2):179-183.

Bhushan S, Kumar A, Malik F, Andotra SS, Sethi VK, Kaur IP, Taneja SC, Qazi GN, Singh J (2007 Oct). "A triterpenediol from Boswellia serrata induces apoptosis through both the intrinsic and extrinsic apoptotic pathways in human leukemia HL-60 cells," Apoptosis. 12(10):1911-26.

Bixby WR, Spalding TW, Haufler AJ, Deeny SP, Mahlow PT, Zimmerman JB, Hatfield BD (2007 Aug). "The unique relation of physical activity to executive function in older men and women," Med Sci Sports Exerc, 39(8):1408-16.

Bixquert JM (2009). "Treatment of irritable bowel syndrome with probiotics: An etiopathogenic approach at last?," Revista Espanola de Enfermadades Digestivas. 101(8):553-64.

Blain EJ, Ali AY, Duance VC (2010 Jun). "Boswellia frereana (frankincense) supresses cytokine-induced matrix metalloproteinase expression and production of pro-inflammatory molecules in articular cartilage," Phytother Res. 24(6):905-12.

Blanes-Mira C, Clemente J, Jodas G, Gil A, Fernandez-Ballester G, Ponsati B, Gutierrez L, Perez-Paya E, Ferrer-Montiel A (2002 Oct). "A synthetic hexapeptide (Argireline) with antiwrinkle activity," Int J Cosmet Sci. 24(5):303-10.

Blumenthal JA, Sherwood A, Babyak MA, Watkins LL, Smith PJ, Hoffman BM, O'Hayer CV, Mabe S, Johnson J, DOraiswamy PM, Jiang W, Schocken DD, Hinderliter AL (2012 Sep). "Exercise and pharmacological treatment of depressive symptoms in patients with coronary heart disease: results from the UPBEAT (Understanding the Prognostic Benefits of Exercise and Antidepressant Therapy study," J Am Coll Cardiol, 60(12):1053-63.

Bobe G et al (2008 Mar). "Flavonoid intake and risk of pancreatic cancer in male smokers (Finland)," Cancer Epidemiol Biomarkers Prev. 17(3):553-62.

Bonan, R.F., Bonan, P.R., Batista, A.U., Sampaio, F.C., Albuquerque, A.J., Moraes, M.C., Mattoso, L.H., Glenn, G.M., Medeiros, E.S., and Oliveira J.E. (2015). "In vitro antimicrobial activity of solution blow spun poly(lactic acid)/polyvinylpyrrolidone nanofibers loaded with Copaiba (Copaifera sp.) oil," Mater Sci Eng C Mater Biol Appl. 48:372-7.

Bone ME, Wilkinson DJ, Young JR, McNeil J, Charlton S (1990 Aug). "Ginger root--a new antiemetic. The effect of ginger root on postoperative nausea and vomiting after major gynaecological surgery," Anaesthesia. 45(8):669-71.

344

Boots AW, Wilms LC, Swennen EL, Kleinjans JC, Bast A, Haenen GR (2008 Jul-Aug). "In vitro and ex vivo anti-inflammatory activity of quercetin in healthy volunteers," Nutrition. 24(7-8):703-10.

Boque, N., Campion, J., de la Iglesia, R., de la Garza, A. L., Milagro, F. I., San Roman, B., . . . Martinez, J. A. (2013 Mar). Screening of polyphenolic plant extracts for anti-obesity properties in Wistar rats. J Sci Food Agric, 93(5), 1226-1232.

Bora, K. S., Arora, S., & Shri, R. (2011 Oct). Role of Ocimum basilicum L. in prevention of ischemia and reperfusion-induced cerebral damage, and motor dysfunctions in mice brain. J Ethnopharmacol, 137(3), 1360-1365.

Borgatti, M., Mancini, I., Bianchi, N., Guerrini, A., Lampronti, I., Rossi, D., . . . Gambari, R. (2011 Apr). Bergamot (Citrus bergamia Risso) fruit extracts and identified components alter expression of interleukin 8 gene in cystic fibrosis bronchial epithelial cell lines. BMC Biochem, 12, 15.

Borkow G (2014). "Using copper to improve the well-being of the skin," Current Chemical Biology. 8:89-102.

Bose M, Lambert JD, Ju J, Reuhl KR, Shapses SA, Yang CS (2008 Sep). "The major green tea polyphenol, (-)-epigallocatechin-3-gallate, inhibits obesity, metabolic syndrome, and fatty liver disease in high-fat-fed mice," J Nutr. 138(9):1677-83.

Boudier D, Breugnot J, Vignau E, Loumonier J, Li L, Closs B (2010 Jun). "Skin care—The refinement of pores," Cosmeticbusiness.com.

Boudier D, Perez E, Rondeau D, Bordes S, Closs B (2008 Mar). "Innovatory approach fights pigment disturbances," Personal Care.

Bounihi A, Hajjaj G, Alnamer R, Cherrah Y, Zellou A (2013). "In vivo potential anti-inflammatory activity of melissa officinalis l. essential oil," Adv Pharmacol Sci.

Bourgou, S., Rahali, F.Z., Ourghemmi, I., and Saïdani Tounsi, M. (2012.) "Changes of peel essential oil composition of four Tunisian citrus during fruit maturation," Scientific World J. 2012:528593.

Boussetta T, Raad H, Lettéron P, Gougerot-Pocidalo MA, Marie JC, Driss F, El-Benna J (2009 Jul 31). "Punicic acid a conjugated linolenic acid inhibits TNFalpha-induced neutrophil hyperactivation and protects from experimental colon inflammation in rats," PLoS One. 4(7):e6458.

Bouwstra J.A., Gooris G.S., Dubbelaar F.E.R., Weeheim A.M., Ijzerman A.P., Ponec M. (1998) Role of ceramide 1 in the molecular organization of the stratum corneum lipids. Journal of Lipid Research. 39: 186-196.

Bouzenna, H., Hfaiedh, N., Giroux-Metges, M.A., Elfeki, A., & Talarmin, H. (2017 May). "Protective effects of essential oil of Citrus limon against aspirin-induced toxicity in IEC-6 cells," Appl Physiol Nutr Metab. 42(5):479-486.

Bowen, R. (2006). The gastrointestinal barrier. In W.E. Wingfield & M.R. Raffe (Eds.), The veterinary ICU book (40-46). Alpine, WY: Teton NewMedia.

Bowles, E. J. (2003). The chemistry of aromatherapeutic oils (3rd ed.). Australia: Allen & Unwin.

Bradley BF, Brown SL, Chu S, Lea RW (2009 Jun). "Effects of orally administered lavender essential oil on responses to anxiety-provoking film clips," Hum Psychopharmacol. 24(4):319-30.

Bradley BF, Starkey NJ, Brown SL, Lea RW (2007 May 22). "Anxiolytic effects of Lavandula angustifolia odour on the Mongolian gerbil elevated plus maze," J Ethnopharmacol. 111(3):517-25.

Brady A, Loughlin R, Gilpin D, Kearney P, Tunney M (2006 Oct). "In vitro activity of tea-tree oil against clinical skin isolates of methicillin-resistant and -sensitive Staphylococcus aureus and coagulase-negative staphylococci growing planktonically and as biofilms," J Med Microbiol. 55(Pt 10):1375-80.

Brand C, Ferrante A, Prager RH, Riley TV, Carson CF, Finlay-Jones JJ, Hart PH. (2001 Apr). "The water-soluble components of the essential oil of Melaleuca alternifolia (tea tree oil) suppress the production of superoxide by human monocytes, but not neutrophils, activated in vitro.," Inflamm Res. 50(4):213-9.

Brand C, Grimbaldeston MA, Gamble JR, Drew J, Finlay-Jones JJ, Hart PH (2002 May). "Tea tree oil reduces the swelling associated with the efferent phase of a contact hypersensitivity response," Inflamm Res. 51(5):236-44.

Brand C, Townley SL, Finlay-Jones JJ, Hart PH (2002 Jun). "Tea tree oil reduces histamine-induced oedema in murine ears," Inflamm Res. 51(6):283-9.

Bras C, Gumilar F, Gandini N, Minetti A, Ferrero A (2011 Oct). "Evaluation of the acute dermal exposure of the ethanolic and hexanic extracts from leaves of Schinus molle var. areira L. in rats," J.Ethnopharmacol. 137 (3):1450-56.

Brass EP, Adler S, Sietsema KE, Hiatt WR, Orlando AM, Amato A; CHIEF Investigators (2001 May). "Intravenous L-carnitine increases plasma carnitine, reduces fatigue, and may preserve exercise capacity in hemodialysis patients," Am J Kidney Dis. 37(5):1018-28.

Brenner, G. M., & Stevens, C. (2009). Pharmacology (3rd ed.). Philadelphia, PA: Saunders Elsevier.

Brien S, Lewith G, Walker A, Hicks SM, Middleton D (2004 Dec). "Bromelain as a Treatment for Osteoarthritis: a Review of Clinical Studies," Evid Based Complement Alternat Med. 1(3):251-257.

Brown AL et al. (2008 Aug). "Effects of dietary supplementation with the green tea polyphenol epigallocatechin-3-gallate on insulin resistance and associated metabolic risk factors: randomized controlled trial," Br J Nutr. 19:1-9.

Brown T.L., LeMay H.E., Bursten B.E. Chemistry: The Central Science. 10th ed. Upper Saddle River: Pearson Prentice Hall, 2006.

Brum LF, Elisabetsky E, Souza D (2001 Aug). "Effects of linalool on [(3) H]MK801 binding and [(3)H] muscimol binding in mouse cortical membranes," Phytother Res. 15(5):422-5.

Brussow, H. (2013). Microbiota and healthy ageing: observational and nutritional intervention studies. Microb Biotechnol, 6(4), 326-334.

Buchbauer G, Jirovetz L, Jäger W, Dietrich H, Plank C (1991 Nov-Dec). "Aromatherapy: evidence for sedative effects of the essential oil of lavender after inhalation," Z Naturforsch C. 46(11-12):1067-72.

Bucheli, P., Vidal, K., Shen, L., Gu, Z., Zhang, C., Miller, L. E., & Wang, J. (2011 Feb). Goji berry effects on macular characteristics and plasma antioxidant levels. Optom Vis Sci, 88(2), 257-262.

Bucher HC, Hengstler P, Schindler C, Meier G (2002 Mar). "N-3 polyunsaturated fatty acids in coronary heart disease: a meta-analysis of randomized controlled trials," Am J Med. 112(4):298-304.

Budiyanto, A., Ahmed, N.U., Wu, A., Bito, T., Nikaido, O., Osawa, T., Ueda, M., Ichihashi, M. (200 Nov). "Protective effect of topically applied olive oil against photocarcinogenesis following UVB exposure of mice," Carcinogenesis, 21(11): 2085-2090.

Buck DS, Nidorf DM, Addino JG (1994 Jun). "Comparison of two topical preparations for the treatment of onychomycosis: Melaleuca alternifolia (tea tree) oil and clotrimazole," J Fam Pract. 38(6):601-5.

Bukovska, A., Cikos, S., Juhas, S., Il'kova, G., Rehak, P., & Koppel, J. (2007 Feb). Effects of a combination of thyme and oregano essential oils on TNBS-induced colitis in mice. Mediators Inflamm, 2007, 23296.

Bulbring E. (1946) Observations on the Isolated Phrenic Nerve Diaphragm Preparation of the Rat. British Journal of Pharmacology. 1: 38-61.

Burke BE, Baillie JE, Olson RD (2004 May). "Essential oil of Australian lemon myrtle (Backhousia citriodora) in the treatment of molluscum contagiosum in children," Biomed Pharmacother. 58(4):245-7.

Bushra, R., Aslam, N., & Khan, A. Y. (2011 Mar). Food-drug interactions. Oman Med J, 26(2), 77-83.

Butte NF, Puyau MR, Adoph AL, Vohra FA, Zakeri I (2007 Aug). "Physical activity in nonoverweight and overweight Hispanic children and adolescents," Med Sci Sports Exerc, 39(8):1257-66.

Cabrera, C., Artacho, R., & Giménez, R. (2006 Apr). Beneficial Effects of Green Tea—A Review. J Am Coll Nutr, 25(2), 79-99.

Cabrera-Vique C, Marfil R, Gimenez R, Martinez-Augustin O (2012 May). "Bioactive compounds and nutritional significance of virgin argan oil—an edible oil with potential as a functional food,' Nutr Rev. 70(5):266-79.

Caccioni DR, Guizzardi M, Biondi DM, Renda A, Ruberto G (1998 Aug 18). "Relationship between volatile components of citrus fruit essential oils and antimicrobial action on Penicillium digitatum and penicillium italicum," Int J Food Microbiol. 43(1-2):73-9.

Caceres, A.I., Liu, B., Jabba S.V., Achanta, S., Morris, J.B., & Jordt, S.E. (2017 May). "Transient Receptor Potential Cation Channel Subfamily M Member 8 channels mediate the anti-inflammatory effects of eucalyptol," Br J Pharmacol. 174(9):867-879.

Cai, X., Zhou, Y. F., & Hu, Z. H. (2008 Apr). Ultrastructure and secretion of secretory canals in vegetative organs of Bupleurum chinense DC. Journal of Molecular Cell Biology, 41(2), 96-106.

Cal K, Janicki S, Sznitowska M (2001 Aug). "In vitro studies on penetration of terpenes from matrix-type transdermal systems through human skin," Int. J. Pharm. 224(1-2):81-88.

Caldefie-Chézet F, Fusillier C, Jarde T, Laroye H, Damez M, Vasson MP, Guillot J (2006 May). "Potential anti-inflammatory effects of Melaleuca alternifolia essential oil on human peripheral blood leukocytes," Phytother Res. 20(5):364-70.

Caldefie-Chézet F, Guerry M, Chalchat JC, Fusillier C, Vasson MP, Guillot J (2004 Aug). "Anti-inflammatory effects of Melaleuca alternifolia essential oil on human polymorphonuclear neutrophils and monocytes," Free Radic Res. 38(8):805-11.

Camarda L, Dayton T, Di Stefano V, Pitonzo R, Schillaci D (2007 Sep). "Chemical composition and antimicrobial activity of some oleogum resin essential oils from Boswellia spp. (Burseraceae)," Ann Chim. 97(9):837-844.

Campelo, L. M., Goncalves, F. C., Feitosa, C. M., & de Freitas, R. M. (2011 Jul). Antioxidant activity of Citrus limon essential oil in mouse hippocampus. Pharm Biol, 49(7), 709-715.

Candan F, Unlu M, Tepe B, Daferera D, Polissiou M, Sökmen A, Akpulat HA (2003 Aug). "Antioxidant and antimicrobial activity of the essential oil and methanol extracts of Achillea millefolium subsp. millefolium Afan. (Asteraceae)," J Ethnopharmacol. 87(2-3):215-20.

Cannas S. et al (2015 Jun). "Essential oils in ocular pathology: an experimental study," J. Infect. Dev. Ctries. 9(6):650-654.

Canyon DV, Speare R (2007 Apr). "A comparison of botanical and synthetic substances commonly used to prevent head lice (Pediculus humanus var. capitis) infestation," Int J Dermatol. 46(4):422-6.

Capasso R, Savino F, Capasso F (2007 Oct). "Effects of the herbal formulation ColiMil on upper gastrointestinal transit in mice in vivo," Phytother. Res. 21(10):999-1101.

Cappello G, Spezzaferro M, Grossi L, Manzoli L, Marzio L (2007 Jun). "Peppermint oil (Mintoil) in the treatment of irritable bowel syndrome: a prospective double blind placebo-controlled randomized trial," Dig Liver Dis. 39(6):530-6.

Capuzzo A, Occhipinti A, Maffei M.E. (2014 Dec). "Antioxidant and radical scavenging activities of chamazulene," Nat. Prod. Res. 28(24):2321-2323.

Carnesecchi S., Bradaia A., Fischer B., Coelho D., Scholler-Guinard M., Gosse F., Raul F. (2002) Perturbation by Geraniol of Cell Membrane Permeability and Signal Transduction Pathways in Human Colon Cancer Cells. The Journal of Pharmacology and Experimental Therapeutics. 303: 711-715.

Carnesecchi S., Bras-Goncalves R., Bradaia A., Zeisel M., Gosse F., Poupon M-F., Raul F. (2004) Geraniol, a component of plant essential oils, modulates DNA synthesis and potentiates 5-fluorouracil efficacy on human colon tumor xenografts. Cancer Letters. 215: 53-59.

Carnesecchi S., Langley K., Exinger F., Gosse F., Raul F. (2002) Geraniol, a Component of Plant Essential Oils, Sensitizes Human Colonic Cancer Cells to 5-Flurouracil Treatment. The Journal of Pharmacology and Experimental Therapeutics. 301: 625-630.

Carnesecchi S, Schneider Y, Ceraline J, Duranton B, Gosse F, Seiler N, Raul F (2001 Jul). "Geraniol, a component of plant essential oils, inhibits growth and polyamine biosynthesis in human colon cancer cells," J Pharmacol Exp Ther. 298(1):197-200.

Carson CF, Cookson BD, Farrelly HD, Riley TV (1995 Mar). "Susceptibility of methicillin-resistant Staphylococcus aureus to the essential oil of Melaleuca alternifolia," J Antimicrob Chemother. 35(3):421-4.

Carvalho-Freitas MI, Costa M (2002 Dec). "Anxiolytic and sedative effects of extracts and essential oil from Citrus aurantium L," Biol Pharm Bull. 25(12):1629-33.

Catalán A, Pacheco JG, Martínez A, Mondaca MA (2008 Mar). "In vitro and in vivo activity of Melaleuca alternifolia mixed with tissue conditioner on Candida albicans," Oral Surg Oral Med Oral Pathol Oral Radiol Endod. 105(3):327-32.

Cavaleiro C, Salgueiro L, Goncalves MJ, Hrimpeng K, Pinto J, Pinto E (2015 Apr). "Antifungal activity of the essential oil of Angelica major against Candida, Cryptococcus, Aspergillus and dermatophyte species," J Nat Med. 69(2):241-248.

Ceccarelli I, Lariviere WR, Fiorenzani P, Sacerdote P, Aloisi AM (2004 Mar 19). "Effects of long-term exposure of lemon essential oil odor on behavioral, hormonal and neuronal parameters in male and female rats," Brain Res. 1001(1-2):78-86.

Cencic A, Chingwaru W (2010). The Role of Functional Foods, Nutraceuticals, and Food Supplements in Intestinal Health. Nutrients, 2(6):611-625.

Cenizo, V., Andre, V., Reymermier, C., Sommer, P., Damour, O., & Perrier, E. (2006 Aug). LOXL as a target to increase the elastin content in adult skin: a dill extract induces the LOXL gene expression. Exp Dermatol, 15(8), 574-581.

Centers for Disease Control and Prevention (CDC) (2004 May 7). "Spina bifida and anencephaly before and after folic acid mandate--United States, 1995-1996 and 1999-2000," MMWR Morb Mortal Wkly Rep. 53(17):362-5.

Ceriotti G, Spandrio L, Gazzaniga A (1967 Jul-Aug). "[Demonstration, isolation and physical and chemical characteristics of narciclasine, a new antimitotic of plant origin]," Tumori. 53(4):359-71.

Cermelli C, Fabio A, Fabio G, Quaglio P (2008 Jan). "Effect of eucalyptus essential oil on respiratory bacteria and viruses," Curr Microbiol. 56(1):89-92.

Cetinkaya B, Basbakkal Z (2012 Apr). "The effectiveness of aromatherapy massage using lavender oil as a treatment for infantile colic," Int. J. Nurs. Pract. 18(2):164-169.

Chaiyana W, Okonogi S (2012 Jun). "Inhibition of cholinesterase by essential oil from food plant," Phytomedicine Int. J. Phytother. Phytopharm. 19(8-9):836-839.

Chaudhuri, R.K., and Bojanowski, K. (2014). "Bakuchiol: a retinol-like functional compound revealed by gene expression profiling and clinically proven to have anti-aging effects," Int J Cosmet Sci. 36(3):221-30.

Cháfer, M., Sanchez-Gonzalez, L., Gonzalez-Martinez, C., & Chiralt, A. (2012 Aug). Fungal decay and shelf life of oranges coated with chitosan and bergamot, thyme, and tea tree essential oils. J Food Sci, 77(8), E182-187.

Chaieb K, Zmantar T, Ksouri R, Hajlaoui H, Mahdouani K, Abdelly C, Bakhrouf A (2007 Sep). "Antioxidant properties of the essential oil of Eugenia caryophyllata and its antifungal activity against a large number of clinical Candida species," Mycoses. 50(5):403-6.

Chaiyakunapruk N, Kitikannakorn N, Nathisuwan S, Leeprakobboon K, Leelasettagool C (2006 Jan). "The efficacy of ginger for the prevention of postoperative nausea and vomiting: a meta-analysis," Am J Obstet Gynecol. 194(1):95-9.

Chakraborty PK, Mustafi SB, Raha S (2008 Sep). "Pro-survival effects of repetitive low-grade oxidative stress are inhibited by simultaneous exposure to resveratrol," Phamacol Res. 2.

Chambers H.F. (2001) The Changing Epidemiology of Staphylococcus aureus?. Emerging Infectious Diseases. 7: 178-182.

Chan YS, Cheng LN, Wu JH, Chan E, Kwan YW, Lee SM, Leung GP, Yu PH, Chan SW (2011 Oct). "A review of the pharmacological effects of Arctium lappa (burdock)," Inflammopharmacology. 19(5):245-54.

Chang, K. S., Tak, J. H., Kim, S. I., Lee, W. J., & Ahn, Y. J. (2006 Nov). Repellency of Cinnamomum cassia bark compounds and cream containing cassia oil to Aedes aegypti (Diptera: Culicidae) under laboratory and indoor conditions. Pest Manag Sci, 62(11), 1032-1038.

Chang SM, Chen CH (2016 Feb). "Effects of an intervention with drinking chamomile tea on sleep quality and depression in sleep disturbed postnatal women: a randomized controlled trial," J Adv Nurs. 72(2):306-15.

Chang WC, Yu YM, Chiang SY, Tseng CY (2008 Apr). "Ellagic acid supresses oxidised low-density lipoprotein-induced aortic smooth muscle cell proliferation: studies on the activation of extracellular signal-regulated kinase ½ and proliferating cell nuclear antigen expression," Br J Nutr. 99(4):709-14.

Chang WL, Cheng FC, Wang SP, Chou ST, Shih Y (2016 Feb). "Cinnamomum cassia essential oil and its major constituent cinnamaldehyde induced cell cycle arrest and apoptosis in human oral squamous cell carcinoma HSC-3 cells," Environ. Toxicol.

Chang YT, Chu FH (2011 Mar). "Molecular cloning and characterization of monoterpene synthases from Litsea cubeba (Lour.) Persoon," Tree Genetics & Genomes. 7(4):835-844.

Chapman A.G. (1998) Glutamate receptors in epilepsy. Progress in Brain Research. 116: 371-383.

Chapman A.G. (2000) Glutamate and Epilepsy. The Journal of Nutrition. 130: 1043S-1045S.

Charles C.A. et al (2014). "Early benefits with daily rinsing on gingival health improvements with an essential oil mouthrinse--post-hoc analysis of 5 clinical trials," J. Dent. Hyg. JDH Am. Dent. Hyg. Assoc. 88L40-50.

Charles CH, Vincent JW, Borycheski L, Amatnieks Y, Sarina M, Qaqish J, Proskin HM (2000 Sep). "Effect of an essential oil-containing dentifrice on dental plaque microbial composition," Am J Dent. 13():26C-30C.

Charrouf Z, Guillaume D (2010 May). "Should the amazigh diet (regular and moderate argan-oil consumption) have a beneficial impact on human health?," Crit Rev Food Sci Nutr. 50(5):473-7.

Chaturvedi AP, Kumar M, Tripathi YB (2013 Dec). "Efficacy of Jasminum grandiflorum L. leaf extract on dermal wound healing in rats," Int Wound J. 10(6):675-82.

Chaudhary S.C., Siddiqui M.S., Athar M, Alam M.S. (2012 Aug). "D-Limonene modulates inflammation, oxidative stress and Ras-ERK pathway to inhibit murine skin tumorigenesis," Hum. Exp. Toxicol. 31(8):798-811.

Chaudhuri RK, Bojanowski K (2014 Jun). "Bakuchiol: a retinol-like functional compound revealed by gene expression profiling and clinically proven to have anti-aging effects," Int J Cosmet Sci. 36(3):221-30.

Checker R, Chatterjee S, Sharma D, Gupta S, Variyar P, Sharma A, Poduval TB (2008 May). "Immunomodulatory and radioprotective effects of lignans derived from fresh nutmeg mace (Myristica fragrans) in mammalian splenocytes," Int Immunopharmacol. 8(5):661-9.

Chee H.Y., Lee M.H. (2007 Dec). "Antifungal activity of clove essential oil and its volatile vapour against dermatophytic fungi," Mycobiology. 35(4):241-243.

Cheeke PR, Piacente S, Oleszek W (2006). "Anti-inflammatory and anti-arthritic effects of yucca schidigera: A review," J Inflamm (Lond). 3:6.

Chen CJ. et al (2012 Dec). "Neuropharmacological activities of fruit essential oil from Litsea cubeba Persoon," Journal of Wood Science. 58(6):538-543.

Chen CJ, Kumar KJ, Chen YT, Tsao NW, Chien SC, Chang ST, Chu FH, Wang SY (2015). "Effect of Hinoki and Meniki Essential Oils on Human Autonomic Nervous System Activity and Mood States," Nat Prod Commun. 10(7):1305-8.

Chen HC et al (2016 Aug). "Immunosuppressive Effect of Litsea cubeba L. Essential Oil on Dendritic Cell and Contact Hypersensitivity Responses," International Journal of Molecular Sciences. 17(8):1319.

Chen M, Zhang J, Yu S, Wang S, Zhang Z, Chen J, Xiao J, Wang Y (2012). "Anti-lung-cancer activity and liposome -based delivery systems of beta-elemene," Evid Based Complement Alternat Med. 2012:259523.

Chen MC, Fang SH, Fang L (2015 Feb). "The effects of aromatherapy in relieving symptoms related to job stress among nurses: Aromatherapy," Int. J. Nurs. Pract. 21(1):87-93.

Chen YC, Chiu WT, Wu MS (2006 Jul). "Therapeutic effect of topical gamma-linolenic acid on refractory uremic pruritus," Am J Kidney Dis. 48(1):69-76.

Chen Y. et al (2013 Oct "Composition and potential anticancer activities of essential oils obtained from myrrh and frankincense," Oncol Lett. 6(4):1140-1146.

Chen, Y., Zeng, H., Tian, J., Ban, X., Ma, B., & Wang, Y. (2014 Apr). Dill (Anethum graveolens L.) seed essential oil induces Candida albicans apoptosis in a metacaspase-dependent manner. Fungal Biol, 118(4), 394-401.

Cheung S, Tai J (2007 Jun). "Anti-proliferative and antioxidant properties of rosemary Rosmarinus officinalis," Oncol Rep. 17(6):1525-31.

Chevrier MR, Ryan AE, Lee DY, Zhongze M, Wu-Yan Z, Via CS (2005 May). "Boswellia carterii extract inhibits TH1 cytokines and promotes TH2 cytokines in vitro," Clin Diagn Lab Immunol. 12(5):575-80.

Chidambara Murthy K.N., Jayaprakasha G.K., Patil B.S. (2012 Oct). "D-limonene rich volatile oil from blood oranges inhibits angiogenesis, metastasis and cell death in human colon cancercells," Life Sci. 91(11-12):429-439.

Chien, L. W., Cheng, S. L., & Liu, C. F. (2012 Aug). The effect of lavender aromatherapy on autonomic nervous system in midlife women with insomnia. Evid Based Complement Alternat Med, 2012.

Chinou IB, Roussis V, Perdetzoglou D, Loukis A (1996 Aug). "Chemical and biological studies on two Helichrysum species of Greek origin," Planta Med. 62(4):377-9.

Chioca L.R., Antunes V.D.C., Ferro M.M., Losso E.M., Andreatini R (2013 May). "Anosmia does not impair the anxiolytic-like effect of lavender essential oil inhalation in mice," Life Sci. 92(20-21):971-975.

Chioca L.R. et al (2013 May). "Anxiolytic-like effect of lavender essential oil inhalation in mice: participation of GABAA/benzodiazepine neurotransmission," J. Ethnopharmacol. 147(2):412-418.

Cho, M. Y., Min, E. S., Hur, M. H., & Lee, M. S. (2013 Feb). Effects of aromatherapy on the anxiety, vital signs, and sleep quality of percutaneous coronary intervention patients in intensive care units. Evid Based Complement Alternat Med, 2013, 1-6.

Cho, S., Choi, Y., Park, S., & Park, T. (2012 Feb). Carvacrol prevents diet-induced obesity by modulating gene expressions involved in adipogenesis and inflammation in mice fed with high-fat diet. J Nutr Biochem, 23(2), 192-201.

Choi, H. Y., Yang, Y. C., Lee, S. H., Clark, J. M., & Ahn, Y. J. (2010 May). Efficacy of spray formulations containing binary mixtures of clove and eucalyptus oils against susceptible and pyrethroid/ malathion-resistant head lice (Anoplura: Pediculidae). J Med Entomol, 47(3), 387-391.

Choi, S. Y., Kang, P., Lee, H. S., and Seol, G. H. (2014). "Effects of Inhalation of Essential Oil of Citrus aurantium L. var. amara on Menopausal Symptoms, Stress, and Estrogen in Postmenopausal Women: A Randomized Controlled Trial," Evid Based Complement Alternat Med. 2014:796518.

Choi, U. K., Lee, O. H., Yim, J. H., Cho, C. W., Rhee, Y. K., Lim, S. I., & Kim, Y. C. (2010 Feb). Hypolipidemic and antioxidant effects of dandelion (Taraxacum officinale) root and leaf on cholesterol-fed rabbits. Int J Mol Sci, 11(1), 67-78.

Choi, Y. Y., Kim, M. H., Han, J. M., Hong, J., Lee, T. H., Kim, S. H., & Yang, W. M. (2014 Feb 8). "The anti-inflammatory potential of Cortex Phellodendron in vivo and in vitro: down-regulation of NO and iNOS through suppression of NF-kappaB and MAPK activation," Int Immunopharmacol, 19(2): 214-220.

Chou ST, Peng HY, Hsu JC, Lin CC, Shih Y (2013 Jun). "Achillea millefolium L. Essential Oil Inhibits LPS-Induced Oxidative Stress and Nitric Oxide Production in RAW 264.7 Macrophages," Int. J. Mol. Sci. 14(7):12978-12993.

Chow H.S., Salazar D, Hakin I.A. (2002 Nov). "Pharmacokinetics of perillic acid in humans after a single dose administration of a citrus preparation rich in d-limonene content," Cancer Epidemiol. Biomark. Prev. Publ. Am. Assoc. Cancer Res. Cosponsored Am. Soc. Prev. Oncol 11(11):1472-1476.

Chung, H. S., Harris, A., Kristinsson, J. K., Ciulla, T. A., Kagemann, C., & Ritch, R. (1999 Jun). Ginkgo biloba extract increases ocular blood flow velocity. J Ocul Pharmacol Ther, 15(3), 233-240.

Chung, M. J., Cho, S. Y., Bhuiyan, M. J., Kim, K. H., & Lee, S. J. (2010 Jul). Anti-diabetic effects of lemon balm (Melissa officinalis) essential oil on glucose- and lipid-regulating enzymes in type 2 diabetic mice. Br J Nutr, 104(2), 180-188.

Chungchunlam, S. M., Henare, S. J., Ganesh, S., & Moughan, P. J. (2014 Apr 5). Effect of whey protein and glycomacropeptide on measures of satiety in normal-weight adult women. Appetite, 78, 172-178.

Chunmuang S, Jitpukdeebodintra S, Chuenarrom C, Benjakul P (2007). "Effect of xylitol and fluoride on enamel erosion in vitro," J. Oral Sci. 49(4):293-297.

Ciacci C, Peluso G, Iannoni E, Siniscalchi M, Iovino P, Rispo A, Tortora R, Bucci C, Zingone F, Margarucci S, Calvani M (2007 Oct). "L-Carnitine in the treatment of fatigue in adult celiac disease patients: a pilot study," Dig Liver Dis. 39(10):922-8.

Cibulka MT, Sinacore DR, Cromer GS, Delitto A (1998). "Unilateral hip rotation range of motion asymmetry in patients with sacroiliac joint regional pain," Spine, 23(9):1009-115.

Ciftci O., Ozdemir I., Tanyildizl S., Yildiz S., Oguzturk H. (2011) Antioxidative effects of curcumin, β-myrcene and 1,8-cineole against 2,3,7,8-tetracholorodibenzo-p-dioxin - induced oxidative stress in rats liver. Toxicology and Industrial Health. 27: 447-453.

Cioanca, O., Hritcu, L., Mihasan, M., Trifan, A., & Hancianu, M. (2014 May). Inhalation of coriander volatile oil increased anxiolytic-antidepressant-like behaviors and decreased oxidative status in beta-amyloid (1-42) rat model of Alzheimer's disease. Physiol Behav, 131, 68-74.

Cioanca, O., Hritcu, L., Mihasan, M., & Hancianu, M. (2013 Aug). Cognitive-enhancing and antioxidant activities of inhaled coriander volatile oil in amyloid beta(1-42) rat model of Alzheimer's disease. Physiol Behav, 120, 193-202.

Cline M, Taylor J.E., Flores J, Bracken S, McCall S, Ceremuga T.E. (2008 Feb). "Investigation of the anxiolytic effects of linalool, a lavender extract, in the male Sprague-Dawley rat," AANA J. 76(1):47-52.

Coderch L., Lopez O., de la Maza A., Parra J.L. (2003) Ceramides and Skin Function. American Journal of Clinical Dermatology. 4: 107-129.

Conrad P, Adams C (2012 Aug). "The effects of clinical aromatherapy for anxiety and depression in the high risk postpartum woman - a pilot study," Complement. Ther. Clin. Pract. 18(3):164-168.

Cooley K, Szczurko O, Perri D, Mills EJ, Bernhardt B, Zhou Q, Seely D (2009 Aug 31). "Naturopathic care for anxiety: a randomized controlled trial ISRCTN78958974," PLoS One. 4(8):e6628.

Corasaniti, M. T., Maiuolo, J., Maida, S., Fratto, V., Navarra, M., Russo, R., . . . Bagetta, G. (2007 Jun). Cell signaling pathways in the mechanisms of neuroprotection afforded by bergamot essential oil against NMDA-induced cell death in vitro. Br J Pharmacol, 151(4), 518-529.

Costalonga M., Herzberg M.C. (2014 Dec). "The oral microbiome and the immunobiology of periodontal disease and caries," Immunol. Lett. 162(200):22-38.

Couse JF, Lindzey J, Grandien K, Gustafsson JA, Korach KS (1997 Nov). "Tissue distribution and quantitative analysis of estrogen reseptor-alpha (ERalpha) and estrogen receptor-beta (ERbeta) messenger ribonucleic acid in the wild-type and ERalpha-knockout mouse," Endocrinology. 138*11):4613-21.

Cowan M.K. Talaro K.P. Microbiology: A Systems Approach. 2nd ed. New York: McGraw Hill, 2009.

Cox SD, Mann CM, Markham JL, Bell HC, Gustafson JE, Warmington JR, Wyllie SG (2000 Jan). "The mode of antimicrobial action of the essential oil of Melaleuca alternifolia (tea tree oil)," J Appl Microbiol. 88(1):170-5.

Cronin H, Draelos Z.D. (2010 Sep). "Top 10 botanical ingredients in 2010 anti-aging creams," J Cosmet Dermatol. 9(3):218-225.

Cross SE, Russell M, Southwell I, Roberts MS (2008 May). "Human skin penetration of the major components of Australian tea tree oil applied in its pure form and as a 20% solution in vitro," Eur J Pharm Biopharm. 69(1):214-22.

Crowell P.L., Chang R.R., Ren Z., Elson C.E., Gould M.N. (1991) Selective Inhibition of Isoprenylation of 21-26kDa Proteins by the Anticarcinogen d-Limonene and Its Metabolites. J. Biol. Chem. 266: 17679-17685.

Crowell P.L., Elson C.E., Bailey H.H., Elegbede A, Haag J.D., Gould M.N. (1994). "Human metabolism of the experimental cancer therapeutic agent d-limonene," Cancer Chemother. Pharmacol. 35 (1):31-37.

Crowell, P.L., & Gould, M.N. (1994). "Chemoprevention and therapy of cancer by d-limonene," Crit Rev Oncog. 5(1):1-22.

Crowell P.L., Lin S, Vedejs E, Gould M.N. (1992). "Identification of metabolites of the antitumor agent d-limonene capable of inhibiting protein isoprenylation and cell growth," Cancer Chemother. 13(3):205-212.

Cuellar, M. J., Giner, R. M., Recio, M. C., Manez, S., & Rios, J. L. (2001 Mar). Topical anti-inflammatory activity of some Asian medicinal plants used in dermatological disorders. Fitoterapia, 72(3), 221-229.

Cui Y et al. (2008 May 15). "Dietary flavonoid intake and lung cancer—a population-based case-control study," Cancer. 112(10):2241-8.

Curi R, Alvarez M, Bazotte RB, Botion LM, Godoy JL, Bracht A (1986). "Effect of Stevia rebaudiana on glucose tolerance in normal adult humans," Braz J Med Biol Res. 19(6):771-4.

Curio M, Jacone H, Perrut J, Pinto AC, Filho VF, Silva RC (2009 Aug). "Acute effect of Copaifera reticulata Ducke copaiba oil in rats tested in the elevated plus-maze: an ethological analysis," J Pharm Pharmacol. 61(8):1105-10.

Dahham S.S. et al (2015). "The Anticancer, Antioxidant and Antimicrobial Properties of the Sesquiterpene β-Caryophyllene from the Essential Oil of Aquilaria crassna," Mol. Basel Switz. 20(7):11808-11829.

Dai ZJ, Tang W, Lu WF, Gao J, Kang HF, Ma XB, Min WL, Wang XJ, Wu WY (2013 Mar 14). "Antiproliferative and apoptotic effects of beta-elemne on human hepatoma HepG2 cells," Cancer Cell Int. 13(1):27.

Dagli N, Dagli R, Mahmoud R.S., Baroudi K (2015). "Essential oils, their therapeutic properties, and implication in dentistry: A review," J. Int. Soc. Prev. Community Dent. 5(5):335-340.

d'Alessio P.A., Mirshani M, Bisson JF, Bene M.C. (2014 Mar). "Skin repair properties of d-Limonene and perillyl alcohol in murine models," Anti-Inflamm. Anti-Allergy Agents Med. Chem. 13(1):29-35.

d'Alessio P.A., Ostan R, Bisson JF, Schulzke J.D., Ursini M.V., Béné M.C (2013 Jul). "Oral administration of d-limonene controls inflammation in rat colitis and displays anti-inflammatory properties as diet supplementation in humans," Life Sci. 92(24-26):1151-1156.

Danner G.R., Muto K.W., Zieba A.M., Stillman C.M., Seggio J.A., Ahmad S.T. (2011 Dec). "Spearmint (1-Carvone) Oil and Wintergreen (Methyl Salicylate) Oil Emulsion Is an Effective Immersion Anesthetic of Fishes," J. Fish Wildl. Manag. 2(2):146-155.

Darmstadt GL, Mao-Qiang M, Chi E, Saha SK, Ziboh VA, Black RE, Santosham M, Elias PM (2002). "Impact of topical oils on the skin barrier: possible implications for neonatal health in developing countries," Acta Paediatr. 91(5):546-54.

Darmstadt GL, Saha SK, Ahmed AS, Chowdhury MA, Law PA, Ahmed S, Alam MA, Black RE, Santosham M (2005 Mar 19-25). "Effect of topical treatment with skin barrier-enhancing emollients on nosocomial infections in preterm infants in Bangladesh: a randomised controlled trial," Lancet. 365(9464):1039-45.

Damiani C.E.N., Rossoni L.V., Vassallo D.V. (2003) Vasorelaxant effects of eugenol on rat thoracic aorta. Vascular Pharmacology. 40: 59-66.

Das, I., Acharya, A., Berry, D. L., Sen, S., Williams, E., Permaul, E., . . . Saha, T. (2012 Sep). Antioxidative effects of the spice cardamom against non-melanoma skin cancer by modulating nuclear factor erythroid-2-related factor 2 and NF-kappaB signalling pathways. Br J Nutr, 108(6), 984-997.

da Silva, A.G., Puziol Pde, F., Leitao, R.N., Gomes, T.R., Scherer, R., Martins, M.L., Cavalcanti, A.S., and Cavalcanti, L.C. (2012). "Application of the essential oil from copaiba (Copaifera langsdori Desf.) for acne vulgaris: a double-blind, placebo-controlled clinical trial," Altern Med Rev. 17(1):69-75.

da Silva E.B.P., Matsuo A.L., Figueiredo C.R., Chaves M.H., Sartorelli P., Lago J.H.G. (2013 Feb). "Chemical constituents and cytotoxic evaluation of essential oils from leaves of Porcelia macrocarpa (Annonaceae)," Nat. Prod. Commun. 8(2):277-279.

D'Auria FD, Laino L, Strippoli V, Tecca M, Salvatore G, Battinelli L, Mazzanti G (2001 Aug). "In vitro activity of tea tree oil against Candida albicans mycelial conversion and other pathogenic fungi," J Chemother. 13(4):377-83.

D'Auria FD, Tecca M, Strippoli V, Salvatore G, Battinelli L, Mazzanti G (2005 Aug). "Antifungal activity of Lavandula angustifolia essential oil against Candida albicans yeast and mycelial form," Med Mycol. 43(5):391-6.

Darvesh S, Hopkins A, Guela C (2003 Feb). "Neurobiology of butyrylcholines-terase," Nat. Rev. Neurosci. 4(2):131-138.

Davaatseren, M., Hur, H. J., Yang, H. J., Hwang, J. T., Park, J. H., Kim, H. J., . . . Sung, M. J. (2013 Aug). Taraxacum official (dandelion) leaf extract alleviates high-fat diet-induced nonalcoholic fatty liver. Food Chem Toxicol, 58, 30-36.

Davenport MH, Hogan DB, Exkes GA, Longman RS, Poulin MJ (2012). "Cerebrovascular Reserve: The LInk Between Fitness and Cognitive Function?," Sport Sci Rev, 40(3):153-8.

Davies K (1995). "Oxidative stress: the paradox of aerobic life," Biochem Soc Symp. 61:1-31.

d'Avila Farias M et al (2014 May). "Eugenol derivatives as potential anti-oxidants: is phenolic hydroxyl necessary to obtain an effect?," J. Pharm. Pharmacol. 66(5):733-746.

Dayan N., Sivalenka R, Chase J (2009 Feb). "Skin Moisturization by hydrogenated polyisobutene - Quantitative and visual evaluation," Journal of Cosmetic Science. 60.

de Almeida R.N., Araujo D.A.M., Goncalvevs J.C.R., Montenegro F.C., de Sousa D.P., Leite J.R., Mattei R., Benedito M.A.C., de Carvalho J.G.B., Cruz J.S., Maia J.G.S. (2009) Rosewood oil induces sedation and inhibits compound action petential in rodents. Journal of Ethanopharmacology. 124: 440-443.

de Almeida R.N., de Sousa D.P., Nobrega F.F.F., Claudino F.S., Araujo D.A.M., Leite J.R., Mattei R. (2008) Anticonvulsant effect of a natural compound α,β-epoxy-carvone and its actioin on the nerve excitability. Neuroscience Letters. 443: 51-55.

de Boer H.J., Lamxay V, Björk L (2011 Dec). "Steam sauna and mother roasting in Lao PDR: practices and chemical constituents of essential oils of plant species used in postpartum recovery," BMC Complement Altern Med. 11:128.

Debersac P, Heydel JM, Amiot MJ, Goudonnet H, Artur Y, Suschetet M, Siess MH (2001 Sep). "Induction of cytochrome P450 and/or detoxication enzymes by various extracts of rosemary: description of specific patterns," Food Chem Toxicol. 39(9):907-18.

de Cássia da Silveira e Sá R, Andrade L.N., de Sousa D.P. (2013). "A review on anti-inflammatory activity of monoterpenes," Mol. Basel Switz. 18(1):1227-1254.

Deeptha K, Kamaleeswari M, Sengottuvelan M, Nalini N (2006 Nov). "Dose dependent inhibitory effect of dietary caraway on 1,2-dimethylhydrazine induced colonic aberrant crypt foci and bacterial enzyme activity in rats," Invest New Drugs. 24(6):479-88.

de la Garza, A. L., Etxeberria, U., Lostao, M. P., San Roman, B., Barrenetxe, J., Martinez, J. A., & Milagro, F. I. (2013 Dec). Helichrysum and grapefruit extracts inhibit carbohydrate digestion and absorption, improving postprandial glucose levels and hyperinsulinemia in rats. J Agric Food Chem, 61(49), 12012-12019.

Delaquis, P. J., Stanich, K., Girard, B., & Mazza, G. (2002 Mar). Antimicrobial activity of individual and mixed fractions of dill, cilantro, coriander and eucalyptus essential oils. Int J Food Microbiol, 74(1-2), 101-109.

DeLeo F.R., Otto M., Kreiswirth B.N., Chambers H.F. (2010) Community associated meticillin-resistant Staphylococcus aureus. The Lancet. 375: 1557-1568.

Del Toro-Arreola S. et al (2005 May). "Effect of D-limonene on immune response in BALB/c mice with lymphoma," Int. Immunopharmacol. 5(5):829-838.

de Mendonça Rocha PM, Rodilla JM, Díez D, Elder H, Guala MS, Silva LA, Pombo EB (2012 Oct). "Synergistic antibacterial activity of the essential oil of aguaribay (Schinus molle L.)," Molecules. 17(10):12023-36.

Department of Environmental Medicine, Odense University, Denmark (1992 Dec). "Ginger (Zingiber officinale) in rheumatism and musculoskeletal disorders," Med Hypotheses. 39(4):342-8.

de Rapper S., Kamatou G., Viljoen, A., & van Vuuren, S. (2013 Jun). The in vitro antimicrobial activity of lavandula angustifolia essential oil in combination with other aroma-therapeutic oils. Evid Based Complement Alternat Med, 2013, 1-10.

de Rapper S, Van Vuuren F, Kamatou G.P.P., Viljoen A.M., Dagne E (2012 Apr). "The additive and synergistic antimicrobial effects of select frankincense and myrrh oils – a combination from the pharaonic pharmacopoeia," Letters in Applied Microbiology. 54(4):352-358.

De S. Aguiar, R. W., Ootani, M. A., Ascencio, S. D., Ferreira, T. P., dos Santos, M. M., & dos Santos, G. R. (2014 Jan). Fumigant antifungal activity of Corymbia citriodora and Cymbopogon nardus essential oils and citronellal against three fungal species. Scientific World Journal, 2014, 1-8.

de Sant'anna J.R. et al (2009 Feb). "Genotoxicity of Achillea millefolium essential oil in diploid cells of Aspergillus nidulans," Phytother. Res. PTR. 23(2):231-235.

De Spirt S, Stahl W, Tronnier H, Sies H, Bejot M, Maurette JM, Heinrich U (2009 Feb). "Intervention with flaxseed and borage oil supplements modulates skin condition in women," Br J Nutr. 101(3):440-5.

de Sousa D.P., Goncalves J.C.R., Quintanas-Junior L., Cruz J.S., Araujo D.A.M., de Almeida R.N. (2006) Study of anticonvulsant effect of citronellol, a monoterpene alcohol, in rodents. Neuroscience Letters. 401: 231-235.

Deters A, Zippel J, Hellenbrand N, Pappai D, Possemeyer C, Hensel A (2010 Jan 8). "Aqueous extracts and polysaccharides from Marshmallow roots (Althea officinalis L.): cellular internalisation and stimulation of cell physiology of human epithelial cells in vitro," J Ethnopharmacol. 127(1):62-9.

Devika PT, Mainzen Prince PS (2008 Jan). "(-) Epigallocatechin gallate (EGCG) prevents isoprenaline-induced cardiac marker enzymes and membrane-bound ATPases," J Pharm Pharmacol. 60(1):125-33.

De Vriendt T, Moreno LA, De Henauw S (2009 Sep). "Chronic stress and obesity in adolescents: scientific evidence and methodological issues for epidemiological research," Nutr Metab Cardiovasc Dis. 19(7):511-9.

Dey, Y. N., Ota, S., Srikanth, N., Jamal, M., & Wanjari, M. (2012 Jan). A phytopharmacological review on an important medicinal plant - Amorphophallus paeoniifolius. Ayu, 33(1), 27-32.

Dhawan K, Dhawan S, Sharma A (2004 Sep). "Passiflora: a review update," Journal of Ethnopharmacology. 94(1):1-23.

Dias, F. M., Leffa, D. D., Daumann, F., Marques Sde, O., Luciano, T. F., Possato, J. C., . . . de Lira, F. S. (2014 Feb). Acerola (Malpighia emarginata DC.) juice intake protects against alterations to proteins involved in inflammatory and lipolysis pathways in the adipose tissue of obese mice fed a cafeteria diet. Lipids Health Dis, 13, 1-9.

Díaz C, Quesada S, Brenes O, Aguilar G, Cicció JF (2008). "Chemical composition of Schinus molle essential oil and its cytotoxic activity on tumour cell lines," Nat Prod Res. 22(17):1521-34.

Diego MA, Jones NA, Field T, Hernandez-Reif M, Schanberg S, Kuhn C, McAdam V, Galamaga R, Galamaga M (1998 Dec). "Aromatherapy positively affects mood, EEG patterns of alertness and math computations," Int J Neurosci. 96(3-4):217-24.

Diggins K.C. (2008) Treatment of mild to moderate dehydration in children with oral rehydration therapy. Journal of the American Academy of Nurse Practitioners. 20: 402-406.

Dikshit A, Naqvi AA, Husain A. (1986 May). "Schinus molle: a new source of natural fungitoxicant," Appl Environ Microbiol. 51(5):1085-8.

Dimas K, Kokkinopoulos D, Demetzos C, Vaos B, Marselos M, Malamas M, Tzavaras T (1999 Mar). "The effect of sclareol on growth and cell cycle progression of human leukemic cell lines," Leuk Res. 23(3):217-34.

Dimpfel W, Pischel I, Lehnfeld R (2004 Sep 29). "Effects of lozenge containing lavender oil, extracts from hops, lemon balm and oat on electrical brain activity of volunteers," Eur J Med Res. 9(9):423-31.

Ding XF, Shen M, Xu LY, Dong JH, Chen G (2013 May). "13,14-bis(-cis-3,5-dimethyl-1-piperazinyl)-beta-elemene, a novel beta-elemene derivative, shows potent antitumor activities via inhibition of mTOR in human breast cancer cells," Oncol Lett. 5(5):1554-1558.

Di Pasqua R, Betts G, Hoskins N, Edwards M, Ercolini D, Mauriello G (2007 Jun). "Membrane toxicity of antimicrobial compounds from essential oils," J. Agric. Food Chem. 55(12):4863-4870.

Djilani, A., & Dicko, A. (2012 Feb). The Therapeutic Benefits of Essential Oils. In J. Bouayed (Ed.), Nutrition, Well-Being and Health (pp. 155-178): InTech.

Do M, Martins R, Arantes S, Candeias F, Tinoco M.T., Cruz-Morais J (2014 Jan). "Antioxidant, antimicrobial and toxicological properties of Schinus molle L. essential oil.," J. Ethnopharmacol. 151(1):485-92.

Dohare P, Garg P, Sharma U, Jagannathan N, Ray M (2008). "Neuroprotective efficacy and therapeutic window of curcuma oil: in rat embolic stroke model," BMC Complement. Altern. Med. 8(1):55.

Dohare P, Varma S, Ray M (2008 Aug). "Curcuma oil modulates the nitric oxide system response to cerebral ischemia/reperfusion injury," Nitric Oxide. 19(1):1-11.

Domitrović R, Jakovac H, Romić Z, Rahelić D, Tadić Z (2010 Aug 9). "Antifibrotic activity of Taraxacum officinale root in carbon tetrachloride-induced liver damage in mice," J Ethnopharmacol. 130(3):569-77.

Doran AL, Morden WE, Dunn K, Edwards-Jones V (2009 Apr). "Vapour-phase activities of essential oils against antibiotic sensitive and resistant bacteria including MRSA," Lett Appl Microbiol. 48(4):387-92.

Dorman H.J., Deans S.G. (2000 Feb). "Antimicrobial agents from plants: antibacterial activity of plant volatile oils," J. Appl. Microbiol. 88(2):308-316.

Dorow P, Weiss T, Felix R, Schmutzler H (1987 Dec). "[Effect of a secretolytic and a combination of pinene, limonene and cineole on mucociliary clearance in patients with chronic obstructive pulmonary disease]," Arzneimittelforschung. 37(12):1378-1381.

Dozmorov M.G. et al (2014). "Differential effects of selective frankincense (Ru Xiang) essential oil versus non-selective sandalwood (Tan Xiang) essential oil on cultured bladder cancer cells: a microarray and bioinformatics study," Chin Med. 9:18.

Drobiova H, Thomson M, Al-Qattan K, Peltonen-Shalaby R, Al-Amin Z, Ali M (2009 Feb 20). "Garlic increases antioxidant levels in diabetic and hypertensive rats determined by a modified peroxidase method," Evid Based Complement Alternat Med. Epub ahead of print.

Duarte MC, Leme EE, Delarmelina C, Soares AA, Figueira GM, Sartoratto A (2007 May 4). "Activity of essential oils from Brazilian medicinal plants on Escherichia coli," J Ethnopharmacol. 111(2):197-201

Duarte, Luiza C, Speakman John R (2014). "Low resting metabolic rate is associated with greater lifespan because of a confounding effect of body fatness," Age, 36:9731.

Dudai N, Weinstein Y, Krup M, Rabinski T, Ofir R (2005 May). "Citral is a new inducer of caspase-3 in tumor cell lines," Planta Med. 71(5):484-8.

Dunn C, Sleep J, Collett D (1995 Jan). "Sensing an improvement: an experimental study to evaluate the use of aromatherapy, massage and periods of rest in an intensive care unit," J Adv Nurs. 21(1):34-40.

Dunstan JA, Mori TA, Barden A, Beilin LJ, Taylor AL, Holt PG, Prescott SL (2003 Dec). "Fish oil supplementation in pregnancy modifies neonatal allergen-specific immune responses and clinical outcomes in infants at high risk of atopy: a randomized, controlled trial," J Allergy Clin Immunol. 112(6):1178-84.

Duwiejua M, Zeitlin IJ, Waterman PG, Chapman J, Mhango GJ, Provan GJ (1993 Feb). "Anti-inflammatory activity of resins from some species of the plant family Burseraceae," Planta Med. 59(1):12-6.

Dwivedi C, Abu-Ghazaleh A (1997 Aug). "Chemopreventive effects of sandalwood oil on skin papillomas in mice," Eur J Cancer Prev. 6(4):399-401.

Dwivedi C, Guan X, Harmsen WL, Voss AL, Goetz-Parten DE, Koopman EM, Johnson KM, Valluri HB, Matthees DP (2003 Feb). "Chemopreventive effects of alpha-santalol on skin tumor development in CD-1 and SENCAR mice," Cancer Epidemiol Biomarkers Prev. 12(2):151-6.

Dwivedi C, Maydew ER, Hora JJ, Ramaeker DM, Guan X. (2005 Oct). "Chemopreventive effects of various concentrations of alpha-santalol on skin cancer development in CD-1 mice," Eur J Cancer Prev. 14(5):473-6.

Dwivedi C, Valluri HB, Guan X, Agarwal R (2006 Sep). "Chemopreventive effects of alpha-santalol on ultraviolet B radiation-induced skin tumor development in SKH-1 hairless mice," Carcinogenesis. 27(9):1917-22.

Dwyer, L., Oh, A., Patrick, H., & Hennessy, E. (2015). Promoting family meals: a review of existing interventions and opportunities for future research. Adolesc Health Med Ther, 6, 115-131.

Dyer J, Cleary L, Ragsdale-Lowe M, McNeill S, Osland C (2014 Nov). "The use of aromasticks at a cancer centre: a retrospective audit," Complement. Ther. Clin. Pract. 20(4):203-206.

Ebihara T, Ebihara S, Maruyama M, Kobayashi M, Itou A, Arai H, Sasaki H (2006 Sep). "A randomized trial of olfactory stimulation using black pepper oil in older people with swallowing dysfunction," J Am Geriatr Soc. 54(9):1401-6.

Edwards-Jones V, Buck R, Shawcross SG, Dawson MM, Dunn K (2004 Dec). "The effect of essential oils on methicillin-resistant Staphylococcus aureus using a dressing model," Burns. 30(8):772-7.

Elaissi A. et al (2012). "Chemical composition of 8 eucalyptus species' essential oils and the evaluation of their antibacterial, antifungal and antiviral activities," BMC Complement. 12:81.

Ellouze I, Abderrabba M, Sabaou N, Mathieu F, Lebrihi A, Bouajila J (2012 Sep). "Season's variation impact on Citrus aurantium leaves essential oil chemical composition and biological activities," J Food Sci. 77(9):T173-80.

ElSalhy M, Sayed Zahid I, Honkala E (2012 Dec). "Effects of xylitol mouthrinse on Streptococcus mutans," J. Dent. 40(12):1151-1154.

Elson CE, Underbakke GL, Hanson P, Shrago E, Wainberg RH, Qureshi AA (1989 Aug). "Impact of lemongrass oil, an essential oil, on serum cholesterol," Lipids. 24(8):677-9.

El-Soud NH, Deabes M, El-Kassem LA, Khalil M (2015 Sep 15). "Chemical composition and antifungal activity of ocimum basilicum l. essential oil," Open Access Maced J Med Sci. 3(3):374-9.

Elwakeel HA, Moneim HA, Farid M, Gohar AA (2007 Jul). "Clove oil cream: a new effective treatment for chronic anal fissure," Colorectal Dis. 9(6):549-52.

Enan E (2001 Nov). "Insecticidal activity of essential oils: octopaminergic sites of action," Comp Biochem Physiol C Toxicol Pharmacol. 130(3):325-37.

Enshaieh S, Jooya A, Siadat AH, Iraji F (2007 Jan-Feb). "The efficacy of 5% topical tea tree oil gel in mild to moderate acne vulgaris: a randomized, double-blind placebo-controlled study," Indian J Dermatol Venereol Leprol. 73(1):22-5.

Eriksson K., Levin J.O. (1996) Gas chromatographic-mass spectrometric identification of metabolites from α-pinene in human urine after occupational exposure to sawing fumes. J. Chromatography B. 677: 85-98.

Erkkilä AT, Lichtenstein AH, Mozaffarian D, Herrington DM (2004 Sep). "Fish intake is associated with a reduced progression of coronary artery atherosclerosis in postmenopausal women with coronary artery disease," Am J Clin Nutr. 80(3):626-32.

Erkkilä AT, Schwab US, de Mello VD, Lappalainen T, Mussalo H, Lehto S, Kemi V, Lamberg-Allardt C, Uusitupa MI (2008 Sep). "Effects of fatty and lean fish intake on blood pressure in subjects with coronary heart disease using multiple medications," Eur J Nutr. 47(6):319-28.

Esfandiary, E., Karimipour, M., Mardani, M., Alaei, H., Ghannadian, M., Kazemi, M., . . . Esmaeili, A. (2014 Apr). Novel effects of Rosa damascena extract on memory and neurogenesis in a rat model of Alzheimer's disease. J Neurosci Res, 92(4), 517-530.

Evandri MG, Battinelli L, Daniele C, Mastrangelo S, Bolle P, Mazzanti G (2005 Sep). "The antimutagenic activity of Lavandula angustifolia (lavender) essential oil in the bacterial reverse mutation assay," Food Chem Toxicol. 43(9):1381-7.

Evangelista M.T.P., Abad-Casintahan F, Lopez-Villafuerte (2014 Jan). "The effect of topical virgin coconut oil on SCORAD index, transepidermal water loss, and skin capacitance in mild to moderate pediatric atopic dermatitis: a randomized, double-blind, clinical trial," Int J Dermatol. 53(1):100-108.

Evans D.L, Miller D.M., Jacobsen K.L., Bush P.B. (1987). "Modulation of immune responses in mice by d-limonene," J. Toxicol. Environ. Health. 20(1-2):51-66.

Evans J.D., Martin S.A. (2000) Effects of Thymol on Ruminal Microorganisms. Current Microbiology. 41: 336-340.

Ezoddini-Ardakani F (2010 May). "Efficacy of Miswak (salvadora persica) in preventing dental caries," Health (N. Y.). 2(5):499.

Fabio A, Cermelli C, Fabio G, Nicoletti P, Quaglio P (2007 Apr). "Screening of the antibacterial effects of a variety of essential oils on microorganisms responsible for respiratory infections," Phytother Res. 21(4):374-7.

Fan AY, Lao L, Zhang RX, Zhou AN, Wang LB, Moudgil KD, Lee DY, Ma ZZ, Zhang WY, Berman BM (2005 Oct 3). "Effects of an acetone extract of Boswellia carterii Birdw. (Burseraceae) gum resin on adjuvant-induced arthritis in lewis rats," J Ethnopharmacol. 101(1-3):104-9.

Fahn, A. (1988). Secretory tissues in vascular plants. New Phytologist, 108(3), 229-257.

Falk A.J., Bauer L., Bell C.L., Smolenski S.J. (1974 Dec). "The constituents of the essential oil from Achillea millefolium L," Lloydia. 37(4):598-602.

Fang, J. Y., Leu, Y. L., Hwang, T. L., & Cheng, H. C. (2004 Nov). Essential oils from sweet basil (Ocimum basilicum) as novel enhancers to accelerate transdermal drug delivery. Biol Pharm Bull, 27(11), 1819-1825.

Fang, Y.-Z., Yang, S., & Wu, G. (2002). Free radicals, antioxidants, and nutrition. Nutrition, 18(10), 872-879.

Farco J.A., Grundmann O. (2013). "Menthol--pharmacology of an important naturally medicinal 'cool,'" Mini Rev. Med. Chem. 13(1):124-131.

Farnsworth, N. R., & Soejarto, D. D. (1985). Potential consequence of plant extinction in the United States on the current and future availability of prescription drugs. Economic botany, 39(3), 231-240.

Farris PK (2005 Jul). "Topical vitamin C: a useful agent for treating photoaging and other dermatologic conditions," Dermatol Surg. 31(7 Pt 2):814-7

Fathiazad, F., Matlobi, A., Khorrami, A., Hamedeyazdan, S., Soraya, H., Hammami, M., . . . Garjani, A. (2012 Jan). Phytochemical screening and evaluation of cardioprotective activity of ethanolic extract of Ocimum basilicum L. (basil) against isoproterenol induced myocardial infarction in rats. Daru, 20(1), 87.

Faturi, C. B., Leite, J. R., Alves, P. B., Canton, A. C., & Teixeira-Silva, F. (2010 May). Anxiolytic-like effect of sweet orange aroma in Wistar rats. Prog Neuropsychopharmacol Biol Psychiatry, 34(4), 605-609.

Fayazi S, Babashahi M, Rezaei M (2011). "The effect of inhalation aromatherapy on anxiety level of the patients in preoperative period," Iran. J. Nurs. Midwifery Res. 16(4):278-283.

Feinblatt HM (1960 Jan). "Cajeput-type oil for the treatment of furunculosis," J Natl Med Assoc. 52:32-4.

Feng J, Zhang S, Shi W, Zubcevik N, Miklossy J, Zhang Y (2017 Oct). "Selective Essential Oils from Spice or Culinary Herbs Have High Activity against Stationary Phase and Biofilm Borrelia burgdorferi," Front Med (Lausanne). 4:169.

Fernandez, L. F., Palomino, O. M., & Frutos, G. (2014 Jan). Effectiveness of Rosmarinus officinalis essential oil as antihypotensive agent in primary hypotensive patients and its influence on health-related quality of life. J Ethnopharmacol, 151(1), 509-516.

Ferrara, L., Naviglio, D., & Armone Caruso, A. (2012). Cytological aspects on the effects of a nasal spray consisting of standardized extract of citrus lemon and essential oils in allergic rhinopathy. ISRN Pharm, 2012, 1-6.

Ferreira B.S. et al (2011 Jul). "Comparative Properties of Amazonian Oils Obtained by Different Extraction Methods," Molecules. 16(7):5875-5885.

Ferrini AM, Mannoni V, Aureli P, Salvatore G, Piccirilli E, Ceddia T, Pontieri E, Sessa R, Oliva B (2006 Jul-Sep). "Melaleuca alternifolia essential oil possesses potent anti-staphylococcal activity extended to strains resistant to antibiotics," Int J Immunopathol Pharmacol. 19(3):539-44.

Field T, Diego M, Hernandez-Reif M, Cisneros W, Feijo L, Vera Y, Gil K, Grina D, Claire He Q (2005 Feb). "Lavender fragrance cleansing gel effects on relaxation," Int J Neurosci. 115(2):207-22.

Filiptsove O.V., Gazzavi-Rogozina L.V., Timoshyna I.A., Naboka O.I., Dyomina Y.V., Ochkur A.V (2018 Mar). "The effect of the essential oils of lavender and rosemary on the human short-term memory," Alex. J. Med. 54(1):41-44.

Filoche SK, Soma K, Sissons CH (2005 Aug). "Antimicrobial effects of essential oils in combination with chlorhexidine digluconate," Oral Microbiol Immunol. 20(4):221-5.

Fine DH, Furgang D, Barnett ML, Drew C, Steinberg L, Charles CH, Vincent JW (2000 Mar). "Effect of an essential oil-containing antiseptic mouthrinse on plaque and salivary Streptococcus mutans levels," J Clin Periodontol. 27(3):157-61.

Fitzhugh DJ, Shan S, Dewhirst MW, Hale LP (2008 Jul). "Bromelain treatment decreases neutrophil migration to sites of inflammation," Clin Immunol. 128(1):66-74.

Flor-Weiler, L. B., Behle, R. W., & Stafford, K. C., 3rd. (2011 Mar). Susceptibility of four tick species, Amblyomma americanum, Dermacentor variabilis, Ixodes scapularis, and Rhipicephalus sanguineus (Acari: Ixodidae), to nootkatone from essential oil of grapefruit. J Med Entomol, 48(2), 322-326.

Force M, Sparks WS, Ronzio RA (2000 May). "Inhibition of enteric parasites by emulsified oil of oregano in vivo," Phytother Res. 14(3):213-4.

Fowke JH, Morrow JD, Motley S, Bostick RM, Ness RM (2006 Oct). "Brassica vegetable consumption reduces urinary F2-isoprostane levels independent of micronutrient intake," Carcinogenesis. 27(10):2096-102.

Franek KJ, Zhou Z, Zhang WD, Chen WY (2005 Jan). "In vitro studies of baicalin alone or in combination with Salvia miltiorrhiza extract as a potential anti-cancer agent," Int J Oncol. 26(1):217-24.

Frangou S, Lewis M, McCrone P (2006 Jan). "Efficacy of ethyl-eicosapentaenoic acid in bipolar depression: randomised double-blind placebo-controlled study," Br J Psychiatry. 188:46-50.

Frank K, Patel K, Lopez G, Willis B (2017 Jun). "Coconut Oil Research Analysis," Examine.com.

Frank M.B. et al (2009). "Frankincense oil derived from Boswellia carteri induces tumor cell specific cytotoxicity," BMC Complement Altern Med. 9:6.

Fraňková A, Marounek M, Mozrová V, Weber J, Klouček P, Lukešová D (2014 Oct). "Antibacterial activities of plant-derived compounds and essential oils toward Cronobacter sakazakii and Cronobacter malonaticus," Foodborne Pathog. Dis. 11(10):795-797.

Freires Ide, A., Murata, R. M., Furletti, V. F., Sartoratto, A., Alencar, S. M., Figueira, G. M., . . . Rosalen, P. L. (2014 Jun). Coriandrum sativum L. (Coriander) Essential Oil: Antifungal Activity and Mode of Action on Candida spp., and Molecular Targets Affected in Human Whole-Genome Expression. PLoS ONE, 9(6), 1-13.

Freise J, Köhler S (1999 Mar). "Peppermint oil-caraway oil fixed combination in non-ulcer dyspepsia--comparison of the effects of enteric preparations," Pharmazie. 54(3):210-5.

Freitas F.P., Freitas S.P., Lemos G.C.S., Vieira I.J.C., Gravina G.A., Lemos F.J.A. (2010) Comparative Larvicial Activity of Essential Oils from Three Medicinal Plants against Aedes aeypti L. Chemistry & Biodiversity. 7: 2801-2807.

Frontera WR, Meredith CN, O'Reilly KP, Knuttgen HG, Evans WJ (1988 Mar). "Strength conditioning in older men: skeletal muscle hypertrophy and improved function," J Appl Physiol, 64(3):1038-44.

Frydman-Marom, A., Levin, A., Farfara, D., Benromano, T., Scherzer-Attali, R., Peled, S., . . . Ovadia, M. (2011 Feb). Orally administered cinnamon extract reduces beta-amyloid oligomerization and corrects cognitive impairment in Alzheimer's disease animal models. PLoS ONE, 6(1), 1-11.

Fu Y. et al (2007 Oct). "Antimicrobial activity of clove and rosemary essential oils alone and in combination," Phytother. Res. PTR. 21(10):989-994.

Fu Y. et al (2009). "The antibacterial activity of clove essential oil against Propionibacterium acnes and its mechanism of action," Arch. Dermatol. 145(1):86-88.

Fukada M, Kano E, Miyoshi M, Komaki R, Watanabe T (2012 May). "Effect of 'Rose Essential Oil' Inhalation on Stress-Induced Skin-Barrier Disruption in Rats and Humans," Chemical Senses. 37(4):347-356.

Fukumoto S, Sawasaki E, Okuyama S, Miyake Y, Yokogoshi H (2006 Feb-Apr). "Flavor components of monoterpenes in citrus essential oils enhance the release of monoamines from rat brain slices," Nutr Neurosci. 9(1-2):73-80.

Furuhjelm C, Warstedt K, Larsson J, Fredriksson M, Böttcher MF, Fälth-Magnusson K, Duchén K (2009 Sep). "Fish oil supplementation in pregnancy and lactation may decrease the risk of infant allergy," Acta Paediatr. 98(9):1461-7.

Gaetani G.F., Ferraris A.M., Rolfo M., Mangerini R., Arena S., Kirkman H.N. (1996) Predominant role of catalase in the disposal of hydrogen peroxide within human erythrocytes. Blood. 87: 1595-1599.

Ganesan B, Buddhan S, Anandan R, Sivakumar R, AnbinEzhilan R. (2010 Mar). "Antioxidant defense of betaine against isoprenaline-induced myocardial infarction in rats," Mol Biol Rep. 37(3):1319-27.

Gauch L.M.R. et al (2014 Jun). "Effects of Rosmarinus officinalis essential oil on germ tube formation by Candida albicans isolated from denture wearers," Rev. Soc. Bras. Med. Trop. 47(3):389-391.

Gaunt L.F., Higgins S.C., Hughes J.F. (2005) Interaction of air ions and bactericidal vapours to control micro-organisms. Journal of Applied Microbiology. 99: 1324-1329.

Gayathri B, Manjula N, Vinaykumar KS, Lakshmi BS, Balakrishnan A (2007 Apr). "Pure compound from Boswellia serrata extract exhibits anti-inflammatory property in human PBMCs and mouse macrophages through inhibition of TNFalpha, IL-1beta, NO and MAP kinases," Int Immunopharmacol. 7(4):473-82.

Gbenou J. D., Ahounou, J. F., Akakpo, H. B., Laleye, A., Yayi, E., Gbaguidi, F., . . . Kotchoni, S. O. (2013 Feb). Phytochemical composition of Cymbopogon citratus and Eucalyptus citriodora essential oils and their anti-inflammatory and analgesic properties on Wistar rats. Mol Biol Rep, 40(2), 1127-1134.

Gershenzon, J. (1994 Jun). Metabolic costs of terpenoid accumulation in higher plants. J Chem Ecol, 20(6), 1281-1328.

Ghelardini C, Galeotti N, Di Cesare Mannelli L, Mazzanti G, Bartolini A (2001 May-Jul). "Local anaesthetic activity of beta-caryophyllene," Farmaco. 56(5-7):387-9.

Ghelardini C, Galeotti N, Mazzanti G (2001 Aug). "Local anaesthetic activity of monoterpenes and phenylpropanes of essential oils," Planta Med. 67(6):564-6.

Ghelardini C, Galeotti N, Salvatore G, Mazzanti G (1999 Dec). "Local anaesthetic activity of the essential oil of Lavandula angustifolia," Planta Med. 65(8):700-3.

Ghersetich I, Lotti T, Campanile G, Grappone C, Dini G (1994 Feb). "Hyaluronic acid in cutaneous intrinsic aging," Int J Dermatol. 33(2):119-22.

Ghods A.A., Abforosh N.H., Ghorbani R, Asgari M.R. (2015 Jun). "The effect of topical application of lavender essential oil on the intensity of pain caused by the insertion of dialysis needles in hemodialysis patients: A randomized clinical trial," Complement. Ther. Med. 23(3):325-330.

Ghosh, V., Saranya, S., Mukherjee, A., & Chandrasekaran, N. (2013 May). Antibacterial microemulsion prevents sepsis and triggers healing of wound in wistar rats. Colloids Surf B Biointerfaces, 105, 152-157.

Gibriel, A., Al-Sayed, H., Rady, A., & Abdelaleem, M. (2013 Jun). Synergistic antibacterial activity of irradiated and nonirradiated cumin, thyme and rosemary essential oils. Journal of Food Safety, 33(2), 222-228.

Gilani, A. H., Jabeen, Q., Khan, A. U., & Shah, A. J. (2008 Feb). Gut modulatory, blood pressure lowering, diuretic and sedative activities of cardamom. J Ethnopharmacol, 115(3), 463-472.

Gillissen A, Wittig T, Ehmen M, Krezdorn H.G., de Mey C (2013 Jan). "A multi-centre, randomised, double-blind, placebo-controlled clinical trial on the efficacy and tolerability of GeloMyrtol® forte in acute bronchitis," Drug Res. 63(1):19-27.

Gnatta J.R., Piason P.P., de C, Lopes L.B.C., Rogenski N.M.B., da Silva M.J.P. (2014 Jun). "[Aromatherapy with ylang ylang for anxiety and self-esteem: a pilot study]," Rev. Esc. Enferm. Ú P. 48(3):492-499.

Göbel H, Schmidt G, Soyka D (1994 Jun). "Effect of peppermint and eucalyptus oil preparations on neurophysiological and experimental algesimetric headache parameters," Cephalalgia. 14(3):228-34.

Goel A, Ahmad FJ, Singh RM, Singh GN (2010 Feb). "3-Acetyl-11-keto-beta-boswellic acid loaded-polymeric nanomicelles for topical anti-inflammatory and anti-arthritic activity," J Pharm Pharmacol. 62(2):273-8.

Goel N, Kim H, Lao R.P. (2005). "An olfactory stimulus modifies nighttime sleep in young men and women," Chronobiol. Int. 22(5):889-904.

Goes, T. C., Antunes, F. D., Alves, P. B., & Teixeira-Silva, F. (2012 Aug). Effect of sweet orange aroma on experimental anxiety in humans. J Altern Complement Med, 18(8), 798-804.

Golab M, Skwarlo-Sonta K (2007 Mar). "Mechanisms involved in the anti-inflammatory action of inhaled tea tree oil in mice," Exp Biol Med (Maywood). 232(3):420-6.

Goldberg, D. R. (2009). Aspirin: Turn of the Century Miracle Drug. Chemical Heritage Magazine, 27.

Gomes NM, Rezende CM, Fontes SP, Matheus ME, Fernandes PD. (2007 Feb 12). "Antinociceptive activity of Amazonian Copaiba oils," J Ethnopharmacol. 109(3):486-92.

Gómez-Rincón, C., Langa, E., Murillo, P., Valero, M. S., Berzosa, C., & López, V. (2014 May). Activity of Tea Tree (Melaleuca alternifolia) Essential Oil against L3 Larvae of Anisakis simplex. 2014, 1-6.

Goncalves J.C.R., Alves A.M.H., de Araujo A.E.V., Cruz J.S., Araujo D.A.M. (2010) Distinct effects of carvone analogues on the isolated nerve of rats. European Journal of Pharmacology. 645: 108-112.

Goncalves J.C.R., Oliveira F.S., Benedito R.B., de Sousa D.P., de Almeida R.N., Araujo D.A.M. (2008) Antinociceptive Activity of (-)-Carvone: Evidence of Association with Decreased Peripheral Nerve Excitability. Biological and Parmaceutical Bulletin. 31: 1017-1020.

Gonzalez-Audino P, Picollo M.I., Gallardo A, Toloza A, Vassena C, Mougabure-Cueto G (2011 Jul). "Comparative toxicity of oxygenated monoterpenoids in experimental hydroalcoholic lotions to permethrin resistant adult head lice," Arch. Dermatol. 303(5):361-366.

Gonzalez-Castejon, M., Garcia-Carrasco, B., Fernandez-Dacosta, R., Davalos, A., & Rodriguez-Casado, A. (2014 May). Reduction of adipogenesis and lipid accumulation by Taraxacum officinale (Dandelion) extracts in 3T3L1 adipocytes: an in vitro study. Phytother Res, 28(5), 745-752.

González-Trujano ME, Peña EI, Martínez AL, Moreno J, Guevara-Fefer P, Déciga-Campos M, López-Muñoz FJ (2007 May 22). "Evaluation of the antinociceptive effect of Rosmarinus officinalis L. using three different experimental models in rodents," J Ethnopharmacol. 111(3):476-82.

Goodpaster, Bret H, Chomentowski, Peter, Ward, Bryan K, Rossi, Andrea, Glynn, Nancy W, Delmonico, Matthew J, Kritchevsky, Stephen B, Pahor, Marco, Newman, Anne B (2008 Sep). "Effects of physical activity on strength and skeletal muscle fat infiltration in older adults: a randomized controlled trial," J Appl Physiol. 105:1498-503.

Goodwin J.S., Atluru D., Sierakowski S., Lianos E.A. (1986) Mechanism of Action of Glucocorticosteroids: Inhibition of T Cell Proliferation and Interleukin 2 Production by Hydrocortisones Is Reversed by Leukotriene B4. Journal of Clinical Investigation. 77: 1244-1250.

Gorwitz R.J., Kruszon-Moran D., McAllister S.K., McQuillan G., McDougal L.K., Fosheim G.E., Jensen B.J., Killgore G., Tenover F.C., Kuehnert M.J. (2008) Changes in the Prevalence of Nasal Colonization with Staphylococcus aureusin the United States, 2001-2004. Journal of Infectious Diseases. 197: 1226-1234.

Gossell-Williams M, Hyde C, Hunter T, Simms-Stewart D, Fletcher H, McGrowder D, Walters CA (2011 Oct). "Improvement in HDL cholesterol in postmenopausal women supplemented with pumpkin seed oil: pilot study," Climacteric. 14(5):558-64.

Goswami, S. K., Inamdar, M. N., Jamwal, R., & Dethe, S. (2014 Jun). Effect of Cinnamomum cassia Methanol Extract and Sildenafil on Arginase and Sexual Function of Young Male Wistar Rats. J Sex Med, 11(6), 1475-1483.

Goswami, S. K., Inamdar, M. N., Jamwal, R., & Dethe, S. (2013 Dec). Efficacy of Cinnamomum cassia Blume. in age induced sexual dysfunction of rats. J Young Pharm, 5(4), 148-153.

Grassmann J, Hippeli S, Dornisch K, Rohnert U, Beuscher N, Elstner EF (2000 Feb). "Antioxidant properties of essential oils. Possible explanations for their anti-inflammatory effects," Arzneimittelforschung. 50(2):135-9.

Grassmann J, Schneider D, Weiser D, Elstner EF (2001 Oct). "Antioxidative effects of lemon oil and its components on copper induced oxidation of low density lipoprotein," Arzneimittelforschung. 51(10):799-805.

Greche, H., Hajjaji, N., Ismaïli-Alaoui, M., Mrabet, N., and Benjilali, B. (2000). "Chemical Composition and Antifungal Properties of the Essential Oil of Tanacetum annuum," J Essential Oil Research. 12(1):122-124.

Greive, K.A., & Barnes T.M. (2017 Mar. 7). "The efficacy of Australian essential oils for the treatment of head lice infestation in children: A randomised controlled trial," Australas J Dermatol. Epub ahead of print.

Grespan, R., Paludo, M., Lemos Hde, P., Barbosa, C. P., Bersani-Amado, C. A., Dalalio, M. M., & Cuman, R. K. (2012 Oct). Anti-arthritic effect of eugenol on collagen-induced arthritis experimental model. Biol Pharm Bull, 35(10), 1818-1820.

Grether-Beck, S., Muhlberg, K., Brenden, H., & Krutmann, J. (2008 Jul). [Topical application of vitamins, phytosterols and ceramides. Protection against increased expression of interstitial collagenase and reduced collagen-I expression after single exposure to UVA irradiation]. Hautarzt, 59(7), 557-562.

Grigoleit HG, Grigoleit P (2005 Aug). "Peppermint oil in irritable bowel syndrome," Phytomedicine. 12(8):601-6.

Grunebaum L.D., Murdock J, Castanedo-Tardan M.P., Basumann L.S. (2011 Jun). "Effects of lavender olfactory input on cosmetic procedures," J. Cosmet. Dermatol. 10(2):89-93.

Gonzalez, J. T., & Stevenson, E. J. (2012 Aug 3). Postprandial glycemia and appetite sensations in response to porridge made with rolled and pinhead oats. J Am Coll Nutr, 31(2), 111-116.

Gross, M., Nesher, E., Tikhonov, T., Raz, O., & Pinhasov, A. (2013 Mar). Chronic food administration of Salvia sclarea oil reduces animals' anxious and dominant behavior. J Med Food, 16(3), 216-222.

Guang, L., Li-Bin, Z., Bing-An, F., Ming-Yang, Q., Li-Hua, Y., and Ji-Hong, X. (2004). "Inhibition of growth and metastasis of human gastric cancer implanted in nude mice by d-limonene," World J. Gastroentero. 10: 2140-2144.

Guerra-Boone L, Alvarez-Román R, Salazar-Aranda R, Torres-Cirio A, Rivas-Galindo VM, Waksman de Torres N, González González GM, Pérez-López LA (2013 Jan). "Chemical compositions and antimicrobial and antioxidant activities of the essential oils from Magnolia grandiflora, Chrysactinia mexicana, and Schinus molle found in northeast Mexico," Nat Prod Commun. 8(1):135-8.

Guillemin J, Rousseau A, Delaveau P (1989). "Neurodepressive effects of the essential oil of Lavandula angustifolia Mill," Ann Pharm Fr. 47(6):337-43.

Guimarães A.G., Quintans J.S.S., Quintans-Júnior L.J. (2013 Jan). "Monoterpenes with Analgesic ActivityA Systematic Review: MONOTERPENES WITH ANALGESIC ACTIVITY," Phytother. Res. 27(1):1-15.

Gumral, N., Doguc Kumbul, D., Aylak, F., Saygin, M., & Savik, E. (2013 Jan). Juniperus communis Linn oil decreases oxidative stress and increases antioxidant enzymes in the heart of rats administered a diet rich in cholesterol. Toxicol Ind Health.

Gundidza M (1993 Nov). "Antimicrobial activity of essential oil from Schinus molle Linn," Cent Afr J Med. 39(11):231-4.

Guo X., Longnecker M.P., Michalek J.E. (2001) Relation of serum tetrachlorodibenzo-p-dioxin concentration to diet among veterans in the Air Force health study with background-level exposure. Journal of Toxicology and Environmental Health, Part A. 63: 159-172.

Guo, X.M., Lu, Q., Liu, Z.J., Wang, L.F., & Feng, B.A. (2006 Aug.). "[Effects of D-limonene on leukemia cells HL-60 and K562 in vitro]," Zhongguo Shi Yan Xue Ye Xue Za Zhi. 14(4):692-5.

Gupta A., Myrdal P.B. (2004) Development of perillyl alcohol topical cream formulation. International Journal of Pharmaceutics. 269: 373-383.

Gurney AM. (1994) Mechanisms of Drug-induced Vasodilation. Journal of Pharmacy and Pharmacology. 46: 242-251.

Guzmán-Gutiérrez S.L., Bonilla-Jaime H., Gómez-Cansino R., Reyes-Chilpa R (2015 May). "Linalool and βpinene exert their antidepressant-like activity through the monoaminergic pathway," Life Sci. 128:24-29.

Haag J.D., Lindstrom M.J., Gould M.N. (1992) Limonene-induced Regression of Mammary Carcinomas. Cancer Research. 52: 4021-4026.

Habashy, R. R., Abdel-Naim, A. B., Khalifa, A. E., & Al-Azizi, M. M. (2005 Feb). Anti-inflammatory effects of jojoba liquid wax in experimental models. Pharmacol Res, 51(2), 95-105.

Hadley SK, Gaarder SM (2005 Dec 15). "Treatment of irritable bowel syndrome," Am Fam Physician. 72(12):2501-6.

Hagen TM, Liu J, Lykkesfeldt J, Wehr CM, Ingersoll RT, Vinarsky V, Bartholomew JC, Ames BN. "Feeding acetyl-L-carnitine and lipoic acid to old rats significantly improves metabolic function while decreasing oxidative stress," Proc Natl Acad Sci U S A. 99(4):1870-5.

Hager K, Kenklies M, McAfoose J, Engel J, Münch G (2007). "Alpha-lipoic acid as a new treatment option for Alzheimer's disease--a 48 months follow-up analysis," J Neural Transm Suppl. (72):189-93.

Hajhashemi V, Abbasi N (2008 Mar). "Hypolipidemic activity of Anethum graveolens in rats," Phytother Res. 22(3):372-5.

Hajhashemi V, Ghannadi A, Sharif B (2003 Nov). "Anti-inflammatory and analgesic properties of the leaf extracts and essential oil of Lavandula angustifolia Mill," J Ethnopharmacol. 89(1):67-71.

Hajhashemi V, Zolfaghari B, Yousefi A (2012). "Antinociceptive and anti-inflammatory activity of Satureja hortensis seed essential oil, hydroalcoholic and polyphenolic extracts in animal models," Med Princ Pract. 21(2):178-82.

Hakim IA, Harris RB, Ritenbaugh C (2000). "Citrus peel use is associated with reduced risk of squamous cell carcinoma of the skin," Nutr Cancer. 37(2):161-8.

Hakim I.A., McClure T, Liebler D (2000 Aug). "Assessing Dietary D-Limonene Intake for Epidemiological Studies," J. Food Compos. Anal. 13(4):329-336.

Halder, S., Mehta, A. K., Kar, R., Mustafa, M., Mediratta, P. K., & Sharma, K. K. (2011 May). Clove oil reverses learning and memory deficits in scopolamine-treated mice. Planta Med, 77(8), 830-834.

Halder, S., Mehta, A. K., Mediratta, P. K., & Sharma, K. K. (2011 Aug). Essential oil of clove (Eugenia caryophyllata) augments the humoral immune response but decreases cell mediated immunity. Phytother Res, 25(8), 1254-1256.

Halm M.A., Baker C, Harshe V (2014 Dec). "Effect of an Essential Oil Mixture on Skin Reactions in Women Undergoing Radiotherapy for Breast Cancer: A Pilot Study," Journal of Holistic Nursing. 32(4):290-303.

Hamada M, Uezu K, Matsushita J, Yamamoto S, Kishino Y (2002 Apr). "Distribution and immune responses resulting from oral administration of D-limonene in rats," J. Nutr. Sci. Vitaminol. (Tokyo) 48(2):155-160.

Hammer KA, Carson CF, Riley TV (2008 Aug). "Frequencies of resistance to Melaleuca alternifolia (tea tree) oil and rifampicin in Staphylococcus aureus, Staphylococcus epidermidis and Enterococcus faecalis," Int J Antimicrob Agents. 32(2):170-3.

Hammer KA, Carson CF, Riley TV (1996 Jun). "Susceptibility of transient and commensal skin flora to the essential oil of Melaleuca alternifolia (tea tree oil)," J Antimicrob Chemother. 24(3):186-9.

Hammer KA, Carson CF, Riley TV (2004 Jun). "Antifungal effects of Melaleuca alternifolia (tea tree) oil and its components on Candida albicans, Candida glabrata and Saccharomyces cerevisiae," J Antimicrob Chemother. 53(6):1081-5.

Hancianu M, Cioanca O, Mihasan M, Hritcu L (2013 Mar). "Neuroprotective effects of inhaled lavender oil on scopolamine-induced dementia via anti-oxidative activities in rats," Phytomedicine Int. J. Phytother. Phytopharm. 20(5):446-452.

Han, S. H., Hur, M. H., Buckle, J., Choi, J., & Lee, M. S. (2006 Aug). Effect of aromatherapy on symptoms of dysmenorrhea in college students: A randomized placebo-controlled clinical trial. J Altern Complement Med, 12(6), 535-541.

Han, X. Gibson, J., Eggett, D.L., & Parker, T.L. "Bergamot (Citrus bergamia) Essential Oil Inhalation Improves Positive Feelings in the Waiting Room of a Mental Health Treatment Center: A Pilot Study," Phytother Res. 31(5):812-816.

Han X, Parker TL (2017 Feb 20). "Arborvitae (thuja plicata) essential oil significantly inhibited critical inflammation—and tissue remodeling—related proteins and genes in human dermal fibroblasts," Biochim Open. 4:56-6.

Han X, Parker TL (2017 Mar 3). "Anti-inflammatory, tissue remodeling, immunomodulatory, and anticancer activities of oregano (origanum vulgare) essential oil in a human skin disease model," Biochim Open. 4:73-77.

Han X, Parker TL (2017 Mar 21). "Lemongrass (cymbopogon flexuosus) essential oil demonstrated anti-inflammatory effect in pre-inflamed human dermal fibroblasts," Biochim Open. 4:107-111.

Han, X., & Parker, T.L. (2017 Jul). "Antiinflammatory Activity of Cinnamon (Cinnamomum zeylanicum) Bark Essential Oil in a Human Skin Disease Model," Phytother Res. 31(7):1034-1038.

Han, X., & Parker, T.L. (2017 Dec.). "Anti-inflammatory activity of clove (Eugenia caryophyllata) essential oil in human dermal fibroblasts," Pharm Biol. 55(1):1619-1622.

Han XJ, Wang YD, Chen YC, Lin LY, Wu QK (2013 Oct). "Transcriptome Sequencing and Expression Analysis of Terpenoid Biosynthesis Genes in Litsea cubeba," PLoS ONE. 8(10):e76890.

Hanus L.O., Rezanka T., Dembitsky V.M., Moussaieff A. (2005 Jun). "Myrrh--Commiphora chemistry," Biomed. Pap. Med. Fac. Univ. Palacký Olomouc Czechoslov. 149(1):3-27.

Haque M.M., Alsareii S.A. (2015 May). "A review of the therapeutic effects of using miswak (Salvadora Persica) on oral health," Saudi Med. J. 36(5):530-543.

Hargreaves IP, Lane A, Sleiman PM (2008 Dec 5). "The coenzyme Q(10) status of the brain regions of Parkinson's disease patients," Neurosci Lett. 447(1):17-9.

Hart PH, Brand C, Carson CF, Riley TV, Prager RH, Finlay-Jones JJ (2000 Nov). "Terpinen-4-ol, the main component of the essential oil of Melaleuca alternifolia (tea tree oil), suppresses inflammatory mediator production by activated human monocytes," Inflamm Res. 49(11):619-26.

Harv Womens Health Watch (2013 Oct). "Staying mentally active throughout life preserves brain health," 21(2):8.

Hastak K. et al (1997). "Effect of turmeric oil and turmeric oleoresin on cytogenetic damage in patients suffering from oral submucous fibrosis," Cancer Lett. 116(2):265-269.

Hayashi N, Togawa K, Yanagisawa M, Hosogi J, Mimura D, Yamamoto Y, (2003). "Effect of sunlight exposure and aging on skin surface lipids and urate," Ex Dermatol. 12 Suppl 2:13-7.

Hay IC, Jamieson M, Ormerod AD (1998 Nov). "Randomized trial of aromatherapy. Successful treatment for alopecia areata," Arch Dermatol. 135(5):1349-52.

Hayes AJ, Markovic B (2002 Apr). "Toxicity of Australian essential oil Backhousia citriodora (Lemon myrtle). Part 1. Antimicrobial activity and in vitro cytotoxicity," Food Chem Toxicol. 40(4):535-43.

Hayflick L (1979 Jul). "The cell biology of aging," J Invest Dermatol. 73(1):8-14.

Hayouni E.A. et al (2008 Jul). "Tunisian Salvia officinalis L. and Schinus molle L. essential oils: their chemical compositions and their preservative effects against Salmonella inoculated in minced beef meat," Int. J. Food Microbiol. 125(3):242-51.

Haze S, Sakai K, Gozu Y (2002 Nov). "Effects of fragrance inhalation on sympathetic activity in normal adults," Jpn J Pharmacol 90(3):247-53.

Haze, S., Sakai, K., Gozu, Y., & Moriyama, M. (2010 Jul). Grapefruit oil attenuates adipogenesis in cultured subcutaneous adipocytes. Planta Med, 76(10), 950-955.

Hazgui S et al. (2008 Apr). "Epigallocatechin-3-gallate (EGCG) inhibits the migratory behavior of tumor bronchial epithelial cells," Respir Res. 9:33.

He M, Du M, Fan M, Bian Z (2007 Mar). "In vitro activity of eugenol against Candida albicans biofilms," Mycopathologia. 163(3):137-143.

Helland IB, Smith L, Saarem K, Saugstad OD, Drevon CA (2003 Jan). "Maternal supplementation with very-long-chain n-3 fatty acids during pregnancy and lactation augments children's IQ at 4 years of age," Pediatrics. 111(1):e39-44.

Herman A, Tambor K (2016 Feb). "Linalool Affects the Antimicrobial Efficacy of Essential Oils," Curr. Microbiol. 72(2):165-172.

Herman, C. P., Roth, D. A., & Polivy, J. (2003). Effects of the presence of others on food intake: a normative interpretation. Psychological Bulletin, 129(6), 873-886.

Herz, R. S., & Engen, T. (1996 Sep). Odor memory: Review and analysis. Psychon Bull Rev, 3(3), 300-313.

Heuberger, E., Hongratanaworakit, T., & Buchbauer, G. (2006 Aug). East Indian sandalwood and alpha-santalol odor increase physiological and self-rated arousal in humans. Planta Med, 72(9), 792-800.

Heydari N, Abootalebi M, Jamalimoghadam N, Kasraeian M, Emamghoreishi M, Akbarzaded M (2018 May 22). "Evaluation of aromatherapy with essential oils of rosa damascena for the management of premenstrual syndrome," Int J Gynaecol Obstet.

Hiramatsu N, Xiufen W, Takechi R, Itoh Y, Mamo J, Pal S (2004). "Antimutagenicity of Japanese traditional herbs, gennoshoko, yomogi, senburi and iwa-tobacco," Biofactors. 22(1-4):123-5.

Hirota R, Roger N.N., Nakamura H, Song HS, Sawamura M, Suganuma N (2010 Apr). "Antiinflammatory effects of limonene from yuzu (Citrus junos Tanaka) essential oil on eosinophils," J. Food Sci. 75(3):H87-92.

Hitokoto H, Morozumi S, Wauke T, Sakai S, Kurata H (1980 Apr). "Inhibitory effects of spices on growth and toxin production of toxigenic fungi," Appl Environ Microbiol. 39(4):818-22.

Ho C, Spence C (2005 Nov). "Olfactory facilitation of dual-task performance," Neurosci. Lett. 389(1):35-40.

Hojsak, I, Snovak N, Abdovic S, Szajewska H, Misak Z, Kolacek S (2009). "Lactobacillus GG in the prevention of gastrointestinal and respiratory tract infections in children who attend day care centers: A randomized, double-blind, placebo-controlled trial," Clin. Nutr. 29(3):312-6.

Holmes C, Hopkins V, Hensford C, MacLaughlin V, Wilkinson D, Rosenvinge H (2002 Apr). "Lavender oil as a treatment for agitated behaviour in severe dementia: a placebo controlled study," Int. J. 17(4):305-308.Geriatr. Psychiatry

Hölzle E (1992 Sep). "Pigmented lesions as a sign of photodamage," Br J Dermatol. 17(Suppl 41):48-50.

Hong SL et al (2014). "Essential oil content of the rhizome of Curcuma purpurascens Bl. (Temu Tis) and its antiproliferative effect on selected human carcinoma cell lines," ScientificWorldJournal. 2014:397430.

Hongratanaworakit T (2009 Feb). "Relaxing effect of rose oil on humans," Nat Prod Commun. 4(2):291-6.

Hongratanaworakit T (2011 Aug). "Aroma-therapeutic effects of massage blended essential oils on humans," Nat. Prod. Commun. 6(8):1199-1204.

Hongratanaworakit T, Buchbauer G (2004 Jul). "Evaluation of the harmonizing effect of ylang-ylang oil on humans after inhalation," Planta Med. 70(7):632-6.

Hongratanaworakit T, Buchbauer G (2006 Sep). "Relaxing effect of ylang ylang oil on humans after transdermal absorption," Phytother Res. 20(9):758-63.

Hongratanaworakit, T., Heuberger, E., & Buchbauer, G. (2004 Jan). Evaluation of the effects of East Indian sandalwood oil and alpha-santalol on humans after transdermal absorption. Planta Med, 70(1), 3-7.

Holloszy JO, (1967 May). "Biochemical adaptations in muscle. Effects of exercise on mitochondrial oxygen uptake and respiratory enzyme activity in skeletal muscle," J Biol Chem, 242(9):2278-82.

Hosseini, M., Ghasemzadeh Rahbardar, M., Sadeghnia, H. R., & Rakhshandeh, H. (2011 Oct). Effects of different extracts of Rosa damascena on pentylenetetrazol-induced seizures in mice. Zhong Xi Yi Jie He Xue Bao, 9(10), 1118-1124.

Hosseini, M., Jafarianheris, T., Seddighi, N., Parvaneh, M., Ghorbani, A., Sadeghnia, H. R., & Rakhshandeh, H. (2012). Effects of different extracts of Eugenia caryophyllata on pentylenetetrazole-induced seizures in mice. Zhong Xi Yi Jie He Xue Bao, 10(12), 1476-1481.

Hosseinzadeh, H., Karimi, G. R., & Ameri, M. (2002 Dec). Effects of Anethum graveolens L. seed extracts on experimental gastric irritation models in mice. BMC Pharmacol, 2, 1-5.

Hostanska K, Daum G, Saller R (2002 Sep-Oct). "Cytostatic and apoptosis-inducing activity of boswellic acids toward malignant cell lines in vitro," Anticancer Res. 22(5):2853-62.

Houicher A, Hechanchna H, Teldji H, Ozogul F (2016). "In vitro study of the antifungal activity of essential oils obtained from mentha spicata thymus vulgaris, and laurus nobilis," Recent Pat Food Nutr Agric. 8(2) 99-106.

Howard J., Hyman A.A. (2003) Dynamics and mechanics of the microtubule plus end. Nature. 422: 753-758.

Hoya Y, Matsumura I, Fujita T, Yanaga K. (2008 Nov-Dec). "The use of nonpharmacological interventions to reduce anxiety in patients undergoing gastroscopy in a setting with an optimal soothing environment," Gastroenterol Nurs. 31(6):395-9.

Hozumi H et al (2017 Oct). "Aromatherapies using osmanthus fragrans oil and grapefruit oil are effective complementary treatments for anxious patients undergoing colonoscopy: a randomized controlled study" Complement Ther Med. 34:165-169.

Hritcu L, Cioanca O, Hancianu M (2012 Apr). "Effects of lavender oil inhalation on improving scopolamine-induced spatial memory impairment in laboratory rats," Phytomedicine Int. J. Phytother. Phytopharm. 19(6):529-534.

Hsieh LC, Hsieh SL, Chen CT, Chung JG, Wang JJ, Wu CC (2015). "Induction of αphellandrene on autophagy in human liver tumor cells," Am. J. Chin. Med. 43(1):121-136.

Hu L, Wang Y, Du M, Zhang J (2011 Jul). "Characterization of the volatiles and active components in ethanol extracts of fruits of Litsea cubeba (Lour.) by gas chromatography-mass spectrometry (GC-MS) and gas chromatography-olfactometry (GC-O)," JMPR. 5(14):3298-3303.

Hu, W., Zhang, N., Chen, H., Zhong, B., Yang, A., Kuang, F., Ouyang, Z., & Chun, J. (2017 Apr. 21). "Fumigant Activity of Sweet Orange Essential Oil Fractions Against Red Imported Fire Ants (Hymenoptera: Formicidae)," J Econ Entomol. [Epub ahead of print].

Huang, C. S., Yin, M. C., & Chiu, L. C. (2011 Sep). Antihyperglycemic and antioxidative potential of Psidium guajava fruit in streptozotocin-induced diabetic rats. Food Chem Toxicol, 49(9), 2189-2195.

Huang L, Abuhamdah S, Howes MJ, Dixon CL, Elliot MS, Ballard C, Holmes C, Burns A, Perry EK, Francis PT, Lees G, Chazot PL (2008 Nov). "Pharmacological profile of essential oils derived from Lavandula angustifolia and Melissa officinalis with anti-agitation properties: focus on ligand-gated channels," J Pharm Pharmacol. 60(11):1515-22.

Huang MT, Badmaev V, Ding Y, Liu Y, Xie JG, Ho CT (2000). "Anti-tumor and anti-carcinogenic activities of triterpenoid, beta-boswellic acid," Biofactors. 13(1-4):225-30.

Hucklenbroich J. et al (2014 Sep). "Aromatic-turmerone induces neural stem cell proliferation in vitro and in vivo," Stem Cell Res. Ther. 5(4).

Hudaib, M., Speroni, E., Di Pietra, A. M., & Cavrini, V. (2002 Jul). GC/MS evaluation of thyme (Thymus vulgaris L.) oil composition and variations during the vegetative cycle. J Pharm Biomed Anal, 29(4), 691-700.

Hunan Yi Ke Da Xue Xue Bao (1999). "Experimental study on induction of apoptosis of leukemic cells by Boswellia carterii Birdw extractive," Hunan Yi Ke Da Xue Xue Bao. 24(1):23-5.

Hudson, J., Kuo, M., & Vimalanathan, S. (2011 Dec). The antimicrobial properties of cedar leaf (Thuja plicata) oil; a safe and efficient decontamination agent for buildings. Int J Environ Res Public Health, 8(12), 4477-4487.

Hull, S., Re, R., Chambers, L., Echaniz, A., & Wickham, M. S. (2014 Sep 3). A mid-morning snack of almonds generates satiety and appropriate adjustment of subsequent food intake in healthy women. Eur J Nutr.

Hur M.H., Han SH (2004 Feb). "[Clinical trial of aromatherapy on postpartum mother's perineal healing]," Taehan Kanho Hakhoe Chi. 34(1):53-62.

Hur M.H., Park J, Maddock-Jennings W, Kim D.O., Lee M.S. (2007 Jul). "Reduction of mouth malodour and volatile sulphur compounds in intensive care patients using an essential oil mouthwash," Phytother. Res. PTR. 21(7):641-643.

Husain F.M., Ahmad I, Asif M, Tahseen Q (2013 Dec). "Influence of clove oil on certain quorumsensing-regulated functions and biofilm of Pseudomonas aeruginosa and Aeromonas hydrophila," J. Biosci. 38(5):835-844.

Hussein G, Miyashiro H, Nakamura N, Hattori M, Kakiuchi N, Shimotohno K (2000 Nov). "Inhibitory effects of sudanese medicinal plant extracts on hepatitis C virus (HCV) protease," Phytother Res. 14(7):510-6.

Hyldgaard, M., Mygind, T., & Meyer, R. L. (2012 Feb). Essential oils in food preservation: mode of action, synergies, and interactions with food matrix components. Frontiers in Microbiology, 3, 1-24.

Idaomar M, El-Hamss R, Bakkali F, Mezzoug N, Zhiri A, Baudoux D, Muñoz-Serrano A, Liemans V, Alonso-Moraga A (2002 Jan 15). "Genotoxicity and antigenotoxicity of some essential oils evaluated by wing spot test of Drosophila melanogaster," Mutat Res. 13(1-2):61-8.

Iamsaard, S., Prabsattroo, T., Sukhorum, W., Muchimapura, S., Srisaard, P., Uabundit, N., . . . Wattanathorn, J. (2013 Mar). Anethum graveolens Linn. (dill) extract enhances the mounting frequency and level of testicular tyrosine protein phosphorylation in rats. J Zhejiang Univ Sci B, 14(3), 247-252.

Ilmberger J, Heuberger E, Mahrhofer C, Dessovic H, Kowarik D, Buchbauer G (2001 Mar). "The influence of essential oils on human attention. I: alertness," Chem. Senses. 26(3):239-248.

Imai H, Osawa K, Yasuda H, Hamashima H, Arai T, Sasatsu M (2001). "Inhibition by the essential oils of peppermint and spearmint on the growth of pathogenic bacteria," Microbios. 106(Suppl 1):31-9.

Imokawa G (2009 Jul). "A possible mechanism underlying the ceramide deficiency in atopic dermatitis: expression of a deacylase enzyme that cleaves the N-acyl linkage of sphingomyelin and glucosylceramide," J Dermatol Sci. 55(1):1-9.

Imura M, Misao H, Ushijima H (2006 Mar). "The Psychological Effects of Aromatherapy-Massage in Healthy Postpartum Mothers," J. Midwifery Womens Health. 51(2):e21-e27.

Inouye S, Nishiyama Y, Uchida K, Hasumi Y, Yamaguchi H, Abe S (2006 Dec). "The vapor activity of oregano, perilla, tea tree, lavender, clove, and geranium oils against a Trichophyton mentagrophytes in a closed box," J Infect Chemother. 12(6):349-54.

Inouye S, Takizawa T, Yamaguchi H (2001 May). "Antibacterial activity of essential oils and their major constituents against respiratory tract pathogens by gaseous contact," J Antimicrob Chemother. 47(5):565-73.

Inouye S, Yamaguchi H, Takizawa T (2001 Dec). "Screening of the antibacterial effects of a variety of essential oils on respiratory tract pathogens, using a modified dilution assay method," J Infect Chemother. 7(4):251-4.

Iori A, Grazioli D, Gentile E, Marano G, Salvatore G (2005 Apr 20). "Acaricidal properties of the essential oil of Melaleuca alternifolia Cheel (tea tree oil) against nymphs of Ixodes ricinus," Vet Parasitol. 129(1-2):173-6.

Iscan G, Kirimer N, Kürkcüoğlu M, Baser K.H.C., Demirci F (2002 Jul). "Antimicrobial screening of Mentha piperita essential oils," J. Agric. Food Chem. 50(14):3943-3946.

Ishida T, Mizushina Y, Yagi S, Irino Y, Nishiumi S, Miki I, Kondo Y, Mizuno S, Yoshida H, Azuma T, Yoshida M (2012). "Inhibitory effects of glycyrrhetinic Acid on DNA polymerase and inflammatory activities," Evid Based Complement Alternat Med. 2012:650514.

Ishikawa H, Matsumoto S, Ohashi Y, Imaoka A, Setoyama H, Umesaki Y, Tanaka R, Otani T (2011 Apr). "Beneficial effects of probiotic bifidobacterium and galacto-oligosaccharide in patients with ulcerative colitis: a randomized controlled study," Digestion. 84(2):128-33.

Itai T, Amayasu H, Kuribayashi M, Kawamura N, Okada M, Momose A, Tateyama T, Narumi K, Uematsu W, Kaneko S (2000 Aug). "Psychological effects of aromatherapy on chronic hemodialysis patients," Psychiatry Clin Neurosci. 54(4):393-7.

Itai T, Amayasu H, Kuribayashi M, Kawamura N, Okada M, Momose A, Tateyama T, Narumi K, Uematsu W, Kaneko S (2000 Aug). "Psychological effects of aromatherapy on chronic hemodialysis patients," Psychiatry Clin Neurosci. 54(4):393-7.

Itkin M. et al (2016 Nov). "The biosynthetic pathway of the nonsugar, high-intensity sweetener mogroside V from Siraitia grosvenorii," Proc. Natl. Acad. Sci. U. S. A. 113(47):E7619-7628.

Ito, Y., Ohnishi, S., & Fujie, K. (1989). Chromosome aberrations induced by aflatoxin B1 in rat bone marrow cells in vivo and their suppression by green tea. Mutation Research/Genetic Toxicology, 222(3), 253-261.

Iwata, J., LeDoux, J. E., Meeley, M. P., Arneric, S., & Reis, D. J. (1986 Sep). Intrinsic neurons in the amygdaloid field projected to by the medial geniculate body mediate emotional responses conditioned to acoustic stimuli. Brain Res, 383(1-2), 195-214.

Jacob J.N., Badyal D.K. (2014 Feb). "Biological studies of turmeric oil, part 3: anti-inflammatory and analgesic properties of turmeric oil and fish oil in comparison with aspirin," Nat. Prod. Commun. 9(2):225-228.

Jacques, P. F., & Wang, H. (2014 Apr 4). Yogurt and weight management. Am J Clin Nutr, 99(5 Suppl), 1229s-1234s.

Jafarzadeh, M., Arman, S., & Pour, F. F. (2013 Aug). Effect of aromatherapy with orange essential oil on salivary cortisol and pulse rate in children during dental treatment: A randomized controlled clinical trial. Adv Biomed Res, 2, 1-10.

Jager, W., Buchbauer, G., Jirovetz, L., & Fritzer, M. (1992). Percutaneous absorption of lavender oil from a massage oil. J Soc Cosmet Chem, 43(1), 49-54.

Jager, W., Nasel, B., Nasel, C., Binder, R., Stimpfl, T., Vycudilik, W., & Buchbauer, G. (1996 Aug). Pharmacokinetic studies of the fragrance compound 1,8-cineol in humans during inhalation. Chem Senses, 21(4), 477-480.

Jamal A, Javed K, Aslam M, Jafri MA (2006 Jan 16). "Gastroprotective effect of cardamom, Elettaria cardamomum Maton. fruits in rats," J Ethnopharmacol. 103(2):149-53.

Janahmadi M, Niazi F, Danyali S, Kamalinejad M (2006 Mar 8). "Effects of the fruit essential oil of Cuminum cyminum Linn. (Apiaceae) on pentylenetetrazol-induced epileptiform activity in F1 neurones of Helix aspersa," J Ethnopharmacol. 104(1-2):278-82.

Jang M, Cai L, Udeani GO, Slowing KV, Thomas CF, Beecher CW, Fong HH, Farnsworth NR, Kinghorn AD, Mehta RG, Moon RC, Pezzuto JM (1997 Jan 10). "Cancer chemopreventive activity of resveratrol, a natural product derived from grapes," Science. 275 (5297):218-20.

Jang SE, Ryu KR, Park SH, Chung S, Teruya Y, Han MJ, Woo JT, Kim DH (2013 Nov). "Nobiletin and tangeretin ameliorate scratching behavior in mice by inhibiting the action of histamine and the activation of NF-κB, AP-1 and p38," Int Immunopharmacol. 17(3):502-7.

Jankasem M, Wuthi-udomlert M, Gritsanapan W (2013). "Antidermatophytic Properties of Ar-Turmerone, Turmeric Oil, and Curcuma longa Preparations," ISRN Dermatol. 2013:1-3.

Jayaprakasha G.K., Jena B.S., Negi P.S., Sakariah K.K. (2002 Jan). "Evaluation of Antioxidant Activities and Antimutagenicity of Turmeric Oil: A Byproduct from Curcumin Production," Z. Für Naturforschung C. 57(9-10).

Jefferies H., Coster J., Khalil A., Bot J., McCauley R.D., Hall J.C. (2003) Glutathione. ANZ Journal of Surgery. 73: 517-522.

Jenkins, D. J., Chiavaroli, L., Wong, J. M., Kendall, C., Lewis, G. F., Vidgen, E., . . . Lamarche, B. (2010 Dec 14). Adding monounsaturated fatty acids to a dietary portfolio of cholesterol-lowering foods in hypercholesterolemia. Canadian Medical Association journal, 182(18), 1961-1967.

Jeon, S., Bose, S., Hur, J., Jun, K., Kim, Y. K., Cho, K. S., & Koo, B. S. (2011 Sep). A modified formulation of Chinese traditional medicine improves memory impairment and reduces Abeta level in the Tg-APPswe/PS1dE9 mouse model of Alzheimer's disease. J Ethnopharmacol, 137(1), 783-789.

Jeong C, Han J, Cho J, Suh K, Nam G (2013 Aug). "Analysis of electrical property changes of skin by oil-in-water emulsion components," Int. J. Cosmet. Sci. 35(4):402-410.

Jeong HU, Kwon SS, Kong T.Y., Kim J.H., Lee H.S. (2014 Dec). "Inhibitory Effects of Cedrol, βCedrene, and Thujopsene on Cytochrome P450 Enzyme Activities in Human Liver Microsomes," Journal of Toxicology and Environmental Health, Part A. 77(22-24):1522-1532.

Jia S. et al (2013 Jan). "Induction of apoptosis by D-limonene is mediated by inactivation of Akt in LS174T human colon cancer cells," Oncol. Rep. 29 (1):349-54.

Jiang, J., Xu, H., Wang, H., Zhang, Y., Ya, P., Yang, C., & Li, F. (2017 Feb.). "Protective effects of lemongrass essential oil against benzo(a)pyrene-induced oxidative stress and DNA damage in human embryonic lung fibroblast cells," Toxicol Mech Methods. 27(2):121-127.

Jiang, Q., Wu, Y., Zhang, H., Liu, P., Yao, J., Chen, J., & Duan, J. (2017 Dec.). "Development of essential oils as skin permeation enhancers: penetration enhancement effect and mechanism of action," Pharm Biol. 55(1):1592-1600.

Jimenez A, Santos A, Alonso G, Vazquez D (1976 Mar 17). "Inhibitors of protein synthesis in eukarytic cells. Comparative effects of some amaryllidaceae alkaloids," Biochim Biophys Acta. 425(3):342-8.

Jiang Z, Akhtar Y, Bradbury R, Zhang X, Isman M.B. (2009 Jun). "Comparative toxicity of essential oils of Litsea pungens and Litsea cubeba and blends of their major constituents against the cabbage looper, Trichoplusia ni," J. Agric. Food Chem. 57(11): 4833-4837.

Jin M.H. et al (2014 Sep). "Cedrol Enhances Extracellular Matrix Production in Dermal Fibroblasts in a MAPK-Dependent Manner," Annals of Dermatology. 24(1):16.

Jing, L., Zhang, Y., Fan, S., Gu, M., Guan, Y., Lu, X., . . . Zhou, Z. (2013 Sep). Preventive and ameliorating effects of citrus D-limonene on dyslipidemia and hyperglycemia in mice with high-fat diet-induced obesity. Eur J Pharmacol, 715(1-3), 46-55.

Jing Y, Nakajo S, Xia L, Nakaya K, Fang Q, Waxman S, Han R (1999 Jan). "Boswellic acid acetate induces differentiation and apoptosis in leukemia cell lines," Leuk Res. 23(1):43-50.

Jing Y, Xia L, Han R (1992 Mar). "Growth inhibition and differentiation of promyelocytic cells (HL-60) induced by BC-4, an active principle from Boswellia carterii Birdw," Chin Med Sci J. 7(1):12-5.

Johannessen B (2013 Nov). "Nurses experience of aromatherapy use with dementia patients experiencing disturbed sleep patterns. An action research project," Complement. Ther. Clin. Pract. 19(4):209-213.

Johnson, K., West, T., Diana, S., Todd, J., Haynes, B., Bernhardt, J., & Johnson, R. (2017 Jun.). "Use of aromatherapy to promote a therapeutic nurse environment," Intensive Crit Care Nurs. 40:18-25.

Johnson, L. R., Ghishan,F.K., Kaunitz, J.D., Merchant, J., Said, H.M., & Wood, J. (Eds.). (2012 Jul). Physiology of the gastrointestinal tract (5th ed.). London: Elsevier.

Johnson, M., Pace, R. D., Dawkins, N. L., & Willian, K. R. (2013 Nov). Diets containing traditional and novel green leafy vegetables improve liver fatty acid profiles of spontaneously hypertensive rats. Lipids Health Dis, 12, 168.

Johny AK, Baskaran SA, Charles AS, Amalaradjou MA, Darre MJ, Khan MI, Hoagland TA, Schreiber DT, Donoghue AM, Donoghue DJ, Venkitarayanan K. (2009 Apr). "Prophylactic supplementation of caprylic acid in feed reduces Salmonella enteritidis colonization in commercial broiler chicks," J. Food Prot. 72(4):722-7.

Jolliff, G.D., Tinsley, I.J., Calhoun, W., and Crane, J.M. (1981). "Meadowfoam (Limnanthes alba): Its Research and Development as a Potential New Oilseed Crop for the Willamette Valley of Oregon," Oregon State University Agricultural Experiment Station. Station Bulletin 648.

Juergens U.R., Dethlefsen U., Steinkamp G., Gillissen A., Repges R., Vetter H. (2003) Anti-inflammatory activity of 1.8-cineol (eucalyptol) in bronchial asthma: a double-blind placebo-controlled trial. Respiratory Medicine. 97: 250-256.

Juergens UR, Stöber M, Schmidt-Schilling L, Kleuver T, Vetter H (1998 Sep 17). "Anti-inflammatory effects of euclyptol (1.8-cineole) in bronchial asthma: inhibition of arachidonic acid metabolism in human blood monocytes ex vivo," Eur J Med Res. 3(9):407-12.

Juergens UR, Stöber M, Vetter H (1998 Dec 16). "The anti-inflammatory activity of L-menthol compared to mint oil in human monocytes in vitro: a novel perspective for its therapeutic use in inflammatory diseases," Eur J Med Res. 3(12):539-45.

Juglal S, Govinden R, Odhav B (2002 Apr). "Spice oils for the control of co-occurring mycotoxin-producing fungi," J Food Prot. 65(4):683-7.

Jun, H. J., Lee, J. H., Jia, Y., Hoang, M. H., Byun, H., Kim, K. H., & Lee, S. J. (2012 Mar). Melissa officinalis essential oil reduces plasma triglycerides in human apolipoprotein E2 transgenic mice by inhibiting sterol regulatory element-binding protein-1c-dependent fatty acid synthesis. J Nutr, 142(3), 432-440.

Jung DL, Cha JY, Kim SE, Ko IG, Jee YS (2013 Apr). "Effects of Ylang-Ylang aroma on blood pressure and heart rate in healthy men," J. Exerc. Rehabil. 9(2):250-255.

Jung K, Kim IH, Han D (2004). "Effect of medicinal plant extracts on forced swimming capacity in mice," J Ethnopharmacol. 93:75-81.

Jung SH, Kang KD, Ju D, Fawcen RJ, Safa R, Kamalden TA, Osborne NN (2008 Sep). "The flavanoid baicalin counteracts ischemic and oxidative insults to retinal cells and lipid peroxidation to brain membranes," Neurochem Int.

Jung, Y. H., Kwon, S. H., Hong, S. I., Lee, S. O., Kim, S. Y., Lee, S. Y., & Jang, C. G. (2012 Dec). 5-HT(1A) receptor binding in the dorsal raphe nucleus is implicated in the anxiolytic-like effects of Cinnamomum cassia. Pharmacol Biochem Behav, 103(2), 367-372.

Kabuto, H., Tada, M., & Kohno, M. (2007 Mar). Eugenol [2-methoxy-4-(2-propenyl)phenol] prevents 6-hydroxydopamine-induced dopamine depression and lipid peroxidation inductivity in mouse striatum. Biol Pharm Bull, 30(3), 423-427.

Kadekaro AL, Kanto H, Kavanagh R, Abdel-Malek ZA (2003 Jun). "Significance of the melanocortin 1 receptor in regulating human melanocyte pigmentation, proliferation, and survival," Ann N Y Acad Sci. 994:359-65.

Kadohisa, M. (2013 Oct). Effects of odor on emotion, with implications. Front Syst Neurosci, 7, 1-6.

Kamatou G.P.P., Vermaak I, Viljoen A.M., Lawrence B.M. (2013 Dec). "Menthol: a simple monoterpene with remarkable biological properties," Phytochemistr. 96:15-25.

Kambara T, Zhou Y, Kawashima Y, Kishida N, Mizutani K, Ikeda T, Kamayama K (2003). "A New Dermatological Availability of the Flavonoid Fraction from Licorice Roots—Effect on Acne," J Soc Cosmet Chem Jpn. 37(3)179-85.

Kamiyama, M., & Shibamoto, T. (2012 Jun). Flavonoids with potent antioxidant activity found in young green barley leaves. J Agric Food Chem, 60(25), 6260-6267.

Kane FM, Brodie EE, Coull A, Coyne L, Howd A, Milne A, Niven CC, Robbins R (2004 Oct 28-Nov 10). "The analgesic effect of odour and music upon dressing change," Br J Nurs. 13(19):S4-12.

Kanehara S, Ohtani T, Uede K, Furukawa F (2007 Dec). "Clinical effects of undershirts coated with borage oil on children with atopic dermatitis: a double-blind, placebo-controlled clinical trial," J Dermatol. 34(12):811-5.

Karadog E, Samanciouglu S, Ozden D, Bakir E (2015 Jul). "Effects of aromatherapy on sleep quality and anxiety of patients," Nurs. Crit. Care.

Kasper S (2013 Nov). "An orally administered lavandula oil preparation (Silexan) for anxiety disorder and related conditions: an evidence based review," Int J Psychiatry Clin Pract. 17 Suppl 1:15-22.

Kasperczyk, S., Dobrakowski, M., Kasperczyk, J., Ostalowska, A., Zalejska-Fiolka, J., & Birkner, E. (2014 Jul). Beta-carotene reduces oxidative stress, improves glutathione metabolism and modifies antioxidant defense systems in lead-exposed workers. Toxicol Appl Pharmacol, 280(1), 36-41.

Katdare M, Singhal H, Newmark H, Osborne MP, Telang NT (1997 Jan 1). "Prevention of mammary preneoplastic transformation by naturally-occurring tumor inhibitors," Cancer Lett. 111(1-2):141-7.

Kato K., Cox A.D., Hisaka M.M., Graham S.M., Buss J.E., Der C.J. (1992) Isoprenoid addition to Ras protein is the critical modification for its membrane association and transforming activity. Proc. Natl. Sci. USA. 89: 6403-6407.

Kato T, Hancock RL, Mohammadpour H, McGregor B, Manalo P, Khaiboullina S, Hall MR, Pardini L, Pardini RS (2002 Dec). "Influence of omega-3 fatty acids on the growth of human colon carcinoma in nude mice," Cancer Lett. 187(1-2):169-77.

Kaur M, Agarwal C, Singh RP, Guan X, Dwivedi C, Agarwal R (2005 Feb). "Skin cancer chemopreventive agent, {alpha}-santalol, induces apoptotic death of human epidermoid carcinoma A431 cells via caspase activation together with dissipation of mitochondrial membrane potential and cytochrome c release," Carcinogenesis. 26(2):369-80.

Kawaski H, Morinushi T, Yakushiji M, Takigawa M (2009 Feb). "Nonlinear dynamical analysis of the effect by six stimuli on electroencephalogram," J. Clin. Neurophysiol. Off. Publ. Am. Electroencephalogr. Soc. 26(1):24-38.

Kawata S, Nagase T, Yamasaki E, Ishiguro H, Matsuzawa Y (1994 Jun). "Modulation of the mevalonate pathway and cell growth by pravastatin and d-limonene in a human hepatoma cell line (Hep G2)," Br. J. Cancer. 69(6):1015-1020.

Kee Y, Lin RC, Hsu SC, Scheller RH (1995 May). "Distinct domains of syntaxin are required for synaptic vesicle fusion complex formation and dissociation," Neuron. 14(5):991-8.

Kéita SM, Vincent C, Schmit J, Arnason JT, Bélanger A (2001 Oct). "Efficacy of essential oil of Ocimum basilicum L. and O. gratissimum L. applied as an insecticidal fumigant and powder to control Callosobruchus maculatus (Fab.)," J Stored Prod Res. 37(4):339-349.

Kennedy DO, Little W, Haskell CF, Scholey AB (2006 Feb). "Anxiolytic effects of a combination of Melissa officinalis and Valeriana officinalis during laboratory induced stress," Phytother Res. 20(2):96-102.

Kennedy DO, Wake G, Savelev S, Tildesley NT, Perry EK, Wesnes KA, Scholey AB (2003 Oct). "Modulation of mood and cognitive performance following acute administration of single doses of Melissa officinalis (Lemon balm) with human CNS nicotinic and muscarinic receptor-binding properties," Neuropsychopharmacology. 28(10):1871-81.

Keogh A, Fenton S, Leslie C, Aboyoun C, Macdonald P, Zhao YC, Bailey M, Rosenfeldt F (2003). "Randomised double-blind, placebo-controlled trial of coenzyme Q therapy in class II and III systolic heart failure," Heart Lung Circ. 12(3):135-41.

Keshavarz Afshar M, Behboodi Moghadam Z, Taghizadeh Z, Bekhradi R, Montazeri A, Mokhtari P (2015 Apr). "Lavender fragrance essential oil and the quality of sleep in postpartum women," Iran. Red Crescent Med. J. 17(4):E25880.

Keskin, I., Gunal, Y., Alya, S., Kolbasi, B., Sakul, A., Kilc, U., Gok, O., Koroglu, K., & Ozbek, H. (2017 Apr. 20). "Effects of Foeniculum vulgare essential oil compounds, fenchone and limonene, on experimental wound healing," Biotech Histochem. 92(4):274-282.

Khachik, F., Beecher, G. R., & Smith, J. C. (1995). Lutein, lycopene, and their oxidative metabolites in chemoprevention of cancer. Journal of Cellular Biochemistry, 59(S22), 236-246.

Khalessi A.M., Pack A.R.C., Thomson W.M, Tomplins G.R. (2004 Oct). "An in vivo study of the plaque control efficacy of Persica: a commercially available herbal mouthwash containing extracts of Salvadora persica," Int. Dent. J. 54(5):279-283.

Khallouki F, Younos C, Soulimani R, Oster T, Charrouf Z, Spiegelhalder B, Bartsch H, Owen RW (2003 Feb). "Consumption of argan oil (Morocco) with its unique profile of fatty acids, tocopherols, squalene, sterols and phenolic compounds should confer valuable cancer chemopreventive effects," Eur J Cancer Prev. 12(1):67-75.

Khan AU, Gilani AH (2009 Dec 10). "Antispasmodic and bronchodilator activities of Artemisia vulgaris are mediated through dual blockade of muscarinic receptors and calcium influx," J Ethnopharmacol. 126(3):480-6.

Khatibi A, Haghparast A, Shams J, Dianati E, Komaki A, Kamalinejad M (2008 Dec 19). "Effects of the fruit essential oil of Cuminum cyminum L. on the acquisition and expression of morphine-induced conditioned place preference in mice," Neurosci Lett. 448(1):94-8.

Kheirkhah A, Casas V, Li W, Raju VK, Tseng SC (2007 May). "Corneal manifestations of ocular demodex infestation," Am J Ophthalmol. 143(5):743-749.

Kheirkhah M, Vali Pour NS, Nisani L, Haghani H (2014 Aug 17). "Comparing the effects of aromatherapy with rose oils and warm foot bath on anxiety in the first stage of labor in nulliparous women," Iran Red Crescent Med J. 16(9):e14455.

Khodabakhsh, P., Shafaroodi, H., and Asgarpanah. J. (2015). "Analgesic and anti-inflammatory activities of Citrus aurantium L. blossoms essential oil (neroli): involvement of the nitric oxide/cyclic-guanosine monophosphate pathway," J Nat Med. 69(3):324-31.

Kiecolt-Glaser JK, Graham JE, Malarkey WB, Porter K, Lemeshow S, Glaser R (2008 Apr). "Olfactory influences on mood and autonomic, endocrine, and immune function," Psychoneuroendocrinology. 33(3):328-39.

Kim D, Suh Y, Lee H, Lee Y (2013 Feb). "Immune activation and antitumor response of ar-turmerone on P388D1 lymphoblast cell implanted tumors," Int. J. Mol. Med. 31(2):386-392.

Kim DS. et al (2015). "Alpha-Pinene Exhibits Anti-Inflammatory Activity Through theSuppression of MAPKs and the NF-κB Pathway in Mouse Peritoneal Macrophages," Am. J. Chin. Med. 43(4):731-742.

Kim ES, Kang SY, Kim YH, Lee YE, Choi NY, You YO, Kim KJ (2015 Apr). "Chamaecyparis obtusa Essential Oil Inhibits Methicillin-Resistant Staphylococcus aureus Biofilm Formation and Expression of Virulence Factors," J Med Food. 18(7):810-7.

Kim, H. J., Yang, H. M., Kim, D. H., Kim, H. G., Jang, W. C., & Lee, Y. R. (2003 Jun). Effects of ylang-ylang essential oil on the relaxation of rat bladder muscle in vitro and white rabbit bladder in vivo. J Korean Med Sci, 18(3), 409-414.

Kim HM, Cho SH (1999 Feb). "Lavender oil inhibits immediate-type allergic reaction in mice and rats," J Pharm Pharmacol. 51(2):221-6.

Kim, I. H., Kim, C., Seong, K., Hur, M. H., Lim, H. M., & Lee, M. S. (2012 Dec). Essential oil inhalation on blood pressure and salivary cortisol levels in prehypertensive and hypertensive subjects. Evid Based Complement Alternat Med, 2012, 1-9.

Kim J.T. et al (2007 Jul). "Treatment with lavender aromatherapy in the post-anesthesia care unit reduces opioid requirements of morbidly obese patients undergoing laparoscopic adjustable gastric banding," Obes. Surg. 17(7):920-925.

Kim JM, Marshall M, Cornell J.A., Iii J.F.P., Wei C.I (1995 Nov). "Antibacterial Activity of Carvacrol, Citral, and Geraniol against Salmonella typhimurium in Culture Medium and on Fish Cubes," Journal of Food Science. 60(6):1364-1368.

Kim MA, Sakong JK, Kim EJ, Kim EH, Kim EH (2005 Feb). "Effect of aromatherapy massage for the relief of constipation in the elderly," Taehan Kanho Hakhoe Chi. 35(1):56-64.

Kim MJ, Nam ES, Paik SI (2005 Feb). "The effects of aromatherapy on pain, depression, and life satisfaction of arthritis patients," Taehan Kanho Hakhoe Chi. 35(1):186-94.

Kim SE, Lee CM, Kim YC (2017 Jan). "Anti-Melanogenic Effect of Oenothera laciniata Methanol Extract in Melan-a Cells," Toxicol Res. 33(1):55-62.

Kim SS, Baik J.S., Oh TH, Yoon WJ, Lee N.H., Hyun CG (2008 Oct). "Biological activities of Korean Citrus obovoides and Citrus natsudaidai essential oils against acne-inducing bacteria," Biosci. Biotechnol. Biochem. 72(10):2507-2513.

Kim, T. H., Kim, H. J., Lee, S. H., & Kim, S. Y. (2012 Jun). Potent inhibitory effect of Foeniculum vulgare Miller extract on osteoclast differentiation and ovariectomy-induced bone loss. Int J Mol Med, 29(6), 1053-1059.

Kim, W., & Hur, M.H. (2016 Dec). "Inhalation Effects of Aroma Essential Oil on Quality of Sleep for Shift Nurses after Night Work," J Korean Acad Nurs. 46(6):769-779.

Kim Y-J, Lee MS, Yang YS, Hur M-H (2011). "Self-aromatherapy massage of the abdomen for the reduction of menstrual pain and anxiety during menstruation in nurses: a placebo-controlled clinical trial," Eur J Integr Med. 3:e165–e168.

Kim Y.W. et al (2013). "Safety evaluation and risk assessment of d-Limonene," J. Toxicol. Environ. Health B Crit. 16 (1):17-38.

Kimura K, Ozeki M, Juneja LR, Ohira H (2007 Jan). "L-Theanine reduces psychological and physiological stress responses," Biol Psychol. 74(1):39-45.

Kite SM, Maher EJ, Anderson K, Young T, Young J, Wood J, Howells N, Bradburn J (1998 May). "Development of an aromatherapy service at a Cancer Centre," Palliat Med. 12(3):171-80.

Klauke AL, Racz I, Pradier B, Markert A, Zimmer AM, Gertsch J, Zimmer A (2014 Apr). "The cannabinoid CB₂ receptor-selective phytocannabinoid beta-caryophyllene exerts analgesic effects in mouse models of inflammatory and neuropathic pain," Eur Neuropsychopharmacol. 24(4):608-20.

Klein A.H., Jpe C.L., Davoodi A., Takechi K., Carstens M.I., Carsents E (2014 Jun). "Eugenol and carvacrol excite first- and second-order trigeminal neurons and enhance their heat-evoked responses," Neuroscience. 271:45-55.

Kline RM, Kline JJ, Di Palma J, Barbero GJ (2001 Jan). "Enteric-coated, pH-dependent peppermint oil capsules for the treatment of irritable bowel syndrome in children," J Pediatr. 138(1):125-8.

Klug W.S., Cummings M.R., Spencer C., Palladino M.A. Concepts of Genetics. San Francisco: Pearson Custom Publishing, 2009.

Knott A, Reuschlein K, Mielke H, Wensorra U, Mummert C, Koop U, Kausch M, Kolbe L, Peters N, Stäb F, Wenck H, Gallinat S (2008 Dec). "Natural Arctium lappa fruit extract improves the clinical signs of aging skin," J Cosmet Dermatol. 7(4):281-9.

Kobayashi Y, Takahashi R, Ogino F (2005 Oct 3). "Antipruritic effect of the single oral administration of German chamomile flower extract and its combined effect with antiallergic agents in ddY mice," J Ethnopharmacol. 101(1-3):308-12.

Kocevski, D., Du, M., Kan, J., Jing, C., Lacanin, I., & Pavlovic, H. (2013 May). Antifungal effect of Allium tuberosum, Cinnamomum cassia, and Pogostemon cablin essential oils and their components against population of Aspergillus species. J Food Sci, 78(5), M731-737.

Kodama R, Yano T, Furukawa K, Noda K, Ide H (1976 Jun). "Studies on the metabolism of d-limonene (p- mentha-1,8-diene). IV. Isolation and characterization of new metabolites and specie differences in metabolism," Xenobiotica Fate Foreign Compd. Biol. Syst. 6(6):337-389.

Koh KJ, Pearce AL, Marshman G, Finlay-Jones JJ, Hart PH (2002 Dec). "Tea tree oil reduces histamine-induced skin inflammation," Br J Dermatol. 147(6):1212-7.

Kohlert, C., van Rensen, I., Marz, R., Schindler, G., Graefe, E. U., & Veit, M. (2000 Aug). Bioavailability and pharmacokinetics of natural volatile terpenes in animals and humans. Planta Med, 66(6), 495-505.

Komiya M, Takeuchi T, Harada E (2006 Sep 25). "Lemon oil vapor causes an anti-stress effect via modulating the 5-HT and DA activities in mice," Behav Brain Res. 172(2):240-9.

Komori T, Fujiwara R, Tanida M, Nomura J (1995 Dec). "Potential antidepressant effects of lemon odor in rats," Eur Neuropsychopharmacol. 5(4):477-80.

Komori T, Fujiwara R, Tanida M, Nomura J, Yokoyama MM (1995 May-Jun). "Effects of citrus fragrance on immune function and depressive states," Neuroimmunomodulation. 2(3):174-80.

Koo HN, Hong SH, Kim CY, Ahn JW, Lee YG, Kim JJ, Lyu YS, Kim HM (2002 Jun). "Inhibitory effect of apoptosis in human astrocytes CCF-STTG1 cells by lemon oil," Pharmacol Res. 45(6):469-73.

Koo HN, Jeong HJ, Kim CH, Park ST, Lee SJ, Seong KK, Lee SK, Lyu YS, Kim HM (2001 Dec). "Inhibition of heat shock-induced apoptosis by peppermint oil in astrocytes," J Mol Neurosci. 17(3):391-6.

Kooncumchoo P, Sharma S, Porter J, Govitrapong P, Ebadi M (2006). "Coenzyme Q(10) provides neuroprotection in iron-induced apoptosis in dopaminergic neurons," J Mol Neurosci. 28(2):125-41.

Kosalec I, Pepeljnjak S, Kustrak D. (2005 Dec). "Antifungal activity of fluid extract and essential oil from anise fruits (Pimpinella anisum L, Apiaceae)," Acta Pharm. 55(4):377-85.

Kotan R, Kordali S, Cakir A (2007 Aug). "Screening of antibacterial activities of twenty-one oxygenated monoterpenes," Z. Für Naturforschung C J. Biosci. 62(7-8):507-513.

Kothiwale S.V., Patwardham V., Ghandi M., Sohoni R., Kumar A. (2014). "A comparative study of antiplaque and antigingivitis effects of herbal mouth-rinse containing tea tree oil, clove, and basil with commercially available essential oil mouthrinse," J. Indian Soc. Periodontol. 18(3):316-320.

Koto R. et al (2006 Jul). "Linalyl acetate as a major ingredient of lavender essential oil relaxes the rabbit vascular smooth muscle through dephosphorylation of myosin light chain," J. Cardiovasc. Pharmacol. 48(1):850-856.

Koutroumanidou, E., Kimbaris, A., Kortsaris, A., Bezirtzoglou, E., Polissiou, M., Charalabopoulos, K., & Pagonopoulou, O. (2013 Aug). Increased seizure latency and decreased severity of pentylenetetrazol-induced seizures in mice after essential oil administration. Epilepsy Res Treat, 2013.

Kozics, K., Srancikova, A., Sedlackova, E., Horvathova, E., Melusova, M., Melus, V., Krajcovicova, Z., & Sramkova, M. (2017). "Antioxidant potential of essential oil from Lavandula angustifolia in in vitro and ex vivo cultured liver cells," Neoplasma. 64(4):485-493.

Krishnakumar A, Abraham PM, Paul J, Paulose CS (2009 Sep 15). "Down-regulation of cerebellar 5-HT(2C) receptors in pilocarpine-induced epilepsy in rats: therapeutic role of Bacopa monnieri extract," J Neurol Sci. 284(1-2):124-8.

Krishnakumar A, Nandhu MS, Paulose CS (2009 Oct). "Upregulation of 5-HT2C receptors in hippocampus of pilocarpine-induced epileptic rats: antagonism by Bacopa monnieri," Epilepsy Behav. 16(2):225-30.

Kritsidima M, Newton T, Asimakopoulou K (2010 Feb). "The effects of lavender scent on dental patient anxiety levels: a cluster randomised-controlled trial," Community Dent. Oral Epidemiol. 38(1):83-87.

Kudryavtseva, A., Krasnov, G., Lipatova, A., Alekseev, B., Maganova, F., Shaposhnikov, M., Fedorova, M., Snexhkina, A., and Moskaley, A. (2016). "Effects of Abies sibirica terpenes on cancer- and aging-associated pathways in human cells," Oncotarget, 7(50), 83744–83754.

Kuettner A, Pieper A, Koch J, Enzmann F, Schroeder S (2005 Feb 28). "Influence of coenzyme Q(10) and cervistatin on the flow-mediated vasodilation of the brachial artery: results of the ENDOTACT study," Int J Cardiol. 98(3):413-9.

Kumar A, Malik F, Bhushan S, Sethi VK, Shahi AK, Kaur J, Taneja SC, Qazi GN, Singh J (2008 Feb 15). "An essential oil and its major constituent isointermedeol induce apoptosis by increased expression of mitochondrial cytochrome c and apical death receptors in human leukaemia HL-60 cells," Chem Biol Interact. 171(3):332-47.

Kumar, D., Nisha, S., Vinay, P. and Ali, S. (2012.) "An Insight To Pullulan: A Biopolymer in Pharmaceutical Approaches," Int J of Basic and Applied Sci. 1(3):202-219.

Kumar P, Kumar A (2003 Jun). "Possible neuroprotective effect of Withania somnifera root extract against 3-nitropropionic acid-induced behavioral, biochemical, and mitochondrial dysfunction in an animal model of Huntington's disease," J Med Food. 12(3):591-600.

Kumaran AM, D'Souza P, Agarwal A, Bokkolla RM, Balasubramaniam M (2003 Sep). "Geraniol, the putative anthelmintic principle of Cymbopogon martinii," Phytother Res. 17(8):957.

Kumari, S., & Dutta, A. (2013 Jul). Protective effect of Eleteria cardamomum (L.) Maton against Pan masala induced damage in lung of male Swiss mice. Asian Pac J Trop Med, 6(7), 525-531.

Kummer R. et al (2013). "Evaluation of Anti-Inflammatory Activity of Citrus latifolia Tanaka Essential Oil and Limonene in Experimental Mouse Models," Evid.-Based Complement. Altern. Med. 859083.

Kuroda K. et al (2005 Oct). "Sedative effects of the jasmine tea odor and (R)-(-)-linalool, one of its major odor components, on autonomic nerve activity and mood states," Eur. J. Appl. Physiol. 95(2-3):107-114.

Kuo YM, Hayflick SJ, Gitschier J (2007 Jun). "Deprivation of pantothenic acid elicits a movement disorder and azoospermia in a mouse model of pantothenate kinase-associated neurodegeneration," J Inherit Metab Dis. 30(3):310-7.

Kusuhara M. et al (2012 Feb). "Fragrant environment with α-pinene decreases tumor growth in mice," Biomed. Res. 33(1):57-61.

Kuttan R, Liju V, Jeena K (2011). An evaluation of antioxidant, anti-inflammatory, and antinociceptive activities of essential oil from Curcuma longa. L," Indian J. Pharmacol. 43(5):526.

Kuwahata, H., Komatsu, T., Katsuyama, S., Corasaniti, M. T., Bagetta, G., Sakurada, S., . . . Takahama, K. (2013 Feb). Peripherally injected linalool and bergamot essential oil attenuate mechanical allodynia via inhibiting spinal ERK phosphorylation. Pharmacol Biochem Behav, 103(4), 735-741.

Kwasniewska M, Jegier A, Kostka T, Dziankowska-Zaborszczyk E, Rebowska E, Kozinska J, Drygas W (2014 Jan). "Long-term effect of different physical activity levels on subclinical atherosclerosis in middle-aged men: a 25-year prospective study," PLoS One, 9(1):e85209.

Kwieciński J, Eick S, Wójcik K (2009 Apr). "Effects of tea tree (Melaleuca alternifolia) oil on Staphylococcus aureus in biofilms and stationary growth phase," Int J Antimicrob Agents. 33(4):343-7.

Kwon Y.S., Lee S.H., Hwang Y.C., Rosa V, Lee K.W., Min K.S. (2015 Dec). "Behaviour of human dental pulp cells cultured in a collagen hydrogel scaffold crosslinked with cinnamaldehyde," Int. Endod. J.

Labib G.S., Aldawsari H. (2015). "Innovation of natural essential oil-loaded Orabase for local treatment of oral candidiasis," Drug Des. Devel. Ther. 9:3349-3359.

Lachowicz, K., Jones, G., Briggs, D., Bienvenu, F., Wan, J., Wilcock, A., & Coventry, M. (1998). The synergistic preservative effects of the essential oils of sweet basil (Ocimum basilicum L.) against acid-tolerant food microflora. Letters in Applied Microbiology, 26(3), 209-214.

Lagouge M et al. (2006 Dec 15). "Resveratrol improves mitochondrial function and protects against metabolic disease by activating SIRT1 and PGC-1alpha," Cell. 127(6):1109-22.

Lahlou S, Figueiredo AF, Magalhães PJ, Leal-Cardoso JH (2002 Dec). "Cardiovascular effects of 1,8-cineole, a terpenoid oxide present in many plant essential oils, in normotensive rats," Can J Physiol Pharmacol. 80(12):1125-31.

Lahlou S., Interaminense L.F.L., Magalhaes P.J.C., Leal-Cardoso J.H., Duarte G.P. (2004) Cardiovascular Effects of Eugenol, a Phenolic Compound Present in Many Plant Essential Oils, in Normotensive Rats. Journal of Cardiovascular Pharmacology. 43: 250-257.

Lai F, Sinico C, De Logu A, Zaru M, Muller R.H., Fadda A.M. (2007). "SLN as a topical delivery system for Artemisia arborescens essential oil: in vitro antiviral activity and skin permeation study," Int. J. Nanomedicine. 2(3):419.

Lai Y. et al (2014 Jun). "In vitro studies of a distillate of rectified essential oils on sinonasal components of mucociliary clearance," Am. J. Rhinol. Allergy. 28(3):224-248.

Lambert R.J.W., Skandamis P.N., Coote P.J., Nychas G-J.E. (2001) A study of the minimun inhibitory concentration and mode of action of oregano essential oil, thymol and carvacrol. Journal of Applied Microbiology. 91: 453-462.

Lampronti I, Saab AM, Gambari R (2006 Oct). "Antiproliferative activity of essential oils derived from plants belonging to the Magnoliophyta division," Int J Oncol. 29(4):989-95.

Langeveld, W. T., Veldhuizen, E. J., & Burt, S. A. (2014 Feb). Synergy between essential oil components and antibiotics: a review. Crit Rev Microbiol, 40(1), 76-94.

Lantry LE, Zhang Z, Gao F, Crist KA, Wang Y, Kelloff GJ, Lubet RA, You M (1997). "Chemopreventive effect of perillyl alcohol on 4-(methylnitrosamino)-1-(3-pyridyl)-1-butanone induced tumorigenesis in (C3H/HeJ X A/J)F1 mouse lung," J Cell Biochem Suppl. 27:20-5.

Lappas C.M., Lappas N.T. (2012 Sep). "D-Limonene modulates T lymphocyte activity and viability," Cell. Immunol. 279(1):30-41.

Larder B.A., Kemp S.D., Harrigan P.R. (1995) Potential Mechanism for Sustained Antiretroviral Efficacy of AZT-3TC Combination Therapy. Science. 269: 696-699.

Laurent TC, Laurent UB, Frazer JR (1995 May). "Functions of hyaluronan," Ann Rheum Dis. 54(5):429-32.

Lawrence, H. A., & Palombo, E. A. (2009 Dec). Activity of essential oils against Bacillus subtilis spores. J Microbiol Biotechnol, 19(12), 1590-1595.

Leaf DA, Parker DL, Schaad D (1997 Sep). "Changes in Vo2max, phsical activity, and body fat with chronic exercise: effects on plasma lipids," Med Sci Sports Exerc, 29(9):1152-9.

LeDoux, J. (2003). The emotional brain, fear, and the amygdala. Cellular and molecular neurobiology, 23(4-5), 727-738.

LeDoux, J. E., Iwata, J., Cicchetti, P., & Reis, D. J. (1988 Jul). Different projections of the central amygdaloid nucleus mediate autonomic and behavioral correlates of conditioned fear. J Neurosci, 8(7), 2517-2529.

Ledoux, J. E., Romanski, L., & Xagoraris, A. (1989 Jul). Indelibility of subcortical emotional memories. J Cogn Neurosci, 1(3), 238-243.

Lee HR, Kim GH, Choi WS, Park IK (2017 Apr 1). "Repellent Activity of Apiaceae Plant Essential Oils and their Constituents Against Adult German Cockroaches," J Econ Entomol. 110(2):552-557.

Lee, H. S. (2002 Dec). Inhibitory activity of Cinnamomum cassia bark-derived component against rat lens aldose reductase. J Pharm Pharm Sci, 5(3), 226-230.

Lee HS (2005 Apr 6). "Cuminaldehyde: Aldose Reductase and alpha-Glucosidase Inhibitor Derived from Cuminum cyminum L. Seeds," J Agric Food Chem. 53(7):2446-50.

Lee, H. S., & Ahn, Y. J. (1998 Jan). Growth-Inhibiting Effects of Cinnamomum cassia Bark-Derived Materials on Human Intestinal Bacteria. J Agric Food Chem, 46(1), 8-12.

Lee IS, Lee GJ (2006 Feb). "Effects of lavender aromatherapy on insomnia and depression in women college students," Taehan Kanho Hakhoe Chi. 36(1):136-43.

Lee K, Lee JH, Kim SI, Cho M.H., Lee J (2014 Nov). "Anti-biofilm, anti-hemolysis, and antivirulence activities of black pepper, cananga, myrrh oils, and nerolidol against Staphylococcus aureus," Appl. Microbiol. Biotechnol. 98(22):9447:9457.

Lee KH et al (2011 Dec). "Essential oil of Curcuma longa inhibits Streptococcus mutans biofilm formation," J. Food Sci. 76(9):H226-230.

Lee SH, Do HS, Min KJ (2015 Dec). Effects of Essential Oil from Hinoki Cypress, Chamaecyparis obtusa, on Physiology and Behavior of Flies. PLoS One. 10(12):e0143450.

Lee SK, Zhang W, Sanderson BJ (2008 Aug). "Selective growth inhibition of human leukemia and human lymphoblastoid cells by resveratrol via cell cycle arrest and apoptosis induction," J Agric Food Chem. 56(16):7572-7.

Lee SU, Shim KS, Ryu SY, Min YK, Kim SH (2009 Feb). "Machilin A isolated from Myristica fragrans stimulates osteoblast differentiation," Planta Med. 75(2):152-7.

Lee, S. Y., Ha, S. A., Seo, J. S., Sohn, C. M., Park, H. R., & Kim, K. W. (2014). Eating habits and eating behaviors by family dinner frequency in the lower-grade elementary school students. Nutr Res Pract, 8(6), 679-687.

Lee, T., Lee, S., Ho Kim, K., Oh, K. B., Shin, J., & Mar, W. (2013 Sep). Effects of magnolialide isolated from the leaves of Laurus nobilis L. (Lauraceae) on immunoglobulin E-mediated type I hypersensitivity in vitro. J Ethnopharmacol, 149(2), 550-556.

Lee Y (2009). "Activation of apoptotic protein in U937 cells by a component of turmeric oil," BMB Rep. 42(2):96-100.

Leffa, D. D., da Silva, J., Daumann, F., Dajori, A. L., Longaretti, L. M., Damiani, A. P., ... de Andrade, V. M. (2013 Dec). Corrective effects of acerola (Malpighia emarginata DC.) juice intake on biochemical and genotoxical parameters in mice fed on a high-fat diet. Mutat Res.

Legault J, Dahl W, Debiton E, Pichette A, Madelmont JC (2003 May). "Antitumor activity of balsam fir oil: production of reactive oxygen species induced by alpha-humulene as possible mechanism of action," Planta Med. 69(5):402-7.

Legault J, Pichette A (2007 Dec). "Potentiating effect of beta-caryophyllene on anticancer activity of alpha-humulene, isocaryophyllene and paclitaxel," J Pharm Pharmacol. 59(12):1643-7.

Leggio B, Mazza A, Cruciani G, Sgorbini L, Publiese M, Bendinin MG, Severi P, Jesi AP (2014 Jul). "Effects of exercise training on systo-diastoli ventricular dysfunction in patients with hypertension: an echocardiographic study with tissue velocity and strain imaging evaluation," Hypertens Res, 37(7):649-54.

Lehrner J, Eckersberger C, Walla P, Pötsch G, Deecke L (2000 Oct 1-15). "Ambient odor of orange in a dental office reduces anxiety and improves mood in female patients," Physiol Behav. 71(1-2):83-6.

Lehrner J, Marwinski G, Lehr S, Johren P, Deecke L. (2005 Sep 15). "Ambient odors of orange and lavender reduce anxiety and improve mood in a dental office," Physiol Behav. 86(1-2):92-5.

Lekshmi P.C., Arimboor R, Indulekha P.S., Nirmala Menon A (2012 Nov). "Turmeric (Curcuma longa L.) volatile oil inhibits key enzymes linked to type 2 diabetes," Int. J. Food Sci. Nutr. 63(7):832-834.

Letawe C, Boone M, Piérard GE (1998 Mar). "Digital image analysis of the effect of topically applied linoleic acid on acne microcomedones," Clin Exp Dermatol. 23(2):56-8.

Leung LH (1995 Jun). "Pantothenic acid deficiency as the pathogenesis of acne vulgaris," Med Hypotheses. 44(6):490-2.

Lewith GT, Godfrey AD, Prescott P (2005 Aug). "A single-blinded, randomized pilot study evaluating the aroma of Lavandula augustifolia as a treatment for mild insomnia," J Altern Complement Med. 11(4):631-7.

Li F, Tao Y, Qiao Y, Li K, Jiang Y, Cao C, Ren S, Chang X, Wang X, Wang Y, Xie Y, Dong Z, Zhao J, Liu K (2017 Sep). "Eupatilin inhibits EGF-induced JB6 cell transformation by targeting PI3K," Int J Oncol. 49(3):1148-54.

Li SP, Li P, Dont TT, Tsim KW (2001). "Anti-oxidation activity of different types of natural Cordyceps sinensis and cultured Cordyceps mycelia," Phytomedicine. 8:207-12.

Li Q, Kobayashi M, Wakayama Y, Inagaki H, Katsumata M, Hirata Y, Hirata K, Shimizu T, Kawada T, Park BJ, Ohira T, Kagawa T, Miyazaki Y. (2009 Oct). "Effect of phytoncide from trees on human natural killer cell function," Int J Immunopathol Pharmacol. 22(4):951-9

Li QQ, Lee RX, Liang H, Zhong Y (2013 Jan). "Anticancer activity of beta-elemene and its synthetic analogs in human malignant brain tumor cells," Anticancer Res. 33(1):65-76.

Li QQ, Wang G, Huang F, Li JM, Cuff CF, Reed E (2013 Mar). "Sensitization of lung cancer cells to cisplatin by beta-elemene is mediated through blockade of cell cycle progression: antitumor efficacies of beta-elemene and its synthetic analogs," Med Oncol. 30(1):488.

Li QQ, Wang G, Liang H, Li JM, Huang F, Agarwal PK, Zhong Y, Reed E (2013). "Beta element promotes cisplatin-induced cell death in human bladder cancer and other carcinomas," Anticancer Res. 33(4):1421-8.

Li, R., Liang, T., Xu, L., Li, Y., Zhang, S., & Duan, X. (2013 Jan). Protective effect of cinnamon polyphenols against STZ-diabetic mice fed high-sugar, high-fat diet and its underlying mechanism. Food Chem Toxicol, 51, 419-425.

Li WR, Shi QS, Liang Q, Xie XB, Huang XM, Chen YB (2014 Nov). "Antibacterial Activity and Kinetics of Litsea cubeba Oil on Escherichia coli," PLoS ONE. 9(11):e110983.

Li, X., Duan, S., Chu, C., Xu, J., Zeng, G., Lam, A. K., . . . Jiang, L. (2013 Aug). Melaleuca alternifolia concentrate inhibits in vitro entry of influenza virus into host cells. Molecules, 18(8), 9550-9566.

Li XJ, Yang YJ, Li YS, Zhang W.K., Tang HB (2015 Dec). "α-Pinene, linalool, and 1-octano contribute to the topical anti-inflammatory and analgesic activities of frankincense by inhibiting COX-2," J Ethnopharmacol.

Li, Y. P., Yuan, S. F., Cai, G. H., Wang, H., Wang, L., Yu, L., . . . Yun, J. (2014 May). Patchouli Alcohol Dampens Lipopolysaccharide Induced Mastitis in Mice. Inflammation.

Liakos I, Rizzello L, Scurr D.J., Pomp P.P., Bayer I.S., Athanassiou A. (2014 Mar). "All-natural composite wound dressing films of essential oils encapsulated in sodium alginate with antimicrobial properties," Int. J. Pharm, 463(2):137-145.

Liao JC, Tsai JC, Liu CY, Huang HC, Wu LY, Peng WH (2013). "Antidepressant-like activity of turmerone in behavioral despair tests in mice," BMC Complement. Altern. Med. 13(1):299.

Liapi C, Anifandis G, Chinou I, Kourounakis AP, Theodosopoulos S, Galanopoulou P (2007 Oct). "Antinociceptive properties of 1,8-Cineole and beta-pinene, from the essential oil of Eucalyptus camaldulensis leaves, in rodents," Planta Med. 73(12):1247-54.

Liju V.B., Jeena K, Kuttan R (2015 Jan). "Gastroprotective activity of essential oils from turmeric and ginger," J. Basic Clin. Physiol. Pharmacol. 26(1):95-103.

Lim W.C., Seo J.M., Lee C.I., Pyo H.B., Lee B.C. (2005 jul). "Stimulative and sedative effects of essential oils upon inhalation in mice," Arch. Pharm. Res. 28(7):770-774.

Lima CF, Azevedo MF, Araujo R, Fernandes-Ferreira M, Pereira-Wilson C (2006 Aug). "Metformin-like effect of Salvia officinalis (common sage): is it useful in diabetes prevention?," Br J Nutr. 96(2):326-33.

Lima DF, Brandao MS, Moura JB, Leitao JM Carvalho FA, Miura LM, Leite JR, Sousa DP, Almeida FR (2012 Feb). "Antinociceptive activity of the monoterpene a-phellandrene in rodents: possible mechanisms of action," J Pharm Pharmacol: 64(2):283-92.

Lima N.G.P.B et al (2013 Jan). "Anxiolytic-like activity and GC-MS analysis of (R)-(+)-limonene fragrance, a natural compound found in foods and plants," Pharmacol. Biochem. Behav. 103(3):450-454.

Lin JJ et al (2013 Dec). "Alpha-phellandrene promotes immune responses in normal mice through enhancing macrophage phagocytosis and natural killer cell activities," Vivo Athens Greece. 27(6):809-814.

Lin JJ, Wu CC, Hsu SC, Weng SW, Ma YS, Huang YP, Lin JG, Chung JG (2014 May). "Alpha-phellandrene-induced DNA damage and affect DNA repair protein expression in WEHI-3 murine leukemia cells in vitro," Environ Toxicol. 30(11):1322-30.

Lin PW, Chan WC, Ng BF, Lam LC (2007 May). "Efficacy of aromatherapy (Lavandula angustifolia) as an intervention for agitated behaviours in Chinese older persons with dementia: a cross-over randomized trial," Int J Geriatr Psychiatry. 22(5):405-10.

Lin RF et al. (2014 Jun 11). "Prevention of UV radiation-induced cutaneous photoaging in mice by topical administration of patchouli oil," J Ethnopharmacol. 154(2):408-18.

Lin SC, Chung TC, Lin CC, Ueng TH, Lin YH, Lin SY, Wang LY (2000). "Hepatoprotective effects of Arctium lappa on carbon tetrachloride- and acetaminophen-induced liver damage," Am J Chin Med. 28(2):163-73.

Lin TK, Zhong L, Santiago J.L. (2017 Dec). "Anti-Inflammatory and Skin Barrier Repair Effects of Topical Application of Some Plant Oils," International Journal of Molecular Sciences. 19(1):70.

Linck V.M., da Silva A.L., Figueiro M., Piato A.L., Herrmann A.P., Birck F.D., Moreno P.R.H., Elisabetsky E. (2009) Inhaled linalool-induced sedation in mice. Phytomedicine. 16: 303-307.

Lipovac M, Chedraui P, Gruenhut C, Gocan A, Stammler M, Imhof M (2010 Mar). "Improvement of postmenopausal depressive and anxiety symptoms after treatment with isoflavones derived from red clover extracts," Maturitas. 65(3):258-61.

Lis-Balchin M, Hart S (1999 Sep). "Studies on the mode of action of the essential oil of lavender (Lavandula angustifolia P. Miller)," Phytother Res. 13(6):540-2.

Lis-Balchin M, Hart S, Wan Hang Lo B (2002 Aug). "Jasmine absolute (Jasminum grandiflora L.) and its mode of action on guinea-pig ileum in vitro," Phytother Res. 16(5):437-9.

Liu, C. T., Raghu, R., Lin, S. H., Wang, S. Y., Kuo, C. H., Tseng, Y. J., & Sheen, L. Y. (2013 Nov). Metabolomics of ginger essential oil against alcoholic fatty liver in mice. J Agric Food Chem, 61(46), 11231-11240.

Liu J, Head E, Gharib AM, Yuan W, Ingersoll RT, Hagen TM, Cotman CW, Ames BN (2002 Feb). "Memory loss in old rats is associated with brain mitochondrial decay and RNA/DNA oxidation: partial reversal by feeding acetyl-L-carnitine and/or R-alpha -lipoic acid," Proc Natl Acad Sci U S A. 99(4):2356-61.

Liu J, Killilea DW, Ames BN (2002 Feb 19). "Age-associated mitochondrial oxidative decay: improvement of carnitine acetyltransferase substrate-binding affinity and activity in brain by feeding old rats acetyl-L- carnitine and/ or R-alpha-lipoic acid," Proc Natl Acad Sci U S A. 99(4):1876-81.

Liu JH, Chen GH, Yeh HZ, Huang CK, Poon SK (1997 Dec). "Enteric-coated peppermint-oil capsules in the treatment of irritable bowel syndrome: a prospective, randomized trial," J Gastroenterol. 32(6):765-8.

Liu JJ, Nilsson A, Oredsson S, Badmaev V, Duan RD (2002 Oct). "Keto- and acetyl-keto-boswellic acids inhibit proliferation and induce apoptosis in Hep G2 cells via a caspase-8 dependent pathway," Int J Mol Med. 10(4):501-5.

Liu JJ, Nilsson A, Oredsson S, Badmaev V, Zhao WZ, Duan RD (2002 Dec). "Boswellic acids trigger apoptosis via a pathway dependent on caspase-8 activation but independent on Fas/Fas ligand interaction in colon cancer HT-29 cells," Carcinogenesis. 23(12):2087-93.

Liu R, Sui X, Laditka JN, Church TS, Colabianchi N, Hussey J, Blair SN, (2012 Feb). "Cardiorespiratory fitness as a predictor of dementia mortality in men and women," Med Sci Sports Exerc, 44(2):253-9.

Liu TT, Yang TS (2012 May). "Antimicrobial impact of the components of essential oil of Litsea cubeba from Taiwan and antimicrobial activity of the oil in food systems," International Journal of Food Microbiology. 156(1):68-75.

Lobo, V., Patil, A., Phatak, A., & Chandra, N. (2010 Jul). Free radicals, antioxidants and functional foods: Impact on human health. Pharmacogn Rev, 4(8), 118-126.

Loew O. (1900) A New Enzyme of General Occurrence in Organisms. Science. 11: 701-702.

Lohidasan S, Paradkar AR, Mahadik KR (2009 Nov). "Nootropic activity of lipid-based extract of Bacopa monniera Linn. compared with traditional preparation and extracts," J Pharm Pharmacol. 61(11):1537-44.

Loizzo MR, Tundis R, Menichini F, Saab AM, Statti GA, Menichini F (2007 Sep-Oct). "Cytotoxic activity of essential oils from labiatae and lauraceae families against in vitro human tumor models," Anticancer Res. 27(5A):3293-9.

Long J, Gao F, Tong L, Cotman CW, Ames BN, Liu J (2009 Apr). "Mitochondrial decay in the brains of old rats: ameliorating effect of alpha-lipoic acid and acetyl-L-carnitine," Neurochem Res. 34(4):755-63.

Longley D.B., Harkin D.P., Johnston P.G. (2003) 5-Fluorouracil: Mechanisms of Action and Clinical Strategies. Nature Reviews. 3: 330-338.

López, V., Nielsen, B., Solas, M., Ramírez, M. J., & Jäger, A. K. (2017 May 19). "Exploring Pharmacological Mechanisms of Lavender (Lavandula angustifolia) Essential Oil on Central Nervous System Targets," Front Pharmacol. 8:280.

Loughlin R, Gilmore BF, McCarron PA, Tunney MM (2008 Apr). "Comparison of the cidal activity of tea tree oil and terpinen-4-ol against clinical bacterial skin isolates and human fibroblast cells.," Lett Appl Microbiol. 46(4):428-33.

Louis M, Kowalski S.D. (2002 Dec). "Use of aromatherapy with hospice patients to decrease pain, anxiety, and depression and to promote an increased sense of well-being," Am. J. Hosp. Palliat. Care. 19(6):381-386.

Lu J. et al (2014 Sep). "Sesquiterpene acids from Shellac and their bioactivities evaluation," Fitoterapia. 97:64-70.

Lu LJ, Cree M, Josyula S, Nagamani M, Grady JJ, Anderson KE (2000 Mar 1). "Increased urinary excretion of 2-hydroxyestrone but not 16alpha-hydroxyestrone in premenopausal women during a soya diet containing isoflavones," Cancer Res. 60(5):1299-305.

Lu M, Battinelli L, Daniele C, Melchioni C, Salvatore G, Mazzanti G (2002 Mar). "Muscle relaxing activity of Hyssopus officinalis essential oil on isolated intestinal preparations," Planta Med. 68(3):213-6.

Lu M, Xia L, Hua H, Jing Y (2008 Feb 15). "Acetyl-keto-beta-boswellic acid induces apoptosis through a death receptor 5-mediated pathway in prostate cancer cells," Cancer Res. 68(4):1180-6.

Lu, T., Sheng, H., Wu, J., Cheng, Y., Zhu, J., & Chen, Y. (2012 Jun). Cinnamon extract improves fasting blood glucose and glycosylated hemoglobin level in Chinese patients with type 2 diabetes. Nutr Res, 32(6), 408-412.

Lu X, Feng B, Zhan L, Yu Z (2003 Jul). "[D-limonene induces apoptosis of gastric cancer cells]," Zhonghua Zhong Liu Za Zhi. 25(4):325-327.

Lu XG, Zhan LB, Feng BA, Qu MY, Yu LH, Xie JH (2004 Jul). "Inhibition of growth and metastasis of human gastric cancer implanted in nude mice by d-limonene," World J. Gastroenterol. 10(14):2140-2144.

Lu XQ, Tang FD, Wang Y, Zhao T, Bian RL (2004 Feb). "Effect of Eucalyptus globulus oil on lipopolysaccharide-induced chronic bronchitis and mucin hypersecretion in rats," Zhongguo Zhong Yao Za Zhi. 29(2):168-71.

Lucas M, Asselin G, Mérette C, Poulin MJ, Dodin S (2009 Feb). "Ethyl-eicosapentaenoic acid for the treatment of psychological distress and depressive symptoms in middle-aged women: a double-blind, placebo-controlled, randomized clinical trial," Am J Clin Nutr. 89(2):641-51.

Luo M, Jiang LK, Zou GL (2005). "Acute and genetic toxicity of essential oil extracted from Litsea cubeba (Lour.) Pers.," Journal of Food Protection®. 68(3):581-588.

Luqman S, Dwivedi G.R., Darokar M.P., Kalra A, Khanuja S.P.S. (2007 Oct). "Potential of rosemary oil to be used in drug-resistant infections," Altern. Ther. Health Med. 13(5):54-59.

Lytle J, Mwatha C, Davis K.K (2014 Jan). "Effect of Lavender Aromatherapy on Vital Signs and Perceived Quality of Sleep in the Intermediate Care Unit: A Pilot Study," Am. J. Crit. Care. 23(1):24-29.

Maatta-Riihinen KR, Kahkonen MP, Torronen AR, Heinonen IM (2005 Nov 2). "Catechins and procyanidins in berries of vaccinium species and their antioxidant activity," J Agric Food Chem. 53(22):8485-91.

Mabrok HB, Klopfleisch R, Ghanem KZ, Clavel T, Blaut M, Loh G (2012 Jan). "Lignan transformation by gut bacteria lowers tumor burden in a gnotobiotic rat model of breast cancer," Carcinogenesis. 33(1):203-8.

Machado, D. G., Cunha, M. P., Neis, V. B., Balen, G. O., Colla, A., Bettio, L. E., . . . Rodrigues, A. L. (2013 Jan). Antidepressant-like effects of fractions, essential oil, carnosol and betulinic acid isolated from Rosmarinus officinalis L. Food Chem, 136(2), 999-1005.

Maddocks-Jennings W, Wilkinson JM, Cavanagh HM, Shillington D (2009 Apr). "Evaluating the effects of the essential oils Leptospermum scoparium (manuka) and Kunzea ericoides (kanuka) on radiotherapy induced mucositis: a randomized, placebo controlled feasibility study," Eur J Oncol Nurs. 13(2):87-93.

Mahboubi M (2017 Feb). "Mentha spicata as natural analgesia for treatment of pain in osteoarthritis patients," Complement Ther Clin Pract. 26:1-4.

Mahesh A, Jeyachandran R, Cindrella L, Thangadurai D, Veerapur VP, Muralidhara Rao D (2010 Jun). "Hepatocurative potential of sesquiterpene lactones of Taraxacum officinale on carbon tetrachloride induced liver toxicity in mice," Acta Biol Hung. 61(2):175-90.

Maickel, R. P., & Snodgrass, W. R. (1973 Oct). Physicochemical factors in maternal-fetal distribution of drugs. Toxicology and Applied Pharmacology, 26(2), 218-230.

Malachowska B, Fendler W, Pomykala A, Suwala S, Mlynarski W (2016 Jan). "Essential oils reduce autonomous response to pain sensation during self-monitoring of blood glucose among children with diabetes," J. Pediatr. Endocrinol. Metab. JPEM. 29(1):47-53.

Mao S, Wang K, Lei Y, Yao S, Lu B, Huang W (2017 Apr). "Antioxidant synergistic effects of Osmanthus fragrans flowers with green tea and their major contributed antioxidant compounds," Sci Rep. 7.

Maiwulanjiang M, Zhu KY, Chen J, Miernisha A, Xu SL, Du CYQ, Lau KKM, Choi, RCY, Dong TTX, Aisa HA, Tsim KWK (2013). "Song bu li decoction, a traditional uyghur medicine, protects cell death by regulation of oxidative stress and differentiation in cultured PC12 cells," Evidence-Based Complementary and Alternative Medicine.

Maiwulanjiang M, Zhu KY, Chen J, Miernisha A, Xu SL, Du CYQ, Lau KKM, Choi, RCY, Dong TTX, Aisa HA, Tsim KWK (2014 Apr). "The volatile oil of Nardostachyos radix et rhizoma inhibits the oxidative stress-induced cell injury via reactive oxygen species scavenging and Akt activation in H9c2 cardiomyocyte," J Ethnopharmacol. 153(2):491-8.

Maiwulanjiang M, Bi CW, Lee, PS, Xin G, Miernisha A, Lau KM, Xiong A, Li N, Dong TTX, Aisa HA, Tsim KWK (2014 Apr). "The volatile oil of nardostachyos radix et rhizoma induces endothelial nitric oxide synthase activity in HUVEC cells," PLOS One.

Malachowska B, Fendler W, Pomykala A, Suwala S, Mlynarski W (2016 Jan). "Essential oils reduce autonomous response to pain sensation during self-monitoring of blood glucose among children with diabetes," J. Pediatr. Endocrinol. Metab. JPEM. 29(1):47-53

Malaguarnera M, Cammalleri L, Gargante MP, Vacante M, Colonna V, Motta M (2007 Dec). "L-Carnitine treatment reduces severity of physical and mental fatigue and increases cognitive functions in centenarians: a randomized and controlled clinical trial," Am J Clin Nutr. 86(6):1738-44.

Manassero C.A., Girotti J.R., Mijailovsky S, García de Bravo M, Polo M (2013). "In vitro comparative analysis of antiproliferative activity of essential oil from mandarin peel and its principal component limonene," Nat. Prod. Res. 27(16):1475-1478.

Mandel S, Stoner GD (1990 Jan). "Inhibition of N-nitrosobenzylmethylamine-induced esophageal tumorigenesis in rats by ellagic acid," Carcinogenisis. 11(1):55-61.

Manohar V, Ingram C, Gray J, Talpur NA, Echard BW, Bagchi D, Preuss HG (2001 Dec). "Antifungal activities of origanum oil against Candida albicans," Mol Cell Biochem. 228(1-2):111-7.

Manosroi J, Dhumtanom P, Manosroi A (2006 Apr). "Anti-proliferative activity of essential oil extracted from Thai medicinal plants on KB and P388 cell lines," Cancer Lett. 235(1):114-120.

Maquart FX, Siméon A, Pasco S, Monboisse JC (1999). "[Regulation of cell activity by the extracellular matrix: the concept of matrikines]," J Soc Biol. 193(4-5):423-8.

Marder M, Viola H, Wasowski C, Fernández S, Medina JH, Paladini AC (2003 Jun). "6-methylapigenin and hesperidin: new valeriana flavonoids with activity on the CNS," Pharmacol Biochem Behav. 75(3):537-45.

Margetts, L., & Sawyer, R. (2007). Transdermal drug delivery: principles and opioid therapy. Continuing Education in Anaesthesia, Critical Care & Pain, 7(5), 171-176.

Marinangeli CP, Jones PJ (2012 Aug). "Pulse grain consumption and obesity: effects on energy expenditure, substrate oxidation, body composition, fat deposition and satiety," Br J Nutr. 108 Suppl 1:246-51.

Marotti M, Piccaglia R, Giovanelli E, Deans S.G., Eaglesham E (1994 May). "Effects of planting time and mineral fertilization on peppermint (mentha x piperita l.) essential oil. 9(3):125-129.

composition and its biological activity," Flavour Fragr. J

Marounek M, Skrivanova E, Rada V, (2003). "Susceptibility of Escherichia coli to C2-C18 fatty acids," Folia Microbiol (Praha). 48(6):731-5.

Martins Mdo R, Arantes S, Candeias F, Tinoco MT, Cruz-Morais J (2013 Nov). "Antioxidant, antimicrobial and toxicological properties of Schinus molle L. essential oil," J Ethnopharmacol. 151(1):485-92.

Maruf FA, Salako BL, Akinpelu AO (2014 Jun). "Can aerobic exercise complement antihypertensive drugs to achieve blood pressure control in individuals with essential hypertension," J Cardiovasc Med (Hagerstown), 15(6):456-62.

Maruyama N, Sekimoto Y, Ishibashi H, Inouye S, Oshima H, Yamaguchi H, Abe S (2005 Feb 10). "Suppression of neutrophil accumulation in mice by cutaneous application of geranium essential oil," J Inflamm (Lond). 2(1):1.

Masago R. et al (2000 Jan). "Effects of inhalation of essential oils on EEG activity and sensory evaluation," J. Physiol. Anthropol. Appl. Human Sci. 19(1):35-42.

Masango, P. (2005). Cleaner production of essential oils by steam distillation. Journal of Cleaner Production, 13(8), 833-839.

Masukawa Y., Narita H., Sato H., Naoe A., Kondo N., Sugai Y., Oba T., Homma R., Ishikawa J., Takagi Y., Kitahara T. (2009) Comprehensive quantification of ceramide species in human stratum corneum. Journal of Lipid Research. 50: 1708-1719.

Masumoto Y, Morinushi T, Kawasaki H, Ogura T, Takigawa M (1999 Feb). "Effects of three principal constituents in chewing gum on electroencephalographic activity," Psychiatry Clin. Neurosci. 53(1):17-23.

Matsubara E et al (2012). "Volatiles emitted from the roots of Vetiveria zizanioides suppress the decline in attention during a visual display terminal task," Biomed. Res. Tokyo Jpn. 33(5):299-308.

Matsubara E., Tsunetsugu Y., Ohira T., & Sugiyama M. (2017 Jan. 21). "Essential Oil of Japanese Cedar (Cryptomeria japonica) Wood Increases Salivary Dehydroepiandrosterone Sulfate Levels after Monotonous Work," Int J Res Public Health. 14(1).

Matsumoto T, Asakura H, Hayashi T (2013). "Does lavender aromatherapy alleviate premenstrual emotional symptoms?: a randomized crossover trial," Biopsychosoc. Med. 7:12.

Matsumoto T, Kimura T, Hayashi T (2016 Apr). "Aromatic effects of a Japanese citrus fruit-yuzu (Citrus junos Sieb. ex Tanaka)-on psychoemotional states and autonomic nervous system activity during the menstrual cycle: a single-blind randomized controlled crossover study," Biopsychosoc Med. 10:11.

Matsumoto T, Kimura T, Hayashi T (2017 May). "Does Japanese Citrus Fruit Yuzu (Citrus junos Sieb. ex Tanaka) Fragrance Have Lavender-Like Therapeutic Effects That Alleviate Premenstrual Emotional Symptoms? A Single-Blind Randomized Crossover Study," J Altern Complement Med. 23(6):461-470.

Matsuo A.L. et al (2011 Jul). "α-Pinene isolated from Schinus terebinthifolius Raddi (Anacardiaceae) induces apoptosis and confers antimetastatic protection in a melanoma model," Biochem. Biophys. Res. Commun. 411(2):449-454.

Matthys H, de Mey C, Carls C, Ryś A, Geib A, Wittig T (2000 Aug). "Efficacy and tolerability of myrtol standardized in acute bronchitis. A multi-centre, randomised, double-blind, placebo-controlled parallel group clinical trial vs. cefuroxime and ambroxol," Arzneimittelforschung. 50(8):700-711.

Maurya, A. K., Singh, M., Dubey, V., Srivastava, S., Luqman, S., Bawankule, D. U. (2014 Jun 5). "α-(-)-bisabolol reduces pro-inflammatory cytokine production and ameliorates skin inflammation," Curr Pharm Biotechnol, 15(2): 173-181.

May B, Kuntz HD, Kieser M, Köhler S (1996 Dec). "Efficacy of a fixed peppermint oil/caraway oil combination in non-ulcer dyspepsia," Arzneimittelforschung. 46(12):1149-53.

McCaffrey R, Thomas D.J., Kinzelman A.O. (2009 Apr). "The effects of lavender and rosemary essential oils on test-taking anxiety among graduate nursing students," Holist. Nurs. Pract. 23(2):88-93.

McKay D.L., Blumberg J.B. (2006 Aug). "A review of the bioactivity and potential health benefits of peppermint tea (Mentha piperita L.)," Phytother. Res. PTR. 20(8):619-633.

McCord J.M., Fridovich I. (1969) Superoxide Dismutase: an enzymic function for erytrocuprein (hemocuprein). The Journal of Biological Chemistry. 244: 6049-6055.

Meamarbashi, A., & Rajabi, A. (2013 Mar). The effects of peppermint on exercise performance. J Int Soc Sports Nutr, 10(1), 15.

Mehta S, Stone D.N. Whitehead H.F. (1998 Jul). "Use of essential oil to promote induction of anaesthesia." Anaesthesia. 53(7):720-721.

Meier B, Berger D, Hoberg E, Sticher O, Schaffner W, (2000). "Pharmacological Activities of Vitex agnus-castus Extracts in Vitro," Phytomedicine. 7(5):373-81.

Meier , L., Stange, R., Michalsen, A., & Uehleke, B. (2012 May). Clay jojoba oil facial mask for lesioned skin and mild acne--results of a prospective, observational pilot study. Forsch Komplementmed, 19(2), 75-79.

Meiller, T. F., Silva, A., Ferreira, S. M., Jabra-Rizk, M. A., Kelley, J. I., & DePaola, L. G. (2005 Apr). Efficacy of Listerine Antiseptic in reducing viral contamination of saliva. J Clin Periodontol, 32(4), 341-346.

Meister R, Wittig T, Beuscher N, de Mey C (1999 Apr). "Efficacy and tolerability of myrtol standardized in long-term treatment of chronic bronchitis. A double-blind, placebo-controlled study. Study Group Investigators," Arzneimittelforschung. 49(4):351-358.

Meldrum B.S. (1994) The role of glutamate in epilepsy and other CNS disorders. Neurology. 44: S14-S23.

Meldrum B.S., Akbar M.T., Chapman A.G. (1999) Glutamate receptors and transporters in genetic and acquired models of epilepsy. Epilepsy Research. 36: 189-204.

Melo, F. H., Venancio, E. T., de Sousa, D. P., de Franca Fonteles, M. M., de Vasconcelos, S. M., Viana, G. S., & de Sousa, F. C. (2010 Aug). Anxiolytic-like effect of Carvacrol (5-isopropyl-2-methylphenol) in mice: involvement with GABAergic transmission. Fundam Clin Pharmacol, 24(4), 437-443.

Melov S., Ravenscroft J., Malik S., Gill M.S., Walker D.W., Clayton P.E., Wallace D.C., Malfroy B., Doctrow S.R., Lithgow G.J. (2000) Extension of Life-Span with Superoxide Dismutase/Catalase Mimetics. Science. 289: 1567-1569.

Mercier B., Prost J., Prost M. (2009) The Essential Oil of Turpentine and Its Major Volatile Fraction (α- and β-Pinenes): A Review. International Journal of Occupational Medicine and Environmental Health. 22: 331-342.

Metwalli K.H., Khan S.A., Krom B.P., Jabra-Rizk M.A. (2013 Oct). "Streptococcus mutans, Candida albicans, and the Human Mouth: A Sticky Situation," PLoS Pathog. 9(10).

Michie C.A., Cooper E (1991). "Frankincense and myrrh as remedies in children," J. R. Soc. Med. 84(10):602-605.

Miguel, M. G. (2010 Dec). Antioxidant and anti-inflammatory activities of essential oils: a short review. Molecules, 15(12), 9252-9287.

Mikhaeil B.R., Maatooq G.T., Badria F.A., Amer M.M.A. (2003 Apr). "Chemistry and immunomodulatory activity of frankincense oil," Z. Naturforsch., C, J. Biosci. 58(3-4):230-238.

Miller J.A. et al (2013 Jun). "Human breast tissue disposition and bioactivity of limonene in women with earlystage breast cancer," Cancer Prev. Res. 6(6):557-84.

Miller J.A. et al (2015 Jan). "Plasma metabolomic profiles of breast cancer patients after short-term limonene intervention," Cancer Prev. Res. 8(1):86-93.

Miller J.A., Hakin I.A., Chew W, Thompson P, Thomson C.A., Chow HS (2010). "Adipose tissue accumulation of d-limonene with the consumption of a lemonade preparation rich in d-limonene content," Nutr. Cancer. 62(6):783-788.

Mills JJ, Chari RS, Boyer IJ, Gould MN, Jirtle RL (1995 Mar 1). "Induction of apoptosis in liver tumors by the monoterpene perillyl alcohol," Cancer Res. 55(5):979-83.

Mimica-Dukić N, Bozin B, Soković M, Mihajlović B, Matavulj M (2003 May). "Antimicrobial and antioxidant activities of three Mentha species essential oils," Planta Med. 69(5):413-9.

Minaiyan, M., Ghannadi, A. R., Afsharipour, M., & Mahzouni, P. (2011 Jan). Effects of extract and essential oil of Rosmarinus officinalis L. on TNBS-induced colitis in rats. Res Pharm Sci, 6(1), 13-21.

Miocinovic R et al. (2005 Jan). "In vivo and in vitro effect of baicalin on human prostate cancer cells," Int J Oncol. 26(1):241-6.

Mishra, A., Bhatti, R., Singh, A., & Singh Ishar, M. P. (2010 Mar). Ameliorative effect of the cinnamon oil from Cinnamomum zeylanicum upon early stage diabetic nephropathy. Planta Med, 76(5), 412-417.

Mishra S, Palanivelu K (2008). "The effect of curcumin (turmeric) on Alzheimer's disease: An overview," Ann. Indian Acad. Neurol. 11(1):13-19.

Misharina TA, Bulakova EB, Fatkullina LD, Terinina MB, Krikunova NI, Vorob'eva AK, Erokhin VN, Goloshchapov AN (2011 Nov–Dec). "Changes in fatty acid composition in the brain and liver in aging mice of high cancer risk AKR strain and effect of savory essential oil administration on leukemic process," biomed Khim. 57(6):604-14.

Mix, J. A., & Crews, W. D., Jr. (2000 Jun). An examination of the efficacy of Ginkgo biloba extract EGb761 on the neuropsychologic functioning of cognitively intact older adults. J Altern Complement Med, 6(3), 219-229.

Miyazawa M, Shindo M, Shimada T (2002 May). "Metabolism of (+)- and (-)-limonenes to respective carveols and perillyl alcohols by CYP2C9 and CYP2C19 in human liver microsomes," Drug Metab. Dispos. Biol. Fate Chem. 30(5):602-607.

Mkolo MN, Magano SR (2007 Sep). "Repellent effects of the essential oil of Lavendula angustifolia against adults of Hyalomma marginatum rufipes," J S Afr Vet Assoc. 78(3):149-52.

Mogosan, C., Vostinaru, O., Operean, R., Heghes, C., Filip, L., Balica, G., & Moldovan R.I. (2017 Feb. 10). "A Comparative Analysis of the Chemical Composition, Anti-Inflammatory, and Antinociceptive Effects of the Essential Oils from Three Species of Mentha Cultivated in Romania," Molecules. 22(2).

Mohamed A.G., Abbas H.M., Kassem J.M., Gafour W.A., Attalah A.G. (2016 Feb). "Impact of Myrrh Essential Oil as a Highly Effective Antimicrobial Agent in Processed Cheese Spreads," Int. J. Dairy Sci. 11(2):41-51.

Mohamed S.A., Khan J.A. (2013 Feb). "Antioxidant capacity of chewing stick miswak Salvadora persica," BMC Complement. Altern. Med. 13:40.

Mohsenzadeh M (2007 Oct 15). "Evaluation of antibacterial activity of selected Iranian essential oils against Staphylococcus aureus and Escherichia coli in nutrient broth medium," Pak J Biol Sci. 10(20):3693-7.

Mondello F, De Bernardis F, Girolamo A, Cassone A, Salvatore G (2006 Nov 3). "In vivo activity of terpinen-4-ol, the main bioactive component of Melaleuca alternifolia Cheel (tea tree) oil against azole-susceptible and -resistant human pathogenic Candida species," BMC Infect Dis. 6:158.

Monfalouti HE, Guillaume D, Denhez C, Charrouf Z (2010 Dec). "Therapeutic potential of argan oil: a review," J Pharm Pharmacol. 62(12):1669-75.

Monsefi, M., Zahmati, M., Masoudi, M., & Javidnia, K. (2011 Dec). Effects of Anethum graveolens L. on fertility in male rats. Eur J Contracept Reprod Health Care, 16(6), 488-497.

Moon HJ, Park KS, Ku MJ, Lee MS, Jeong SH, Imbs TI, Zvyagintseva TN, Ermakova SP, Lee YH (2009 Oct). "Effect of Costaria costata fucoidan on expression of matrix metalloproteinase-1 promoter, mRNA, and protein," J Nat Prod. 72(10):1731-4.

Moon SE, Kim HY, Cha JD (2011 Sep). "Synergistic effect between clove oil and its major compounds and antibiotics against oral bacteria," Arch. Oral Biol. 56(9):907-916.

Moon T, Wilkinson JM, Cavanagh HM (2006 Nov). "Antiparasitic activity of two Lavandula essential oils against Giardia duodenalis, Trichomonas vaginalis and Hexamita inflata," Parasitol Res. 99(6):722-8.

Moore LE, Brennan P, Karami S, Hung RJ, Hsu C, Boffetta P, Toro J, Zaridze D, Janout V, Bencko V, Navratilova M, Szeszenia-Dabrowska N, Mates D, Mukeria A, Holcatova I, Welch R, Chanock S, Rothman N, Chow WH (2007 Sep). "Glutathione S-transferase polymorphisms, cruciferous vegetable intake and cancer risk in the Central and Eastern European Kidney Cancer Study," Carcinogenesis. 28(9):1960-4.

Moraes T.M. et al (2009 Aug). "Effects of limonene and essential oil from Citrus aurantium on gastric mucosa: role of prostaglandins and gastric mucus secretion," Chem. Biol. Interact. 180(3):499-505.

Moreno S, Scheyer T, Romano CS, Vojnov AA (2006 Feb). "Antioxidant and antimicrobial activities of rosemary extracts linked to their polyphenol composition," Free Radic Res. 40(2):223-31.

Moretti MD, Sanna-Passino G, Demontis S, Bazzoni E (2002). "Essential oil formulations useful as a new tool for insect pest control," AAPS PharmSciTech. 3(2):E13.

Mori TA, Bao DQ, Burke V, Puddey IB, Beilin LJ (1999 Aug). "Docosahexaenoic acid but not eicosapentaenoic acid lowers ambulatory blood pressure and heart rate in humans," Hypertension. 34(2):253-60.

Morris N (2002 Dec). "The effects of lavender (Lavendula angustifolium) baths on psychological well-being: two exploratory randomised control trials," Complement. Ther. Med. 10(4):223-228.

Morinobu A et al. (2008 Jul). "-Epigallocatechin-3-gallate suppresses osteoclast differentiation and ameliorates experimental arthritis in mice," Arthritis Rheum. 58(7):2012-8.

Morowitz, M. J., Carlisle, E. M., & Alverdy, J. C. (2011). Contributions of intestinal bacteria to nutrition and metabolism in the critically ill. Surg Clin North Am, 91(4), 771-785, viii.

Morris MC, Sacks F, Rosner B (1993 Aug). "Does fish oil lower blood pressure? A meta-analysis of controlled trials," Circulation. 88(2):523-33.

Morris N (2002 Dec). "The effects of lavender (Lavendula angustifolium) baths on psychological well-being: two exploratory randomised control trials," Complement. Ther. Med. 10(4):223-228.

Morse M.A., Stoner G.D. (1993) Cancer chemoprevention: principles and prospects. Carcinogenesis. 14: 1737-1746.

Mosaffa F, Behravan J, Karimi G, Iranshahi M (2006 Feb). "Antigenotoxic effects of Satureja hortensis L. on rat lymphocytes exposed to oxidative stress," Arch Pharm Res. 29(2):159-64.

Moss M, Cook J, Wesnes K, Duckett P (2003 Jan). "Aromas of rosemary and lavender essential oils differentially affect cognition and mood in healthy adults," Int J Neurosci. 113(1):15-38.

Moss M, Hewitt S, Moss L, Wesnes K (2008 Jan). "Modulation of cognitive performance and mood by aromas of peppermint and ylang-ylang," Int J Neurosci. 118(1):59-77.

Moss M, Oliver L (2012). "Plasma 1, 8-cineole correlates with cognitive performance following exposure to rosemary essential oil aroma," Ther. Adv. Psychopharmacol. 2(3):103-113.

Motomura N, Sakurai A, Yotsuya Y (2001 Dec). "Reduction of mental stress with lavender odorant," Percept Mot Skills. 93(3):713-8.

Moussaieff A. et al (2008 Aug). "Incensole acetate, an incense component, elicits psychoactivity by activating TRPV3 channels in the brain," FASEB J. 22(8):3024-3034.

Moussaieff A, Rimmerman N, Bregman T, Straiker A, Felder CC, Shoham S, Kashman Y, Huang SM, Lee H, Shohami E, Mackie K, Caterina MJ, Walker JM, Fride E, Mechoulam R (2008 Aug). "Incensole acetate, an incense component, elicits psychoactivity by activating TRPV3 channels in the brain," FASEB J. 22(8):3024-34.

Moussaieff A, Shein NA, Tsenter J, Grigoriadis S, Simeonidou C, Alexandrovich AG, Trembovler V, Ben-Neriah Y, Schmitz ML, Fiebich BL, Munoz E, Mechoulam R, Shohami E (2008 Jul). "Incensole acetate: a novel neuroprotective agent isolated from Boswellia carterii," J Cereb Blood Flow Metab. 28(7):1341-52.

Moustafa, A. H., Ali, E. M., Moselhy, S. S., Tousson, E., & El-Said, K. S. (2012 Oct). Effect of coriander on thioacetamide-induced hepatotoxicity in rats. Toxicol Ind Health, 1-10.

Moy KA, Yuan JM, Chung FL, Wang XL, Van Den Berg D, Wang R, Gao YT, Yu MC (2009 Dec 1). "Isothiocyanates, glutathione S-transferase M1 and T1 polymorphisms and gastric cancer risk: a prospective study of men in Shanghai, China," Int J Cancer. 125(11):2652-9.

Mugnaini, L., Nardoni, S., Pinto, L., Pistelli, L., Leonardi, M., Pisseri, F., & Mancianti, F. (2012 Jun). In vitro and in vivo antifungal activity of some essential oils against feline isolates of Microsporum canis. J Mycol Med, 22(2), 179-184.

Muhlbauer, R. C., Lozano, A., Palacio, S., Reinli, A., & Felix, R. (2003 Apr). Common herbs, essential oils, and monoterpenes potently modulate bone metabolism. Bone, 32(4), 372-380.

Mukherjee P.K., Chandra J., Kuhn D.M., Ghannoum M.A. (2003) Mechanism of Fluconazole Resistance in Candida albicansBiofilms: Phase-Specific Role of Efflux Pumps and Membrane Sterols. Infection and Immunity. 71: 4333-4340.

Mumcuoglu KY, Magdassi S, Miller J, Ben-Ishai F, Zentner G, Helbin V, Friger M, Kahana F, Ingber A (2004 Dec). "Repellency of citronella for head lice: double-blind randomized trial of efficacy and safety," Isr Med Assoc J. 6(12):756-9.

Munzel T., Feil R., Mulsch A., Lohmann S.M., Hofmann F., Walter U. (2003) Physiology and Pathophysiology of Vascular Signaling Controlled by Cyclic Guanosine 3',5' –Cyclic Monophospate—Dependent Protein Kinase. Circulation. 108: 2172-2183.

Muzzarelli L, Force M, Sebold M (2006 Dec). "Aromatherapy and reducing preprocedural anxiety: A controlled prospective study," Gastroenterol. Nurs. Off. J. Soc. Gastroenterol. Nurses Assoc. 29(6):466-471.

Na HJ, Koo HN, Lee GG, Yoo SJ, Park JH, Lyu YS, Kim HM (2001 Dec). "Juniper oil inhibits the heat shock-induced apoptosis via preventing the caspase-3 activation in human astrocytes CCF-STTG1 cells," Clin Chim Acta. 314(1-2):215-20.

Nadeem M, Anjum FM, Kah MI, Tehseen S, El-Ghorab A, sultan JI (2013 May). "Nutritional and medicinal aspects of coriander (Coriandrum sativum L.)," British Food Journal. 115(5):743-55.

Nadim M.M., Malink A.A., Ahmad J, Bakshi S.K. (2011). "The essential oil composition of Achillea millefolium L. cultivated under tropical condition in India," World J Agric Sci. 7(5):561-565.

Nagashyana N, Sankarankutt P, Nampoothiri MRV, Moahan P, Mohan Kumar P (2000). "Association of L-dopa with recovery following Ayurvedic medication in Parkinson's disease," J Neurol Sci. 176:1121-7.

Naguib YM (2000 Apr). "Antioxidant activities of astaxanthin and related carotenoids," J Agric Food Chem. 48(4):1150-4.

Nair B (2001). "Final report on the safety assessment of Mentha Piperita (Peppermint) Oil, Mentha Piperita (Peppermint) Leaf Extract, Mentha Piperita (Peppermint) Leaf, and Mentha Piperita (Peppermint) Leaf Water," Int J Toxicol. 20(Suppl 3):61-73..

Nair B, Joy J, Vasudevan P, Hinckley L, Hoagland TA, Venkitanarayanan KS (2009 Mar 30). "Antibacterial effect of caprylic acid and monocaprylin on major bacterial mastitis pathogens," Vet Microbiol. 135(3-4):358-62.

Nair, V., Singh, S., & Gupta, Y. K. (2012 Mar). Evaluation of disease modifying activity of Coriandrum sativum in experimental models. Indian J Med Res, 135, 240-245.

Nakayama, S., Kishimoto, Y., Saita, E., Sugihara, N., Toyozaki, M., Taguchi, C., . . . Kondo, K. (2015 Jan). Pine bark extract prevents low-density lipoprotein oxidation and regulates monocytic expression of antioxidant enzymes. Nutr Res, 35(1), 56-64.

Nanthakomon T, Pongrojpaw D (2006 Oct). "The efficacy of ginger in prevention of postoperative nausea and vomiting after major gynecologic surgery," J Med Assoc Thai. 89:S130-6.

Nardoni, S., Mugnaini, L., Pistelli, L., Leonardi, M., Sanna, V., Perrucci, S., . . . Mancianti, F. (2014 Apr). Clinical and mycological evaluation of an herbal antifungal formulation in canine Malassezia dermatitis. J Mycol Med.

Nascimento CM, Pereira JR, de Andrade LP, Garuffi M, Talib LL, Forlenza OV, Cancela JM, Cominetti MR, Stella F, (2014). "Physical exercise in MCI elderly promotes reduction of pro-inflammatory cytokines and improvements on cognition and BDNF peripheral levels," Curr Alzheimer Res, 11(8):799-805.

Narishetty S.T.K., Panchagnula R. (2004) Transdermal delivery of zidovudine: effect of terpenes and their mechanism of action. Journal of Controlled Release. 95: 367-379.

Narishetty S.T.K., Panchagnula R. (2005) Effects of L-menthol and 1,8-cineole on phase behavior and molecular organization of SC lipids and skin permeation of zidovudine. Journal of Controlled Release. 102: 59-70.

Nasel C, Nasel B, Samec P, Schindler E, Buchbauer G (1994 Aug). "Functional imaging of effects of fragrances on the human brain after prolonged inhalation," Chem Senses. 19(4):359-64.

Naseri, M., Mojab, F., Khodadoost, M., Kamalinejad, M., Davati, A., Choopani, R., . . . Emtiazy, M. (2012 Nov). The Study of Anti-Inflammatory Activity of Oil-Based Dill (Anethum graveolens L.) Extract Used Topically in Formalin-Induced Inflammation Male Rat Paw. Iran J Pharm Res, 11(4), 1169-1174.

Nasiri, A., Mahmodi, M.A., & Nobakht, Z. (2016 Nov). "Effect of aromatherapy massage with lavender essential oil on pain in patients with osteoarthritis of the knee: A randomized controlled clinical trial," Complement Ther Clin Pract. 25:75-80.

Navarra M., Mannucci C., Delbò M, Calapai G (2015 Mar). "Citrus bergamia essential oil: from basic research to clinical application," Front Pharmacol. 6.

Navarra, M., Ursino, M. R., Ferlazzo, N., Russo, M., Schumacher, U., & Valentiner, U. (2014 Jun). Effect of Citrus bergamia juice on human neuroblastoma cells in vitro and in metastatic xenograft models. Fitoterapia, 95, 83-92.

Navarro SL, Chang JL, Peterson S, Chen C, King IB, Schwarz Y, Li SS, Li L, Potter JD, Lampe JW (2009 Nov). "Modulation of human serum glutathione S-transferase A1/2 concentration by cruciferous vegetables in a controlled feeding study is influenced by GSTM1 and GSTT1 genotypes," Cancer Epidemiol Biomarkers Prev. 18(11):2974-8.

Navarro SL, Peterson S, Chen C, Makar KW, Schwarz Y, King IB, Li SS, Li L, Kestin M, Lampe JW. (2009 Apr). "Cruciferous vegetable feeding alters UGT1A1 activity: diet- and genotype-dependent changes in serum bilirubin in a controlled feeding trial," Cancer Prev Res (Phila Pa). 2(4):345-52.

Nayak P.A., Nayak U.A., Khandelwal (2014 Nov). "The effect of xylitol on dental caries and oral flora," Clin. Cosmet. Investig. Dent. 6:89-94.

Nevin K.G., Rajamohan T (2010). "Effect of topical application of virgin coconut oil on skin components and antioxidant status during dermal wound healing in young rats," Skin Pharmacol Physiol. 23(6):290-297.

Ngan A, Conduit R (2011 Aug). "A double-blind, placebo-controlled investigation of the effects of Passiflora incarnata (passionflower) herbal tea on subjective sleep quality," Phytother Res. 25(8):1153-9.

Ni X et al (2012). "Frankincense essential oil prepared from hydrodistillation of Boswellia sacra gum resins induces human pancreatic cancer cell death in cultures and in a xenograft murine model," BMC complementary and alternative medicine. 12(1):253.

Nielsen FH, Hunt CD, Mullen LM, Hunt JR (1987 Nov). "Effect of dietary boron on mineral, estrogen, and testosterone metabolism in postmenopausal women," FASEB J. 1(5):394-7.

Nikolaevski VV, Kononova NS, Pertsovski AI, Shinkarchuk IF (1990 Sep-Oct). "Effect of essential oils on the course of experimental atherosclerosis," Patol Fiziol Eksp Ter. (5):52-3.

Ninomiya K, Matsuda H, Shimoda H, Nishida N, Kasajima N, Yoshino T, Morikawa T, Yoshikawa M (2004 Apr 19). "Carnosic acid, a new class of lipid absorption inhibitor from sage," Bioorg Med Chem Lett. 14(8):1943-6.

Ni Raghallaigh S, Bender K, Lacey N, Brennan L, Powell FC (2012 Feb). "The fatty acid profile of the skin surface lipid layer in papulopustular rosacea," Br J Dermatol. 166(2):279-87.

Nishio M, Kawmata H, Fujita K, Ishizaki T, Hayman R, Idemi T (2004). "A new enamel restoring agent for use after PMTC," Journal of Dental Research 83(1920):SpclIssueA.

Nomicos E.Y.H. (2007 Dec). "Myrrh: medical marvel or myth of the Magi?," Holist. Nurs. Pract. 21(6):308-323.

Noori, S., Hassan, Z. M., & Salehian, O. (2013 Mar). Sclareol reduces CD4+ CD25+ FoxP3+ Treg cells in a breast cancer model in vivo. Iran J Immunol, 10(1), 10-21.

Norazmir, M. N., Jr., & Ayub, M. Y. (2010 Apr). Beneficial lipid-lowering effects of pink guava puree in high fat diet induced-obese rats. Malays J Nutr, 16(1), 171-185.

Noreikaitė, A., Ayupova, R., Satbayeva, E., Seitaliyeva, A., Amirkulova, M., Pichkhadze, G., Datkhayev, U., and Stankevičius, E. (2017). "General Toxicity and Antifungal Activity of a New Dental Gel with Essential Oil from Abies Sibirica L.," Med Sci Monit. 23:521-527.

Nord D, Belew J (2009 Oct). "Effectiveness of the essential oils lavender and ginger in promoting children's comfort in a perianesthesia setting," J. Perianesthesia Nurs. Off. J. Am. Soc. PeriAnesthesia Nurses Am. Soc. PeriAnesthesia Nurses. 24(5):307-312.

Nostro A, Bisignano G, Angela Cannatelli M, Crisafi G, Paola Germanò M, Alonzo V (2001 Jun). "Effects of Helichrysum italicum extract on growth and enzymatic activity of Staphylococcus aureus," Int J Antimicrob Agents. 17(6):517-20.

Nostro A, Blanco AR, Cannatelli MA, Enea V, Flamini G, Morelli I, Sudano Roccaro A, Alonzo V (2004 Jan 30). "Susceptibility of methicillin-resistant staphylococci to oregano essential oil, carvacrol and thymol," FEMS Microbiol Lett. 230(2):191-5.

Nostro A, Cannatelli MA, Marino A, Picerno I, Pizzimenti FC, Scoglio ME, Spataro P (2003 Jan). "Evaluation of antiherpesvirus-1 and genotoxic activities of Helichrysum italicum extract," New Microbiol. 26(1):125-8.

Nothlings U, Murphy SP, Wilkens LR, Henderson BE, Kolonel LN (2007 Oct). "Flavonols and pancreatic cancer risk: the multiethnic cohort study," Am J Epidemiol. 166(8):924-31.

Nuñez L, Aquino M.D. (2012). "Microbicide activity of clove essential oil (Eugenia caryophyllata)," Braz. J. Microbiol. 43(4):1255-1260.

Nyadjeu, P., Nguelefack-Mbuyo, E. P., Atsamo, A. D., Nguelefack, T. B., Dongmo, A. B., & Kamanyi, A. (2013 Feb). Acute and chronic antihypertensive effects of Cinnamomum zeylanicum stem bark methanol extract in L-NAME-induced hypertensive rats. BMC Complement Altern Med, 13, 1-10.

Oboh, G., Olasehinde, T. A., & Ademosun, A. O. (2014 Mar). Essential oil from lemon peels inhibit key enzymes linked to neurodegenerative conditions and pro-oxidant induced lipid peroxidation. J Oleo Sci, 63(4), 373-381.

O'Bryan C.A., Crandall P.G., Chalova V.I., Ricke S.C. (2008 Aug). "Orange Essential Oils Antimicrobial Activities against Salmonella spp.," J. Food Sci. 73(6):M264-M267.

Ogeturk, M., Kose, E., Sarsilmaz, M., Akpinar, B., Kus, I., & Meydan, S. (2010 Oct). Effects of lemon essential oil aroma on the learning behaviors of rats. Neurosciences (Riyadh), 15(4), 292-293.

Oh M.J. (2017 Sep). "Novel phytoceramides containing fatty acids of diverse chain lengths are better than a single C18-ceramide N-stearoyl phytosphingosine to improve the physiological properties of human stratum corneum," Clin Cosmet Investig Dermatol. 10:363-371.

Oh S. et al (2014 Jul). "Suppression of Inflammatory cytokine production by ar-Turmerone isolated from Curcuma phaeocaulis," Chem. Biodivers. 11(7):1034-1041.

Ohkawara S, Tanaka-Kagawa T, Furukawa Y, Nishimura T, Jinno H (2010). "Activation of the Human Transient Receptor Potential Vanilloid Subtype 1 by Essential Oils," Biological and Pharmaceutical Bulletin. 33(8):1434-1437.

Ohno T, Kita M, Yamaoka Y, Imamura S, Yamamoto T, Mitsufuji S, Kodama T, Kashima K, Imanishi J (2003 Jun). "Antimicrobial activity of essential oils against Helicobacter pylori," Helicobacter. 8(3):207-15.

Ohta T, Imagawa T, Ito S (2009 Feb). "Involvement of Transient Receptor Potential Vanilloid Subtype 1 in Analgesic Action of Methylsalicylate," Mol. Pharmacol. 75(2):307-317.

Okugawa, H., Ueda, R., Matsumoto, K., Kawanishi, K., & Kato, K. (2000 Oct). Effects of sesquiterpenoids from Oriental incenses on acetic acid-induced writhing and D2 and 5-HT2A receptors in rat brain. Phytomedicine, 7(5), 417-422.

Olajide OA, Ajayi FF, Ekhelar AI, Awe SO, Makinde JM, Alada AR (1999 Jun). "Biological effects of Myristica fragrans (nutmeg) extract," Phytother Res. 13(4):344-5.

Olapour, A., Behaeen, K., Akhondzadeh, R., Soltani, F., Al Sadat Razavi, F., & Bekhradi, R. (2013 Nov). The Effect of Inhalation of Aromatherapy Blend containing Lavender Essential Oil on Cesarean Postoperative Pain. Anesth Pain Med, 3(1), 203-207.

Onawunmi GO, Yisak WA, Ogunlana EO (1984 Dec). "Antibacterial constituents in the essential oil of Cymbopogon citratus (DC.) Stapf.," J Ethnopharmacol. 12(3):279-86.

Onocha, P., Oloyede, G., & Afolabi, Q. (2011). Chemical composition, cytotoxicity and antioxidant activity of essential oils of Acalypha hispida flowers. Inter J Pharm, 7(1), 144-148.

Opalchenova G, Obreshkova D (2003 Jul). "Comparative studies on the activity of basil--an essential oil from Ocimum basilicum L.--against multidrug resistant clinical isolates of the genera Staphylococcus, Enterococcus and Pseudomonas by using different test methods," J Microbiol Methods. 54(1):105-10.

Orafidiya LO, Agbani EO, Abereoje OA, Awe T, Abudu A, Fakoya FA (2003 Oct). "An investigation into the wound-healing properties of essential oil of Ocimum gratissimum linn," J Wound Care. 12(9):331-4.

Orav A, Arak E, Raal A (2006 Oct). "Phytochemical analysis of the essential oil of Achillea millefolium L. from various European Countries," Nat. Prod. Res. 20(12):1082-1088.

Orellana-Paucar A.M. et al (2013 Dec). "Insights from Zebrafish and Mouse Models on the Activity and Safety of Ar-Turmerone as a Potential Drug Candidate for the Treatment of Epilepsy," PLoS ONE. 8(12):e81634.

Ornano L. et al (2013 Aug). "Chemopreventive and Antioxidant Activity of the Chamazulene-Rich Essential Oil Obtained from Artemisia arborescens L. Growing on the Isle of La Maddalena, Sardinia, Italy," Chem. Biodivers. 10(8):1464-1474.

Osawa K, Saeki T, Yasuda H, Hamashima H, Sasatsu M, Araj T (1999). "The Antibacterial Activities of Peppermint Oil and Green Tea Polyphenols, Alone and in Combination, against Enterohemorrhagic <I>Escherichia coil</I>," Biocontrol Sci. 4(1):1-7.

Osher Y, Bersudsky Y, Belmaker RH (2005 Jun). "Omega-3 eicosapentaenoic acid in bipolar depression: report of a small open-label study," J Clin Psychiatry. 66(6):726-9.

Ostad SN, Soodi M, Shariffzadeh M, Khorshidi N, Marzban H (2001 Aug). "The effect of fennel essential oil on uterine contraction as a model for dysmenorrhea, pharmacology and toxicology study," J Ethnopharmacol. 76(3):299-304.

Ou, M. C., Hsu, T. F., Lai, A. C., Lin, Y. T., & Lin, C. C. (2012 May). Pain relief assessment by aromatic essential oil massage on outpatients with primary dysmenorrhea: a randomized, double-blind clinical trial. J Obstet Gynaecol Res, 38(5), 817-822.

Ou-Yang, D.W., Wu, L., Li, Y.L., Yang, P.M., Kong, D.Y., Yang, X.W., and Zhang, W.D. (2011). "Miscellaneous terpenoid constituents of Abies nephrolepis and their moderate cytotoxic activities," Phytochemistry. 72(17):2197-204.

Palmefors H, DuttaRoy S, Rundqvist B, Borjesson M (2014 Jul). "The effect of physical activity or exercise on key biomarkers in atherosclerosis—a systematic review," Atherosclerosis, 235(1):150-61.

Paliwal S, J Sundaram and S Mitragotri (2005). "Induction of cancer-specific cytotoxicity towards human prostate and skin cells using quercetin and ultrasound," British Journal of Cancer. 92:499-502.

Palozza P, Krinsky NI (1992 Sep). "Astaxanthin and canthaxanthin are potent antioxidants in a membrane model," Arch Biochem Biophys. 297(2):291-5.

Pandey, A., Bigoniya, P., Raj, V., & Patel, K. K. (2011 Jul). Pharmacological screening of Coriandrum sativum Linn. for hepatoprotective activity. J Pharm Bioallied Sci, 3(3), 435-441.

Paoletti P., Neyton J. (2007 Jun). NMDA receptor subunits: functions and pharmacology. Current Opinion in Pharmacology. 7: 39-47.

Pardridge, W. M. (2003 Mar). Blood-brain barrier drug targeting: the future of brain drug development. Mol Interv, 3(2).

Pardridge, W. M. (2009 Sep). Alzheimer's disease drug development and the problem of the blood-brain barrier. Alzheimers Dement, 5(5), 427-432.

Parimoo, H. A., Sharma, R., Patil, R. D., Sharma, O. P., Kumar, P., & Kumar, N. (2014 Apr). Hepatoprotective effect of Ginkgo biloba leaf extract on lantadenes-induced hepatotoxicity in guinea pigs. Toxicon, 81, 1-12.

Park, G., Kim, H. G., Kim, Y. O., Park, S. H., Kim, S. Y., & Oh, M. S. (2012 Feb). Coriandrum sativum L. protects human keratinocytes from oxidative stress by regulating oxidative defense systems. Skin Pharmacol Physiol, 25(2), 93-99.

Park, H. J., Kim, S. K., Kang, W. S., Woo, J. M., & Kim, J. W. (2014 Feb). Effects of essential oil from Chamaecyparis obtusa on cytokine genes in the hippocampus of maternal separation rats. Can J Physiol Pharmacol, 92(2), 95-101.

Park H.M., Lee J.H., Yaoyao J, Jun H.J., Lee S.J. (2011 Jan). "Limonene, a natural cyclic terpene, is an agonistic ligand for adenosine A(2A) receptors," Biochem. Biophys. Res. Commun. 404(1):345-348.

Park S.Y., Kim HS, Cho EK, Kwon BY, Phark S, Hwang KW, Sul D (2008 Aug). "Curcumin protected PC12 cells against beta-amyloid-induced toxicity through the inhibition of oxidative damage and tau hyperphosphorylation," Food Chem Toxicol. 46(8):2881-7.

Park S.Y., Kim Y.H., Kim Y, Lee SJ (2012 Dec). "Aromatic-turmerone attenuates invasion and expression of MMP-9 and COX-2 through inhibition of NF-κB activation in TPA-induced breast cancer cells," J. Cell. Biochem. 113(12):3653-3662.

Park S.Y., Jin M.L., Kim Y.H., Kim Y., Lee S.J. (2012 Sep). "Anti-inflammatory effects of aromatic-turmerone through blocking of NF-κB, JNK, and p38 MAPK signaling pathways in amyloid β-stimulated microglia," Int. Immunopharmacol. 14(1):13-20.

Patel, B. P., Bellissimo, N., Luhovyy, B., Bennett, L. J., Hurton, E., Painter, J. E., & Anderson, G. H. (2013 Jun 29). An after-school snack of raisins lowers cumulative food intake in young children. J Food Sci, 78 Suppl 1, A5-A10.

Patrick L (2011 Jun). "Gastroesophageal reflux disease (GERD): a review of conventional and alternative treatments," Altern. Med. Rev. J. Clin. Ther. 16(2):116-133.

Pattnaik S, Subramanyam V.R., Bapaji M, Kole C.R. (1997). "Antibacterial and antifungal activity of aromatic constituents of essential oils," Microbios. 89(358):39-46.

Pattnaik S, Subramanyam V.R., Kole C.R., Sahoo S (1995). "Antibacterial activity of essential oils from Cymbopogon: inter- and intra-specific differences," Microbios. 84(341):239-245.

Pause, B. M., Raack, N., Sojka, B., Goder, R., Aldenhoff, J. B., & Ferstl, R. (2003 Mar). Convergent and divergent effects of odors and emotions in depression. Psychophysiology, 40(2), 209-225.

Pavela R (2005 Dec). "Insecticidal activity of some essential oils against larvae of Spodoptera littoralis," Fitoterapia. 76(7-8):691-6.

Pavela R (2008 Feb). "Insecticidal properties of several essential oils on the house fly (Musca domestica L.)," Phytother Res. 22(2):274-8.

Peana AT, D'Aquila PS, Panin F, Serra G, Pippia P, Moretti MD (2002 Dec). "Anti-inflammatory activity of linalool and linalyl acetate constituents of essential oils," Phytomedicine. 9(8):721-6.

Peana A.T., D'Aquila P.S., Chessa M. L., Moretti M.D.L., Serra G., Pippia P. (2003) (-)-Linalool produces antinociception in two experimental models of pain. European Journal of Pharmacology. 460: 37-41.

Peana A.T., Marzocco S, Popola A, Pinto A (2006 Jan). "(-)-Linalool inhibits in vitro NO formation: Probable involvement in the antinociceptive activity of this monoterpene compound," Life Sci. 78(7):719-723.

Pearce AL, Finlay-Jones JJ, Hart PH (2005 Jan). "Reduction of nickel-induced contact hypersensitivity reactions by topical tea tree oil in humans," Inflamm Res. 54(1):22-30.

Pemberton E, Turpin PG (2008 Mar-Apr). "The effect of essential oils on work-related stress in intensive care unit nurses," Holist Nurs Pract. 22(2):97-102.

Penalvo JL, Lopez-Romero P (2012 Feb 29). "Urinary enterolignan concentrations are positively associated with serum HDL cholesterol and negatively associated with serum triglycerides in U.S. adults," J Nutr. [Epub ahead of print].

Peng SM, Koo M, Yu ZR (2009 Jan). "Effects of music and essential oil inhalation on cardiac autonomic balance in healthy individuals," J Altern Complement Med. 15(1):53-7.

Pengelly, A. (2004). The Constituents of Medicinal Plants (2nd ed.). Singapore: Allen and Unwin.

Perry N, Perry E (2006). "Aromatherapy in the management of psychiatric disorders: clinical and neurological perspectives," CNS Drugs. 20(4):257-80.

Peters G.J., Backus H.H.J., Freemantle S., van Triest B., Codacci-Pisanelli G., van der Wilt C.L., Smid K., Lunec J., Calvert A.H., Marsh S., McLeod H.L., Bloemena E., Meijer S., Jansen G., van Groeningen C.J., Pinedo H.M. (2002) Induction of thymidylate synthase as a 5-fluorouracil resistance mechanism. Biochimica et Biophysica Acta. 1587: 194-205.

Pevsner J, Hsu SC, Braun JE, Calakos N, Ting AE, Bennett MK, Scheller RH (1994 Aug). "Specificity and regulation of a synaptic vesicle docking complex," Neuron. 13(2):353-61.

Philippe M, Garson JC, Gilard P, Hocquaux M, Hussler G, Leroy F, Mahieu C, Semeria D, Vanlerberghe G (1994 Aug). "Synthesis of 2-N-oleoylamino-octadecane-1,3-diol: a new ceramide highly effective for the treatment of skin and hair," Int J Cosmet Sci. 17(4):133-46.

Phillips L.R., Malspeis L., Supko J.G. (1995 Jul.) "Pharmacokinetics of active drug metabolites after oral administration of perillyl alcohol, an investigational antineoplastic agent, to the dog," Drug Metab. Dispos. Biol. Fate Chem. 23(7):676-680.

Piazza GA, Ritter JL, Baracka CA (1995 Jan). "Lysophosphatidic acid induction of transforming growth factors alpha and beta: modulation of proliferation and differentiation in cultured human keratinocytes and mouse skin," Exp Cell Res. 216(1):51-64.

Piccinelli A.C. et al "Antihyperalgesic and antidepressive actions of (R)-(+)-limonene, αphellandrene, and essential oil from Schinus terebinthifolius fruits in a neuropathic pain model," Nutr. Neurosci. 18(5):217-224.

Pichette A, Larouche PL, Lebrun M, Legault J (2006 May). "Composition and antibacterial activity of Abies balsamea essential oil," Phytother Res. 20(5):371-3.

Pietruck F, Busch S, Virchow S, Brockmeyer N, Siffert W (1997 Jan). "Signalling properties of lysophosphatidic acid in primary human skin fibroblasts: role of pertussis toxin-sensitive GTP-binding proteins," Naunyn Schmiedebergs Arch Pharmacol. 355(1):1-7.

Pinker, S. (2010 May). Colloquium paper: the cognitive niche: coevolution of intelligence, sociality, and language. Proc Natl Acad Sci USA, 107 Suppl 2, 8993-8999.

Pina-Vaz C, Gonçalves Rodrigues A, Pinto E, Costa-de-Oliveira S, Tavares C, Salgueiro L, Cavaleiro C, Gonçalves MJ, Martinez-de-Oliveira J (2004 Jan). "Antifungal activity of Thymus oils and their major compounds," J Eur Acad Dermatol Venereol. 18(1):73-8.

Ping H, Zhang G, Ren G (2010 Aug-Sep). "Antidiabetic effects of cinnamon oil in diabetic KK-Ay mice," Food Chem Toxicol. 48(8-9):2344-9.

Pinto E, Vale-Silva L, Cavaleiro C, Salgueiro L (2009 Nov). "Antifungal activity of the clove essential oil from Syzygium aromaticum on Candida, Aspergillus and dermatophyte species," J. Med. Microbiol. 58(11):1454-62.

Pistone G, Marino A, Leotta C, Dell'Arte S, Finocchiaro G, Malaguarnera M (2003). "Levocarnitine administration in elderly subjects with rapid muscle fatigue: effect on body composition, lipid profile and fatigue," Drugs Aging. 20(10):761-7.

P. M. de Mendonça Rocha et al. (2012 Oct). "Synergistic antibacterial activity of the essential oil of aguaribay (Schinus molle L.)," Mol. Basel Switz., vol. 17(10):12023-12036.

Porres-Martínez M, González-Burgos E, Carretero M.E., Gómez-Serranillos M.P. (2015 Jun). "Major selected monoterpenes α-pinene and 1,8-cineole found in Salvia lavandulifolia (Spanish sage) essential oil as regulators of cellular redox balance," Pharm Biol. 53(6):921-929.

Portincasa P et al (2016 June). "Curcumin and fennel essential oil improve symptoms and quality of life," J Gastrointestin Liver Dis. 25(2):151-7.

Pouresalmi H.R., Makarem A, Mojab F (2007). "Paraclinical Effects of Miswak Extract on Dental Plaque," Dent. Res. J. 4(2):5.

Pouvreau L, Gruppen H, Piersma SR, van den Broek LA, van Koningsveld GA, Voragen AG (2001 Jun). "Relative abundance and inhibitory distribution of protease inhibitors in potato juice from cv. Elkana," J Agric Food Chem. 49(6):2864-74.

Prabuseenivasan S, Jayakumar M, Ignacimuthu S (2006). "In vitro antibacterial activity of some plant essential oils," BMC Complement. Altern. Med. 6(1):39.

Prakash P. et al (2011 Feb). "Anti-platelet effects of Curcuma oil in experimental models of myocardial ischemia-reperfusion and thrombosis," Thromb. Res. 127(2):111-118.

Pramod K., Ansari S.H., Ali J (2010 Dec). "Eugenol: a natural compound with versatile pharmacological actions," Nat. Prod. Commun. 5(12):1999-2006.

Prasad M. et al (2016 May "The Clinical Effectiveness of Post-Brushing Rinsing in Reducing Plaque and Gingivitis: A Systematic Review," J. Clin. Diagn. 10(5):ZE01-ZE07.

Preuss HG, Echard B, Enig M, Brook I, Elliott TB (2005 Apr). "Minimum inhibitory concentrations of herbal essential oils and monolaurin for gram-positive and gram-negative bacteria," Mol Cell Biochem. 272(1-2):29-34.

Prins, C. L., Vieira, I. J., & Freitas, S. P. (2010). Growth regulators and essential oil production. Brazilian Journal of Plant Physiology, 22(2), 91-102.

Prottey C, Hartop C.J., Press M (1975 Apr). "Correction of the cutaneous manifestations of essential fatty acid deficiency in man by application of sunflower-seed oil to the skin," J. Invest. Dermatol. 64(4):228-234.

Puatanachokchai R, Kishida H, Denda A, Murata N, Konishi Y, Vinitketkumnuen U, Nakae D (2002 Sep 8). "Inhibitory effects of lemon grass (Cymbopogon citratus, Stapf) extract on the early phase of hepatocarcinogenesis after initiation with diethylnitrosamine in male Fischer 344 rats," Cancer Lett. 183(1):9-15.

Qiu Y, Du GH, Qu ZW, Zhang JT (1995). "Protective effects of ginsenoside on the learning and memory impairment induced by transient cerebral ischemia-reperfusion in mice," Chin Pharmacol Bull. 11:299-302.

Quiroga P.R., Asensio C.M., Nepote V (2015 Feb). "Antioxidant effects of the monoterpenes carvacrol, thymol and sabinene hydrate on chemical and sensory stability of roasted sunflower seeds," J. Sci. Food Agric. 95(3):471-479.

Qureshi A.A., Mangels W.R., Din A.A., Elson C.E. (1988) Inhibition of Hepatic Mevalonate Biosynthesis by the Monoterpene, d-Limonene. J. Agric. Food Chem. 36: 1220-1224.

Ragho R., Postlethwaite AE, Keski-Oja J, Moses HL, Kang AH (1987 Apr). "Transforming growth factor-beta increases steady state levels of type I procollagen and fibronectin messenger RNAs posttranscriptionally in cultured human dermal fibroblasts," J Clin Invest. 79(4):1285-8.

Rahimikian F, Rahimi R, Golzareh P, Bekhradi R, Mehran A (2017 Sep). "Effect of Foeniculum vulgare Mill. (fennel) on menopausal symptoms in postmenopausal women: a randomized, triple-blind, placebo-controlled trial," Menopause. 24(9):1017-1021.

Rahman MM, Ichiyanagi T, Komiyama T, Sato S, Konishi T (2008 Aug). "Effects of anthocyanins on psychological stress-induced oxidative stress and neurotransmitter status," J Agric Food Chem. 56(16):7545-50.

Raisi Dehkordi Z, Hosseini Baharanchi F.S., Bekhardi R (2014 Apr). "Effect of lavender inhalation on the symptoms of primary dysmenorrhea and the amount of menstrual bleeding: A randomized clinical trial," Complement. Ther. Med. 22(2):212-219.

Ra Kovi A., Milanovi I., Pavlovi, N. A., Ebovi, T., Vukmirovi, S. A., & Mikov, M. (2014 Jul). Antioxidant activity of rosemary (Rosmarinus officinalis L.) essential oil and its hepatoprotective potential. BMC Complement Altern Med, 14(1), 1-20.

Raman A, Weir U, Bloomfield SF (1995 Oct). "Antimicrobial effects of tea-tree oil and its major components on Staphylococcus aureus, Staph. epidermidis and Propionibacterium acnes," Lett Appl Microbiol. 21(4):242-5.

Ramezani R, Moghimi A., Rakhshandeh H., Ejtehadi, H., & Kheirabadi, M. (2008 Mar). The effect of Rosa damascena essential oil on the amygdala electrical kindling seizures in rat. Pak J Biol Sci, 11(5), 746-751.

Rana I.S., Rana A.S., Rajak R.C. (2011 Oct). "Evaluation of antifungal activity in essential oil of the Syzygium aromaticum (L.) by extraction, purification and analysis of its main component eugenol," Braz. J. Microbiol. Publ. Braz. Soc. Microbiol. 42(4):1269-1277.

Ranasinghe L, Jayawardena B, Abeywickrama K (2002 Sep). "Fungicidal activity of essential oils of Cinnamomum zeylanicum (L.) and Syzygium aromaticum (L.) Merr et L.M.Perry against crown rot and anthracnose pathogens isolated from banana," Lett. Appl. Microbiol. 35(3):208-211.

Ranzato, E., Martinotti, S. & Burlando, B. (2011 Mar). Wound healing properties of jojoba liquid wax: an in vitro study. J Ethnopharmacol, 134(2), 443-449.

Rao S., Krauss N.E., Heerding J.M., Swindell C.S., Ringel I., Orr G.A., Horwitz S.B. (1994) 3'-(p-Azidobenzamido)taxol Photolabels the N-terminal 31 AminoAcids of β-Tubulin. The Journal of Biological Chemistry. 269: 3132-3134.

Rao S., Orr G.A., Chaudhary A.G., Kingston D.G.I., Horwitz S.B. (1995) Characterization of the Taxol Binding Site on the Microtubule. The Journal of Biological Chemistry. 270: 20235-20238.

Raphael T.J., Kuttan G (2003 May). "Immunomodulatory activity of naturally occurring monoterpenes carvone, limonene, and perillic acid," Immunopharmacol. Immunotoxicol. 25(2):285-294.

Rashidi-Fakari F, Tabatabaeichehr M, Mortazavi H (2015 Dec). "The effect of aromatherapy by essential oil of orange on anxiety during labor: A randomized clinical trial," Iran J Nurs Midwifery Res. 20(6):661-664.

Rasooli I, Fakoor MH, Yadegarinia D, Gachkar L, Allameh A, Rezaei MB (2008 Feb 29). "Antimycotoxigenic characteristics of Rosmarinus officinalis and Trachyspermum copticum L. essential oils," Int J Food Microbiol. 122(1-2):135-9.

Rasooli I, Shayegh S, Taghizadeh M, Astaneh SD (2008 Sep). "Phytotherapeutic prevention of dental biofilm formation," Phytother Res. 22(9):1162-7.

Rates, S. M. K. (2001). Plants as source of drugs. Toxicon, 39(5), 603-613.

Rathi, B., Bodhankar, S., Mohan, V., & Thakurdesai, P. (2013 Jun). Ameliorative Effects of a Polyphenolic Fraction of Cinnamomum zeylanicum L. Bark in Animal Models of Inflammation and Arthritis. Sci Pharm, 81(2), 567-589.

Raudenbush B, Meyer B, Eppich B (2002). "The Effects of Odors on Objective and Subjective Measures of Athletic Performance," Int. Sports J. 6(1):14.

Raut J.S., Shinde R.B., Chauhan N.M., Karuppayil S.M. (2013). "Terpenoids of plant origin inhibit morphogenesis, adhesion, and biofilm formation by Candida albicans," Biofouling. 29(1):87-96.

Reddy AC, Lokesh BR (1994). "Studies on anti-inflammatory activity of spice principles and dietary n-3 polyunsaturated fatty acids on carrageenan-induced inflammation in rats," Ann Nutr Metab. 38(6):349-58.

Reddy BS, Wang CX, Samaha H, Lubet R, Steele VE, Kelloff GJ, Rao CV (1997 Feb 1). "Chemoprevention of colon carcinogenesis by dietary perillyl alcohol," Cancer Res. 57(3):420-5.

Rekka E.A., Kourounakis A.P., Kourounakis P.N. (1996 Jun). "Investigation of the effect of chamazulene on lipid peroxidation and free radical processes," Res. Commun. Mol. Pathol. Pharmacol. 92(3):361-364.

Rees WD, Evans BK, Rhodes J (1979 Oct 6). "Treating irritable bowel syndrome with peppermint oil," Br Med J. 2(6194):835-6.

Reeve, V. E., Allanson, M., Arun, S. J., Domanski, D., & Painter, N. (2010 Apr). Mice drinking goji berry juice (Lycium barbarum) are protected from UV radiation-induced skin damage via antioxidant pathways. Photochem Photobiol Sci, 9(4), 601-607. Reichling J, Fitzi J, Hellmann K, Wegener T, Bucher S, Saller R (2004 Oct). "Topical tea tree oil effective in canine localised pruritic dermatitis--a multi-centre randomised double-blind controlled clinical trial in the veterinary practice," Dtsch Tierarztl Wochenschr. 111(10):408-14.

Reichling J, Koch C, Stahl-Biskup E, Sojka C, Schnitzler P (2005 Dec). "Virucidal activity of a beta-triketone-rich essential oil of Leptospermum scoparium (manuka oil) against HSV-1 and HSV-2 in cell culture," Planta Med. 71(12):1123-7.

Renimel I, Andre P (Inventors) (1995). "Method for treatment of allergic disorders and cosmetic compositions using cucurbitine," USPTO 5714164.

Rhee SG (2006 Jun). "Cell signaling. H2O2, a necessary evil for cell signaling," Science. 312(5782):1882–3.

Rigano D, Dell'Acqua G, Leporatti R (2000). "Benefits of Trimethylglycine (Betaine) in Personal-Care Formulations," Cosm Toil. 115(12):47-54.

Ritschel, W. A., Brady, M. E., & Tan, H. S. (1979 Mar). First-pass effect of coumarin in man. Int J Clin Pharmacol Biopharm, 17(3), 99-103.

Rivas da Silva A.C., Lopes P.M., Barros de Azevedo M.M, Costa D.C.M., Alviano C.S., Alviano D.S. (2012). "Biological activities of α-pinene and β-pinene enantiomers," Molecules. 17(6):6305-6316.

Rivero-Cruz B, Rojas MA, Rodríguez-Sotres R, Cerda-García-Rojas CM, Mata R (2005 Apr). "Smooth muscle relaxant action of benzyl benzoates and salicylic acid derivatives from Brickellia veronicaefolia on isolated guinea-pig ileum," Planta Med. 71(4):320-5.

Rocha, N. F., Rios, E. R., Carvalho, A. M., Cerqueira, G. S., Lopes Ade, A., Leal, L. K., . . . de Sousa, F. C. (2011 Aug 27). "Anti-nociceptive and anti-inflammatory activities of (-)-alpha-bisabolol in rodents," Naunyn Schmiedebergs Arch Pharmacol, 384(6): 525-533.

Rochel I.D. et al (2011). "Effect of experimental xylitol and fluoride-containing dentifrices on enamel erosion with or without abrasion in vitro," J. Oral Sci. 53(2):163-168.

Rodriguez J, Yáñez J, Vicente V, Alcaraz M, Benavente-García O, Castillo J, Lorente J, Lozano JA (2002 Apr). "Effects of several flavonoids on the growth of B16F10 and SK-MEL-1 melanoma cell lines: relationship between structure and activity," Melanoma Res. 12(2):99-107.

Rombolà, L., Tridico, L., Scuteri, D., Sakurada, T., Sakurada, S., Mizoquchi, H., Avato, P., Corasaniti, M.T., Bagetta, G., & Morrone, L.A. (2017 Apr. 11). "Bergamot Essential Oil Attenuates Anxiety-Like Behaviour in Rats," Molecules. 22(4).

Romero-Jiménez M, Campos-Sánchez J, Analla M, Muñoz-Serrano A, Alonso-Moraga A (2005 Aug 1). "Genotoxicity and anti-genotoxicity of some traditional medicinal herbs," Mutat Res. 585(1-2):147-55.

Romijn JA, Coyle EF, Sidossis LS, Gastaldelli A, Horowitz JF, Endert E, Wolfe RR (1993 Sep.). "Regulation of endogenous fat and carbohydrate metabolism in relation to exercise intensity and duration," Am J Physiol, 265(3 Pt 1):E380-91.

Rosa A, Deiana M, Atzeri A, Corona G, Incani A, Melis MP, Appendino G, Dessi MA (2007 Jan 30). "Evaluation of the antioxidant and cytotoxic activity of arzanol, a prenylated alpha-pyrone-phloroglucinol etherodimer from Helichrysum italicum subsp.microphyllum," Chem Biol Interact. 165(2):117-26.

Rose JE, Behm FM (1994 Feb). "Inhalation of vapor from black pepper extract reduces smoking withdrawal symptoms," Drug Alcohol Depend. 34(3):225-9.

Ross R, Freeman JA, Janssen I (2000 Oct). "Exercise alone is an effective strategy for reducing obesity and related comorbidities," Exerc Sport Sci Rev, 28(4):165-70.

Rowinsky E.K., Donehower R.C. (1995) Paclitaxel (Taxol). The New England Journal of Medicine. 332: 1004-1014.

Roy S, Khanna S, Krishnaraju AV, Subbaraju GV, Yasmin T, Bagchi D, Sen CK (2006 Mar-Apr). "Regulation of vascular responses to inflammation: inducible matrix metalloproteinase-3 expression in human microvascular endothelial cells is sensitive to antiinflammatory Boswellia," Antioxid Redox Signal. 8(3-4):653-60.

Roy S, Khanna S, Shah H, Rink C, Phillips C, Preuss H, Subbaraju GV, Trimurtulu G, Krishnaraju AV, Bagchi M, Bagchi D, Sen CK (2005 Apr). "Human genome screen to identify the genetic basis of the anti-inflammatory effects of Boswellia in microvascular endothelial cells," DNA Cell Biol. 24(4):244-55.

Roy S, Khanna S, Alessio HM, Vider J, Bagchi D, Bagchi M, Sen CK (2002 Sep). "Anti-angiogenic property of edible berries," Free Radic Res. 36(9):1023-31.

Rozza, A. L., Moraes Tde, M., Kushima, H., Tanimoto, A., Marques, M. O., Bauab, T. M., . . . Pellizzon, C. H. (2011 Jan). Gastroprotective mechanisms of Citrus lemon (Rutaceae) essential oil and its majority compounds limonene and beta-pinene: involvement of heat-shock protein-70, vasoactive intestinal peptide, glutathione, sulfhydryl compounds, nitric oxide and prostaglandin E(2). Chem Biol Interact, 189(1-2), 82-89.

Ruthig DJ, Meckling-Gill KA (1999 Oct). "Both (n-3) and (n-6) fatty acids stimulate wound healing in the rat intestinal epithelial cell line, IEC-6," J Nutr. 129(10):1791-8.

Sabzghabaee AM, Davoodi N, Ebadian B, Aslani A, Ghannadi A (2012 Mar). "Clinical evaluation of the essential oil of "Saturejo hortensis" for the treatment of denture stomatitis," Dent Res J (isfahan). 9(2):198-202.

Sacchetti G. et al (2005 Aug). "Comparative evaluation of 11 essential oils of different origin as functional antioxidants, antiradicals and antimicrobials in foods," Food Chem. 91(4):621-632.

Sadraei, H., Asghari, G., & Emami, S. (2013 Jan). Inhibitory effect of Rosa damascena Mill flower essential oil, geraniol and citronellol on rat ileum contraction. Res Pharm Sci, 8(1), 17-23.

Sadraei H, Asghari GR, Hajhashemi V, Kolagar A, Ebrahimi M. (2001 Sep). "Spasmolytic activity of essential oil and various extracts of Ferula gummosa Boiss. on ileum contractions," Phytomedicine. 8(5):370-6.

Saeed M.A., Sabir A.W. (2004 Mar). "Antibacterial activities of some constituents from oleo-gumresin of Commiphora mukul," Fitoterapia. 75(2):204-208.

Saeed SA, Gilani AH (1994 May). "Antithrombotic activity of clove oil," J Pak Med Assoc. 44(5):112-5.

Saeedi M, Morteza, Semnani K, Ghoreishi MR (2003 Sep). "The treatment of atopic dermatitis with licorice gel," J Dermatolog Treat. 14(3):153-7.

Saeki Y, Ito Y, Shibata M, Sato Y, Okuda K, Takazoe I (1989 Aug). "Antimicrobial action of natural substances on oral bacteria," Bull. Tokyo Dent. Coll. 30(3):129-135.

Saerens KM, Zhang J, Saey L, Van Bogaert IN, Soetaert W (2011 Apr). "Cloning and functional characterization of the UDP-glucosyltransferase UgtB1 involved in sophorolipid production by Candida bombicola and creation of a glucolipid-producing yeast strain,' Yeast. 28(4):279-92.

Safayhi H, Sabieraj J, Sailer ER, Ammon HP (1994 Oct). "Chamazulene: an antioxidant-type inhibitor of leukotriene B4 formation," Planta Med. 60(5):410-3.

Saha SS, Ghosh M (2009 Jul 18). "Comparative study of antioxidant activity of alpha-eleostearic acid and punicic acid against oxidative stress generated by sodium arsenite," Food Chem Toxicol. [Epub ahead of print].

Saharkhiz M.J., Motamedi M, Zomorodian K, Pakshir K, Miri R, Hemyari K (2012). "Chemical Composition, Antifungal and Antibiofilm Activities of the Essential Oil of Mentha piperita L," ISRN Pharm. 2012:718645.

Said T, Dutot M, Martin C, Beaudeux JL, Boucher C, Enee E, Baudouin C, Warnet JM, Rat P (2007 Mar). "Cytoprotective effect against UV-induced DNA damage and oxidative stress: role of new biological UV filter," Eur J Pharm Sci. 30(3-4):203-10.

Saikia, D., Parveen, S., Gupta, V. K., & Luqman, S. (2012 Dec). Anti-tuberculosis activity of Indian grass KHUS (Vetiveria zizanioides L. Nash). Complement Ther Med, 20(6), 434-436.

Saiyudthong, S., & Marsden, C. A. (2011 Jun). Acute effects of bergamot oil on anxiety-related behaviour and corticosterone level in rats. Phytother Res, 25(6), 858-862.

Saiyudthong S, Pongmayteegul S, Marsden C.A., Phansuwan-Pujito P (2015 Nov). "Anxiety-like behaviour and c-fos expression in rats that inhaled vetiver essential oil," Nat. Prod. Res. 29(22):2141-2144.

Salmalian, H., Saghebi, R., Moghadamnia, A. A., Bijani, A., Faramarzi, M., Nasiri Amiri, F., . . . Bekhradi, R. (2014 Apr). Comparative effect of thymus vulgaris and ibuprofen on primary dysmenorrhea: A triple-blind clinical study. Caspian J Intern Med, 5(2), 82-88.

Samani Keihan, G., Gharib M.H., Momeni, A., Hemati Z., & Sedighin R. (2017 Jan. 24). "A Comparison Between the Effect of Cuminum Cyminum and Vitamin E on the Level of Leptin, Paraoxonase 1, HbA1c and Oxidized LDL in Diabetic Patients," Int J Mol Cel Med. 5(4):229-235.

Samarth RM (2007 Nov). "Protection against radiation induced hematopoietic damage in bone marrow of Swiss albino mice by Mentha piperita (Linn)," J Radiat Res (Tokyo). 48(6):523-8.

Samarth RM, Goyal PK, Kumar A (2004 Jul). "Protection of swiss albino mice against whole-body gamma irradiation by Mentha piperita (Linn.).," Phytother Res. 18(7):546-54.

Samarth RM, Kumar A (2003 Jun). "Radioprotection of Swiss albino mice by plant extract Mentha piperita (Linn.)," J Radiat Res (Tokyo). 44(2):101-9.

Samarth RM, Panwar M, Kumar M, Kumar A (2006 May). "Radioprotective influence of Mentha piperita (Linn) against gamma irradiation in mice: Antioxidant and radical scavenging activity," Int J Radiat Biol. 82(5):331-7.

Samarth RM, Samarth M (2009 Apr). "Protection against radiation-induced testicular damage in Swiss albino mice by Mentha piperita (Linn.).," Basic Clin Pharmacol Toxicol. 104(4):329-34.

Samber N, Khan A, Varma A, Manzoor (2015). "Synergistic anti-candidal activity and mode of action of Mentha piperita essential oil and its major components," Pharm. Biol. 53(10):1496-1504.

Samman S, Naghii MR, Lyons Wall PM, Verus AP (1998 Winter). "The nutritional and metabolic effects of boron in humans and animals," Biol Trace Elem Res. 66(1-3):227-35.

Sándor Z et al (2018 Apr 5). "Evidence support tradition: the in vitro effects of roman chamomile on smooth muscles," Front Pharmacol. 9:323.

Sanguinetti, M., Posteraro, B., Romano, L., Battaglia, F., Lopizzo, T., De Carolis, E., & Fadda, G. (2007 Feb). In vitro activity of Citrus bergamia (bergamot) oil against clinical isolates of dermatophytes. J Antimicrob Chemother, 59(2), 305-308.

Santamaria, M., Jr., Petermann, K. D., Vedovello, S. A., Degan, V., Lucato, A., & Franzini, C. M. (2014 Feb). Antimicrobial effect of Melaleuca alternifolia dental gel in orthodontic patients. Am J Orthod Dentofacial Orthop, 145(2), 198-202.

Santos AO, Ueda-Nakamura T, Dias Filho BP, Veiga Junior VF, Pinto AC, Nakamura CV (2008 May). "Antimicrobial activity of Brazilian copaiba oils obtained from different species of the Copaifera genus," Mem Inst Oswaldo Cruz. 103(3):277-81.

Santos AO, Ueda-Nakamura T, Dias Filho BP, Veiga Junior VF, Pinto AC, Nakamura CV (2008 Nov 20). "Effect of Brazilian copaiba oils on Leishmania amazonensis," J Ethnopharmacol. 120(2):204-8.

Santos FA, Rao VS (2000 Jun). "Anti-inflammatory and antinociceptive effects of 1,8-cineole a terpenoid oxide present in many plant essential oils," Phytother Res. 14(3):240-4.

Santos, R.C., dos Santos Alves, C.F., Schneider, T., Lopes, L.Q., Aurich, C., Giongo, J.L., Brandelli, A., and de Almeida Vaucher, R. (2012). "Antimicrobial activity of Amazonian oils against Paenibacillus species," J Invertebr Pathol. 109(3):265-8.

Sarahroodi, S., Esmaeili, S., Mikaili, P., Hemmati, Z., & Saberi, Y. (2012 Apr). The effects of green Ocimum basilicum hydroalcoholic extract on retention and retrieval of memory in mice. Anc Sci Life, 31(4), 185-189.

Sarrau E, Chatzopoulou P, Dimassi-Theriou K, Therios I (2013). "Volatile constituents and antioxidant activity of peel, flowers, and leaf oils of Citrus aurantium L. growing in Greece," Molecules 18:10639-47.

Sasannejad, P., Saeedi, M., Shoeibi, A., Gorji, A., Abbasi, M., & Foroughipour, M. (2012 Apr). Lavender essential oil in the treatment of migraine headache: a placebo-controlled clinical trial. Eur Neurol, 67(5), 288-291.

Satchell AC, Saurajen A, Bell C, Barnetson RS (2002 Aug). "Treatment of interdigital tinea pedis with 25% and 50% tea tree oil solution: a randomized, placebo-controlled, blinded study," Australas J Dermatol. 43(3):175-8.

Satou, T., Takahashi, M., Kasuya, H., Murakami, S., Hayashi, S., Sadamoto, K., & Koike, K. (2013 Feb). Organ accumulation in mice after inhalation of single or mixed essential oil compounds. Phytother Res, 27(2), 306-311.

Savelev SU, Okello EJ, Perry EK (2004 Apr). "Butyryl- and acetyl-cholinesterase inhibitory activities in essential oils of Salvia species and their constituents," Phytother Res. 18(4):315-24.

Savino F, Cresi F, Castagno E, Silvestro L, Oggero R (2005 Apr). "A randomized double-blind placebo-controlled trial of a standardized extract of Matricariae recutita, Foeniculum vulgare and Melissa officinalis (ColiMil) in the treatment of breastfed colicky infants," Phytother Res. 19(4):335-40.

Sayorwan W (2013). "Effects of Inhaled Rosemary Oil on Subjective Feelings and Activities of the Nervous System," Sci. Pharm. 81(2):531-542.

Sayorwan W, Siripornpanich V, Piriyapunyaporn T, Hongratanaworakit T, Kotchabhakdi N, Ruangrungsi N (2012 Apr). "The effects of lavender oil inhalation on emotional states, autonomic nervous system, and brain electrical activity," J. Med. Assoc. Thail. Chotmaihet Thangphaet. 95(4):598-606.

Sayyah M, Nadjafnia L, Kamalinejad M (2004 Oct). "Anticonvulsant activity and chemical composition of Artemisia dracunculus L. essential oil," J Ethnopharmacol. 94(2-3):283-7.

Sayyah M, Saroukhani G, Peirovi A, Kamalinejad M (2003 Aug). "Analgesic and anti-inflammatory activity of the leaf essential oil of Laurus nobilis Linn," Phytother. Res. 17(7):733-6.

Sayyah M, Valizadeh J, Kamalinejad M (2002 Apr). "Anticonvulsant activity of the leaf essential oil of Laurus nobilis against pentylenetetrazole- and maximal electroshock-induced seizures," Phytomedicine. 9(3):212-6.

Scalbert A, Johnson IT, and Saltmarsh M (2005 Jan). "Polyphenols: antioxidants and beyond," Presented at the 1st International Conference on Polyphenols and Health, Vichy, France. Am J Clin Nut. 81(1):215S-7S.

Schecter A, Birnbaum L., Ryan J.J., Constable J.D. (2006) Dioxins: An overview. Environmental Research. 101: 419-428.

Scheinfeld NS, Mones J (2005 May). "Granular parakeratosis: pathologic and clinical correlation of 18 cases of granular parakeratosis," J Am Acad Dermatol. 52(5):863-7.

Schellack, G. (2011). Series on nursing pharmacology and medicine management part 3: drug dosage forms and the routes of drug administration. Profession Nurse Today, 15(6), 10-15.

Schelz Z, Molnar J, Jojmann J (2006 Jun). "Antimicrobial and antiplasmid activities of essential oils," Fitoterapia. 77(4):279-285.

Schillaci D, Arizza V, Dayton T, Camarda L, Di Stefano V (2008 Nov). "In vitro anti-biofilm activity of Boswellia spp. oleogum resin essential oils," Lett. Appl. Microbiol. 47(5):433-438.

Schlachterman A et al. (2008 Mar). "Combined resveratrol, quercetin, and catechin treatment reduces breast tumor growth in a nude mouse model," Transl Oncol. 1(1):19-27.

Schmid, D., Schürch, C., and Zülli, F. (2006.) "Mycosporine-like Amino Acids from Red Algae Protect against Premature Skin-Aging," Euro Cosmetics.

Schmitt, S., Schaefer, U. F., Doebler, L., & Reichling, J. (2009 Oct). Cooperative interaction of monoterpenes and phenylpropanoids on the in vitro human skin permeation of complex composed essential oils. Planta Med, 75(13), 1381-1385.

Schnitzler P, Schön K, Reichling J (2001 Apr). "Antiviral activity of Australian tea tree oil and eucalyptus oil against herpes simplex virus in cell culture," Pharmazie. 56(4):343-7.

Schnitzler P, Schuhmacher A, Astani A, Reichling J (2008 Sep). "Melissa officinalis oil affects infectivity of enveloped herpesviruses," Phytomedicine. 15(9):734-40.

Schreckinger, M. E., Lotton, J., Lila, M. A., & de Mejia, E. G. (2010 Apr). Berries from South America: a comprehensive review on chemistry, health potential, and commercialization. J Med Food, 13(2), 233-246.

Schroter A., Kessner D., Kiselev M.A., Haub T., Dante S., Neubert R.H.H. (2009) Basic Nanostructure of Stratum Corneum Lipid Matrices Based on Ceramides [EOS] and [AP]: A Neutron Diffraction Study. Biophysical Journal. 97: 1104-1114.

Schuhmacher A, Reichling J, Schnitzler P (2003). "Virucidal effect of peppermint oil on the enveloped viruses herpes simplex virus type 1 and type 2 in vitro," Phytomedicine. 10(6-7):504-10.

Scott, Sophie (2015). "Peanut allergies: Australian study into probiodics offers hope for possible cure," abc.net.au.

Seifi Z, Beikmoradi A, Oshvandi K, Poorolajal J, Araghchian M, Safiaryan R (2014 Nov). "The effect of lavender essential oil on anxiety level in patients undergoing coronary artery bypass graft surgery: A double-blinded randomized clinical trial," Iran. J. Nurs. Midwifery Res. 19(6):574-580.

Selim, S. A., Adam, M. E., Hassan, S. M., & Albalawi, A. R. (2014). Chemical composition, antimicrobial and antibiofilm activity of the essential oil and methanol extract of the Mediterranean cypress (Cupressus sempervirens L.). BMC Complement Altern Med, 14(1), 1-8.

Sell, C. (Ed.). (2006). The Chemistry of Fragrances From Perfumer to Consumer (2nd ed.). Dorchester, UK: The Royal Society of Chemistry.

Senapati S, Banerjee S, Gangopadhyay DN (2008 Sep-Oct). "Evening primrose oil is effective in atopic dermatitis: a randomized placebo-controlled trial," Indian J Dermatol Venereol Leprol. 74(5):447-52.

Senni K, Gueniche F, Foucault-Bertaud A, Igondjo-Tchen S, Fioretti F, Colliec-Jouault S, Durand P, Guezennec J, Godeau G, Letourneur D (2006 Jan 1). "Fucoidan a sulfated polysaccharide from brown algae is a potent modulator of connective tissue proteolysis," Arch Biochem Biophys. 445(1):56-64.

Seo Y.M., Jeong S.H. (2015 Jun). "[Effects of Blending Oil of Lavender and Thyme on Oxidative Stress, Immunity, and Skin Condition in Atopic Dermatitis Induced Mice]," J. Korean Acad. Nurs. 45(3):367-377.

Seol, G. H., Shim, H. S., Kim, P. J., Moon, H. K., Lee, K. H., Shim, I., . . . Min, S. S. (2010 Jul). Antidepressant-like effect of Salvia sclarea is explained by modulation of dopamine activities in rats. J Ethnopharmacol, 130(1), 187-190.

Serafino, A., Sinibaldi Vallebona, P., Andreola, F., Zonfrillo, M., Mercuri, L., Federici, M., . . . Pierimarchi, P. (2008 Apr). Stimulatory effect of eucalyptus essential oil on innate cell-mediated immune response. BMC Immunol, 9, 17.

Shaikh IA, Brown I, Schofield AC, Wahle KW, Heys SD (2008 Nov). "Docosahexaenoic acid enhances the efficacy of docetaxel in prostate cancer cells by modulation of apoptosis: the role of genes associated with the NF-kappaB pathway," Prostate. 68(15):1635-46.

Shaltiel-Karyo R., Davidi D., Frenkel-Pinter, M., Ovadia, M., Segal, D., & Gazit, E. (2012 Oct). Differential inhibition of alpha-synuclein oligomeric and fibrillar assembly in parkinson's disease model by cinnamon extract. Biochim Biophys Acta, 1820(10), 1628-1635.

Sharma N., Tripathi A. (2008 May). "Effects of Citrus sinensis (L.) Osbeck epicarp essential oil on growth and morphogenesis of Aspergillus niger (L.) Van Tieghem," Microbiol. Res. 163(3):337-344.

Shankar GM, Li S, Mehta TH, Garcia-Munoz A, Shepardson NE, Smith I, Brett FM, Farrell MA, Rowan MJ, Lemere CA, Regan CM, Walsh DM, Sabatini BL, Selkoe DJ (2008 Jun 22). "Amyloid-protein dimers isolated directly from Alzheimer's brains impair synaptic plasticity and memory," Nat Med. 14(8):837-42.

Shankar S, Ganapathy S, Hingorani SR, Srivastava RK (2008 Jan). "EGCG inhibits growth, invasion, angiogenesis and metastasis of pancreatic cancer," Front Biosci. 13:440-52.

Shimada K. et al (2011 Feb). "Aromatherapy alleviates endothelial dysfunction of medical staff after night-shift work: preliminary observations," Hypertens. Res. Off. J. Jpn. Soc. Hypertens. 34(2):264-267.

Santha S, Dwivedi C (2015 Jun). "Anticancer Effects of Sandalwood (Santalum album)," Anticancer Res. 35(6):3137-45.

Shapiro S., Guggenheim B. (1995) The action of thymol on oral bacteria. Oral Microbiology and Immunology. 10: 241-246.

Shapiro S, Meier A, Guggenheim B (1994 Aug). "The antimicrobial activity of essential oils and essential oil components towards oral bacteria," Oral Microbiol Immunol. 9(4):202-8.

Shao Y, Ho CT, Chin CK, Badmaev V, Ma W, Huang MT (1998 May). "Inhibitory activity of boswellic acids from Boswellia serrata against human leukemia HL-60 cells in culture," Planta Med. 64(4):328-31.

Sharma JN, Srivastava KC, Gan EK (1994 Nov). "Suppressive effects of eugenol and ginger oil on arthritic rats," Pharmacology. 49(5):314-8.

Sharma M et al (2014 June). "Suppression of lipopolysaccharide-stimulated cytokine/chemokine production in skin cells by sandalwood oils and purified α-santalol and β-santalol," Phytother Res. 28(6).925-32.

Sharma PR, Mondhe DM, Muthiah S, Pal HC, Shahi AK, Saxena AK, Qazi GN (2009 May 15). "Anticancer activity of an essential oil from Cymbopogon flexuosus," Chem Biol Interact. 179(2-3):160-8.

Shaw D, Norwood K, Leslie J.C. (2011 Oct). "Chlordiazepoxide and lavender oil alter unconditioned anxiety-induced c-fos expression in the rat brain," Behav. Brain Res. 224(1):1-7.

Shayegh S, Rasooli I, Taghizadeh M, Astaneh SD (2008 Mar 20). "Phytotherapeutic inhibition of supragingival dental plaque," Nat Prod Res. 22(5):428-39.

Sheikhan F, Jahdi D, Khoei E.M., Shamsalizadeh N, Sheikhan M, Haghani H (2012 Feb). "Episiotomy pain relief: Use of Lavender oil essence in primiparous Iranian women," Complement. Ther. Clin. Pract. 18(1):66-70.

Shen J, Niijima A, Tanida M, Horii Y, Maeda K, Nagai K (2005 Jun 3). "Olfactory stimulation with scent of grapefruit oil affects autonomic nerves, lipolysis and appetite in rats," Neurosci Lett. 380(3):289-94.

Shen J, Niijima A, Tanida M, Horii Y, Maeda K, Nagai K (2005 Jul 22-29). "Olfactory stimulation with scent of lavender oil affects autonomic nerves, lipolysis and appetite in rats," Neurosci Lett. 383(1-2):188-93.

Sherry E, Boeck H, Warnke PH (2001). "Percutaneous treatment of chronic MRSA osteomyelitis with a novel plant-derived antiseptic," BMC Surg. 1:1.

Shetty AV, Thirugnanam S, Dakshinamoorthy G, Samykutty A, Zheng G, Chen A, Bosland MC, Kajdacsy-Balla A, Gnanasekar M (2011 Sep). "18α-glycyrrhetinic acid targets prostate cancer cells by down-regulating inflammation-related genes," Int J Oncol. 39(3):635-40.

Shibata M., Ohkubo T., Takahashi H., Inoki R. (1989) Modified formalin test: characteristic biphasic pain response. Pain. 38: 347-352.

Shieh PC, Tsao CW, Li JS, et al (2008). "Rp;e pf [otiotaru ademu;ate cuc;ase=actovatomg [p;u[e[tode)[ACA{ om tje actopm pf gomsempsode Rj2 agaomst beta=a,u;pod=omdiced omjobotopm pf rat braom astrpcutes. Meirpsoc :ett/ 434"1=5/

Shiina Y. et al (2008 Sep). "Relaxation effects of lavender aromatherapy improve coronary flow velocity reserve in healthy men evaluated by transthoracic Doppler echocardiography," Int. J. Cardiol. 129(2):193-197.

Shimada K. et al (2011 Feb). "Aromatherapy alleviates endothelial dysfunction of medical staff after night-shift work: preliminary observations," Hypertens. Res. Off. J. Jpn. Soc. Hypertens. 34(2):264-267.

Shimizu K. et al (2008 Jul). "Essential oil of lavender inhibited the decreased attention during a long-term task in humans," Biosci. Biotechnol. Biochem. 72(7):1944-1947.

Shinohara, K., Doi, H., Kumagai, C., Sawano, E., & Tarumi, W. (2017 Jan.). "Effects of essential oil exposure on salivary estrogen concentration in perimenopausal women," Neuro Endocrinol Lett. 37(8):567-572.

Shirazi M et al (2017 Jan). "The effect of topical rosa damascena (rose) oil on pregnancy-related low back pain: a randomized controlled clinical trial," J Evid Based Complementary Altern Med. 22(1):120-126.

Shrivastav P, George K, Balasubramaniam N, Jasper MP, Thomas M, Kanagasabhapathy AS (1988 Feb). "Suppression of puerperal lactation using jasmine flowers (Jasminum sambac)," Aust N Z J Obstet Gynaecol. 28(1):68-71.

Shoskes DA, Zeitlin SI, Shahed A, Rajfer J (1999 Dec). "Quercetin in men with category III prostatitis: a preliminary prospective, double-blind, placebo-controlled trial," Urology. 54(6):960-3.

Shukla, V., Vashistha, M., & Singh, S. N. (2009 Jan). Evaluation of antioxidant profile and activity of amalaki (Emblica officinalis), spirulina and wheat grass. Indian J Clin Biochem, 24(1), 70-75.

Shukla, Y. M., Dhruve, J. J., Patel, N. J., Bhatnagar, R., Talati, J. G., & Kathiria, K. B. (2009). Plant Secondary Metabolites. New Delhi, India: New India Publishing Agency.

Shyam, R., Singh, S. N., Vats, P., Singh, V. K., Bajaj, R., Singh, S. B., & Banerjee, P. K. (2007 Aug). Wheat grass supplementation decreases oxidative stress in healthy subjects: a comparative study with spirulina. J Altern Complement Med, 13(8), 789-791.

Si L. et al (2012 Jun). "Chemical Composition of Essential Oils of Litsea cubeba Harvested from Its Distribution Areas in China," Molecules. 17(12):7057-7066.

Sienkiewicz M, Glowacka A, Poznańska-Kurowska K, Kaszuba A, Urbaniak A, Kowalczyk E (2015 Feb). "The effect of clary sage oil on staphylococci responsible for wound infections," Postepy Dermatol Alergol. 32(1):21-6.

Sies H (1997). "Oxidative stress: oxidants and antioxidants," Exp Physiol. 82(2):291–5.

Sikkema J., de Bont J.A.M., Poolman B. (1995) Mechanisms of Membrane Toxicity of Hydrocarbons. Microbiological Reviews. 59: 201-222.

Sikora, E., & Bodziarczyk, I. (2012). Composition and antioxidant activity of kale (Brassica oleracea L. var. acephala) raw and cooked. Acta Sci Pol Technol Aliment, 11(3), 239-248.

Silva Brum L.F., Emanuelli T., Souza D.O., Elisabetsky E. (2001) Effects of Linalool on Glutamate Release and Uptake in Mouse Cortical Synaptosomes. Neurochemical Research. 26: 191-194

Silva Brum L.F., Elisabetsky E., Souza D. (2001) Effects of Linalool on [3H] MK801 and [3H] Muscimol Binding in Mouse Cortical Membranes. Phytotherapy Research. 15: 422-425.

Silva J, Abebe W, Sousa SM, Duarte VG, Machado MI, Matos FJ (2003 Dec). "Analgesic and anti-inflammatory effects of essential oils of Eucalyptus," J Ethnopharmacol. 89(2-3):277-83.

Siméon A, Monier F, Emonard H, Gillery P, Birembaut P, Hornebeck W, Maquart FX (1999 Jun). "Expression and activation of matrix metalloproteinases in wounds: modulation by the tripeptide-copper complex glycyl-L-histidyl-L-lysine-Cu2+," J Invest Dermatol. 112(3):957-64.

Singh, D., Rao, S. M., & Tripathi, A. K. (1984 May). Cedarwood oil as a potential insecticidal agent against mosquitoes. Naturwissenschaften, 71(5), 265-266.

Singh G, Maurya S, deLampasona M.P., Catalan C.A.N. (2007 Sep). "A comparison of chemical, antioxidant and antimicrobial studies of cinnamon leaf and bark volatile oils, oleoresins and their constituents," Food Chem. Toxicol. 45(9):1650-1661.

Singh HB, Srivastava M, Singh AB, Srivastava AK (1995 Dec). "Cinnamon bark oil, a potent fungitoxicant against fungi causing respiratory tract mycoses," Allergy. 50(12):995-9.

Singh, K. K., Mridula, D., Rehal, J., & Barnwal, P. (2011). Flaxseed: a potential source of food, feed and fiber. Crit Rev Food Sci Nutr, 51(3), 210-222.

Singh N, Bhalla M, deJager P, Gilca M (2011). "An overview on ashwagandha: a rasayana (rejuvenator) of ayurveda," Afr J Tradit Complement Altern Med. 8(s):208-13.

Singh RH, Udupa KN (1993). "Clinical and experimental studies on rasayana drugs and rasayana therapy," Special Research Monograph, Central Council for Research in Ayurveda and Siddha (CCRAS), Ministry of Health and Family Welfare, New Delhi.

Singh V. et al (2013 Aug). "Curcuma oil ameliorates hyperlipidaemia and associated deleterious effects in golden Syrian hamsters," Br. J. Nutr. 110(3):437-446.

Singletary K, MacDonald C, Wallig M (1996 Jun 24). "Inhibition by rosemary and carnosol of 7,12-dimethylbenz[a]anthracene (DMBA)-induced rat mammary tumorigenesis and in vivo DMBA-DNA adduct formation," Cancer Lett. 104(1):43-8.

Siqueira H.D.S. et al (2016 Sep). "α-Phellandrene, a cyclic monoterpene, attenuates inflammatory response through neutrophil migration inhibition and mast cell degranulation," Life Sci. 160:27-33.

Siu KM, Mak DH, CHiu PY, Poon MK, Du Y, Ko KM "2004). "Pharmacological basis of "Yin-nourishing" and "Yang-invigorating" actions of Cordyceps, a Chinese tonifying herb," Life Sci. 76:385-95.

Siurin SA (1997). "Effects of essential oil on lipid peroxidation and lipid metabolism in patients with chronic bronchitis," Klin Med (Mosk). 75(10):43-5.

Siveen K.S., Kuttan G. (2011 Dec). "Augmentation of humoral and cell mediated immune responses by Thujone," Int. Immunopharmacol. 11(12):1967-1975.

Skocibusic M, Bezić N (2004 Dec). "Phytochemical analysis and in vitro antimicrobial activity of two Satureja species essential oils," Phytother Res. 18(12):967-70.

Skold M., Borje A., Matura M., Karlberg A-T. (2002) Studies on the autoxidation and sensitizing capacity of the fragrance chemical linalool, identifying a linalool hydroperoxide. Contact Dermatitis. 46: 267-272.

Skrivanova E, Savka OG, Marounek M (2004). "In vitro effect of C2-C18 fatty acids on Salmonellas," Folia Microbiol (Praha). 49(2):199-202.

Slamenova D, Kuboskova K, Horvathova E, Robichova S. (2002 Mar 28). "Rosemary-stimulated reduction of DNA strand breaks and FPG-sensitive sites in mammalian cells treated with H2O2 or visible light-excited Methylene Blue," Cancer Lett. 177(2):145-53.

Slima, A. B., Ali, M. B., Barkallah, M., Traore, A. I., Boudawara, T., Allouche, N., & Gdoura, R. (2013 Mar). Antioxidant properties of Pelargonium graveolens L'Her essential oil on the reproductive damage induced by deltamethrin in mice as compared to alpha-tocopherol. Lipids Health Dis, 12(1), 30.

Smith DG, Standing L, de Man A (1992 Apr). "Verbal memory elicited by ambient odor," Percept Mot Skills. 74(2):339-43.

Smith-Palmer A, Stewart J, Fyfe L (2004 Oct). "Influence of subinhibitory concentrations of plant essential oils on the production of enterotoxins A and B and alpha-toxin by Staphylococcus aureus," J Med Microbiol. 53(Pt 10):1023-7.

Smith PJ, Potter GG, McLaren ME, Blumenthal JA (2013 Oct). "Impact of aerobic exercise on neurobehavioral outcomes," Ment Health Phys Act, 6(3):139-53.

Soares SF, Borges LM, de Sousa Braga R, Ferreira LL, Louly CC, Tresvenzol LM, de Paula JR, Ferri PH (2009 Oct 7). "Repellent activity of plant-derived compounds against Amblyomma cajennense (Acari: Ixodidae) nymphs," Vet Parasitol. Epub ahead of print.

Soković M, Glamočlija J, Marin P.D., Brkić D, van Griensven L.J.L.D (2010 Nov). "Antibacterial effects of the essential oils of commonly consumed medicinal herbs using an in vitro model," Mol. Basel Switz. 15 (11):7532-7546.

Soltani R, Soheilipour S, Hajhashemi V, Asghari G, Bagheri M, Molavi M (2013 Sep). "Evaluation of the effect of aromatherapy with lavender essential oil on post-tonsillectomy pain in pediatric patients: a randomized controlled trial," Int. J. Pediatr. Otorhinolaryngol. 77(9):1579-1581.

Sorentino S., Landmesser U. (2005) Nonlipid-lowering Effects of Statins. Current Treatment Options to Cardiovascular Medicine. 7: 459-466.

Spirduso WW (1975 Jul). "Reaction and movement time as a function of age and physical activity level," J Gerontol, 30(4):435-40.

Sriram N, Kalayarasan S, Sudhandiran G (2008 Jul). "Enhancement of antioxidant defense system by epigallocatechin-3-gallate during bleomycin induced experimental Pulmonary Fibrosis," Biol Pharm Bull. 31(7):1306-11.

Stanzl K, Zastrow L, Röding J, Artmann C (1996 Jun). "The effectiveness of molecular oxygen in cosmetic formulations," Int J Cosmet Sci. 18(3):137-50.

Stefanick ML, Mackey S, Sheehan M, Ellsworth N, Haskell WL, Wood PD (1998 Jul). "Effects of diet and exercise in men and postmenopausal women with low levels of HDL cholesterol and high levels of LDL cholesterol," N Engl J Med, 339(1):12-20.

Stefanovits-Bányai E, Tulok M.H., Hegedűs A, Renner C, Varga I.S. (2003). "Antioxidant effect of various rosemary (Rosmarinus officinalis L.) clones," Acta Biol. Szeged. 47(1-4):111-113.

Steiner M, Priel I, Giat J, Levy J, Sharoni Y, Danilenko M (2001). "Carnosic acid inhibits proliferation and augments differentiation of human leukemic cells induced by 1,25-dihydroxyvitamin D3 and retinoic acid," Nutr Cancer. 41(1-2):135-44.

Steiner JL, Murphy EA, McClellan JL, Carmichael MD, Davis JM (2011 Oct). "Exercise training increases mitochondrial biogenesis in the brain," J Appl Physiol. 111(4):1066-71.

Strati A, Papoutsi Z, Lianidou E, Moutsatsou P (2009 Sep). "Effect of ellagic acid on the expression of human telomerase reverse transcriptase (hTERT) alpha+Beta+ transcript in estrogen receptor-positive MCF-7 breast cancer cells," Clin Biochem. 42(13-14):1358-62.

Stratton S.P., Alberts D.S., Einspahr J.G. (2010) A Phase 2a Study of Topical Perillyl Alcohol Cream for Chemoprevention of Skin Cancer. Cancer Prevention Research. 3: 160-169.

Stratton S.P., Saboda K.L., Myrdal P.B., Gupta A., McKenzie N.E., Brooks C., Salasche S.J., Warneke J.A., Ranger-Moore J., Bozzo P.D., Blanchard J., Einspahr J.G. (2008) Phase 1 Study of Topical Perillyl Alcohol Cream for Chemoprevention of Skin Cancer. Nutrition and Cancer. 60: 325-330.

Su KP, Huang SY, Chiu TH, Huang KC, Huang CL, Chang HC, Pariante CM (2008 Apr). "Omega-3 fatty acids for major depressive disorder during pregnancy: results from a randomized, double-blind, placebo-controlled trial," J Clin Psychiatry. 69(4):644-51.

Subash Babu P, Prabuseenivasan S, Ignacimuthu S. (2007 Jan). "Cinnamaldehyde--a potential antidiabetic agent," Phytomedicine.14(1):15-22.

Subramenium G.A., Vijayakumar K, Pandian S.K. (2015 Aug). "Limonene inhibits streptococcal biofilm formation by targeting surface-associated virulence factors," J. Med. Microbiol. 64(8):879-890.

Südhof TC (1995 Jun 22). "The synaptic vesicle cycle: a cascade of protein-protein interactions," Nature. 375(6533):645-53.

Sugimoto, H., Watanabe, K., Toyama, T., Takahashi, S. S., Sugiyama, S., Lee, M. C., & Hamada, N. (2015 Feb). Inhibitory effects of French pine bark extract, pycnogenol((R)), on alveolar bone resorption and on the osteoclast differentiation. Phytother Res, 29(2), 251-259.

Suhail M.M. et al (2011). "Boswellia sacra essential oil induces tumor cell-specific apoptosis and suppresses tumor aggressiveness in cultured human breast cancer cells," BMC Complement Altern Med. 11:129.

Suneetha, W. J., & Krishnakantha, T. P. (2005 May). Cardamom extract as inhibitor of human platelet aggregation. Phytother Res, 19(5), 437-440.

Sun J (2007 Sep). "D-Limonene: safety and clinical applications," Altern. Med. Rev. J. Clin. Ther. 12(3):259-64.

Sun J, Qian J, Zhao J, Liu L (2011 Oct). "[Clinical observation of mucoregulatory agents' application after chronic rhinosinusitis surgery]," Lin Chuang Er Bi Yan Hou Tou Jing Wai Ke Za Zhi J. Clin. Otorhinolaryngol. Head Neck Surg. 25(20):922-24.

Sun L et al (2016 Dec 24). "The essential oil from the twigs of cinnamomum cassia presl alleviates pain and inflammation in mice," J Ethnopharmacol. 194:904-912.

Svoboda, K. P., Svoboda, T. G., & Syred, A. (2001). A Closer Look: Secretory Structures of Aromatic and Medicinal Plants HerbalGram: The Journal of the Amercian Botanical Council (53), 34-43.

Taavoni S, Darsareh F, Jooalee S, Haghani H (2013 Jun). "The effect of aromatherapy massage on the psychological symptoms of postmenopausal Iranian women," Complement. Ther. Med. 21(3):158-63.

Tabanca, N., Wang, M., Avonto, C., Chittiboyina, A. G., Parcher, J. F., Carroll, J. F., . . . Khan, I. A. (2013 May). Bioactivity-guided investigation of geranium essential oils as natural tick repellents. J Agric Food Chem, 61(17), 4101-4107.

Tadtong S, Suppawat S, Tintawee A, Saramas P, Jareonvong S, Hongratanaworakit T (2012 Oct). "Antimicrobial activity of blended essential oil preparation," Nat. Prod. Commun. 7(10):1401-1404.

Taguchi Y, Hasumi Y, Hayama K, Arai R, Nishiyama Y, Abe S (2012). "Effect of cinnamaldehyde on hyphal growth of C. albicans under various treatment conditions," Med. Mycol. J. 53(3):199-204.

Taher Y.A. et al (2015). "Experimental evaluation of anti-inflammatory, antinociceptive and antipyretic activities of clove oil in mice," Libyan J. Med. 10:28685.

Taherian, A. A., Vafaei, A. A., & Ameri, J. (2012 Apr). Opiate System Mediate the Antinociceptive Effects of Coriandrum sativum in Mice. Iran J Pharm Res, 11(2), 679-688.

Takahashi M, et al (2012 Nov). "Effects of inhaled lavender essential oil on stress-loaded animals: changes in anxiety-related behavior and expression levels of selected mRNAs and proteins," Nat. Prod. Commun. 7(11):1539-1544.

Takahashi M, Satou T, Ohashi M, Hayahi S, Sadamoto K, Koike K (2011 Nov). "Interspecies comparison of chemical composition and anxiolytic-like effects of lavender oils upon inhalation," Nat. Prod. Commun. 6(11):1769-1774.

Takahashi, N., Yao, L., Kim, M., Sasako, H., Aoyagi, M., Shono, J., . . . Kawada, T. (2013 Jul). Dill seed extract improves abnormalities in lipid metabolism through peroxisome proliferator-activated receptor-alpha (PPAR-alpha) activation in diabetic obese mice. Mol Nutr Food Res, 57(7), 1295-1299.

Takaki I, Bersani-Amado LE, Vendruscolo A, Sartoretto SM, Diniz SP, Bersani-Amado CA, Cuman RK (2008 Dec). "Anti-inflammatory and antinociceptive effects of Rosmarinus officinalis L. essential oil in experimental animal models," J Med Food. 11(4):741-6.

Takarada K, Kimizuka R, Takahashi N, Honma K, Okuda K, Kato T (2004 Feb). "A comparison of the antibacterial efficacies of essential oils against oral pathogens," Oral Microbiol Immunol. 19(1):61-4.

Tan P, Zhong W, Cai W (2000 Sep). "Clinical study on treatment of 40 cases of malignant brain tumor by elemene emulsion injection," Zhongguo Zhong Xi Yi Jie He Za Zhi. 20(9):645-8.

Tan X.C., Chua K.H., Ravishankar Ram M, Kuppusamy U.R. (2016 Apr). "Monoterpenes: Novel insights into their biological effects and roles on glucose uptake and lipid metabolism in 3T3-L1 adipocytes," Food Chem. 196:242-250.

Tang J, Wingerchuk DM, Crum BA, Rubin DI, Demaerschalk BM (2007 May). "Alpha-lipoic acid may improve symptomatic diabetic polyneuropathy," Neurologist. 12(3):164-7.

Tanida M, Niijima A, Shen J, Nakamura T, Nagai K (2005 Oct 5). "Olfactory stimulation with scent of essential oil of grapefruit affects autonomic neurotransmission and blood pressure," Brain Res. 1058(1-2):44-55.

Tanida M, Niijima A, Shen J, Nakamura T, Nagai K (2006 May 1). "Olfactory stimulation with scent of lavender oil affects autonomic neurotransmission and blood pressure in rats," Neurosci Lett. 398(1-2):155-60.

Tanida M, Niijima A, Shen J, Nakamura T, Nagai K (2008 Jul). "Day-night difference in thermoregulatory responses to olfactory stimulation," Neurosci. Lett. 439(2):192-197.

Tanida M. et al (2008 May). "Effects of olfactory stimulations with scents of grapefruit and lavender oils on renal sympathetic nerve and blood pressure in Clock mutant mice," Auton. Neurosci. Basic Clin. 139(1-2):1-83.

Tantaoui-Elaraki A, Beraoud L (1994). "Inhibition of growth and aflatoxin production in Aspergillus parasiticus by essential oils of selected plant materials," J Environ Pathol Toxicol Oncol. 13(1):67-72.

Tao L, Zhou L, Zheng L, Yao M (2006 Jul). "Elemene displays anti-cancer ability on laryngeal cancer cells in vitro and in vivo," Cancer Chemother Pharmacol. 58(1):24-34.

Tare V, Deshpande S, Sharma RN (2004 Oct). "Susceptibility of two different strains of Aedes aegypti (Diptera: Culicidae) to plant oils," J Econ Entomol. 97(5):1734-6.

Tavares AC, Gonçalves MJ, Cavaleiro C, Cruz MT, Lopes MC, Canhoto J, Salgueiro LR (2008 Sep 2). "Essential oil of Daucus carota subsp. halophilus: composition, antifungal activity and cytotoxicity," J Ethnopharmacol. 119(1):129-34.

Tayarani-Najaran, Z., Talasaz-Firoozi, E., Nasiri, R., Jalali, N., & Hassanzadeh, M. (2013 Jan). Antiemetic activity of volatile oil from Mentha spicata and Mentha x piperita in chemotherapy-induced nausea and vomiting. Ecancermedicalscience, 7, 1-6.

Terzi V, Morcia C, Faccioli P, Valè G, Tacconi G, Malnati M (2007 Jun). "In vitro antifungal activity of the tea tree (Melaleuca alternifolia) essential oil and its major components against plant pathogens," Lett Appl Microbiol. 44(6):613-8.

Thavara U, Tawatsin A, Bhakdeenuan P, Wongsinkongman P, Boonruad T, Bansiddhi J, Chavalittumrong P, Komalamisra N, Siriyasatien P, Mulla MS (2007 Jul). "Repellent activity of essential oils against cockroaches (Dictyoptera: Blattidae, Blattellidae, and Blaberidae) in Thailand," Southeast Asian J Trop Med Public Health. 38(4):663-73.

Thompson, J. D., Chalchat, J. C., Michet, A., Linhart, Y. B., & Ehlers, B. (2003). Qualitative and quantitative variation in monoterpene co-occurrence and composition in the essential oil of Thymus vulgaris chemotypes. Journal of Chemical Ecology, 29(4), 873.

Thukham-Mee, W., & Wattanathorn, J. (2012). Evaluation of Safety and Protective Effect of Combined Extract of Cissampelos pareira and Anethum graveolens (PM52) against Age-Related Cognitive Impairment. Evid Based Complement Alternat Med, 2012, 1-10.

Tian X, Sun L, Gou L, Ling X, Feng Y, Wang L, Yin X, Liu Y (2013 Mar 29). "Protective effect of l-theanine on chronic restraint stress-induced cognitive impairments in mice," Brain Res. 1503:24-32.

Tiano L, Belardinelli R, Carnevali P, Principi F, Seddaiu G, Littarru GP (2007 Sep). "Effect of coenzyme Q10 administration on endothelial function and extracellular superoxide dismutase in patients with ischaemic heart disease: a double-blind, randomized controlled study," Eur Heart J. 28(18):2249-55.

Tildesley NT, Kennedy DO, Perry EK, Ballard CG, Wesnes KA, Scholey AB (2005 Jan 17). "Positive modulation of mood and cognitive performance following administration of acute doses of Salvia lavandulaefolia essential oil to healthy young volunteers," Physiol Behav. 83(5):699-709.

Tipton DA, Hamman NR, Dabbous MKh (2006 Mar). "Effect of myrrh oil on IL-1beta stimulation of NF-kappaB activation and PGE(2) production in human gingival fibroblasts and epithelial cells," Toxicol In Vitro. 20(2):248-55.

Tipton DA, Lyle B, Babich H, Dabbous MKh (2003 Jun). "In vitro cytotoxic and anti-inflammatory effects of myrrh oil on human gingival fibroblasts and epithelial cells," Toxicol In Vitro. 17(3):301-10.

Tisserand, R. & Young, R. (2014). Essential oil safety a guide for health care professionals (2nd ed.). China: Churchill Livingstone Elsevier.

Tognolini M, Ballabeni V, Bertoni S, Bruni R, Impicciatore M, Barocelli E (2007 Sep). "Protective effect of Foeniculum vulgare essential oil and anethole in an experimental model of thrombosis," Pharmacol Res. 56(3):254-60.

Thompson A. et al (2013). "Comparison of the antibacterial activity of essential oils and extracts of medicinal and culinary herbs to investigate potential new treatments for irritable bowel syndrome," BMC Complement. Altern. Med. 13:338.

Thompson, Dixie L, Rakow, Jennifer, Perdue, Sara M (2004 May). "Relationship between Accumulated Walking and Body Composition in Middle-Aged Women," Med Sci Sports Exerc, 36(5):911-4.

Toda M, Morimoto K (2008 Oct). "Effect of lavender aroma on salivary endocrinological stress markers," Arch. Oral Biol. 53(10):964-968.

Todd J, Friedman M, Patel J, Jaroni D, Ravishankar S (2013 Aug). "The antimicrobial effects of cinnamon leaf oil against multi-drug resistant Salmonella Newport on organic leafy greens," Int. J. Food Microbiol. 166(1):193-199.

Tortora G.J., Funke B.R., Case C.L. Microbiology: An Introduction. 9th ed. San Francisco: Pearson Benjamin Cummings, 2007.

Traka M, Gasper AV, Melchini A, Bacon JR, Needs PW, Frost V, Chantry A, Jones AM, Ortori CA, Barrett DA, Ball RY, Mills RD, Mithen RF (2008 Jul 2). "Broccoli consumption interacts with GSTM1 to perturb oncogenic signalling pathways in the prostate," PLoS One. 3(7):e2568.

Tran KT, Griffith L, Wells A (2004 May-Jun). "palmitoyl-glycyl-histidyl-lysine," Wound Repair Regen. 12(3):262-8.

Trautmann M, Peskar BM, Peskar BA (1991 Aug 16). "Aspirin-like drugs, ethanol-induced rat gastric injury and mucosal eicosanoid release," Eur J Pharmacol. 201(1):53-8.

Trigg JK (1996 Jun). "Evaluation of a eucalyptus-based repellent against Anopheles spp. in Tanzania," J Am Mosq Control Assoc. 12(2 Pt 1):243-6.

Tripathi, P., Tripathi, R., Patel, R. K., & Pancholi, S. S. (2013 Jan). Investigation of antimutagenic potential of Foeniculum vulgare essential oil on cyclophosphamide induced genotoxicity and oxidative stress in mice. Drug Chem Toxicol, 36(1), 35-41.

Trisonthi P, Sato A, Nishiwaki H, Tamura H (2014 May). "A New Diterpene from Litsea cubeba Fruits: Structure Elucidation and Capability to Induce Apoptosis in HeLa Cells," Molecules. 19(5):6838-6850.

Trongtokit Y, Rongsriyam Y, Komalamisra N, Apiwathnasorn C (2005 Apr). "Comparative repellency of 38 essential oils against mosquito bites," Phytother Res. 19(4):303-9.

Trovato, A., Taviano, M. F., Pergolizzi, S., Campolo, L., De Pasquale, R., & Miceli, N. (2010 Apr). Citrus bergamia Risso & Poiteau juice protects against renal injury of diet-induced hypercholesterolemia in rats. Phytother Res, 24(4), 514-519.

Truan JS, Chen JM, Thompson LU (2012). "Comparative effects of sesame seed lignan and flaxseed lignan in reducing the growth of human breast tumors (MCF-7) at high levels of circulating estrogen in athymic mice," Nutr Cancer. 64(1):65-71.

Tsiri, D., Graikou, K., Poblocka-Olech, L., Krauze-Baranowska, M., Spyropoulos, C., & Chinou, I. (2009 Nov). Chemosystematic value of the essential oil composition of Thuja species cultivated in Poland-antimicrobial activity. Molecules, 14(11), 4707-4715.

Tso MOM, Lam TT (1994 Oct 27). "Method of retarding and ameliorating central nervous system and eye damage," University of Illinois: USPatent #5527533.

Tsuda H et al (2004 Aug). "Cancer prevention by natural compounds," Drug Metab. Pharmacokinet. 19(4):245-263.

Tumen, I., Suntar, I., Eller, F. J., Keles, H., & Akkol, E. K. (2013 Jan). Topical wound-healing effects and phytochemical composition of heartwood essential oils of Juniperus virginiana L., Juniperus occidentalis Hook., and Juniperus ashei J. Buchholz. J Med Food, 16(1), 48-55.

Turley, S.M. (2009). Understanding pharmacology for health professionals (4th ed.). Prentice Hall.

Turrens J.F. (2003) Mitochondrial formation of reactive oxygen species. Journal of Physiology.552: 335-344.

Tuzcu M, Sahin N, Karatepe M, Cikim G, Kilinc U, Sahin K (2008 Sep). "Epigallocatechin-3-gallate supplementation can improve antioxidant status in stressed quail," Br Poult Sci. 49(5):643-8.

Tyagi, A., & Malik, A. (2010). Antimicrobial action of essential oil vapours and negative air ions against Pseudomonas fluorescens. Int J Food Microbiol, 143(3), 205-210.

Tyagi, A. K., & Malik, A. (2012). Bactericidal action of lemon grass oil vapors and negative air ions. Innovative Food Science & Emerging Technologies, 13(0), 169-177.

Tysoe P (2000). "The effect on staff of essential oil burners in extended care settings," Int. J. Nurs. Pract. 6(2):110-112.

Uchida, N., Silva-Filho, S.E., Aguiar, R.P., Wiirzler, L.A.M., Cardia, G.F.E., Cavalcante, H.A.O., Silva-Comar, F.M.S., Becker, T.C.A., Silva E.L., Bersani-Amado, C.A., & Cuman, R.K.N. (2017). "Title: Protective Effect of Cymbopogon citratus Essential Oil in Experimental Model of Acetaminophen-Induced Liver Injury," Am J Chin Med. 45(3):515-532.

Ueno-Iio, T., Shibakura, M., Yokota, K., Aoe, M., Hyoda, T., Shinohata, R., . . . Kataoka, M. (2014 Jun). Lavender essential oil inhalation suppresses allergic airway inflammation and mucous cell hyperplasia in a murine model of asthma. Life Sci.

Ulusoy S, Boşgelmez-Tinaz G, Seçilmiş-Canbay H (2009 Nov). "Tocopherol, carotene, phenolic contents and antibacterial properties of rose essential oil, hydrosol and absolute," Curr Microbiol. 59(5):554-8.

Umezu T (2000 Jun). "Behavioral effects of plant-derived essential oils in the geller type conflict test in mice," Jpn J Pharmacol. 83(2):150-3.

Umezu T (1999 Sep). "Anticonflict effects of plant-derived essential oils," Pharmacol Biochem Behav. 64(1):35-40.

Umezu T (2012 Jun). "Evaluation of the Effects of Plant-derived Essential Oils on Central Nervous System Function Using Discrete Shuttle-type Conditioned Avoidance Response in Mice: ESSENTIAL OILS AND AVOIDANCE RESPONSE," Phytother. Res. 26(6):884-891.

Umezu T, Ito H, Nagano K, Yamakoshi M, Oouchi H, Sakaniwa M, Morita M (2002 Nov 22). "Anticonflict effects of rose oil and identification of its active constituents," Life Sci. 72(1):91-102.

Uribe S., Ramirez J., Pena A. (1985) Effects of β-Pinene on Yeast Membrane Functions. Journal of Bacteriology. 161: 1195-1200.

Urso, M. L., & Clarkson, P. M. (2003). Oxidative stress, exercise, and antioxidant supplementation. Toxicology, 189(1), 41-54.

Vakilian K, Atarha M, Bekhradi R, Chaman R (2011 Feb). "Healing advantages of lavender essential oil during episiotomy recovery: a clinical trial," Complement. Ther. Clin. Pract. 17(1):50-53.

Valente J. et al (2013 Dec). "Antifungal, antioxidant and anti-inflammatory activities of Oenanthe crocata L. essential oil," Food Chem. Toxicol. 62:349-354.

Vallianou, I., Peroulis, N., Pantazis, P., & Hadzopoulou-Cladaras, M. (2011 Nov). Camphene, a plant-derived monoterpene, reduces plasma cholesterol and triglycerides in hyperlipidemic rats independently of HMG-CoA reductase activity. PLoS ONE, 6(11), e20516.

Vanderhoof, J.A. (1999). "Lactobacillus GG in the prevention of antibiotic-associated diarrhea in children," The Journal of Pediatrics. 135:564-8.

van Lieshout E.M., Posner G.H., Woodard B.T., Peters W.H. (1998 Mar). "Effects of the sulforaphane analog compound 30, indole-3-carbinol, D-limonene or relafen on glutathione S-transferases and glutathione peroxidase of the rat digestive tract," Biochim. Biophys. 1379(3): 325-336.

van Poppel G, Verhoeven DT, Verhagen H, Goldbohm RA (1999). "Brassica vegetables and cancer prevention. Epidemiology and mechanisms," Adv Exp Med Biol. 472:159-68.

van Tol RW, Swarts HJ, van der Linden A, Visser JH (2007 May). "Repellence of the red bud borer Resseliella oculiperda from grafted apple trees by impregnation of rubber budding strips with essential oils," Pest Manag Sci. 63(5):483-90.

Van Vuuren S.F., Kamatou G.P.P., Vilijoen A.M (2010 Oct). "Volatile composition and antimicrobial activity of twenty commercial frankincense essential oil samples," South African Journal of Botany. 76(4):686-691.

Varga J, Jimenez SA (1986 Jul 31). "Stimulation of normal human fibroblast collagen production and processing by transforming growth factor-beta," Biochem Biophys Res Commun. 138(2):974-80.

Vazquez JA, Arganoza MT, Boikov D, Akins RA, Vaishampayan JK (2000 Jun). "In vitro susceptibilities of Candida and Aspergillus species to Melaleuca alternafolia (tea tree) oil," Rev Iberoam Micol. 17(2):60-3.

Velaga, M. K., Yallapragada, P. R., Williams, D., Rajanna, S., & Bettaiya, R. (2014 Jun). Hydroalcoholic Seed Extract of Coriandrum sativum (Coriander) Alleviates Lead-Induced Oxidative Stress in Different Regions of Rat Brain. Biol Trace Elem Res, 159(1-3), 351-363.

Venegas C, Cabrera-Vique C, Garcia-Corzo L, Escames G, Acuna-Castroviejo D, Lopez LC (2011 Nov). "Determination of coenzyme Q10, coenzyme Q9, and melatonin contents in virgin argan oils: comparison with other edible vegetable oils," J Agric Food Chem. 59(22):12102-8.

Veratti E, Rossi T, Giudice S, Benassi L, Bertazzoni G, Morini D, Azzoni P, Bruni E, Giannnetti A, MaqnoniC. (2011 Jun). "18beta-glycyrrhetinic acid and glabridin prevent oxidative DNA fragmentation in UVB-irradiated human keratinocyte cultures," Anticancer Res. 31(6):2209-15.

Verma, S. K., Jain, V., & Katewa, S. S. (2009 Dec). Blood pressure lowering, fibrinolysis enhancing and antioxidant activities of cardamom (Elettaria cardamomum). Indian J Biochem Biophys, 46(6), 503-506.

Vertuani S, Angusti A, Manfredini S (2004). "The antioxidants and pro-antioxidants network: an overview," Curr Pharm Des. 10(14):1677-94.

Vigo E, Cepeda A, Gualillo O, Perez-Fernandez R (2005 Mar). "In-vitro anti-inflammatory activity of Pinus sylvestris and Plantago lanceolata extracts: effect on inducible NOS, COX-1, COX-2 and their products in J774A.1 murine macrophages," J Pharm Pharmacol. 57(3):383-91.

Victor Antony Santiago J, Jayachitra J, Shenbagam M, Nalini N (2012 Feb). "Dietary d-limonene alleviates insulin resistance and oxidative stress-induced liver injury in high-fat diet and L-NAME-treated rats," Eur. J. Nutr. 51(1):57-68.

Vigo E, Cepeda A, Gualillo O, Perez-Fernandez R (2004 Feb). "In-vitro anti-inflammatory activity of Eucalyptus globulus and Thymus vulgaris: nitric oxide inhibition in J774A.1 murine macrophages," J Pharm Pharmacol. 56(2):257-63.

Vigushin DM, Poon GK, Boddy A, English J, Halbert GW, Pagonis C, Jarman M, Coombes RC (1998). "Phase I and pharmacokinetic study of D-limonene in patients with advanced cancer. Cancer Research Campaign Phase I/II Clinical Trials Committee," Cancer Chemother Pharmacol. 42(2):111-7.

Villareal MO, Ikeya A, Sasaki K, Arfa AB, Neffatic M, Isoda H (2017 Dec 22). "Anti-stress and neuronal cell differentiation induction effects of rosmarinus officinalis l. essential oil," BMC Complement Altern Med. 17(1):549.

Votava-Rai A. et al (2003). "ACTA DERMATOVENEROLOGICA CROATICA".

Vujosević M, Blagojević J (2004). "Antimutagenic effects of extracts from sage (Salvia officinalis) in mammalian system in vivo," Acta Vet Hung. 52(4):439-43.

Vuković-Gacić B, Nikcević S, Berić-Bjedov T, Knezević-Vukcević J, Simić D (2006 Oct). "Antimutagenic effect of essential oil of sage (Salvia officinalis L.) and its monoterpenes against UV-induced mutations in Escherichia coli and Saccharomyces cerevisiae," Food Chem Toxicol. 44(10):1730-8.

Vutyavanich T, Kraisarin T, Ruangsri R (2001 Apr). "Ginger for nausea and vomiting in pregnancy: randomized, double-masked, placebo-controlled trial," Obstet Gynecol. 97(4):577-82.

Walker AF, Bundy R, Hicks SM, Middleton RW (2002 Dec). "Bromelain reduces mild acute knee pain and improves well-being in a dose-dependent fashion in an open study of otherwise healthy adults," Phytomedicine. 9(8):681-6.

Walker TB, Smith J, Herrera M, Lebegue B, Pinchak A, Fischer J (2010 Oct). "The influence of 8 weeks of whey-protein and leucine supplementation on physical and cognitive performance," Int J Sport Nutr Exerc Metab. 20(5):409-17.

Wallerius S, Rosmond R, Ljung T, Holm G, Björntorp P (2003 Jul). "Rise in morning saliva cortisol is associated with abdominal obesity in men: a preliminary report," J Endocrinol Invest. 26(7):616-9. Walter BM, Bilkei G (2004 Mar 15). "Immunostimulatory effect of dietary oregano etheric oils on lymphocytes from growth-retarded, low-weight growing-finishing pigs and productivity," Tijdschr Diergeneeskd. 129(6):178-81.

Wang H, Liu Y (2010 Jan). "Chemical composition and antibacterial activity of essential oils from different parts of Litsea cubeba," Chem. Biodivers. 7(1):229-235.

Wang, K., & Su, C. Y. (2000 Oct). Pharmacokinetics and disposition of beta-elemene in rats. Yao Xue Xue Bao, 35(10), 725-728.

Wang, L., Li, W. G., Huang, C., Zhu, M. X., Xu, T. L., Wu, D. Z., & Li, Y. (2012 Nov). Subunit-specific inhibition of glycine receptors by curcumol. J Pharmacol Exp Ther, 343(2), 371-379.

Wang L. et al (2017 Dec). "Analysis of the main active ingredients and bioactivities of essential oil from Osmanthus fragrans Var. thunbergii using a complex network approach," BMC Syst Biol. 11.

Wang, W., Zu, Y., Fu, Y., Reichling, J., Suschke, U., Nokemper, S., & Zhang, Y. (2009 Feb). In vitro antioxidant, antimicrobial and anti-herpes simplex virus type 1 activity of Phellodendron amurense Rupr. from China. Am J Chin Med, 37(1), 195-203.

Wang, Y.W., Zeng, W.C., Xu, P.Yp., Lan, Y.J., Zhu, R.X., Zhong, K., Huang, Y.N., and Gao, H. (2012). "Chemical composition and antimicrobial activity of the essential oil of kumquat peel," Int J Molecular Sci. 13:3382-3393.

Warskulat U, Brookmann S, Felsner I, Brenden H, Grether-Beck S, Haussinger D (2008 Dec). "Ultraviolet A induces transport of compatible organic osmolytes in human derman fibroblasts," Exp Dermatol. 17(12):1031-6.

Warskulat U, Reinen A, Grether-Beck S, Krutmann J, Haussinger D (2004Sep). "The osmolyte strategy of normal human keratinocyts in maintaining cell homeostasis," J Invest Dermatol. 123(3):516-21.

Watanabe, S., Hara, K., Ohta, K., Iino, H., Miyajima, M., Matsuda, A., . . . Matsushima, E. (2013 Jan). Aroma helps to preserve information processing resources of the brain in healthy subjects but not in temporal lobe epilepsy. Seizure, 22(1), 59-63.

Weaver CM, Martin BR, Jackson GS, McCabe GP, Nolan JR, McCabe LD, Barnes S, Reinwald S, Boris ME, Peacock M (2009 Oct). "Antiresorptive effects of phytoestrogen supplements compared with estradiol or risedronate in postmenopausal women using (41)Ca methodology," J Clin Endocrinol Metab. 94(10):3798-805.

Weaver R.F. Molecular Biology. 4th ed. New York: McGraw Hill, 2008.

Wee, JJ, Park, KM, Chug A (2011). "Biological Activities of Ginseng and Its Application to Human Health," Herbal Medicine: Biomolecular and Clinical Aspects. 2nd ed.

Wei A, Shibamoto T (2007). "Antioxidant activities of essential oil mixtures toward skin lipid squalene oxidized by UV irradiation," Cutan Ocul Toxicol. 26(3):227-33.

Whitehouse PJ, Rajcan JL, Sami SA, Patterson MB, Smyth KA, Edland SD, George DR (2006 Oct). "ADCS Prevention Instrument Project: pilot testing of a book club as a psychosocial intervention and recruitment and retention strategy," Alzheimer Dis Assoc Disord, 20(4 Suppl 3):S203-8.

Wierniuk, A., & Wlodarek, D. (2013). Estimation of energy and nutritional intake of young men practicing aerobic sports. Rocz Panstw Zakl Hig, 64(2), 143-148.

Wiig, H., & Swartz, M. A. (2012). Interstitial fluid and lymph formation and transport: physiological regulation and roles in inflammation and cancer. Physiological Reviews, 92(3), 1005-1060.

Wilkinson JM, Hipwell M, Ryan T, Cavanagh HM (2003 Jan 1). "Bioactivity of Backhousia citriodora: antibacterial and antifungal activity," J Agric Food Chem. 51(1):76-81.

Wilkinson S, Aldridge J, Salmon I, Cain E, Wilson B (1999 Sep). "An evaluation of aromatherapy massage in palliative care," Palliat Med. 13(5):409-17.

Wilkinson, S. M., Love, S. B., Westcombe, A. M., Gambles, M. A., Burgess, C. C., Cargill, A., . . . Ramirez, A. J. (2007 Feb). Effectiveness of aromatherapy massage in the management of anxiety and depression in patients with cancer: a multicenter randomized controlled trial. Journal of Clinical Oncology, 25(5), 532-539.

Wille JJ, Kydonieus A (2003 May-Jun). "Palmitoleic acid isomer (c15:1delta6) in human skin sebum is effective against gram-positive bacteria," Ski Pharmacol Appl Skin Physiol. 16(3):176-87.

Williams R.M. (2004 Apr). "Fragrance Alters Mood and Brain Chemistry," Townsend Lett. Dr. Patients. 249:36-38

Williamson EM, Priestley CM, Burgess IF (2007 Dec). "An investigation and comparison of the bioactivity of selected essential oils on human lice and house dust mites," Fitoterapia. 78(7-8):521-5.

Winkler-Stuck K, Wiedemann FR, Wallesch CW, Kunz WS (2004 May 15). "Effect of coenzyme Q10 on the mitochondrial function of skin fibroblasts from Parkinson patients," J Neurol Sci. 220(1-2):41-8.

Witvrouw E, Danneels L, Asselman P, D'Have T, Cambier D (2003). "Muscle flexibility as a risk factor for developing muscle injuries in male professional soccer players. A prospective study," Am J Sports Med, 31(1):41-46.

Woelk H, Schläfke S (2010 Feb). "A multi-center, double-blind, randomised study of the Lavender oil preparation Silexan in comparison to Lorazepam for generalized anxiety disorder." Phytomedicine. 17 (2):94-9.

Woodruff J (2002 Mar). "Improving Hair Strength," Cosm Toil. :33-5.

Woollard A.C., Tatham K.C., Barker S (2007 Jun). "The influence of essential oils on the process of wound healing: a review of the current evidence," J. Wound Care. 16(6):255-257.

Wu LL, Wang KM, Liao PI, Kao YH, Huang YC (2015 Jul). "Effects of an 8-Week Outdoor Brisk Walking Program on Fatigue in Hi-Tech Industry Employees: A Randomized Control Trial," Workplace Health Saf.

Wu Y. et al (2012). "The metabolic responses to aerial diffusion of essential oils," PloS One. 7(9):e44830.

Xia L, Chen D, Han R, Fang Q, Waxman S, Jing Y (2005 Mar). "Boswellic acid acetate induces apoptosis through caspase-mediated pathways in myeloid leukemia cells," Mol Cancer Ther. 4(3):381-8.

Xiao D, Powolny AA, Barbi de Moura M, Kelley EE, Bommareddy A, Kim SH, Hahm ER, Normolle D, Van Houten B, Singh SV (2010 Jun 22). "Phenethyl isothiocyanate inhibits oxidative phosphorylation to trigger reactive oxygen species-mediated death of human prostate cancer cells," J Biol Chem Epub ahead of print. Epub ahead of print.

Xie P, Lu J, Wan H, Hao Y (2010 Aug). "Effect of toothpaste containing d-limonene on natural extrinsic smoking stain: a 4-week clinical trial," Am. J. Dent. 23(4):196-200.

Xiufen W, Hiramatsu N, Matsubara M (2004). "The antioxidative activity of traditional Japanese herbs," Biofactors. 21(1-4):281-4.

Xu F. et al (2008 Oct). "Pharmaco-physio-psychologic effect of Ayurvedic oil-dripping treatment using an essential oil from Lavendula angustifolia," J. Altern. Complement. Med. N. Y. N. 14(8):947-956.

Xu, J., Guo, Y., Zhao, P., Xie, C., Jin, D. Q., Hou, W., & Zhang, T. (2011 Dec). Neuroprotective cadinane sesquiterpenes from the resinous exudates of Commiphora myrrha. Fitoterapia, 82(8), 1198-1201.

Xu J., Zhou F., Ji B-P., Pei R-S., Xu N. (2008) The antibacterial mechanism of carvacrol and thymol against Escherichia coli. Letters in Applied Microbiology. 47: 174-179.

Xu, P., Wang, K., Lu, C., Dong, L., Gao, L., Yan, M., Aibai, S., Yang, Y., & Liu, X. (2017). "The Protective Effect of Lavender Essential Oil and Its Main Component Linalool against the Cognitive Deficits Induced by D-Galactose and Aluminum Trichloride in Mice," Evid Based Complement Alternat Med. 2017:7426538.

Xu X, Duncan AM, Merz BE, Kurzer MS (1998 Dec). "Effects of soy isoflavones on estrogen and phytoestrogen metabolism in premenopausal women," Cancer Epidemiol Biomarkers Prev. 7(12):1101-8.

Xu X, Duncan AM, Wangen KE, Kurzer MS (2000 Aug). "Soy consumption alters endogenous estrogen metabolism in postmenopausal women," Cancer Epidemiol biomarkers Prev. 9(8):781-6.

Yamada, K., Mimaki, Y., & Sashida, Y. (2005 Feb). Effects of inhaling the vapor of Lavandula burnatii super-derived essential oil and linalool on plasma adrenocorticotropic hormone (ACTH), catecholamine and gonadotropin levels in experimental menopausal female rats. Biol Pharm Bull, 28(2), 378-379.

Yamaguchi M, Tahara Y, Kosaka S (2009 Oct). "Influence of concentration of fragrances on salivary alphaamylase," Int. J. Cosmet. Sci. 31(5):391-395.

Yan, H., Sun, X., Sun, S., Wang, S., Zhang, J., Wang, R., . . . Kang, W. (2011 Jun). Anti-ultraviolet radiation effects of Coptis chinensis and Phellodendron amurense glycans by immunomodulating and inhibiting oxidative injury. Int J Biol Macromol, 48(5), 720-725.

Yang E.J., Kim, S.S., Moon, Y.J., Oh, T.H., Baik, J.S., Lee, N.H., and Hyun, C.G. (2010). "Inhibitory effects of Fortunella japonica var. margarita and Citrus sunki essential oils on nitric oxide production and skin pathogens," Acta Microbiol Immunol Hung. 57(1):15-27.

Yang F. et al. (2005 Feb 18). "Curcumin inhibits formation of amyloid beta oligomers and fibrils, binds plaques, and reduces amyloid in vivo," J Biol Chem. 280(7):5892-901.

Yang GY, Wang W (1994 Sep). "Clinical studies on the treatment of coronary heart disease with Valeriana officinalis var latifolia," Zhongguo Zhong Xi Yi Jie He Za Zhi. 14(9):540-2.

Yang L, Hao J, Zhang J (2009). "Ginsenoside Rg3 promotes beta-amyloid peptide degradation by enhancing gene expression of neprilysin," J Pharm Pharmacol. 61:375-80.

Yang SA, Jeon SK, Lee EJ, Im NK, Jhee KH, Lee SP, Lee IS (2009 May). "Radical Scavenging Activity of the Essential Oil of Silver Fir (Abies alba)," J Clin Biochem Nutr. 44(3):253-9.

Yang SA, Jeon SK, Lee EJ, Shim CH, Lee IS (2010 Jan). "Comparative study of the chemical composition and antioxidant activity of six essential oils and their components," Nat. Prod. Res. 24(2):140-151.

Yano H, Tatsuta M, Iishi H, Baba M, Sakai N, Uedo N (1999 Aug). "Attenuation by d-limonene of sodium chloride-enhanced gastric carcinogenesis induced by N-methyl-N'-nitro-N-nitrosoguanidine in Wistar rats," Int. J. Cancer. 82(5):665-668.

Yap, P. S., Krishnan, T., Yiap, B. C., Hu, C. P., Chan, K. G., & Lim, S. H. (2014 May). Membrane disruption and anti-quorum sensing effects of synergistic interaction between Lavandula angustifolia (lavender oil) in combination with antibiotic against plasmid-conferred multi-drug-resistant Escherichia coli. J Appl Microbiol, 116(5), 1119-1128.

Yates, D. (2014). Study: Many in U.S. have poor nutrition, with the disabled doing worst [Press release]. Retrieved from http://news.illinois.edu/news/14/1023DisabledNutrition_RuopengAn.html

Yavari Kia, P., Safajou, F., Shahnazi, M., & Nazemiyeh, H. (2014 Mar). The effect of lemon inhalation aromatherapy on nausea and vomiting of pregnancy: a double-blinded, randomized, controlled clinical trial. Iran Red Crescent Med J, 16(3).

Yazdanparast R, Shahriyary L (2008 Jan). "Comparative effects of Artemisia dracunculus, Satureja hortensis and Origanum majorana on inhibition of blood platelet adhesion, aggregation and secretion," Vascul Pharmacol. 48(1):32-7.

Yazdkhasti, M., & Pirak, A. (2016 Nov.). "The effect of aromatherapy with lavender essence on severity of labor pain and duration of labor in primiparous women," Complement Ther Clin Pract. 25:81-86.

Yiengprugsawan, V., Banwell, C., Takeda, W., Dixon, J., Seubsman, S. A., & Sleigh, A. C. (2015). Health, Happiness and Eating Together: What Can a Large Thai Cohort Study Tell Us? Glob J Health Sci, 7(4), 270-277.

Yip YB, Tam AC. (2008 Jun). "An experimental study on the effectiveness of massage with aromatic ginger and orange essential oil for moderate-to-severe knee pain among the elderly in Hong Kong," Complement Ther Med. 16(3):131-8.

Yip YB, Tse S. H. M. (2006 Feb). "An experimental study on the effectiveness of acupressure with aromatic lavender essential oil for sub-acute, non-specific neck pain in Hong Kong," Complement. Ther. Clin. Pract. 12(1):18-26.

Yip YB, Tse S. H. M. (2004 Mar). "The effectiveness of relaxation acupoint stimulation and acupressure with aromatic lavender essential oil for non-specific low back pain in Hong Kong: a randomised controlled trial," Complement. Ther. Med. 12(1):28-37.

Yoo, C. B., Han, K. T., Cho, K. S., Ha, J., Park, H. J., Nam, J. H., . . . Lee, K. T. (2005 Jul). Eugenol isolated from the essential oil of Eugenia caryophyllata induces a reactive oxygen species-mediated apoptosis in HL-60 human promyelocytic leukemia cells. Cancer Lett, 225(1), 41-52.

Yoshizaki N, Hashizume R, Masaki H. (2017 Jun). "A polymethoxyflavone mixture extracted from orange peels, mainly containing nobiletin, 3,3',4',5,6,7,8-heptamethoxyflavone and tangeretin, suppresses melanogenesis through the acidification of cell organelles, including melanosomes," J Dematol Sci. S0923-1811(16)31097-0.

Yosipovitch G, Szolar C, Hui X.Y., Maibach H (1996 May). "Effect of topically applied menthol on thermal, pain and itch sensations and biophysical properties of the skin," Arch. Dermatol. Res. 288(5-6):245-248.

Youdim KA, Deans SG (1999 Sep 8). "Dietary supplementation of thyme (Thymus vulgaris L.) essential oil during the lifetime of the rat: its effects on the antioxidant status in liver, kidney and heart tissues," Mech Ageing Dev. 109(3):163-75.

Youdim KA, Deans SG (2000 Jan). "Effect of thyme oil and thymol dietary supplementation on the antioxidant status and fatty acid composition of the ageing rat brain," Br J Nutr. 83(1):87-93.

Youn L.J., Yoon J.W., Hovde C.J. (2010) A Brief Overview of Escherichia coli O157:H7 and Its Plasmid O157. Journal of Microbiology and Biotechnology. 20: 1-10.

Younis F, Mirelman D, Rabinkov A, Rosenthal T (2010 Jun). "S-allyl-mercapto-captopril: a novel compound in the treatment of Cohen-Rosenthal diabetic hypertensive rats," J Clin Hypertens (Greenwich) 12(6):451-5.

Yu B.P. (1994) Cellular Defenses Against Damage From Reactive Oxygen Species. Physiological Reviews. 74: 139-162.

Yu D, Wang J, Shao X, Xu F, Wang H (2015 Nov). "Antifungal modes of action of tea tree oil and its two characteristic components against Botrytis cinerea," J. Appl. Microbiol. 119(5):1253-1262.

Yu YM, Chang WC, Wu CH, Chiang SY (2005 Nov). "Reduction of oxidative stress and apoptosis in hyperlipidemic rabbits by ellagic acid," J Nutr Biochem. 16(11):675-81.

Yu Z, Wang R, Xu L, Xie S, Dong J, Jing Y (2011 Jan 25). "β-Elemene piperazine derivatives induce apoptosis in human leukemia cells through downregulation of c-FLIP and generation of ROS," PLos One 6(1)e15843.

Yuan HQ, Kong F, Wang XL, Young CY, Hu XY, Lou HX (2008 Jun 1). "Inhibitory effect of acetyl-11-keto-beta-boswellic acid on androgen receptor by interference of Sp1 binding activity in prostate cancer cells," Biochem Pharmacol. 75(11):2112-21.

Yuan YV, Walsh NA (2006 Jul). "Antioxidant and antiproliferative activities of extracts from a variety of edible seaweeds," Food Chem Toxicol. 44(7):1144-50.

Yüce, A., Turk, G., Ceribasi, S., Guvenc, M., Ciftci, M., Sonmez, M., . . . Aksakal, M. (2014 Apr). Effectiveness of cinnamon (Cinnamomum zeylanicum) bark oil in the prevention of carbon tetrachloride-induced damages on the male reproductive system. Andrologia, 46(3), 263-272.

Yue G.G.L. et al (2012 Mar). "The Role of Turmerones on Curcumin Transportation and P-Glycoprotein Activities in Intestinal Caco-2 Cells," J. Med. Food. 15(3):242-252.

Yue G.G.L. et al (2010 Aug). "Evaluation of in vitro anti-proliferative and immunomodulatory activities of compounds isolated from Curcuma longa," Food Chem. Toxicol. 48(8-9):2011-2020.

Yun, J. (2014 Jan). Limonene inhibits methamphetamine-induced locomotor activity via regulation of 5-HT neuronal function and dopamine release. Phytomedicine. Retrieved from http://dx.doi.org/10.1016/j.phymed.2013.12.004

Zabirunnisa M, Gadagi J.S., Gadde P, Myla N, Koneru J, Thatimatla C (2014 Jul). "Dental patient anxiety: Possible deal with Lavender fragrance," J. Res. Pharm. Pract. 3(3):100-103.

Zaim, A., Benjelloun, M., El Harchli, E.H., Farah, A., Meni Mahzoum, A., Alaoui Mhamdi, M., and El Ghadraoui, L. (2015). "Chemical Composition And Acridicid Properties Of The Morrocan Tanacetum Annuum L. Essential Oils," Int J Eng and Sci. 5(5):13-19.

Zeidán-Chuliá F. et al (2012 Jun). "Bioinformatical and in vitro approaches to essential oil-induced matrix metalloproteinase inhibition," Pharm. Biol. 50(6):675-686.

Zembron-Lacny A, Szyszka K, Szygula Z (2007 Dec). "Effect of cysteine derivatives administration in healthy men exposed to intense resistance exercise by evaluation of pro-antioxidant ratio," J Physiol Sci. 57(6):343-8.

Zha C., Brown G.B., Brouillette W.J. (2004) Synthesis and Structure-Activity Relationship Studies for Hydantoins and Analogues as Voltage-Gasted Sodium Channel Ligands. Journal of Medicinal Chemistry. 47: 6519-6528.

Zhan L. et al (2012 Jul). "Effects of Xylitol Wipes on Cariogenic Bacteria and Caries in Young Children," J. Dent. Res. 91(7):S85-S90.

Zhao J, Zhang J, Yang B, Lv GP, Li SP (2010 Oct). "Free Radical Scavenging Activity and Characterization of Sesquiterpenoids in Four Species of Curcuma Using a TLC Bioautography Assay and GC-MS Analysis," Molecules. 15(11):7547-7557.

Zhang, J., Kang, M. J., Kim, M. J., Kim, M. E., Song, J. H., Lee, Y. M., & Kim, J. I. (2008 Jan). Pancreatic lipase inhibitory activity of taraxacum officinale in vitro and in vivo. Nutr Res Pract, 2(4), 200-203.

Zhang, L.L., Lv, S., Xu, J.G., and Xhang, L.F. (2017) "Influence of drying methods on chemical compositions, antioxidant and antibacterial activity of essential oil from lemon peel," Natural Product Research. 0(0):1-5.

Zhang, R., Wang, B., Zhao, H., Wei, C., Yuan, G., & Guo, R. (2009). Tissue distribution of curcumol in rats after intravenous injection of zedoary turmeric oil fat emulsion. Asian Journal of Pharmacodynamics and Pharmacokinetics, 1608, 51-57.

Zhang W, Wang X, Liu Y, Tian H, Flickinger B, Empie MW, Sun SZ (2008 Jun). "Dietary flaxseed lignan extract lowers plasma cholesterol and glucose concentrations in hypercholesterolaemic subjects," Br J Nutr. 99(6):1301-9.

Zhang X, Zhang Y, Li Y (2013 Aug). "Beta element decreases cell invasion by upregulating E-cadherin expression in MCF-7 human breast cancer cells," Oncol Rep. 30(2):745-50.

Zhang X-Z., Wang L, Liu D.W., Tang G.Y., Zhang H.Y. (2014 Sep). "Synergistic inhibitory effect of berberine and d-limonene on human gastric carcinoma cell line MGC803," J. Med. 17(9):955-962.

Zhang Z, Li Y, Zhang Y, Song J, Wang Q, Zheng L, Liu D. (2013). "Beta-element blocks epithelial mesenchymal transition in human breast cancer cell line MCF-7 through Smad3-mediated down-regulation of nuclear transcription factors," PLoS One 8(3):e58719.

Zhang, Z., Liu, X., Zhang, X., Liu, J., Hao, Y., Yang, X., & Wang, Y. (2011 May). Comparative evaluation of the antioxidant effects of the natural vitamin C analog 2-O-beta-D-glucopyranosyl-L-ascorbic acid isolated from Goji berry fruit. Arch Pharm Res, 34(5), 801-810.

Zhao W, Entschladen F, Liu H, Niggemann B, Fang Q, Zaenker KS, Han R (2003). "Boswellic acid acetate induces differentiation and apoptosis in highly metastatic melanoma and fibrosarcoma cells," Cancer Detect Prev. 27(1):67-75.

Zheng GQ, Kenney PM, Lam LK. (1992 Aug). "Anethofuran, carvone, and limonene: potential cancer chemopreventive agents from dill weed oil and caraway oil," Planta Med. 58(4):338-41.

Zheng GQ, Kenney PM, Zhang J, Lam LK (1993). "Chemoprevention of benzo[a]pyrene-induced forestomach cancer in mice by natural phthalides from celery seed oil," Nutr Cancer. 19(1):77-86.

Zhou BR, Luo D, Wei FD, Chen XE, Gao J (2008 Jul). "Baicalin protects human fibroblasts against ultraviolet B-induced cyclobutane pyrimidine dimers formation," Arch Dermatol Res. 300(6):331-4.

Zhou J, Ma X, Qiu BH, Chen J, Bian L, Pan L (2013 Jan). "Parameters optimization of supercritical fluid-CO2 extracts of frankincense using response surface methodology and its pharmacodynamics effects," J Sep Sci. 36(2):383-390.

Zhou, J., Tang F., Bian R. (2004) Effect of α-pinene on nuclear translocation of NF-κB in THP-1 cells. Acta Pharmacol Sin. 25: 480-484.

Zhou J, Zhou S, Tang J, Zhang K, Guang L, Huang Y, Xu Y, Ying Y, Zhang L, Li D (2009 Mar 15). "Protective effect of berberine on beta cells in streptozotocin- and high-carbohydrate/high-fat diet-induced diabetic rats," Eur J Pharmacol. 606(1-3):262-8.

Zhou W, Fukumoto S, Yokogoshi H (2009 Apr). "Components of lemon essential oil attenuate dementia induced by scopolamine," Nutr. Neurosci. 12(2):57-64.

Zhou, X. M., Zhao, Y., He, C. C., & Li, J. X. (2012 Feb). Preventive effects of Citrus reticulata essential oil on bleomycin-induced pulmonary fibrosis in rats and the mechanism. Zhong Xi Yi Jie He Xue Bao, 10(2), 200-209.

Zhu BC, Henderson G, Chen F, Fei H, Laine RA (2001 Aug). "Evaluation of vetiver oil and seven insect-active essential oils against the Formosan subterranean termite," J Chem Ecol. 27(8):1617-25.

Zhu BC, Henderson G, Yu Y, Laine RA (2003 Jul 30). "Toxicity and repellency of patchouli oil and patchouli alcohol against Formosan subterranean termites Coptotermes formosanus Shiraki (Isoptera: Rhinotermitidae)," J Agric Food Chem. 51(16):4585-8

Zhu JS, Halpern GM, Jones K (1998). "The scientific rediscovery of a precious ancient Chinese herbal regimen: Cordyceps sinensis. Part I," J Altern Complement Med. 4:289-303.

Ziegler D, Ametov A, Barinov A, Dyck PJ, Gurieva I, Low PA, Munzel U, Yakhno N, Raz I, Novosadova M, Maus J, Samigullin R (2006 Nov). "Oral treatment with alpha-lipoic acid improves symptomatic diabetic polyneuropathy: the SYDNEY 2 trial," Diabetes Care. 29(11):2365-70.

Ziegler G, Ploch M, Miettinen-Baumann A, Collet W (2002 Nov 25). "Efficacy and tolerability of valerian extract LI 156 compared with oxazepam in the treatment of non-organic insomnia--a randomized, double-blind, comparative clinical study," Eur J Med Res. 7(11):480-6.

Zore G.B., Thakre A.D., Jadhav S., Karuppayil S.M. (2011) Terpenoids inhibit Candida albicans growth by affecting membrane integrity and arrest of cell cycle. Phytomedicine. doi: 10.1016/j.phymed.2011.03.008.

Zou B, Li QQ, Zhao J, Li JM, Cuff CF, Reed E (2013 Mar). "Beta-Elemene and taxanes synergistically induce cytotoxicity and inhibit proliferation in ovarian cancer and other tumor cells," Anticancer Res. 33(3):929-40.

Zu Y. et al (2010 Apr). "Activities of Ten Essential Oils towards Propionibacterium acnes and PC-3, A-549 and MCF-7 Cancer Cells," Molecules. 15(5):3200-3210.

Bibliography

Balch, M.D., James, and Phyllis Balch, C.N.C. *Prescription for Nutritional Healing.* Garden City Park, NY: Avery Publishing Group, 1990.

Başer, Kemal Hüsnü Can & Gerhard Buchbauer. *Handbook of Essential Oils: Science, Technology, and Applications.* Florida: CRC Press, 2010. Print.

Bear, M. F., Connors, B. W., Paradiso, M. A. (2007). Neuroscience: Exploring the Brain (3rd ed.). Baltimore, MD: Lippincott Williams & Wilkins.

Bendich, A., & Deckelbaum, R. J. (Eds.). (2010). Preventive Nutrition: The Comprehensive Guide for Health Professionals (4th ed.). New York, NY: Springer Science & Business Media.

Berg, J. M., Tymoczko, J. L., Stryer, L. (2002). Biochemistry (Section 30.2, Each Organ Has a Unique Metabolic Profile) (5th ed.). New York, NY: W H Freeman.

Becker, M.D., Robert O. *The Body Electric.* New York, NY: Wm. Morrow, 1985.

Brown, J. E. (1991). Everywoman's Guide to Nutrition. Minneapolis, MN: University of Minnesota Press.

Brown T.L., LeMay H.E., Bursten B.E. *Chemistry: The Central Science. 10th ed.* Upper Saddle River: Pearson Prentice Hall, 2006.

Burroughs, Stanley. *Healing for the Age of Enlightenment.* Auburn, CA: Burroughs Books, 1993.

Burton Goldberg Group, The. *Alternative Medicine: The Definitive Guide.* Fife, WA: Future Medicine Publishing, Inc., 1994.

Can Baser, K Husnu, Buchbauer, Gerhard. Handbood of Essential Oils: Science Technology, and Applications. Boca Raton, FL: Taylor & Francis Group, 2010.

Carter, Howard. *The Tomb of Tutankhamen.* Washington, D.C.: National Geographic Society, 2003. Print.

Chemical Engineering Research Trends. (2007). (L. P. Berton Ed.). New York, New York: Nova Science Publishers, Inc.

Chevallier, Andrew. *Encyclopedia of Herbal Medicine*, 2nd Ed.. New York, NY: Dorling Kindersley Limited, 2000.

"Chilblains." Mayo Clinic, Mayo Foundation for Medical Education and Research, 17 Aug. 2017.

Clark, Micheal A; Sutton, Brian G; and Lucett, Scott C. *NASM Essentials of Personal Fitness Training.* Burlington, MA: Jones & Bartlett Learning, 2014.

Clark, Micheal A; Lucett, Scott C; and Sutton, Brian G. *NASM Essentials of Corrective Exercise Training.* Burlington, MA: Jones & Bartlett Learning, 2014.

Cowan M.K., Talaro K.P. *Microbiology: A Systems Approach. 2nd ed.* New York: McGraw Hill, 2009.

Fischer-Rizzi, Suzanne. *Complete Aromatherapy Handbook.* New York, NY: Sterling Publishing, 1990.

Gattefosse, Rene-Maurice. *Gattefosse's Aromatherapy.* Essex, England: The C.W. Daniel Company Ltd., 1937 English translation.

Gawronski, Donald. *Medical Choices.* Lincoln, Nebraska: Authors Choice Press, 2002. Print.

Guyton A.C., Hall J.E. *Textbook of Medical Physiology. 10th ed.* Philadelphia: W.B. Saunders Company, 2000.

Green, Mindy. *Natural Perfumes: Simple Aromatherapy Recipes.* Loveland CO: Interweave Press Inc., 1999.

Hill, David K. *Frankincense.* Spanish Fork, UT: AromaTools, 2010.

Integrated Aromatic Medicine. Proceedings from the First International Symposium, Grasse, France. Essential Science Publishing, March 2000.

Kraak, V. I., Liverman, C. T., & Koplan, J. P. (Eds.). (2005). Preventing Childhood Obesity: Health in the Balance. Washington, DC: National Academies Press.

Keville, Kathi. "A History of Fragrance." Healthy.net. 1995. Web. 9 Aug. 2012.

Lis-Balchin, Maria. *Aromatherapy Science: A Guide for Healthcare Professionals.* London, UK: Pharmaceutical Press, 2006.

Lawless, Julia. *The Encyclopaedia of Essential Oils.* Rockport, MA: Element, Inc., 1992.

L. H. Bailey and E. Z. Bailey, Hortus Third: A Concise Dictionary of Plants Cultivated in the United States and Canada, 1 edition. New York: Macmillan, 1976.

Maughan, R. J., Burke L. M. (Eds.). (2002). Sports Nutrition: Handbook of Sports Medicine and Science. Bodmin, England: Blackwell Science Publishing.

Maury, Marguerite. *Marguerite Maury's Guide to Aromatherapy.* C.W. Daniel, 1989.

McArdle, William D.; Katch, Frank I.; and Katch, Victor L. *Exercise Physiology: Nutrition, Energy, and Human Performance, Eighth Edition.* Baltimore, MD: Wolters Kluwer Health, 2015.

Muscolino, Joseph E. Kinesiology: *The Skeletal System and Muscle Function, 2nd Edition.* St. Louis, MO: Elsevier Mosby, 2011.

Pènoël, M.D., Daniel and Pierre Franchomme. L'aromatherapie exactement. Limoges, France: Jollois, 1990.

Petrovska, Biljana Bauer. "Historical Review of Medicinal Plants' Usage." *Pharmacognosy Reviews* 2012 (6:11): 1–5. Print.

Porter, Stephen. *The Great Plague.* Stroud, Gloucestershire: Amberly Publishing, 2009. Print.

Price, Shirley, and Len Price. *Aromatherapy for Health Professionals.* New York, NY: Churchill Livingstone Inc., 1995.

Price, Shirley, and Penny Price Parr. *Aromatherapy for Babies and Children.* San Francisco, CA: Thorsons, 1996.

Rose, Jeanne. *375 Essential Oils and Hydrosols.* Berkeley, CA: North Atlantic Books, 1999.

Rose, Jeanne. *The Aromatherapy Book: Applications and Inhalations.* Berkeley, CA: North Atlantic Books, 1992.

Ryman, Danièle. *Aromatherapy: The Complete Guide to Plant & Flower Essences for Health and Beauty.* New York: Bantam Books, 1993.

Seigler, D. (2002). Plant Secondary Metabolism (Second Printing ed.). Norwell, Massachusetts: Kluwer Academic Publishers.

Sheppard-Hanger, Sylla. *The Aromatherapy Practitioner Reference Manual.* Tampa, FL: Atlantic Institute of Aromatherapy, Twelfth Printing February 2000.

Singh, M. A. F. (Ed.). (2000). Exercise, Nutrition, and the Older Woman: Wellness for Women over Fifty. Boca Raton, FL: CRC Press.

Sizer, F. S. & Whitney, E. (2014). Nutrition: Concepts and Controversies (13th ed.). Belmont, CA: Wadsworth, Cengage Learning.

Tisserand, Maggie. *Aromatherapy for Women: a Practical Guide to Essential Oils for Health and Beauty.* Rochester, VT: Healing Arts Press, 1996.

Tisserand, Robert. *Aromatherapy: to Heal and Tend the Body.* Wilmot, WI: Lotus Press, 1988.

Tisserand, Robert. *The Art of Aromatherapy.* Rochester, VT: Healing Arts Press, 1977.

Tisserand, Robert, and Tony Balacs. *Essential Oil Safety: A Guide for Health Care Professionals.* New York, NY: Churchill Livingstone, 1995.

Tortora G.J., Funke B.R., Case C.L. *Microbiology: An Introduction. 9th ed.* San Francisco: Pearson Benjamin Cummings, 2007.

Valnet, M.D., Jean. *The Practice of Aromatherapy: a Classic Compendium of Plant Medicines and their Healing Properties.* Rochester, VT: Healing Arts Press, 1998.

Valnet, Jean. *The Practice of Aromatherapy.* Rochester Vermont: Healing Arts Press, 1982. Print.

Watson, Franzesca. *Aromatherapy Blends & Remedies.* San Francisco, CA: Thorsons, 1995.

Weaver R.F. *Molecular Biology. 4th ed.* New York: McGraw Hill, 2008.

Wilson, Roberta. *Aromatherapy for Vibrant Health and Beauty: a practical A-to-Z reference to aromatherapy treatments for health, skin, and hair problems.* Honesdale, PA: Paragon Press, 1995.

Worwood, Valerie Ann. *The Complete Book of Essential Oils & Aromatherapy.* San Rafael, CA: New World Library, 1991.

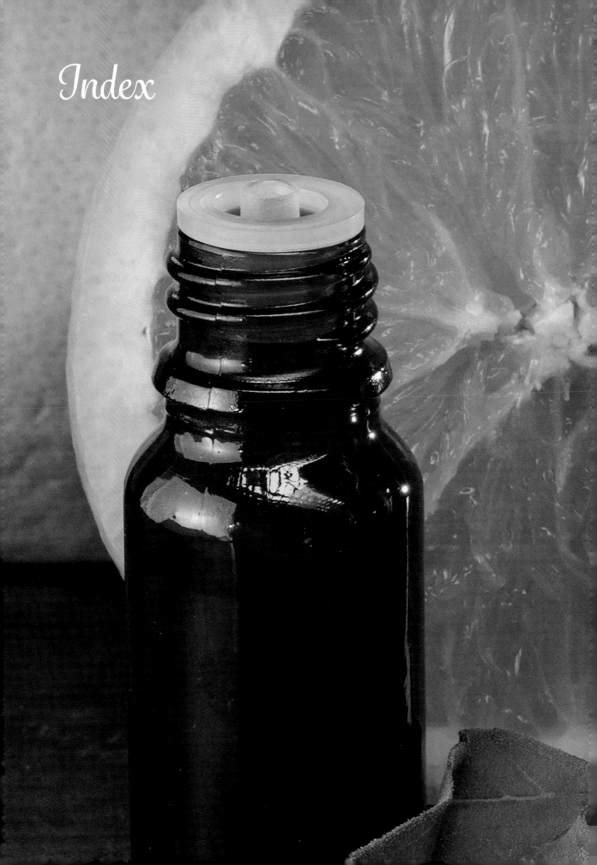

Index

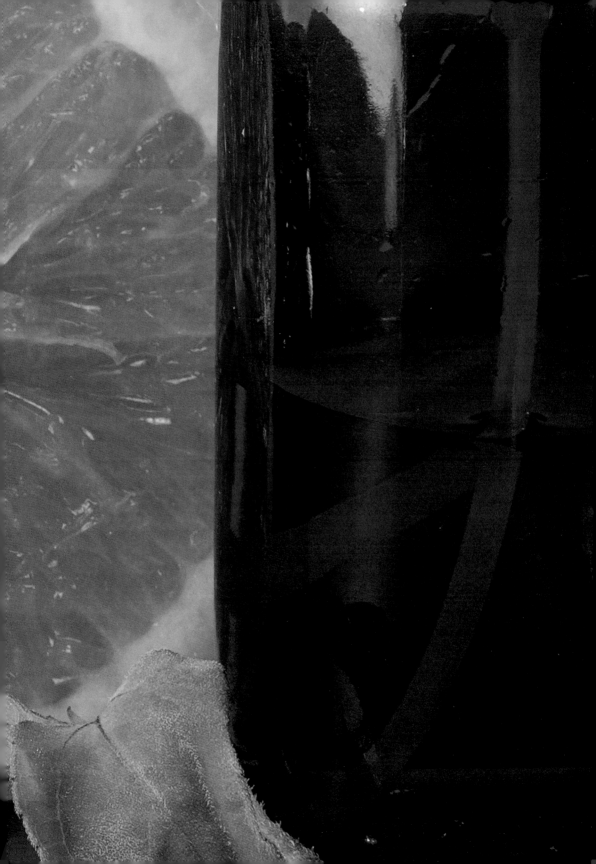

Index

X

Y

Z

Discover Even More about Essential Oils with the Complete *Modern Essentials*

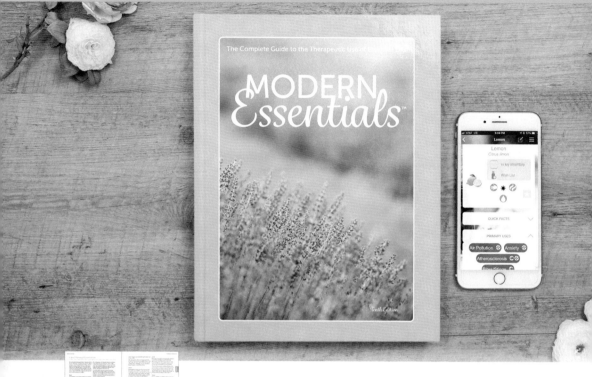

History—Go in depth on the use of aromatic plants and essential oils as medicine throughout history.

Science—How essential oils are created and stored by plants, how they interact with the body, and how they are tested to ensure purity and quality.

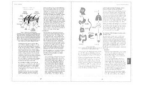

Research—Access over 1,000 references to research studies supporting the therapeutic use of essential oils.

Chemistry—The many chemical constituents that make up essential oils and how they can affect the body.

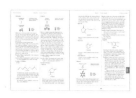

For on-the-go access, discover the new **ME Plus** app at your app store today!

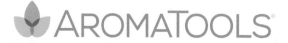

Visit aromatools.com for more details.